Manipal Manual of
Medical
Physiology

Revised First Edition

As per the latest CBME Guidelines | Competency Based
Undergraduate Curriculum for the Indian Medical Graduate

Manipal Manual of
Medical
Physiology

Revised First Edition

As per the latest CBME Guidelines | Competency Based
Undergraduate Curriculum for the Indian Medical Graduate

CN Chandra Shekar

Former Professor of Physiology and Neurosciences
American University of Antigua College of Medicine
Coolidge, Antigua

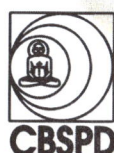

CBSPD

CBS Publishers & Distributors Pvt Ltd

New Delhi • Bengaluru • Chennai • Kochi • Kolkata • Lucknow • Mumbai
Hyderabad • Jharkhand • Nagpur • Patna • Pune • Uttarakhand

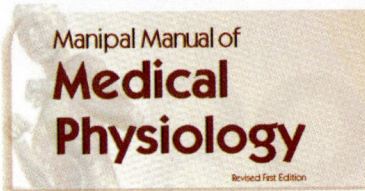

Manipal Manual of
Medical Physiology
Revised First Edition

ISBN: 978-81-239-2890-6

Copyright © Author and Publisher

Revised First Edition: 2018, **2024**
First Edition: 2016
Reprint: 2017

Published by Satish Kumar Jain and produced by Varun Jain for

CBS Publishers & Distributors Pvt Ltd
4819/XI Prahlad Street, 24 Ansari Road, Daryaganj, New Delhi 110 002
Ph: 011-23289259, 23266861   Website: www.cbspd.com
                                    e-mail: delhi@cbspd.com

Corporate Office: 204 FIE, Industrial Area, Patparganj, Delhi 110 092
Ph: 011-4934 4934   Fax: 011-4934 4935   e-mail: publishing@cbspd.com; publicity@cbspd.com

Branches

• **Bengaluru:** Seema House 2975, 17th Cross, KR Road, Banasankari 2nd Stage, Bengaluru 560 070, Karnataka, India
  Ph: +91-80-26771678/79   Fax: +91-80-26771680   e-mail: bangalore@cbspd.com
• **Chennai:** 7, Subbaraya Street, Shenoy Nagar, Chennai 600 030, Tamil Nadu, India
  Ph: +91-44-26680620, 26681266   Fax: +91-44-42032115   e-mail: chennai@cbspd.com
• **Kochi:** 42/1325, 1326, Power House Road, Opp KSEB, Power House, Ernakulum Kochi 682 018, Kerala, India
  Ph: +91-484-4059061-65,67   Fax: +91-484-4059065   e-mail: kochi@cbspd.com
• **Kolkata:** 147, Hind Ceramics Compound, 1st Floor, Nilgunj Road, Belghoria, Kolkata-700056, West Bengal, India
  Ph: +91-9096713055/7798394118, 9836841399   e-mail: kolkata@cbspd.com
• **Lucknow:** Basement, Khushnuma Complex, 7 Meerabai Marg (Behind Jawahar Bhawan), Lucknow-226001, UP, India
  Ph: +0522-4000032   e-mail: tiwari.lucknow@cbspd.com
• **Mumbai:** PWD Shed, Gala no 25/26, Ramchandra Bhatt Marg, Next to JJ Hospital Gate no. 2, Opp. Union Bank of India, Noorbaug, Mumbai-400009, Maharashtra, India
  Ph: 022-66661880/89   e-mail: mumbai@cbspd.com

Representatives

• Hyderabad	0-9885175004	• Jharkhand	0-9811541605	• Nagpur	0-8692091830
• Patna	0-9334159340	• Pune	0-9664372571	• Uttarakhand	0-9716462459

Printed at Goyal Offset Works Pvt. Ltd., Haryana (INDIA)

to

---

my beloved mother
late Smt Shivamma
who pampered me the most and encouraged me to become what I am

and

my most beloved guru, philosopher and guide
Dr P Lakshminarayan Rao
former Dean, Kasturba Medical College, Manipal
and incumbent Registrar, Evaluations, Manipal University

Acknowledgements

I whole heartedly thank Dr P Lakshminarayan Rao, former Dean of Kasturba Medical College, Manipal, whose immense support, guidance and encouragement has shaped my destiny and whatever I have achieved or achieve in the academic field, the credit he deserves the most.

I take this opportunity to thank Mr SK Jain (CMD) and Mr YN Arjuna (Senior Vice President—Publishing, Editorial and Publicity), CBS Publishers & Distributors, New Delhi, for all the efforts and cooperation for enabling me to publish this book.

Last but not the least, the persons who deserve my utmost thanks are: 1. Mrs Nanidini Shekar, my spouse; 2. Mr Shashank Shekar, elder son; 3. Mrs Divi Sharma-Shekar, DIL; and 4. Mr. Shubhank Shekar, the younger son. They withstood all the trials and tribulations at home during the compilation of the material for this venture and supported me immensely.

CN Chandra Shekar

Preface

My earlier book *Manipal Manual of Physiology* was mainly intended to cater to the needs of dental, nursing and paramedical students. The overwhelming response I got even from the medical students inspired me to present the material more in detail to the students of medicine and the result of which is this book *Manipal Manual of Medical Physiology*.

For various reasons, it took almost six years to compile the material. However, a lot more attention has been paid for inclusion of materials more in details in each chapter so that the students would find it very convenient to peruse. Systems like endocrinology, CNS, CVS and renal physiology, etc., have been dealt more in detail with more emphasis on pathophysiology. Due emphasis has been laid to drive home the concepts so that the students would understand easily rather than memorizing. In many chapters, calculations have been explained with representative values for easy comprehension.

Hope and wish that the endeavor is going to benefit the students who really need help when they are crammed with many subjects when they just step into the professional course that is quite demanding and strenuous.

It is my sincere request to the students and all others concerned to send in their constructive criticism and comments to the email id shekardon@yahoo.com/chanss4@gmail.com.

Wish you all the best.

CN Chandra Shekar

Contents

Preface   *vii*

0. General Physiology   xi

Cell xi
Transport of substances across cell xiv
Connection between the adjacent cells xv
Body fluids compartments xvi
Measurement of body fluid volume xix
Body fluid compartments xix
Alterations in the body fluid compartments during certain conditions xx
Dehydration xxii

1. Blood   1

Hematology 1
Functions of blood 1
Composition of blood 1
Plasma 2
Plasma proteins 2
Formed elements 4
Red blood cells (erythrocytes) 4
Leukocytes (white blood cells) 13
Platelets (thrombocytes) 17
Hemostasis and coagulation or clotting of
    blood 19
Blood group 23
Blood volume 27
Lymph 29
Body fluid pH regulation 30

2. Nerve Muscle Physiology   33

Neuron 33
Nerve fiber or axon 34
Strength duration curve 36
Potentials 37
Nerve injuries 40
Myesthenia gravis—disease of neuro
    muscular junction 44

Motor nerve fibers and motor units 44
Muscles 44
Skeletal muscles 45
Smooth muscle 49

3. Cardiovacular System   50

Blood vessels 51
Cardiac muscle 51
Properties of the cardiac muscle 51
Conducting system of human heart 53
Cardiac muscle action potential 55
Biophysical aspects of circulation 57
Peripheral resistance 59
Extrinsic control of peripheral blood flow 60
Venous return 62
Electrocardiogram (ECG/EKG) 64
Lead system 64
Cardiac cycle 67
Heart rate and its regulation 71
Cardiac output 74
Cardiac catheterization 79
Blood pressure 79
Regulation of blood pressure 81
Regional circulations 86
Cardiovascular shock 89
Autoregulation of blood flow 92

4. Respiratory System   94

Respiratory tract 94
Intrapleural and intra-alveolar pressure 98
Lung compliance 99
Spirogram 100
Ventilation perfusion ratio 101
Oxygen transport 104
Carbon dioxide transport 107

Regulation of respiration 109
Hypoxia 114
Dyspnea 115
Cyanosis 115
Mountain sickness 115
Acclimatization 115
Decompression sickness/Caisson's disease/ dysbarism 116
Apnea 116
Asphyxia 116
Periodic breathing 116
Artificial respiration 117

5. Digestive System 118

Gastrointestinal tract 118
Salivary secretion 119
Mastication or chewing 124
Deglutition or swallowing 124
Gastric secretion 127
Motor functions of stomach 134
Pancreas 136
Liver and bile secretion 140
Movements of small intestine 143
Ileocecal junction 145
Large intestine 146
Defecation 147

6. Endocrinology 149

Anterior pituitary gland 153
Posterior pituitary hormones 157
Endocrine function of adrenal cortex 161
Adrenal cortex 161
Adrenal androgens 165
Aldosterone 165
Endocrine function of adrenal medulla 167
Thyroid gland 170
Endocrine pancreas 177
Insulin 177
Glucagon 181
Glucose homeostasis 182
Parathyroid gland and calcium and phosphate metabolism 183
Parathyroid glands 184
Calcitonin 188

7. Reproduction 190

Reproductive physiology 190
Sex differentiation and development 190
Male reproductive system 192
Semen 196
Female reproductive system 197
Placenta 202
Growth of population and contraception 204
Lactation 206
Gonadal dysgenesis 208

8. Renal Physiology 211

Structure of kidney 211
Renal blood flow 212
Glomerular filtration rate 214
Effective filtration pressure (EFP) or net filtration pressure 215
Functions of renal tubules 218
Concept of tubular reabsorption and secretion 218
Substances reabsorbed in PCT 219
Reabsorption of substances in DCT 222
Diuresis 223
Concentration of urine 223
Secretion 225
Regulation of pH by kidney 225
Juxtaglomerular apparatus 227
Nerve supply to urinary bladder and urinary tract 228
Micturition 229
Cystometrogram 229
Composition of urine 230
Skin and thermoregulation 232

9. Central Nervous System 235

Receptors 235
Synapse 238
Mechanism of synaptic transmission 239
Properties of synapse 239
Synaptic inhibitions 240
Reflex 241
Spinal cord 243
Pain 246

Pathway for crude touch from peripheral
   parts of body 251
Motor system overview 251
Muscle tone maintenance and regulation 256
Cerebellum 263
Basal ganglia 267
Reticular formation 269
Vestibular apparatus 271
Cerebrospinal fluid (CSF) 273
Thalamus 275
Hypothalamus 276
Limbic system 280
Electroencephalogram (EEG) 281
Autonomic nervous system 282
Sleep and wakefulness 283
Learning and memory 285

Memory 285
Cerebral cortex 286

10. Special Senses   **289**

Vision 289
Neurophysiological basis of vision 297
Refractive errors 300
Hearing or audition 301
Theories of hearing 306
Auditory pathway 307
Types of deafness 307
Chemical senses 308
Taste/gustation 308
Pathway for taste 309
Sense of smell (olfaction) 310

Index   *313*

Index of Competencies
Competency Based Curriculum for the Indian Medical Graduate

Code	Competency	Page number
General Physiology		
PY1.1	Describe the structure and functions of a mammalian cell	xi
PY1.2	Describe and discuss the principles of homeostasis	182, 211, 276
PY1.3	Describe intercellular communication	34, 272
PY1.5	Describe and discuss transport mechanisms across cell membranes	xiv, 35, 104, 107, 150, 219
PY1.6	Describe the fluid compartments of the body, its ionic composition and measurements	xvi
PY1.7	Describe the concept of pH and Buffer systems in the body	30, 225, 26, 227
PY1.8	Describe and discuss the molecular basis of resting membrane potential and action potential in excitable tissue	37, 38, 51
Haematology (Blood)		
PY2.1	Describe the composition and functions of blood components	1
PY2.2	Discuss the origin, forms, variations and functions of plasma proteins	2, 117, 140, 214
PY2.3	Describe and discuss the synthesis and functions of Haemoglobin and explain its breakdown. Describe variants of haemoglobin	106, 107, 108
PY2.4	Describe RBC formation (erythropoiesis and its regulation) and its functions	23, 27, 30
PY2.5	Describe different types of anaemias	2, 6, 7
PY2.6	Describe WBC formation (granulopoiesis) and its regulation	1, 30, 90
PY2.8	Describe the physiological basis of hemostasis and, anticoagulants. Describe bleeding and clotting disorders (Hemophilia, purpura)	19, 20, 21
PY2.9	Describe different blood groups and discuss the clinical importance of blood grouping, blood banking and transfusion	26
PY2.10	Define and classify different types of immunity. Describe the development of immunity and its regulation	15, 16, 163, 176, 207
PY2.11	Estimate Hb, RBC, TLC, RBC indices, DLC, Blood groups, BT/CT	15, 105, 106
PY2.12	Describe test for ESR, Osmotic fragility, Hematocrit. Note the findings and interpret the test results, etc. (Note ESR: Chapter 9, pages 62–64)	5, 22
PY2.13	Describe steps for reticulocyte and platelet count (Refer to Chapter 12, page 83)	6, 7, 8, 27
Nerve and Muscle Physiology		
PY3.1	Describe the structure and functions of a neuron and neuroglia; Discuss nerve growth factor and other growth factors/cytokines	33, 34, 35, 38
PY3.2	Describe the types, functions and properties of nerve fibers	33
PY3.3	Describe the degeneration and regeneration in peripheral nerves	41
PY3.4	Describe the structure of neuromuscular junction and transmission of impulses	183, 186
PY3.5	Discuss the action of neuromuscular blocking agents	43
PY3.6	Describe the pathophysiology of Myasthenia gravis	44
PY3.7	Describe the different types of muscle fibres and their structure	118
PY3.8	Describe action potential and its properties in different muscle types (skeletal and smooth)	44, 45, 49
PY3.9	Describe the molecular basis of muscle contraction in skeletal and in smooth muscles	143
PY3.10	Describe the mode of muscle contraction (isometric and isotonic)	46, 259
PY3.11	Explain energy source and muscle metabolism	215
PY3.12	Explain the gradation of muscular activity	267
PY3.13	Describe muscular dystrophy: myopathies	231
PY3.14	Perform Ergography	48
PY3.15	Demonstrate effect of mild, moderate and severe exercise and record changes in cardiorespiratory parameters	48–49
PY3.17	Describe Strength-duration curve	36
Gastro-intestinal Physiology		
PY4.1	Describe the structure and functions of digestive system	118
PY4.2	Describe the composition, mechanism of secretion, functions, and regulation of saliva, gastric, pancreatic, intestinal juices and bile secretion	119, 124, 140
PY4.3	Describe GIT movements, regulation and functions. Describe defecation reflex. Explain role of dietary fibre.	9
PY4.4	Describe the physiology of digestion and absorption of nutrients	119, 202
PY4.5	Describe the source of GIT hormones, their regulation and functions	119

Code	Competency	Page number

Cardiovascular Physiology (CVS)

PY5.1 Describe the functional anatomy of heart including chambers, sounds; and Pacemaker tissue and conducting system. — 53

PY5.2 Describe the properties of cardiac muscle including its morphology, electrical, mechanical and metabolic functions — 51

PY5.3 Discuss the events occurring during the cardiac cycle — 67

PY5.4 Describe generation, conduction of cardiac impulse — 645

PY5.10 Describe and discuss regional circulation including microcirculation, lymphatic circulation, coronary, cerebral, capillary, skin, foetal, pulmonary and splanchnic circulation — 57

PY5.11 Describe the patho-physiology of shock, syncope and heart failure — 79

Respiratory Physiology

PY6.1 Describe the functional anatomy of respiratory tract — 94

PY6.2 Describe the mechanics of normal respiration, pressure changes during ventilation, lung volume and capacities, alveolar surface tension, compliance, airway resistance, ventilation, V/P ratio, diffusion capacity of lungs — 98

PY6.3 Describe and discuss the transport of respiratory gases: Oxygen and carbon dioxide — 104, 107

PY6.6 Describe and discuss the pathophysiology of dyspnoea, hypoxia, cyanosis asphyxia; drowning, periodic breathing — 114, 115, 99

PY6.7 Describe and discuss lung function tests and their clinical significance — 100

Renal Physiology

PY7.1 Describe structure and function of kidney — 211

PY7.2 Describe the structure and functions of juxtaglomerular apparatus and role of reninangiotensin system — 85, 93, 213, 227

PY7.3 Describe the mechanism of urine formation involving processes of filtration, tubular reabsorption and secretion; concentration and diluting mechanism — 214, 216

PY7.4 Describe and discuss the significance and implication of renal clearance — 213

PY7.5 Describe the renal regulation of fluid and electrolytes and acid–base balance — 211

PY7.6 Describe the innervations of urinary bladder, physiology of micturition and its abnormalities — 229, 231

PY7.7 Describe artificial kidney, dialysis and renal transplantation — 231

PY7.8 Describe and discuss renal function tests — 231

PY7.9 Describe cystometry and discuss the normal cystometrogram — 229–230

Integrated Physiology

PY11.1 Describe and discuss mechanism of temperature regulation — 48

Endocrine Physiology

PY8.1 Describe the physiology of bone and calcium metabolism — 170, 183

PY8.2 Describe the synthesis, secretion, transport, physiological actions, regulation and effect of altered (hypo and hyper) secretion of pituitary gland, thyroid gland, parathyroid gland, adrenal gland, pancreas and hypothalamus — 117, 164, 183–185

PY8.4 Describe function tests: Thyroid gland; Adrenal cortex, Adrenal medulla and pancreas (Vol 1, GIT for Pancreatic Function Test) — 161, 167, 283

PY8.5 Describe the metabolic and endocrine consequences of obesity and metabolic syndrome, stress response. Outline the psychiatry component pertaining to metabolic syndrome — 278

PY8.6 Describe and differentiate the mechanism of action of steroid, protein and amine hormones — 150

Reproductive Physiology

PY9.1 Describe and discuss sex determination; sex differentiation and their abnormities and outline psychiatry and practical implication of sex determination. — 190

PY9.2 Describe and discuss puberty: Onset, progression, stages; early and delayed puberty and outline adolescent clinical and psychological association. — 191, 197

PY9.3 Describe male reproductive system: Functions of testis and control of spermatogenesis and factors modifying it and outline its association with psychiatric illness — 192

PY9.4 Describe female reproductive system: (a) Functions of ovary and its control; (b) menstrual cycle—hormonal, uterine and ovarian changes — 197

Code	Competency	Page number
PY9.6	Enumerate the contraceptive methods for male and female. Discuss their advantages and disadvantages	204
PY9.8	Describe and discuss the physiology of pregnancy, parturition and lactation and outline the psychology and psychiatry-disorders associated with it.	206
PY9.10	Discuss the physiological basis of various pregnancy tests	203
PY9.12	Discuss the common causes of infertility in a couple and role of IVF in managing a case of infertility	208

Neurophysiology

Code	Competency	Page number
PY10.1	Describe and discuss the organization of nervous system	236
PY10.2	Describe and discuss the functions and properties of synapse, reflex, receptors	239, 240
PY10.5	Describe and discuss structure and functions of reticular activating system, autonomic nervous system (ANS)	282
PY10.6	Describe and discuss spinal cord, its functions, lesion and sensory disturbances	243
PY10.7	Describe and discuss functions of cerebral cortex, basal ganglia, thalamus, hypothalamus, cerebellum and limbic system and their abnormalities	243, 252, 263, 267, 276, 280
PY10.8	Describe and discuss behavioural and EEG characteristics during sleep and mechanism responsible for its production	281
PY10.9	Describe and discuss the physiological basis of memory, learning and speech	285
PY10.10	Describe and discuss chemical transmission in the nervous system (outline the psychiatry element)	35
PY10.12	Identify normal EEG forms	281
PY10.13	Describe and discuss perception of smell and taste sensation	311
PY10.15	Describe and discuss functional anatomy of ear and auditory pathways and physiology of hearing	307
PY10.17	Describe and discuss functional anatomy of eye, physiology of image formation, physiology of vision including colour vision, refractive errors, colour blindness, physiology of pupil and light reflex	169, 300
PY10.20	Demonstrate (i) Testing of visual acuity, colour and field of vision and (ii) hearing (iii) Testing for smell and (iv) taste sensation in volunteer/ simulated environment	291, 301, 310

Integrated Physiology

Code	Competency	Page number
PY11.1	Describe and discuss mechanism of temperature regulation	95
PY11.2	Describe and discuss adaptation to altered temperature (heat and cold)	278
PY11.4	Describe and discuss cardio-respiratory and metabolic adjustments during exercise; physical training effects	48
PY11.8	Discuss and compare cardio-respiratory changes in exercise (isometric and isotonic) with that in the resting state and under different environmental conditions (heat and cold)	46, 259
PY11.11	Discuss the concept, criteria for diagnosis of Brain death and its implications	282
PY11.12	Discuss the physiological effects of meditation	134

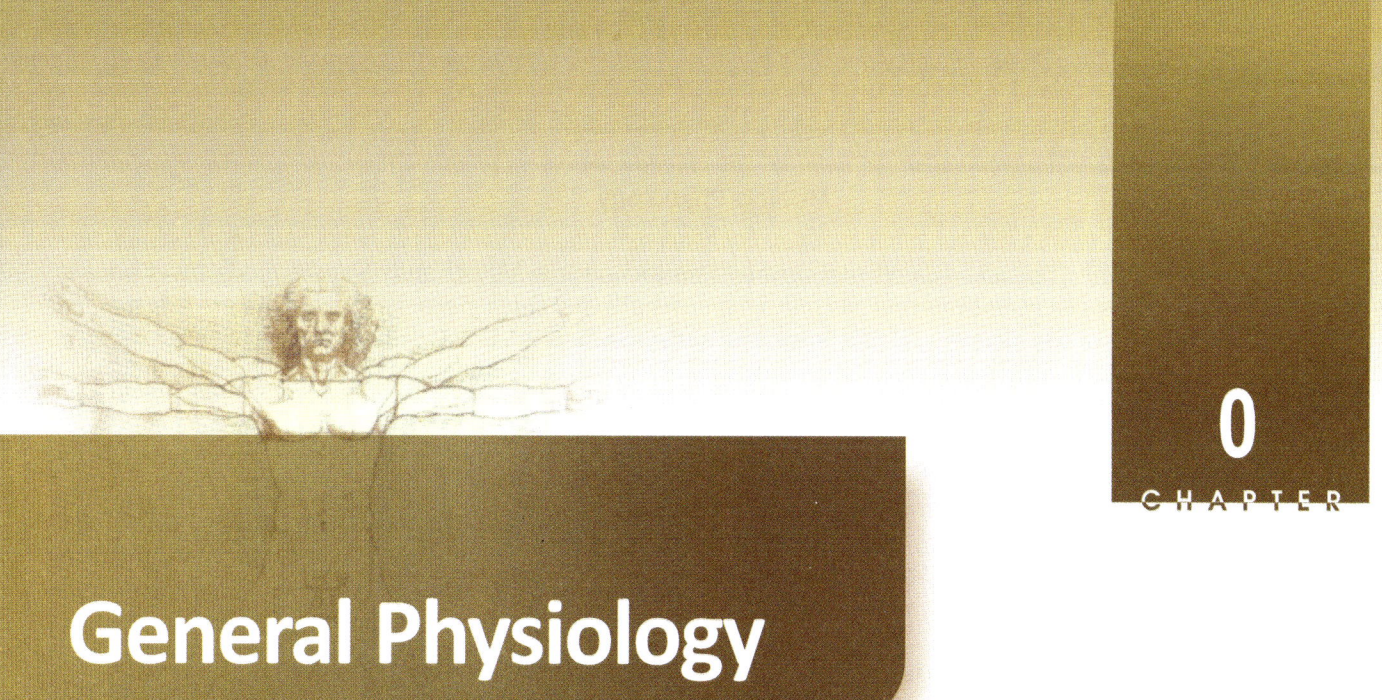

General Physiology

Introduction

What is physiology? Physiology is the study of how the various organs in our body function. Unless one understands the intricacies of the organs function, he will not be able to understand the derangements of the function that drives the body to pathological states. Hence, physiology forms the basis of medicine.

During the process of evolution that might have taken millions of years, human beings have evolved from primitive unicellular organisms. Several trillions of cells have been organized in systematic and diversified way to bring about the complex organs development that have divergent functions to carryout in human body.

Having known that trillions and trillions of cells are going to take part in the formation and function of various organs and tissues, it is quite pertinent to know something more in detail about cell and its components.

CELL

Any cell that is eukaryotic (membrane bound organelle cell) state has the following parts, namely:

a. Cell membrane
b. Cytoplasm
c. Nucleus
d. Other cell organelle like mitochondria, Golgi apparatus, lysosome, ribosome, etc.

Inside the cell, some of the important chemical substances present are:

a. Carbohydrates
b. Charged electrolytes (sodium, potassium, chloride, bicarbonate, etc.)
c. Lipids
d. Proteins
e. Water, etc.

The biologic system has evolved on earth from one of the important substances available on earth that is water. Human beings are no exception to it. All cells have large amount of water and most of the chemical substances are able to be present in dissolved state. In addition to water being present within the cells, water is also present outside between cells and other places. Some of the electrolytes that are abundant on earth are sodium, calcium, potassium, chloride, bicarbonate, etc. These electrolytes are also distributed both within and outside the cells. The distribution of various electrolytes within and outside the cells is not to the same level. Electrolyte like potassium is more within the cells when compared to sodium, chloride, bicarbonate, etc., that are present in higher level outside the cells. This type of differential distribution of electrolytes is essential for maintaining the excitability and normal function of the cells and organs.

The important organic substances inside cells are proteins, lipids and carbohydrates. Proteins form building blocks in the body. Proteins are not only present within the cells, but also in cell membrane. Proteins present in the cell membrane act as channels through which some of the electrolytes like sodium, potassium, calcium can diffuse across from extra cellular compartment into intracellular compartments and vice versa. In addition to this, some of the proteins in the cell membrane act as receptor to which specific chemical substances (ligands) can bind for actions to be brought about in the organelles of cells. Nutrition to the cells is provided by carbohydrates and lipids are insoluble in water. The cell membrane is composed of lipid substances in which proteins and carbohydrates are scattered. The position of most of the proteins are not fixed but in labile state. Hence, the cell membrane presents a fluid mosaic model (Fig. 0.1A).

Some of the important intracellular other than nucleus (Fig. 0.1B)

Mitochondria: The structure of mitochondrion varies from cell to cell. Despite this, the function of the mitochondria within cells remains the same. They are the power generating structures of the cells and depending on the cellular activity the number of the mitochondria differs from cell to cell. Conversion of food products into carbon dioxide and water is brought about by a number of enzymes present in mitochondria. Mitochondria are termed power houses of cells as they help in high energy adenosine triphosphate (ATP) synthesis.

Lysosomes are irregular large structures present in the cytoplasm. They are acidic by nature when compared to other units of the cytoplasm. They contain many of the enzymes like collagenase, ribonuclease, deoxyribonuclease and so on. These enzymes have the ability to cause destruction of the cellular components like vesicles. The lysosomes function within the cells is comparable to the function of the digestive system of the body. Lysosomes function is very important for the digestion of the bacteria that are engulfed by phagocytosis.

Golgi apparatus: Multiple layers of thin flat vesicles contribute for the formation of Golgi apparatus. Vesicles consist of couple of hundred enzymes. Polarized structure of Golgi apparatus has two different sides, namely *cis* and *trans*. Functions of Golgi apparatus include concentration of proteins, contribute for the formation of glycoproteins and lysosomal enzymes.

Ribosome: They are spherical shaped present both in free and bound form. Ribonucleic acid and proteins are abundant in ribosome. Ribosome helps in

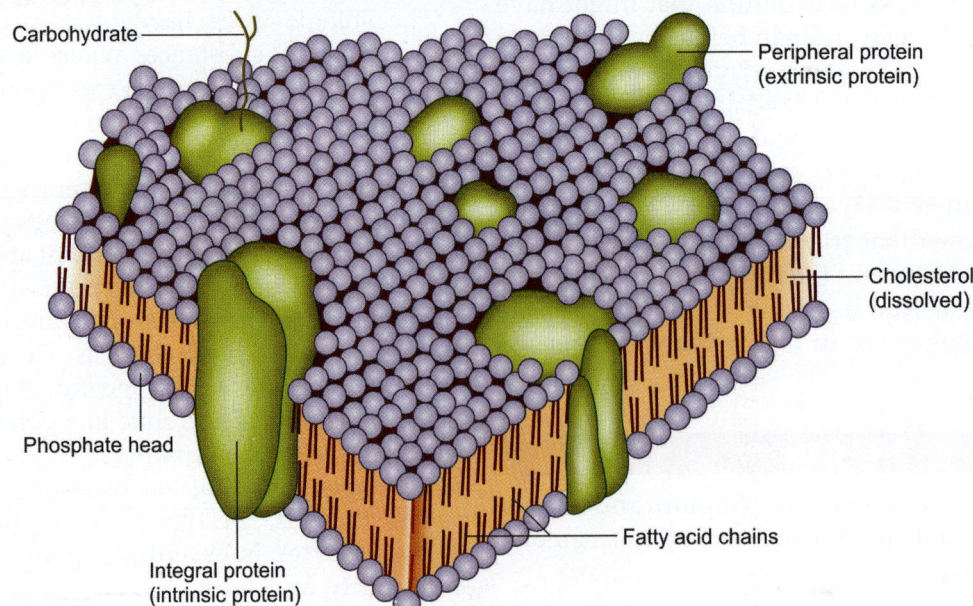

Fig. 0.1A: Biologic membrane. The phospholipid molecules have two fatty acid chains attached to a phosphate head (open circle). Proteins are integral proteins, which extend through the membrane, but peripheral proteins are attached to the inside (not shown) and outside of the membrane, are shown as colored globules (*Courtesy:* Surrinder H Singh: *Principles of Human Physiology.* Reproduced with permission)

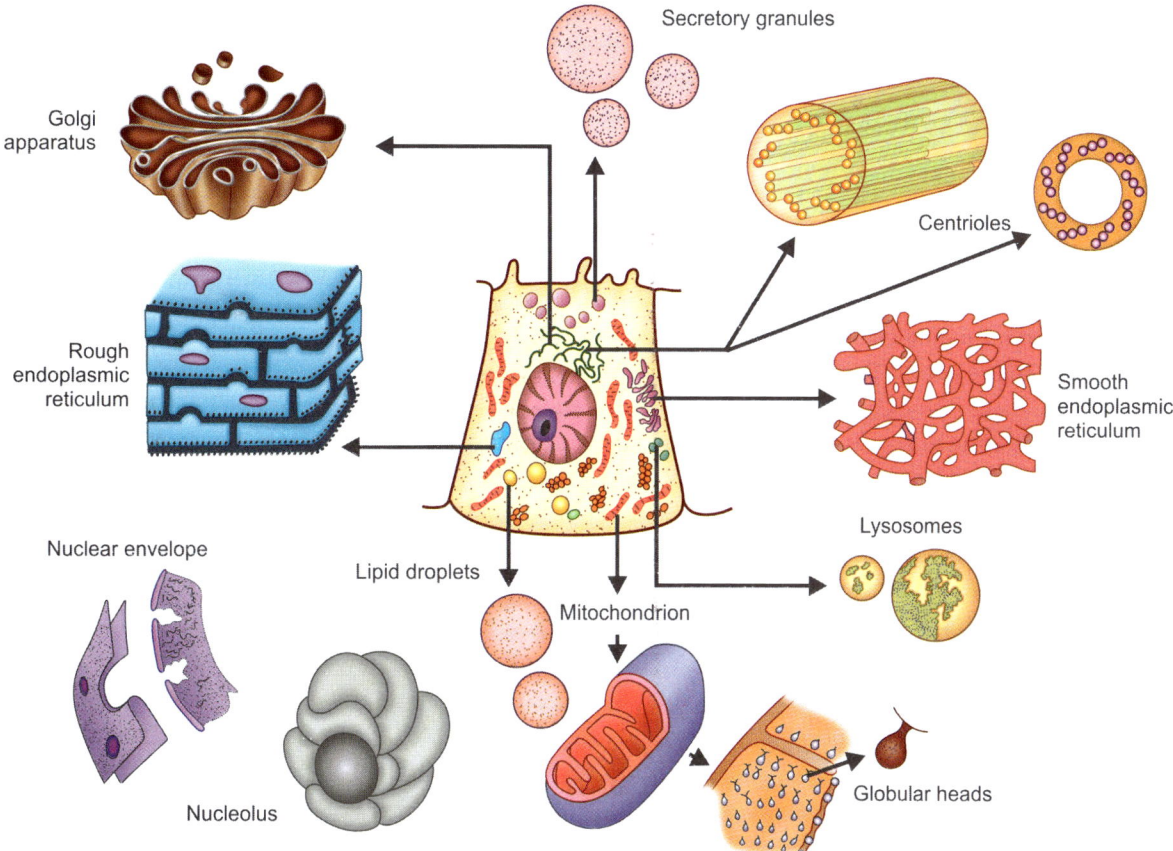

Fig. 0.1B: Diagram showing a hypothetical cell in the center, as seen with the light microscope. Various organelles of the cell are shown (*Courtesy:* Surrinder H Singh: *Principles of Human Physiology*. Reproduced with permission)

synthesis of proteins. One of the cytoplasmic proteins, namely hemoglobin is synthesized in ribosome.

Cytoskeleton: The system of fibers that try to maintain the structure of the cell is termed cytoskeleton. Cytoskeleton is made up of:
a. Intermediate filaments
b. Microfilaments and
c. Microtubules

Intermediate filaments: Connect nuclear membrane with cell membrane. Since they form flexible folds, any pressure on the cell is resisted without damage to cells.

Microfilaments: Provide elastic support to cell membrane. They are made up of actin proteins. Actin interacts with cell membrane bound proteins.

Microtubules are made up of proteins and hollow in structure. They can transport many substances in either direction within the cells.

Cytoskeleton also provides ability of the cells to change their shape.

Nucleus: One of the most important structures within cells is nucleus. It is covered by nuclear membrane. Within nucleus, chromosomes are present. In human beings the number of chromosomes present is 46 (diploid state) of which 44 are termed autosomes and a pair of sex chromosomes. In male, sex chromosomes present are X and Y and in female these are X and X. During the gametogenesis (formation of spermatozoan or ovum), there will be halving of the number of chromosomes and each gamete will have 22 autosomes and one sex chromosome (haploid state) either X or Y in male gamete (spermatozoan) and 22 autosomes and one X chromosome in female gamete (ovum). One of the important components of chromosome is presence of deoxyribonucleic acid (DNA). DNA possesses genes that are going to determine the hereditary characteristics in an organism. In addition to DNA, the other nucleic acid present in nucleus is ribonucleic acid (RNA).

Transport of Substances Across Cell

Not only water, many substances solutes like sodium, potassium, chloride, organic substances like glucose, proteins, neurotransmitters like acetyl choline (ACh), noradrenalin (NA), are transported across cell membrane. There are many mechanisms like osmosis, diffusion, and carrier mediated transport, etc., by which these substances move across the cell membrane.

1. Diffusion
2. Facilitated diffusion
3. Osmosis
4. Passive transport
5. Active transport
6. Carrier mediated transport
7. Exocytosis
8. Endocytosis/phagocytosis
9. Transcellular movement

Diffusion is the process by which any gas or substance in solution move across the electrical and/or chemical gradient without expenditure of energy. Classical example is oxygen and carbon dioxide diffusion in lungs along pressure gradients. When compared to oxygen diffusion (diffuses along a pressure gradient of 64 mm Hg), carbon dioxide diffusion (diffuses along a pressure gradient of only 6 mm Hg) across the respiratory membrane is more easy because of solubility of carbon dioxide across respiratory membrane is 24 times to that of oxygen.

Facilitated diffusion: When special carrier proteins are involved in the transport of substances along electrical and/or chemical gradient without expenditure of energy is termed facilitated diffusion. Facilitated diffusion enables faster rate of transport. It is also dependent on number of carrier proteins available. The carrier proteins are very specific to movement of certain substance. Classical example for facilitated diffusion is transport of glucose from ECF to ICF involving glucose transporter (GLUT) protein. Facilitated diffusion can be inhibited by administering certain chemical substance.

Osmosis is a process by which water is able to diffuse along a semi-permeable membrane. Between the ICF and ECF, there is constant movement of water in either direction across cell membrane. When water moves from ECF to ICF, it is termed endosmosis and when the converse happens, it is called exosmosis. For example, in osmoreceptor cells of hypothalamus when water moves from ICF to ECF is termed exosmosis and converse movement (water movement from ECF into ICF) when occurs is known as endosmosis.

Passive transport: When substances move across the cell membrane along concentration and/or electrical gradient, it is termed passive transport. Movement substance will always be along the down-hill. While the substance is passively transported, there is no expenditure of energy. For example, sodium concentration in the ICF is less when compared to ECF and inside the cell is negative when compared to exterior. Sodium being a cation (positively charged ion) moves along the electro-chemical gradient from ECF to ICF without any expenditure of energy.

Active transport: When substances move across cell membrane against electrical and/or concentration gradient and the process since it is up-hill movement, it needs expenditure of energy. Sodium that has moved in (from ECF to ICF) by passive transport has to be moved back into ECF from ICF. Sodium–potassium pump facilitates return of sodium to ECF from ICF. This is essential to maintain concentration of sodium ion at normal level both in ECF and ICF to maintain homeostasis.

Carrier mediated transport: Movement of certain substances across the cell membrane needs mediation of special proteins that act as carrier. For example, in the intestine, sodium movement from lumen into epithelial cells lining intestine involves the special carrier protein called sodium dependent glucose transporter (SGLT).

Symport or co-transport: When carrier proteins have the ability to transport more than one substance at a time, it is termed symport. For example, protein that transports sodium from tubular lumen in kidney into epithelial cells has the ability to also transport glucose from tubular lumen into epithelial cells. This type of carrier mediated transport that has the ability to transport more than one substance simultaneously in the same direction is termed symport or co-transport.

Antiport or counter transport: As opposed to symport, when a carrier protein has the ability to transport two substances simultaneously but in opposing directions is termed antiport or counter transport. For example, in the renal epithelial cells, when sodium is transported by carrier protein from renal tubular lumen into epithelial cells, the same carrier protein will be facilitating movement of hydrogen ion from epithelial cells into renal tubular lumen.

Exocytosis is the process by which certain substances are able to move from cell to ECF. For example, at neuromuscular junctions, ACh containing synaptic vesicles bind to the membrane of motor neuron terminals and ACh is finally released from motor neuron terminals into synaptic cleft by exocytosis.

Endocytosis or phagocytosis is the process by which substance moves from exterior into cell across cell membrane. Classical example is bacteria are made to move into WBCs (white blood cells/leucocytes) from the exterior by phagocytosis (cell eating) and when solution is ingested by cell it is termed pinocytosis (cell drinking).

Transcellular movement is when substance moves from ECF to ICF or vice versa across the cell membrane. Most of the substances movement across the cells are transcellular (oxygen and carbon dioxide diffusion across cell membrane).

Paracellular movement is when the substance moves not across the cell but between the junctions of cells without passing through the cell membrane. Example is water movement from the interstitium of kidney into lumen of renal tubules at the tight junctions.

Connection between the Adjacent Cells

These connections permit transfer the ions and other molecules from one cell to another. There are two types of intercellular connections, namely:
1. Tight junctions
2. Gap junctions

Tight junctions: Characteristically found in the intestinal mucosa, renal tubules, brain, etc. Ions and solutes pass through epithelia at these junctions. Tissues are able to derive strength by holding the adjacent cells together. There will be selective permeability for ions and solutes. The junction also contributes for the formation of blood–brain barrier.

Gap junctions: Between the adjacent cells there will be narrow intercellular space. This gap permits substance to pass between the cells (paracellular transport) from one cell to another without encountering extra cellular fluid. Diameter of these junctions is regulated by intra-cellular calcium ions.

Communication between the cells: There are certain other ways by which cells can communicate with each other. They are known as intercellular communications. The communication is mediated through a special chemical substance/first messenger (hormones) secreted by cells. Chemical messengers help to modulate opening or closure of ion channels, intracellular production of inositol triphosphate (IP3), increasing transcription of mRNA, etc. The chemical messengers are termed ligands which when bind to the receptors trigger intracellular mediators. The intracellular mediators are called second messengers and examples are inositol triphosphate, diaceyl glycerol, cAMP, etc.

The intercellular communications can be established by:
a. Autocrine
b. Endocrine
c. Neural
d. Paracrine communications

Autocrine communication: The chemical messengers secreted by cells themselves bind to the receptor of the cell itself and pass on the communication for further actions to be brought about. An example of an autocrine agent is cytokine interleukin-1 in monocytes.

Endocrine communication: The special chemical substances/messengers secreted by endorcrine/ductless glands are poured into blood stream. These messengers travel throughout the body along blood stream and pass on the relevant information to the target organs and tissues in almost all parts of body. Hormones secreted by endocrine glands fall into this category.

Neural communication: The chemical substances secreted by the nerve terminals are called neurotransmitters. Neurotransmitters are secreted at synaptic regions and they are able to pass on the information either from one neuron to another or from motor neuron to muscles.

Paracrine communication: In this type of communication, the chemical substances secreted by cells into ECF will be able to act on the cells in the adjacent region without entering circulation. Example is regulation of secretion of insulin from beta cells and glucagon from alpha cells by somatostatin secreted by delta cells of islets of Langerhans.

Body Fluids Compartments

ECF: Fluid present outside the cells is termed ECF. The regions that contribute for ECF are: Plasma, CSF, tubular filtrate in kidneys, intrapleural fluid (fluid present between parietal and visceral pleurae), and interstitial fluid (fluid present between cells), etc.

ICF: Fluid present inside the cells in all organs and tissues.

In an adult body weighing about 60 kg, volume of water present is about 42 liters. Of this, 28 liters water is present in ICF and remaining 14 liters in ECF. Except for about 3 liters of water present in plasma, remaining 11 liters of water is present in regions like interstitial fluid, cerebrospinal fluid (CSF), tubular filtrate in renal tubules, peritoneal and pericardial fluid, etc. It is not just water that is present both in ECF and ICF; there is also presence of organic molecules and inorganic ions.

	ICF	ECF
Sodium (mEqv/L of water)	15	150
Potassium (mEqv/L of water)	150	5
Chloride (mEqv/L of water)	10	110

In addition to the above, one of the anions present in large quantity in ICF is protein anion. Due to relatively least permeability for protein anions proteins remain in ICF and hence ICF is always negative when compared to ECF.

The above distribution of both water and ions has to be regulated for normal functioning of tissues and organs. The differential distribution of the charged ions across cell membrane creates electrical gradient. This is termed trans-membrane potential or to be more precise, resting membrane potential (RMP) when the tissue is at rest. Maintenance of RMP is mandatory for excitable tissues like neuron and muscles to exert normal functions.

Body water balance: Water balance is mainly achieved by function of kidneys. During day-to-day life, body gains water from ingested food and water taken in the form of fluids. In addition to this, some amount of water is endogenously produced during metabolic reactions in body. Body loses water in the form of insensible water loss, along with urine and feces, as sweat, etc. The fine tuning of volume of water present in body is controlled by thirst center present in hypothalamus and osmolarity regulatory mechanisms that alter thirst center activity mediated by secretion of hormone, namely anti-diuretic hormone (ADH).

Electrolyte balance: This is regulated by hormones like aldosterone that tries to maintain plasma sodium and potassium levels, parathormone and calcitonin that maintain plasma calcium level. Sodium depletion associated with water loss brings about volume contraction. This occurs in conditions like diarrhea, vomiting, etc. Excess of sodium retention in body results in person developing hypertension as increased retention of sodium will also increase water retention in the body as sodium is an osmotically active substance. One of the diseases wherein body retains more sodium is decreased ability of kidney function. Plasma potassium level is mainly regulated by aldosterone and hence in renal diseases, hypoaldosteronism (Addison's disease), etc., plasma potassium level increases and brings about alterations in excitability of tissues. In diarrhea, vomiting, etc., not only there will be decrease in plasma sodium level, there will also be decrease in plasma potassium level. This causes decreased excitability of neurons and muscles resulting in muscular weakness and cardiac arrhythmias. In conditions like diarrhea and vomiting, it is not just water content of body should be replenished, sodium and potassium ions also should be compensated, otherwise the imbalance in ions persist affecting normal functioning of neurons and muscles.

Plasma calcium level increases in hyperparathyroidism and this results in decreased excitability of neurons and skeletal muscles. However, increase in plasma calcium level increases the excitability of cardiac muscle and leads to calcium rigor. Decrease in plasma calcium level occurs in hypoparathyroidism and excitability of neurons and skeletal muscles increases leading to hypocalcemic tetany. However, the cardiac muscle activity suffers and hence person may develop hypotension.

Homeostasis is termed maintenance of internal environment constant. Claude Bernard was the first person to coin the word 'milieu interieur', that is maintenance of internal environment constant. For all organs to function properly and for life to become viable, it is a prerequisite that hydrogen ion concentration (pH of ECF), inorganic ion levels, body temperature, blood glucose level, etc., have to be maintained within the normal limitations. Hormones secreted by endocrine glands, neural mechanisms mediated by hypothalamus have significant role to play for maintaining constancy of the internal environment.

Some of the examples of homeostatic regulatory mechanisms are:

1. Negative feedback
2. Positive feedback

Cybernetics is more popular word in 21st century because of the advent of technology. What does cybernetics mean? Cybernetics means "Science of control system and communication". In biologic system, this system is very well organized. Both negative and positive feedback mechanisms are included in this.

Negative feedback: This can be best explained with the following example that tries to bring about restoration of normal heart rate and blood pressure consequent to increase in blood pressure.

1. *Controller neurons in brainstem* refer to the groups of neurons present in medulla oblongata. The groups of neurons are going to constitute a. vasomotor center, b. cardioinhibitory center and c. Respiratory center.

a. *Vasomotor center* (VMC) sends constant excitatory influence to vascular smooth muscle through sympathetic system which takes origin from lateral horn cells in thoraco-lumbar segments of spinal cord. Sympathetic system is responsible for arteriolar tone and venomotor tone. Arteriolar tone is constant excitatory influence by sympathetics on vascular smooth muscle in arterial compartment. This is essential to maintain diastolic blood pressure. Venomotor tone is constant excitatory influence by sympathetics on vascular smooth muscle in venous compartment. This is essential to maintain adequate venous return to the heart from peripheral parts of body.

Apart from this, sympathetic fibers also innervate the cardiac muscle and hence can alter cardiac muscle activity. The influence on cardiac muscle results in increased heart rate and increased stroke volume.

b. *Cardioinhibitory center* has collection of neurons which is generally referred to as dorsal motor nucleus of vagus. From these neurons, vagal fibers take origin. Vagal fibers supplying heart are responsible for vagal tone. Vagal tone is constant inhibitory influence exerted by vagus

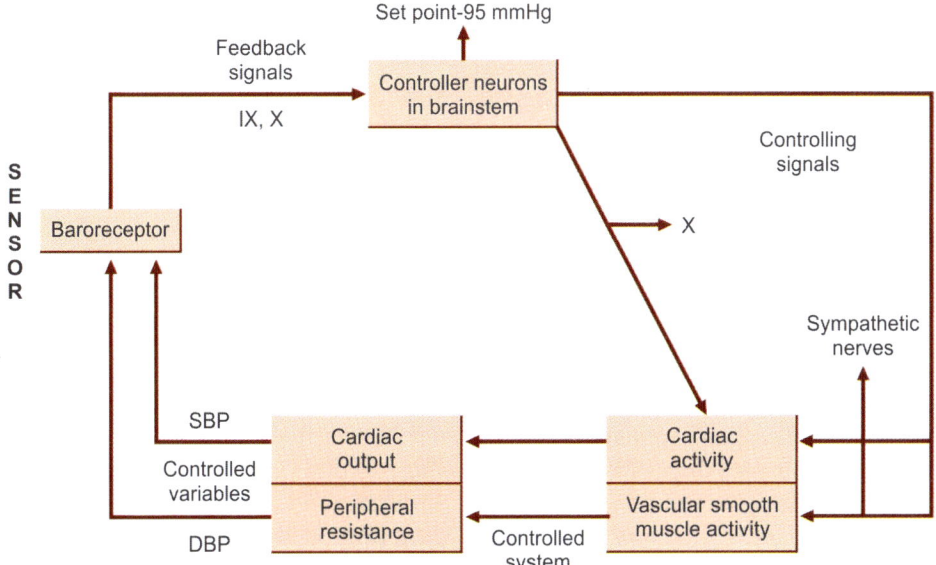

Fig. 0.2: Cardiovascular regulation

on heart. Even under resting conditions, vagal tone is dominant over the sympathetic influence and hence heart is maintained around 75 beats per minute. Increased vagal tone results in decreased heart rate and cardiac output.

c. *Respiratory center* also has influence on cardio-vascular regulation because changes in respiratory activity can lead to alterations in venous return. During respiratory activity, intra-pleural pressure is changed because of which venous return to heart is altered.

2. *Cardiac activity:* This has two components, namely frequency of heart beating and volume of blood pumped out during every beating of heart. The former is referred to as heart rate and the latter is termed stroke volume. Product of heart rate and stroke volume constitutes cardiac output. Cardiac output is the determinant for systolic blood pressure and generally cardiac output and systolic pressure have direct relationship.

3. *Vascular smooth muscle activity:* The smooth muscle present in the tunica media of vascular wall is supplied by sympathetic fibers. Vascular smooth muscle present in the walls of arterioles is constantly in contractile state because of the impulses impinging on them by sympathetic fibers. This maintains the arteriolar tone. Arteriolar tone and diastolic blood pressure also have a direct relationship.

4. *Sensor:* The baroreceptors present in carotid sinus and arch of aorta are able to sense blood pressure prevalent in arterial compartment. They are able to make out pressure termed mean arterial pressure. Mean arterial pressure is diastolic pressure plus 1/3 of pulse pressure. (Pulse pressure is difference between systolic and diastolic pressure.) The normal mean arterial pressure is around 95 mm Hg. If there is any alteration in mean arterial pressure, it is faithfully informed to the controller neurons in brainstem as feedback signals with the help of sinus nerve (branch of IX cranial nerve) and aortic nerve (branch of X cranial nerve).

Positive feedback: As opposed to negative feedback there is also positive feedback mechanism operating in body. One of the examples of positive feedback mechanism is the process of formation of clot which reduces volume of blood loss from body when blood vessel is damaged. This mechanism tries to minimize volume reduction of blood in body.

The positive feedback mechanism operating when there is injury to blood vessel is as detailed:

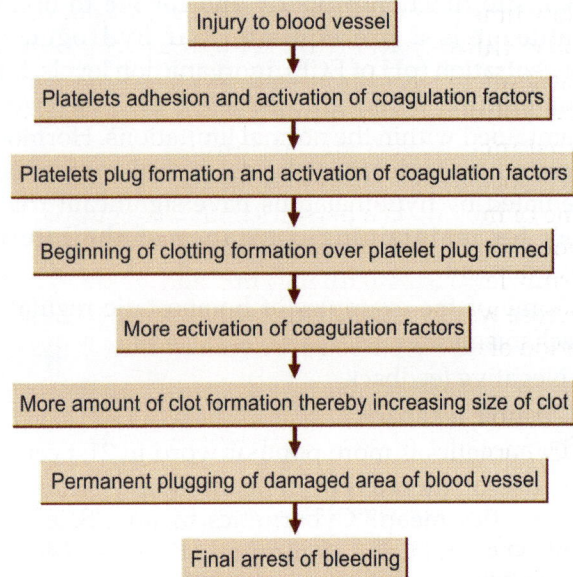

Other than the above mechanisms, certain other responses also help in homeostasis. Biological rhythms like circadian rhythm (variations in activity in 24 hours), circlunar (variation in activity in a month) and circannual (variation in activity in years). Hormones like ADH and steroid secretion rate is altered based on 24 hours time. Estrogen and progesterone hormone secretion varies in a month leading to cyclical changes in female reproductive system. Growth hormone and sex hormone secretion changes as per years which bring about linear growth of body and also attainment puberty.

Prolonged exposure of body to altered atmosphere brings about certain alterations in body to adjust for altered atmosphere. This is termed acclimatization. When person is exposed to high altitude due to fall in atmospheric pressure, in the initial few days, respiration is affected, thereby the person suffers from hypoxia (decreased supply of oxygen to tissues). However, when person has continued to remain in the altitude, changes in respiratory regulatory mechanism and alterations brought about in the intracellular regions like increase in myoglobin content, mitochondria number, cytochrome oxidase, etc., will slowly facilitate person to overcome the hardship and adjust to the altitude with almost normal function. However, the changes that have occurred in body return to normal state when person returns to normal altitude.

Measurement of Body Fluid Volume

It is measured by administering the test substance, allow time for the distribution of the substance in the body fluid. After this, calculate the volume distribution in which the test substance has got into. The volume distribution is equal to amount of substance administered minus the amount of substance metabolized and/or excreted during the time of mixing. In a person's body weighing 70 kg, if about 75 mg of sucrose was injected and the plasma serum level was 0.01 mg/mL and about 5 mg of sucrose was excreted along with the urine during the period of mixing, the sucrose volume distribution will be:

Amount of substance administered – Amount of substance lost and/or metabolized

$$\text{Volume distribution} = \frac{\begin{array}{c}\text{Amount of substance administered}\end{array} - \begin{array}{c}\text{Amount of substance lost and/or metabolized}\end{array}}{\text{Plasma concentration of the substance}}$$

$$= \frac{75 - 5}{0.01} = 7000 \, \text{mL}$$

Since sucrose has been used for measurement, this space is known as sucrose space.

Many substances can be used to measure volume distribution. Some of the criteria any substance should obey are:

1. Should be non-toxic
2. Must get distributed evenly
3. Should not have any effect on the body, etc.

ECF volume can be measured by using some of the following substances like:

a. Inulin
b. Mannitol
c. Sucrose

ICF volume can be measured by subtracting the ECF volume from the total body water (TBW). Deutrium oxide (heavy water) most often preferred to measure the TBW. Aminoprine can also be used to measure TBW.

Body Fluid Compartments

Body fluid volume and/or osmolarity variations may occur in the patient's body for various reasons. These variations will disrupt the functions of many of the vital organs in the body like heart, brain, kidney, etc.

When functions of any of these organs are compromised, it can lead to irreparable loss of functions of the organs in general. In some conditions, variations can lead to fatal situations as well. Hence, it is very pertinent to understand normal body fluid compartments and osmolarity, so that appropriate remedial measures can be resorted at the earliest so that function of the vital organs in the body can be restored and life of the patient is salvaged.

In an adult body, about 42 liters of water is present. Of this, about 28 L (2/3rd) is within the cells and is termed intracellular fluid (ICF) and the remaining 14 L (1/3rd) is outside the cells and is known as extracellular fluid (ECF). The ECF collectively refers to the fluid present in various regions of the body like: Within blood vessels (plasma), interstitial regions of neurons in central nervous system (cerebrospinal fluid), fluid present between the cells in all the parts of body (interstitial fluid), peritoneal fluid, pericardial fluid, etc. Plasma is considered to be the ideal representative of ECF.

It is not just water present both in ICF and ECF, but many of the solutes like: Sodium, potassium, chloride, etc, are also present. The solutes exert pressure termed crystalloid osmotic/oncotic pressure. Many a time, relative proportion between water and solutes is also called Osmolarity/Osmolality (Osmolarity/Osmolality, refers to the concentration of solution in terms of osmoles of solute per kilogram of solvent (water)). Normally, osmolarity of the body fluids is about 300 mOsm/L water or 300 mOsm/kg water (isotonic fluid). Whatever is the osmolarity in the ECF, ICF equalizes the osmolarity of ECF by appropriate directional movement of solvent (water).

The separating structure/membrane between the ICF and ECF is the cell membrane. Cell membrane acts as a semi-permeable membrane (water is able to easily move across the membrane when compared to solutes movement). Movement of water across the semipermeable membrane is termed Osmosis. Even in normal conditions, water keeps moving all the time across the membrane in either direction. Since number of molecules of water moved across (from ECF to ICF and vice versa) the membrane is equal and opposite, net movement of water will be zero in normal conditions.

However, when ECF osmolarity is altered for any reason, ICF osmolarity will also change and equals to that of ECF. How is this possible? For example, if the

ECF osmolarity is increased (either by addition of solutes to ECF, or by decrease in water content of the ECF), the number of molecules of water moving out of ICF into ECF will be more than the number of molecules of water moving from ECF to ICF. This is termed Exosmosis. Because of this, the osmolarity of the ICF matches with that of ECF, leading to reduction of fluid volume present in ICF (volume contraction of ICF).

Conversely, when the ECF osmolarity is decreased (either by entry of more water into ECF or loss of more solutes than water from ECF), number of molecules of water moving from ECF to ICF will be more than the number of molecules of water moving from ICF to ECF. This is termed Endosmosis. Because of this, osmolarity of the ICF is equalized with that of ECF osmolarity. Since more water is gained by ICF, the ICF volume increases (volume expansion of ICF).

Volume contraction or expansion can also occur in ECF in various conditions. Some of the conditions in which volume expansion of ECF occurs are in conditions like: Drinking of large volume of fresh water, infusion of isotonic saline, etc. Some of the conditions in which there will be volume contraction of ECF are: Dehydration for any reason, hemorrhage, diarrhea, etc.

The following diagram is termed Darrow-Yonnet diagram. It is indicating the proportionality of the body fluid compartments by volume and the osmolarity of body fluids.

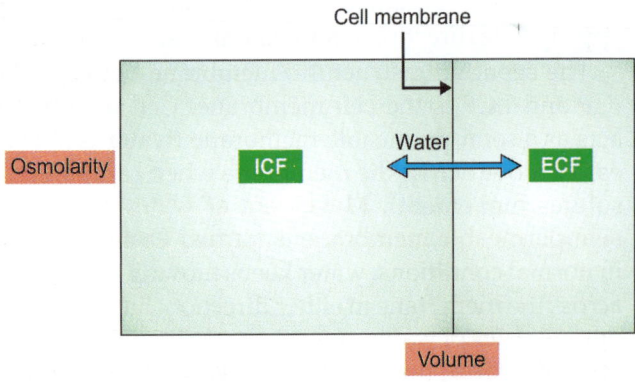

The line separating the ECF from the ICF is presumed as the cell membrane. Across the cell membrane water molecules will be moving from ECF to ICF and vice versa. However, in normal conditions net movement of water is zero.

Alterations in the Body Fluid Compartments during Certain Conditions

1. *In conditions like:* Hemorrhage, diarrhea, etc., there will be loss of isotonic fluid (water and solutes loss in proper/ideal proportion) from the body. Though there will be volume contraction of ECF, but there will not be any change in the volume and/or osmolarity of the ICF as the osmolarity of the ECF continues to be normal. The fluid that has been lost from the body is isotonic.

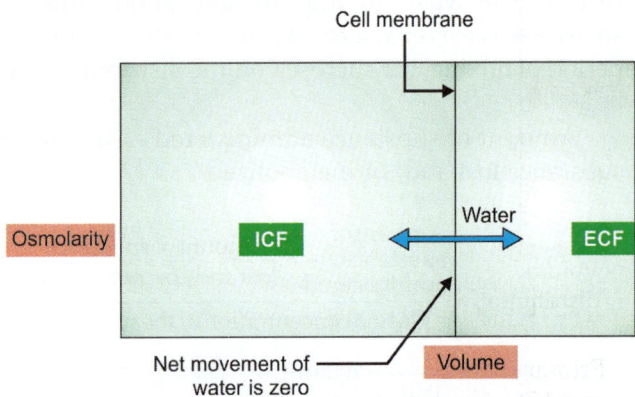

There will be loss of water and solutes in ideal proportion, and ECF contracts.

2. When there is infusion of isotonic saline (0.9% sodium chloride solution), there will be gain of isotonic fluid in ECF. Though there will be expansion of ECF, there will not be any change in the volume and/or osmolarity of ICF as the osmolarity of the ECF has continued to be normal since the fluid that has been gained is isotonic.

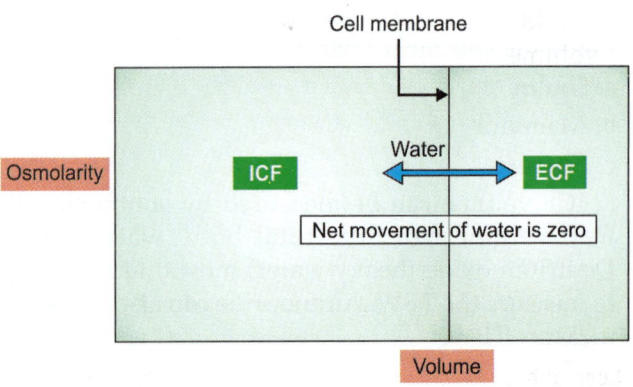

Gain of isotonic fluid, ECF expands but no change in osmolarity.

3. *In conditions like:* Dehydration, diabetes insipidus, etc., there will be loss of hypotonic fluid (more loss of water from ECF when compared to solutes). This

leads to volume contraction of ECF and increase of osmolarity of ECF. Since ECF osmolarity is more than that of ICF, there will be more water molecules movement from ICF to ECF (exosmosis) to equalize the osmolarity of ICF with that of ECF. Hence osmolarity of both ECF and ICF is increased. In addition to this, there will be volume contraction of both ECF and ICF also.

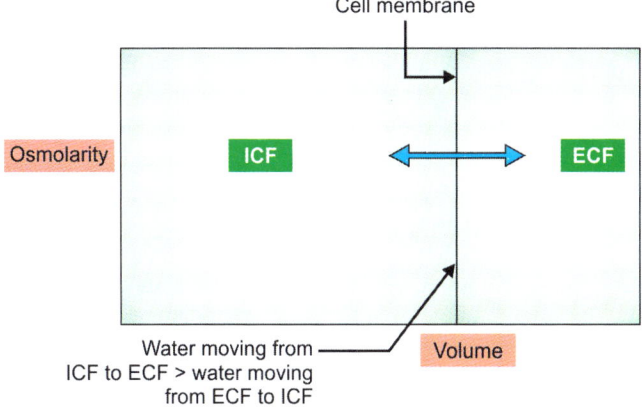

Primary loss of water from ECF leading to both ECF and ICF contraction.

4. *In conditions like:* Hypotonic saline infusion, drinking lot of fresh water, water intoxication, etc., there will be gain of hypotonic fluid in ECF. This leads to expansion of ECF and decrease of osmolarity of ECF. Since, ECF osmolarity is less than normal, there will be more molecules of water movement from ECF to ICF (endosmosis) to equalize the osmolarity of ICF with that of ECF. Hence osmolarity of both ECF and ICF decreased. In addition to this, there will be expansion of ICF volume as well.

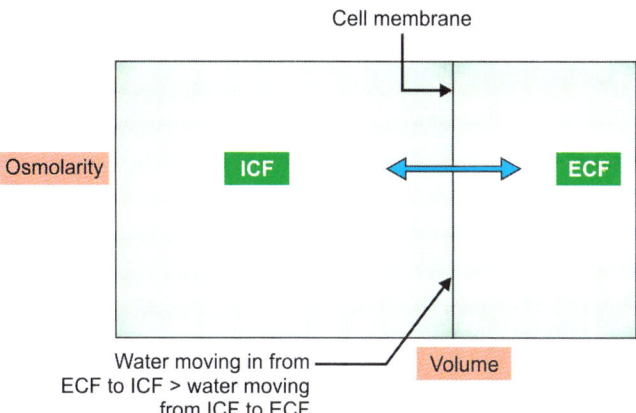

Primary gain of water into ECF leading to both ECF and ICF expansion.

5. When there is gain of hypertonic fluid in conditions like hypertonic saline infusion (more than 0.9% saline solution), ingestion of salt tablets, etc., leads to increase of osmolarity of ECF. Because of this, there will be more molecules of water movement from ICF to ECF (exosmosis). Increased movement of water from ICF to ECF will increase the osmolarity of ICF also. However, there will be expansion of ECF with concomitant contraction of ICF.

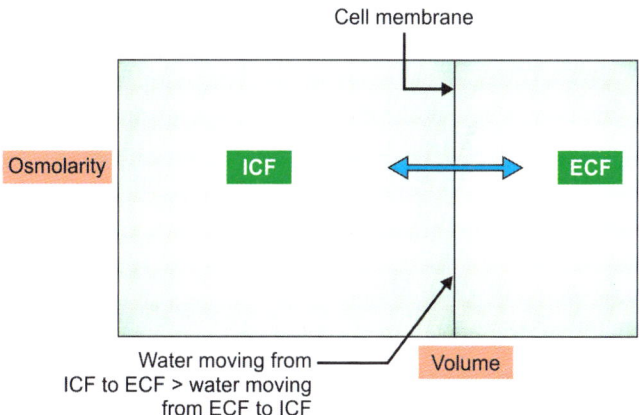

Primary gain of solutes into ECF finally leading to ECF expansion and ICF contraction.

Table 0.1: Changes in volume of ECF and ICF and/or body fluids osmolarity in altered states

	ECF volume	*Body osmolarity*	*ICF volume*
Loss of hypotonic fluid	Contracts/decreased	Increased	Contracts/decreased
Loss of isotonic fluid	Contracts/decreased	No change	No change
Gain of hypotonic fluid	Expands/increased	Decreased	Expands/increased
Gain of isotonic fluid	Expands/increased	No change	No change
Gain of hypertonic fluid/ ingestion of salt tablets	Expands/increased	Increased	Contracts/decreased

Dehydration

1. Isosmotic Dehydration

Causes of isosmotic dehydration include hemorrhage, plasma exudation through burnt skin, and gastrointestinal fluid loss (e.g. vomiting, diarrhea). No major change occurs in the osmolarity of ECF; therefore no fluid shifts into or out ICF compartment.

2. Hyperosmotic Dehydration

Causes of hyperosmotic dehydration includes water deficits caused by decreased intake, diabetes insipidus, diabetes mellitus, fever (through excessive evaporation of the sweat from the skin—sweat is hypotonic). Initially, water is lost from plasma, which becomes hyperosmotic, causing water shift from the ICF into the plasma. Because of increased movement of water from ICF to ECF, the osmolarity of ICF will also increase to match with that of ECF. Finally, both the ECF and ICF compartments contract and the osmolarity increased in both.

3. Hyposmotic Dehydration

Causes of hyposmotic dehydration include renal loss of NaCl because of adrenal insufficiency (e.g. primary adrenal insufficiency—Addison's disease). In Addison's disease, there will be decreased secretion of cortisol and aldosterone, because of which there will be marked loss of salts from the body when compared to volume of water lost.

Over Hydration States

1. Isosmotic Over Hydration

Causes of isosmotic over hydration are oral or parenteral administration of a large volume of isotonic NaCl. This type of over hydration is characterized by an overall expansion of the ECF without any change in the osmolarity of the ECF and ICF compartments.

Table 0.2: Applied aspects—alterations in hydration state

Conditions	Examples
Isomotic dehydration	Hemorrhage
	Burns
	Diarrhea
	Vomiting
Hyperosmotic dehydration	Diabetes insipidus
	Diabetes mellitus
	Severe sweating
	Water deprivation
Hyposmotic dehydration	Addison's disease
Isosmotic over hydration	0.9% saline infusion
Hyperosmotic over hydration	Sea water drinking
	Salt tablets ingestion
	Mannitol administration
Hyposmotic over hydration	Fresh water drinking
	SIADH (syndrome of inappropriate ADH secretion—secretion of ADH is more than what is required by the body)

2. Hyperosmotic Over Hydration

Causes are oral or parenteral intake of large amounts of hypertonic fluid. Intravenous infusion of hypertonic saline solution leads to an increase in plasma/ECF osmolarity. Increase in osmolarity of ECF causes water to move out of ICF into ECF, which eventually decreases the volume of ICF and increases the volume of the ECF. The osmolarity of both compartments is increased.

3. Hyposmotic Over Hydration

There are usually two reasons: 1. ingestion of a large volume of water and 2. renal retention of water due to syndrome of inappropriate antidiuretic hormone (SIADH) secretion. This leads to decrease of ECF osmolarity. Decrease in osmolarity causes more water shift to ICF from ECF. Finally, both ECF and ICF volume expand and osmolarity of both the compartments will be decreased.

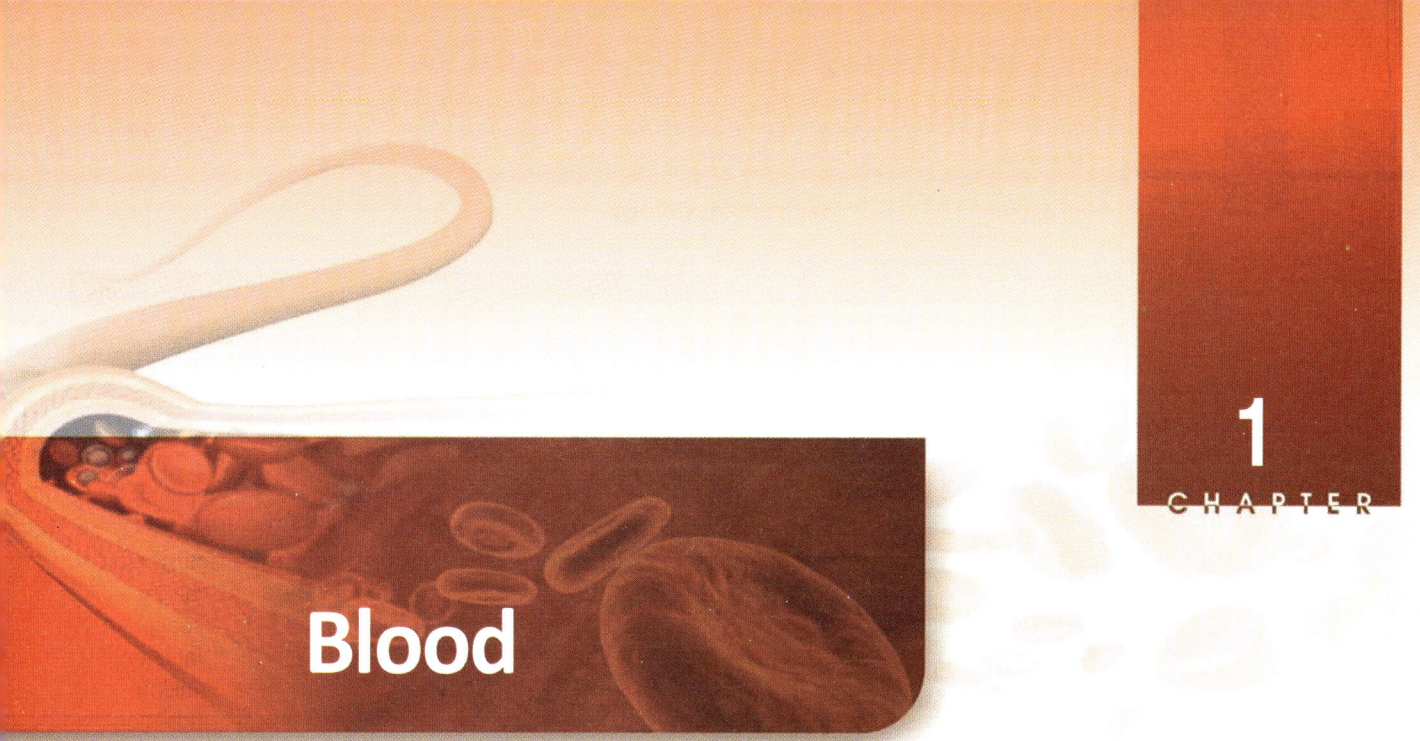

Blood

HEMATOLOGY

Hematology is the study of components and functions of blood. In an adult male of 70 kg body weight, the normal blood volume is about 5 liters. In relation to body weight, it is about:

- 70 ml/kg in adult
- 90 ml/kg in children

Functions of Blood

- Respiratory function includes supply of oxygen from lungs to tissues and removal of carbon dioxide from the tissues to lungs for elimination.
- Excretory function refers to transport of metabolic waste products, urea, uric acid and creatinine, from the tissue to the kidneys for excretion.
- Nutritive function, which includes supply of all the materials, required by the tissues to obtain their energy demands to carry on the metabolic activities.
- Regulation of body temperature by helping in heat transfer mechanism from one body to another along the thermal gradient by physical processes, like convection, radiation, conduction and vaporization.
- Protective function is brought about by the presence of leukocytes and immunoglobulin (gamma globulins). These cells and proteins respectively protect the body from infections. Platelets also help in the prevention of blood loss

from the body when there is any breach in the blood vessel by the processes namely hemostasis and blood coagulation.

- Buffers present in blood help to maintain the pH around 7.4 which is essential for the normal functioning of enzymes.

Composition of Blood

Blood is the fluid connective tissue, which is in constant circulation throughout the body. It is composed of plasma and formed elements.

The formed element of blood is made up of RBCs (erythrocytes), WBCs (leukocytes) and platelets (thrombocytes). The percentage volume of the formed element in 100 ml of blood is about 45, which is known as packed cell volume (PCV) or hematocrit value. Normally, hematocrit refers to the % volume of RBCs alone. Buffy coat contains WBCs and platelets and will be about 1%. The remaining part of blood is made up of plasma, which is about 55%. The formed elements are suspended in plasma.

Method to determine hematocrit value: Wintrobe's technique.

- Collect about 5 ml of blood from a vein.
- Mix it with proper anticoagulant (double oxalate mixture in powder form (ammonium oxalate and potassium oxalate).
- Fill the Wintrobe's tube with the blood sample (taking care to avoid air bubbles).

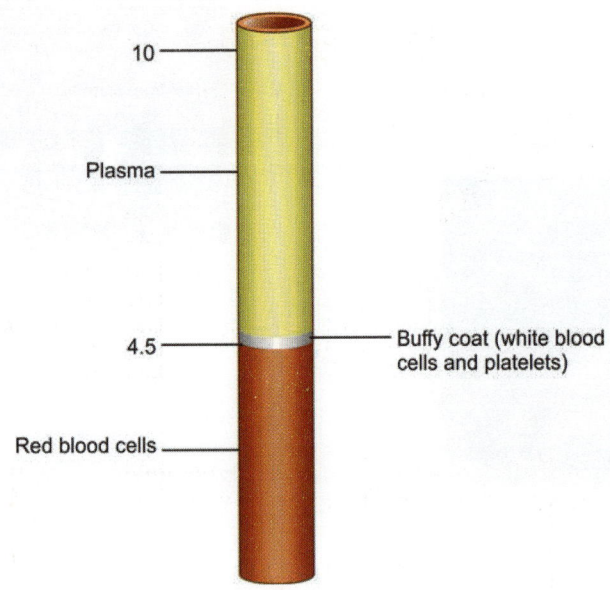

Fig. 1.1: Blood sample after centrifugation showing RBCs, buffy coat and plasma columns

- Centrifuge the tube at 3000 rpm (revolutions per minute) for half an hour.
- Take the reading (note down the height of packed RBC column)

As stated already, the normal packed cell volume in adult is 45% (Fig. 1.1). There are many conditions in which it may either increase or decrease.

Increase in PCV is known as hemoconcentration: It occurs when body water content is decreased for any reason, like severe vomiting, diarrhea, burns and excessive sweating. In hemoconcentration, there will be only a relative increase in the erythrocyte count. In polycythemia, there will be an absolute increase in the erythrocyte count and an increase in PCV.

Decrease in PCV is known as hemodilution: It occurs in all types of anemias, immediately after blood loss, pregnancy and administration of intravenous fluids.

Specific Gravity

Specific gravity is the relative density of blood when compared to water (assuming specific gravity of water as 1000). The specific gravity of blood is as follows:

a. Whole blood   1055–1060
b. Plasma alone   1025–1030
c. Red blood cells alone 1085–1090

When there is hemoconcentration, specific gravity of blood increases and it is reduced in hemodilution.

PLASMA

Plasma is the fluid part of blood that keeps the formed elements suspended for easy circulation throughout the cardiovascular system.

Composition

- It is composed of water (91–92%) and solids (7–9%).
- Solids can be divisible into organic and inorganic components.

Some of the important organic components are:
a. Plasma proteins 6–8 g%
b. Urea 15–40 mg%
c. Glucose 60–90 mg% (fasting)
d. Cholesterol 150–250 mg%
e. Uric acid
f. Creatinine

Some of the important inorganic constituents are:
Na^+, K^+, Ca^{++}, Cl^-, HCO_3^- (Table 1.1 wherein ECF refers to plasma)

Table 1.1: Indicating the relative content of some of the important substances in ECF and ICF

Substance (mEq/L)	ECF	ICF
Na^+	145	12
K^+	4	150
Ca^{2+}	5	0.001
Cl^-	105	5
HCO_3^-	25	12
Pi	2	100
pH	7.4	7.1

Plasma Proteins

Plasma proteins are of different types namely albumin, globulin, fibrinogen and prothrombin.
a. *Albumin:* 4–4.8 g%—Mol. wt. 68,000
b. *Globulin:* 2.3 g%—Mol. wt. ranges from 90,000 to 13,00,000
c. *Fibrinogen:* 0.3 g%—Mol. wt. 3,30,000
d. *Prothrombin:* 15–40 mg%

The globulin can be further divided into α, β and γ (immunoglobulin) fractions.

Normal albumin globulin ratio is about 2:1. Reversal of the ratio occurs in diseases of liver and kidney.

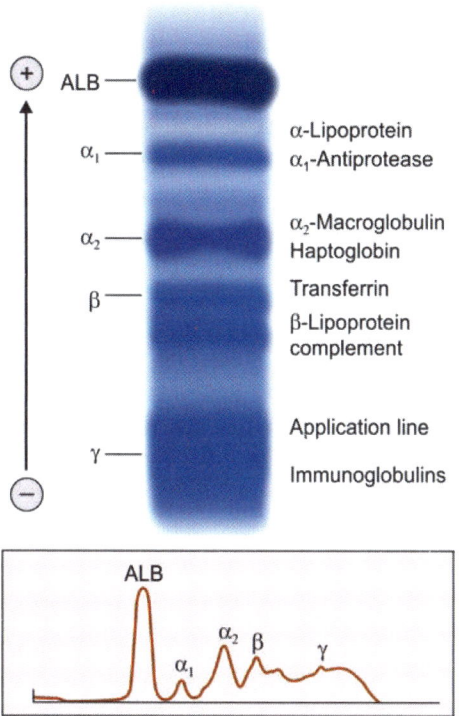

Fig. 1.2: Various plasma proteins separated after electrophoresis

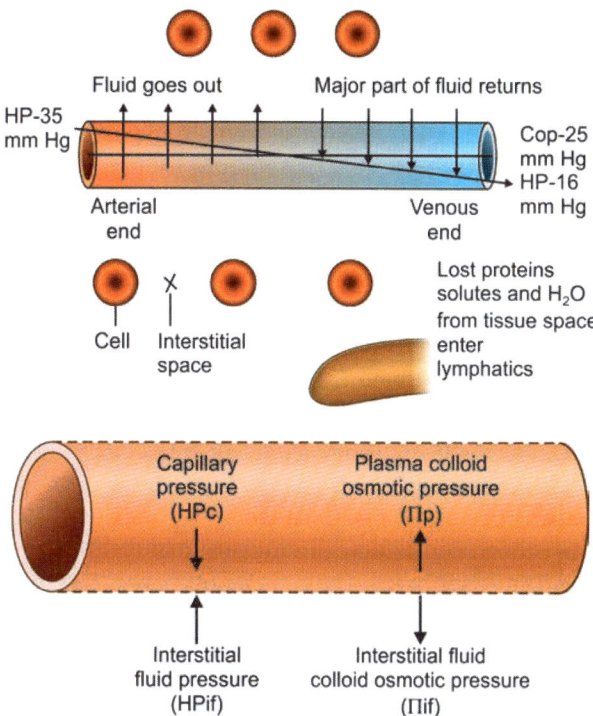

Fig. 1.3: Capillary with the fluid exchange mechanism (Starling's hypothesis)

Separation of the plasma proteins: It can be achieved by various techniques, like:

a. Electrophoresis (commonly employed)
b. Immunoelectrophoresis
c. Salting out method
d. Svedberg ultracentrifugation method

Because the plasma proteins are charged molecules, from the line of application, the proteins move either towards negative or positive pole of an electrical field and at different velocity (Fig. 1.2).

Functions of Plasma Proteins

1. *Maintenance of colloidal osmotic pressure*: Colloidal osmotic pressure is about 25 mm Hg and 80% of this is contributed by albumin alone. Since albumin concentration is more and has low molecular weight, its contribution is more for the maintenance of colloidal osmotic pressure. Maintenance of colloidal osmotic pressure is essential to maintain the fluid balance between the intravascular compartment and interstitial spaces.

   Capillary dynamics (Fig. 1.3): At the level of capillaries, hydrostatic pressure, which is about 35 mm Hg at the arterial end, tries to drive out water from the intravascular compartment into interstitial spaces. This is opposed by the colloidal osmotic pressure, which is about 25 mm Hg. However, since the hydrostatic pressure at the arterial end is greater than the colloidal osmotic pressure, some volume of fluid goes out into the tissue spaces.

   At the venous end of the capillary, the colloidal osmotic pressure remains the same because the capillary is almost impermeable to plasma proteins. But the hydrostatic pressure is reduced to 16 mm Hg due to resistance offered by the capillary wall and gradual decrease of blood volume in the capillary due to leaking out of the fluid into tissue spaces. Therefore, at the venous end of the capillary, the colloidal osmotic pressure remains high compared to hydrostatic pressure. Because of this, some volume of fluid from the tissue spaces returns to the intravascular compartment. However, a small volume of fluid left behind in the tissue spaces. This volume is brought back into circulation by lymphatic so as to maintain the blood volume. When plasma protein level especially that of albumin decreases, it leads to the fall in the colloidal osmotic pressure thereby leads to accumulation of more than normal fluid in tissue spaces. *Edema* is defined as excess of fluid accumulation in the interstitial spaces.

Edema occurs in diseases of the liver, kidney, and in malnutrition (due to decrease in plasma albumin content). Edema can also be due to increase in the hydrostatic pressure in capillaries as happens in hypertension.

2. *Helps in the process of blood coagulation:* When there is bleeding, if the bleeding continues, the person may lose large volume of blood and this will lead to serious consequences. One of the important mechanisms by which the arrest of bleeding is brought about is by coagulation of blood. For coagulation to be brought about, the role of some of the plasma proteins, like fibrinogen, prothrombin and antihemophilic globulin, is very much essential (for details refer to Blood Coagulation).

3. *Protective function:* It helps the body to fight against any micro-organism that may cause disease. Protection is brought about due to presence of immunoglobulin (gamma globulin) which acts as antibodies against bacterial antigen. By this way plasma proteins provide specific immunity throughout the lifespan of the person.

4. *Regulation of pH of blood:* The pH of blood has to be regulated at 7.4 ± 0.04 for smooth functioning of the tissue enzymes. It is essential to maintain the H^+ concentration within this critical range. Plasma proteins have free NH_2 and COOH terminals, which can either, accept or donate H^+ readily for the maintenance of pH of blood within the narrow range. When pH falls below 7.4 is known as acidosis and above 7.4 is termed as alkalosis.

5. *Transport function:* Plasma proteins help to transport many of the substances in the circulation. Some of the important substances transported are carbon dioxide; hormones, like cortisol, thyroxin; metals, like iron and copper.

6. *Maintenance of viscosity of blood:* Blood is more viscous than water by about 4–6 times. Plasma proteins and formed elements contribute equally for maintenance of viscosity. Among the plasma proteins, fibrinogen is most important in the maintenance of viscosity as it has got irregular shape. Viscosity plays an important role in the maintenance of blood pressure.

Synthesis of Plasma Proteins

  i. Plasma proteins are produced in the liver.

 ii. Albumin, fibrinogen, and prothrombin are produced exclusively in the liver.

iii. 80% of globulins also are produced in the liver.

iv. About 20% of globulins are produced from the cells belonging to reticuloendothelial system.

 v. Rate of plasma protein production in liver is about 30 g/day.

Plasma proteins content markedly decreases in:

a. Liver diseases due to decreased rate of synthesis.

b. Kidney diseases due to excretion of proteins along with urine.

c. Malnutrition due to lack of protein material in the diet.

FORMED ELEMENTS

The formed elements are erythrocytes, leukocytes and platelets. Among the three types of cells, in terms of number, erythrocytes are most followed by platelets and least in number are leukocytes.

Red Blood Cells (Erythrocytes)

a. Non-nucleated, biconcave disk or dumb-bell-shaped bodies (Fig. 1.4).

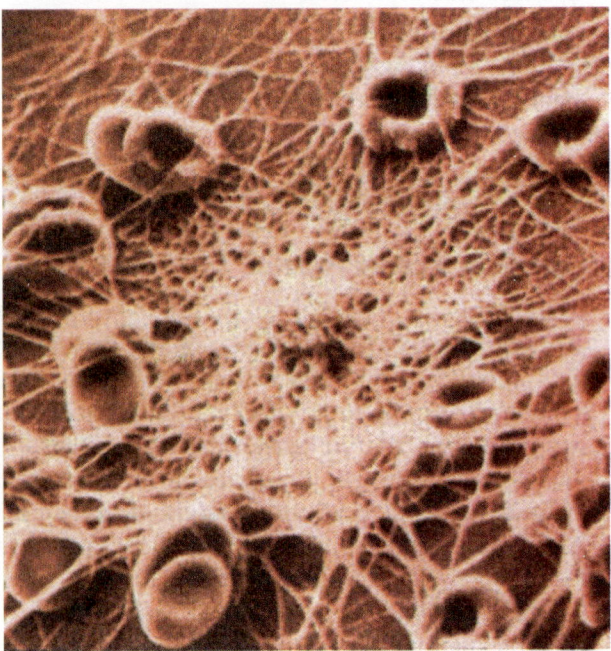

Fig. 1.4: Red blood cell as observed under the microscope

b. Have a mean diameter of about 7.2 μ.

c. Cell volume is 78 to 94 cuμ or fL.

d. Normal count is about 5.5 million/cu mm of blood in adult male. In females, it is about 4.5 million/cu mm and in newborn infant, it is about 6–7 million/cu mm.

e. One of the most important components of this cell is hemoglobin (Hb). All the functions attributed to red blood cells are because of this pigment present in the cell.

Oligocythemia

- Refers to decrease in red blood cell count.
- Can occur in physiological conditions, like exposure to high barometric pressure (deep sea diving, deep mines, etc.).
- Can also occur in pathological condition, like anemia.

Polycythemia (Erythrocytosis)

- Refers to an increase in red blood cell count.
- Occurs in physiological conditions, like high altitude.
- Also occurs in pathological conditions, like chronic diseases of lung and congenital heart diseases associated with cyanosis, in certain endocrine disorders, like hyperthyroidism, Cushing's syndrome, etc.

Functions of red blood cells are as good as functions of hemoglobin:

1. Help to transport oxygen from lungs to tissues for their metabolic needs and carbon dioxide from the tissues to the lungs for elimination purposes.

2. Help to regulate the pH of blood, since the globin part of hemoglobin is made up of proteins, which can either accept or donate H^+ as the situation demands.

Rouleaux Formation

- Surface of erythrocytes carry negative charge.
- As the blood is drawn out from the body, some cells lose the negative charge and hence the cells start adhering to one another. When this happens the cells pile up one above the other like the stack of coins. This is known as rouleaux formation.

Factors influencing rouleaux formation:

- Rouleaux formation is increased by an increase in the fibrinogen concentration.
- Biconcave shape of the cells also facilitates rouleaux formation.
- In spherocytosis (red blood cells will be spherical in shape), rouleaux formation is decreased.

Erythrocyte Sedimentation Rate (ESR)

- It is the rate at which erythrocytes settle down when blood is mixed with a proper anticoagulant and is kept undisturbed in a vertically fixed narrow glass pipette.
- Method adopted is known as Westergren's.
- In Westergren's pipette, numeral 0 is at the top and 200 at the bottom. The graduations are in mm.
- Blood obtained by venepuncture is mixed with anticoagulant in the ratio of 4:1 is drawn into the pipette.
- The anticoagulant of choice is 3.8% sodium citrate solution
- At the end of the unit time, in the tube the cells would have settled down due to the mass of the cells and gravity.
- At the top, the plasma part will have got separated out.
- The height of this plasma column is taken as the rate at which sedimentation of erythrocyte has taken place.
- Result is expressed as mm at the end of first hour, as normally the result is observed at the end of first hour.

Normal values of erythrocyte sedimentation rate:

- In adult male   1–4 mm at the end of 1st hour
- In adult female   4–10 mm at the end of 1st hour
- In children   <1 mm at the end of 1st hour

Significance of erythrocyte sedimentation rate:

It has more of prognostic value than diagnostic, as ESR is increased in many disease states. Some of the conditions in which it is increased are:

- Pulmonary tuberculosis
- In any acute or chronic disease
- Anemia
- Many of the cancerous state
- Rheumatoid arthritis
- Rheumatic fever

Erythrocyte sedimentation rate is also increased in some of the physiological conditions, like menstruation and pregnancy.

Prognostic importance is where, after the diagnosis of the disease while on treatment, if erythrocyte sedimentation rate is determined at regular intervals, show a gradual decrease (that is towards the normal value), it will indicate that the person's health is improving. If the rate goes on increasing in spite of treatment, it signals that the diagnosis may be wrong or the treatment given is not appropriate.

Factors influencing rate of sedimentation of red blood cells:
a. Fibrinogen content of plasma.
b. Shape of the red blood cells.
c. Albumin globulin ratio
d. Cholesterol lecithin ratio.
e. RBC count and temperature.

Hemolysis

- Hemolysis is the process in which the erythrocytes breakdown, leading to the hemoglobin release from the cell.
- When the cells lose hemoglobin, the functional ability of the cell is lost.
- There are many agents, like snake venom, infection by microorganisms, malaria, increased activity of the reticuloendothelial system (RES), chemicals like bile salts and saponin, can bring about hemolysis.
- Hemolysis also occurs in any incompatible blood transfusion.
- It can also be brought about by endosmosis when the cells are surrounded by hypotonic saline solution or water.
- The reminder part of RBC, which has lost its Hb, is known as ghost cell.

Erythropoiesis

The average lifespan of red blood cell is about 120 days. Everyday, billions of senile red blood cells are destroyed and new cells have to replace them. In order to take care of the function in the body, a fine balance has to be maintained between the numbers of cells destroyed to the number of cells produced.

- The process by which mature erythrocytes are produced from the precursor stem cells is known as erythropoiesis.
- The time required for the mature cell to get formed from the stem is about 5–10 days (average 7 days).

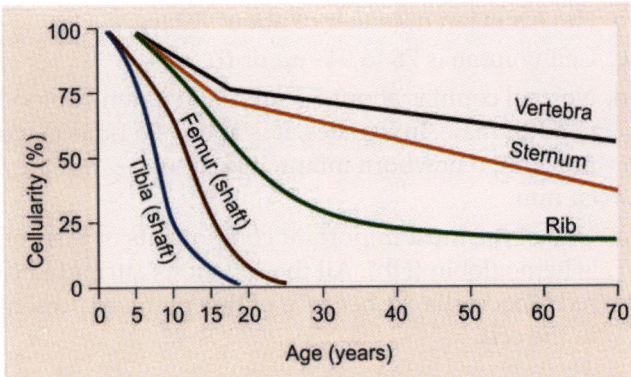

Fig. 1.5: Presence of red bone marrow at different ages in various bones

The site of erythropoiesis varies:
a. From the mesoderm of yolk sac in the first 3 months of intrauterine life (mesoblastic stage)
b. In the liver and spleen from 3rd to 5th month of intrauterine life (hepatic stage)
c. From the red bone marrow from 5th month of intrauterine life and throughout the lifespan of the person (myeloid stage).

Red bone marrow is present in all the bones during childhood. As age advances, by adult age (20 years) it is confined to the proximal ends of long bones and in all the flat bones (Fig. 1.5).

Functions of red bone marrow are:
1. Production of RBCs, WBCs and platelets.
2. Destruction of senile RBCs (by the reticuloendothelial cells).

For any laboratory investigation, a sample of the red bone marrow can be obtained from one of the following regions:
a. In males from sternum by sternal puncture.
b. In female—iliac crest.
c. In child—tibial tuberosity.

The various stages during erythropoiesis are:
- Stem cell/hemocytoblast
- Proerythroblast
- Early normoblast
- Intermediate normoblast
- Late normoblast
- Reticulocyte.
- Mature erythrocyte

During the development of mature cell from the precursor stem cell, a number of changes occur and the cells accordingly have different names (Fig. 1.6).

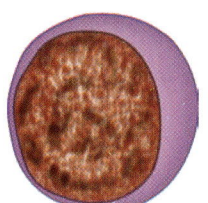

Proerythroblast

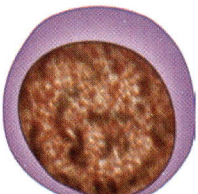

Early normoblast

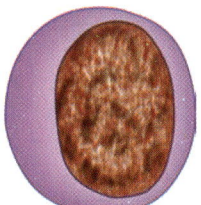

Intermediate
normoblast

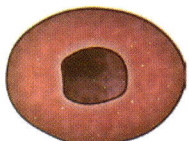

Late normoblast

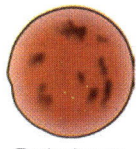

Reticulocyte

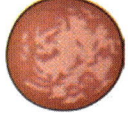

Erythrocyte

Fig. 1.6: The changes in precursor cells in respect of size, staining, etc. during erythropoiesis

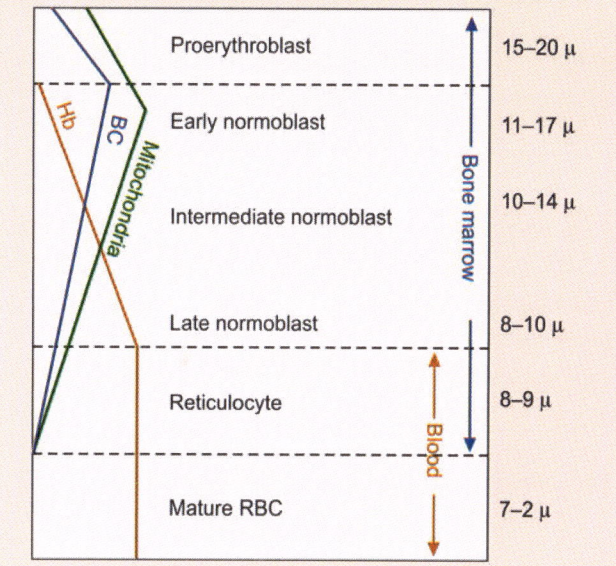

Fig. 1.7: Some of the important intracellular and morphologic changes occurring during erythropoiesis and the presence of the precursor cells in bone marrow and peripheral blood

Some of the common features during erythropoiesis are (Table 1.2 and Fig. 1.7):

a. Gradual reduction in cell size.
b. Increase in hemoglobin concentration.
c. Disappearance of nucleolus and nucleus.
d. Arrest of mitosis after loss of nucleus.
e. Change in the staining property of the cytoplasm (basophilic to polychormatophilic to eosinophilic).

Reticulocyte

- It is an immature erythrocyte.
- Size is about 8–9 (1.12 to 1.16 times bigger than RBC)
- It is also non-nucleated like red blood cell.
- It has reticulum, which is remnant of RNA.
- Normal % in adult will be around 0.5–1.0. In newborn infant, it is more (2–6).

Reticulum can be stained when the cells are treated with brilliant cresyl blue—supravital stain (stains the cells in living condition outside the body).

When count is more than normal it is known as reticulocytosis.

Reticulocytosis occurs in conditions like:

a. Hemolytic anemia.
b. Anemias after treatment with vitamin B_{12}, folic acid and iron.

Table 1.2: Change in cells at different stages during erythropoiesis

Stage	Approx. size of cell in μ	Presence of nucleus and nucleoli	Chromatin material	Conc. of hemoglobin	Staining nature of cytoplasm	Mitotic cell division	Cells are seen in
Proerythroblast	20–22	Both present	Stippled and fine	Nil	Basophilic	Only under stress	Bone marrow
Early normoblast	12–16	Nucleoli - disappears	Stippled and fine	Almost nil	Basophilic	Yes active	Bone marrow
Intermediate normoblast	10–14	Only nucleus	Condensation starts	Starts appearing	Polychro-matophilic	Yes active	Bone marrow
Late normoblast	8–10	Nucleus starts regressing becomes pyknotic	Further condensation occurs	Increases	Eosinophilic	Stops	Bone marrow
Reticulocyte	8	No nucleus	--	Increases further	Eosinophilic	--	Bone marrow and in blood
Erythrocyte	6–9 (7.2 on an average)	No nucleus	--	Maximum	Eosinophilic	--	Bone marrow and in blood

c. After hemorrhage.

d. Erythroblastosis foetalis

In a sample of bone marrow, if 30% of cells are nucleated and 70% non-nucleated, it is known as normoblastic pattern of development of RBCs. If there is reversal of the percentage (70% nucleated and 30% non-nucleated), it is known as megaloblastic pattern.

Stimulus for erythropoiesis is hypoxia (hypoxia means decreased supply of oxygen to the tissues).

Regulation of Erythropoiesis

Flow chart 1.1 indicating the role of pO_2 in blood in the regulation of erythropoiesis.

Factors influencing erythropoiesis are:

a. Hypoxia and erythropoietin.

b. Vitamin B_{12} and folic acid.

c. Metals, like iron and copper.

d. Endocrine factors, like testosterone, growth hormone and thyroxin. Testosterone increases the erythropoietin formation. Estrogen decreases erythropoietin formation and inhibits the bone marrow and hence the red blood cell count is less in females.

e. Good protein diet.

Flow chart 1.1: Regulation of erythropoiesis

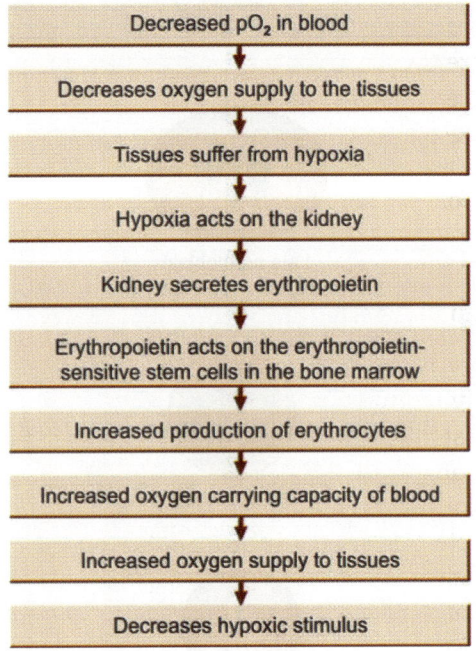

1. Erythropoietin

• Kidneys are essential for the formation of erythropoietin.

- Erythropoietin is the substance that stimulates stem cells to induce erythropoiesis.
- In renal failure, since kidneys are damaged, there will be deficiency of erythropoietin production. This leads to anemia.
- Hence in chronic renal diseases, erythropoietin has to be injected in order to prevent anemia.

2. Iron

- It is necessary for synthesis of hemoglobin.
- Daily requirement is about 10 mg in male, 20 mg in female and children.
- During pregnancy and lactation, the iron requirement by the mother is more, as the mother has to supply iron to the developing fetus and the neonate.
- Site of absorption is duodenum.
- Acid pH and vitamin C facilitate iron absorption. Vitamin C acts as a reducing agent and converts ferric iron to ferrous iron.
- Iron is absorbed in ferrous state.
- Phytic acid, oxalates inhibit absorption.
- Deficiency of iron leads to microcytic anemia.

In microcytic anemia, there will be:
a. Decrease in MCV
b. Decrease in MCH
c. Decrease in MCHC.

Some of the common causes for iron deficiency anemia are bleeding from the gums, piles, peptic ulcer and hookworm infestation of intestine.

3. Maturation Factors

Vitamin B$_{12}$ and folic acid.

Vitamin B$_{12}$

- Daily requirement is about 1 μg.
- It is stored in the liver to the extent of 1000 μg.
- It is absorbed at the ileum.
- Absorption in the intestine requires intrinsic factor secreted by the parietal cells of gastric glands.
- Deficiency may be due to either lack of intrinsic factor or the vitamin itself in the diet. Anemia caused due to the deficiency of intrinsic factor is known as pernicious anemia.

Folic acid daily requirement is about 75–100 μg.

The above two factors in general are referred to as maturation factors. Hence when they are lacking, it will lead to delayed maturation of RBC, decreased cell division and this type of anemia is called as megaloblastic anemia.

Pernicious anemia: In this type of anemia, vitamin B$_{12}$ deficiency due to lack of intrinsic factor, changes are observed in many parts of body namely:

- Peripheral blood
- Bone marrow
- Central nervous system (CNS)
- Peripheral nervous system (PNS)
- Gastrointestinal tract (GIT)

a. *Peripheral blood smear changes are:*
  - Size of red blood cells will be more than normal (macrocytes).
  - More hemoglobin will be present per cell—mean corpuscular hemoglobin (MCH) increases. Normal is 28–32 pg.
  - Mean corpuscular volume (MCV) is more than normal. Normal is 78–94 cuμ or fL.
  - The average volume of RBC occupied by hemoglobin alone or the average amount of Hb present in 100 ml of RBCs only, is known as mean corpuscular hemoglobin (MCHC) and this will remain normal. Normal range is 32–38 g% or 32–38%.
  - Red blood cell count will be markedly decreased.
  - Apart from the decreased red blood cell count, even leukocytes and platelet count also will be decreased and hence the term pancytopenia.

b. *Bone marrow changes are:*
  - Instead of the normoblastic type now it will be of megaloblastic type.
  - There will be hyperplasia of bone marrow (marrow extends to the shaft of long bones).
  - Red bone marrow can be observed in the shafts of long bones even in the adult.

c. *Gastrointestinal tract changes are:*
  - No hydrochloric acid secretion in the stomach (histamine fast achlorhydria).
  - Atrophy of gastric mucosa.
  - Tongue becomes more smooth and glistening.

d. *The changes in the central nervous system:* Tracts in the spinal cord are affected especially in the lateral white matter area of spinal cord and lead to subacute combined degeneration of the cord (both ascending and descending tracts are affected).

e. *Peripheral nervous system changes:* Degeneration of myelin sheath in the nerves leads to numbness and tingling sensation.

Hemoglobin

- Hemoglobin is the pigment present in red blood cells.
- Molecular weight is about 64500.
- Made up of two parts namely heme (iron containing protoporphyrin ring) and globin (polypeptide chains 4 in number of which two are α and two β chains)
- Adult male has approximately 15 g%, in a female it is slightly less and in children it is about 18–22 g%.
- All the functions of red blood cells (transport of respiratory gases in blood and regulation of pH of blood) are due to the hemoglobin present in the cell. 1g of hemoglobin can carry about 1.34 ml of oxygen when fully saturated. This is known as oxygen combining capacity of Hb.

$$Hb + O_2 \rightleftharpoons HbO_2$$
$$Hb + CO \rightarrow HbCO$$
$$Hb + CO_2 \rightarrow HbNH\,COOH$$

Percentage Saturation of Hemoglobin

- It is the ratio between the actual volume of oxygen transported to the maximum ability of Hb to carry oxygen and is expressed as %.
- Normally, it is around 97% in arterial blood and 70% in the venous blood.

Types of Hemoglobin

- There are two different types of hemoglobin namely HbA and HbF.
- In any type of hemoglobin, the two α chains are same, but the difference lies in the other two chains which can be either β (in HbA) or γ (in HbF).
  a. HbA type has two α and two β chains. (98% of adult have this type)
  b. HbF type has two α and two γ chains (present in fetus).
- Heme part is same in all types of Hb.

Functions of Hemoglobin

- Transport of oxygen
- Transport of carbon dioxide.
- Regulation of pH of blood.

Method of Estimation of Hemoglobin Concentration

- Colorimetry (color comparison technique) is one of the easy and popular methods but not very accurate.
- There will be formation of acid hematin when Hb is made to react with N/10 HCl.
- Wait for sufficient time (at least 10 minutes for the formation of acid hematin).
- The contents are diluted by addition of water.
- The color of this solution is matched with the standard amber-colored plates to get the reading.

Anemia

- Anemia can be defined as qualitative or quantitative decrease in either red blood cells or hemoglobin concentration or both.
- Cause can be due to deficiency of iron, vitamin B_{12}, folic acid, depression of bone marrow, total renal failure, hemolysis and repeated blood loss.
- The blood indices (MCV, MCH and MCHC) vary depending on the cause for anemia.

Classification of Anemia

a. Based on blood indices.
b. Based on the cause (clinical classification).

Based on blood indices, it can be classified as (Table 1.3):
- Microcytic (MCV < normal) hypochromic (MCHC < normal), which occurs in iron deficiency (MCH is also less than normal).
- Normocytic (MCV is normal) normochromic (MCHC is normal), which occurs in hemolysis, acute hemorrhage, etc. (MCH will be within normal range).
- Macrocytic (MCV > normal) normochromic (MCHC is within normal range) occurs in vitamin B_{12} and folic acid deficiency (MCH will be more than normal).

Based on the cause
- Hemolytic anemia where the cause is increased hemolysis.

Table 1.3: The blood indices in different types of anemia

Type	MCV	MCH	MCHC	Seen in
Microcytic hypochromic	Decreased	Decreased	Decreased	Iron deficiency, infestation of intestine by worms
Normocytic normochromic	Normal	Normal	Normal	Hemorrhage, hemolysis
Macrocytic normochormic	Increased	Increased	Normal or decreased (if associated with iron deficiency also)	Vitamin B_{12}/ folic acid deficiency

PS: Nowadays color index is not considered for classification of anemia.

- Deficiency anemia when it is due to deficiency of iron, vitamin B_{12}, folic acid or depression of bone marrow.
- Hemorrhagic type when it is due to loss of blood in considerable quantity for whatever reasons, like surgery, delivery, road accidents, bleeding in GI tract, etc.

Following tests results will help to identify the probable cause of anemia:
- PCV determination.
- RBC counts.
- Hb estimation and calculation of blood indices.
- Observing peripheral blood smear/bone marrow studies.

Fate of Hemoglobin

When senile red blood cells are destroyed in the reticuloendothelial system, hemoglobin is liberated from the cells, which will be metabolized as detailed below. The metabolic end product so formed will be excreted from the body in the form of bilinogen.

Steps in Degradation of Hemoglobin

Steps in degradation of hemoglobin are shown in Flow chart 1.2 and Fig. 1.8.

A part of it is excreted along with feces as stercobilinogen. Some part of bilinogen is absorbed from the intestine and enters enterohepatic circulation to reach liver. Then it gets resecreted with bile. The absorbed bilinogen also reaches systemic circulation. In the kidneys, it is filtered and excreted from the body along with urine in the form of urobilinogens. These bilinogens are oxidized to bilins when exposed to the environment.

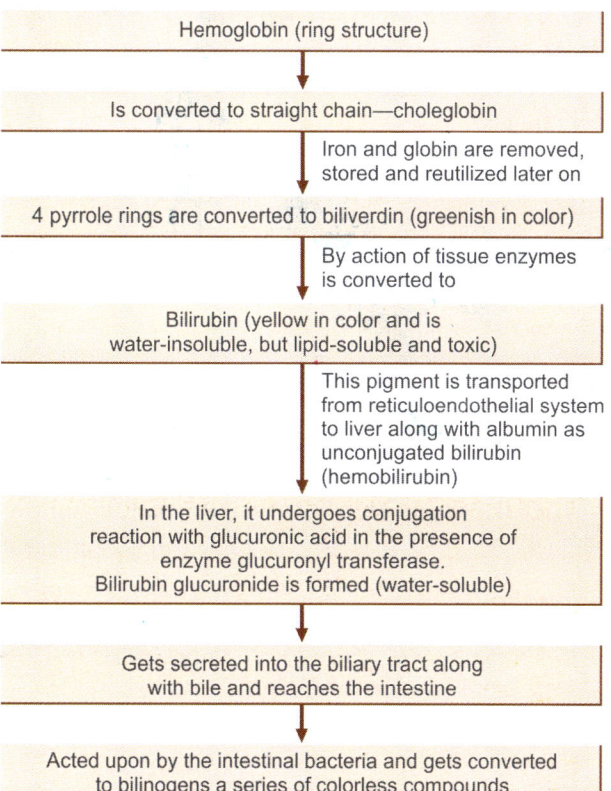

Flow chart 1.2: The major steps and compounds formed during the catabolism and excretion of Hb

Amount of bilinogens excreted per day will be:
- Along with feces about 80 to 240 mg.
- Along with urine will be 0.5 to 2.0 mg.

Jaundice

- Jaundice refers to yellow discoloration of skin, mucous membrane and sclera of the eyes.
- It is due to increase in the serum bilirubin level in circulation.

Reticuloendothelial system

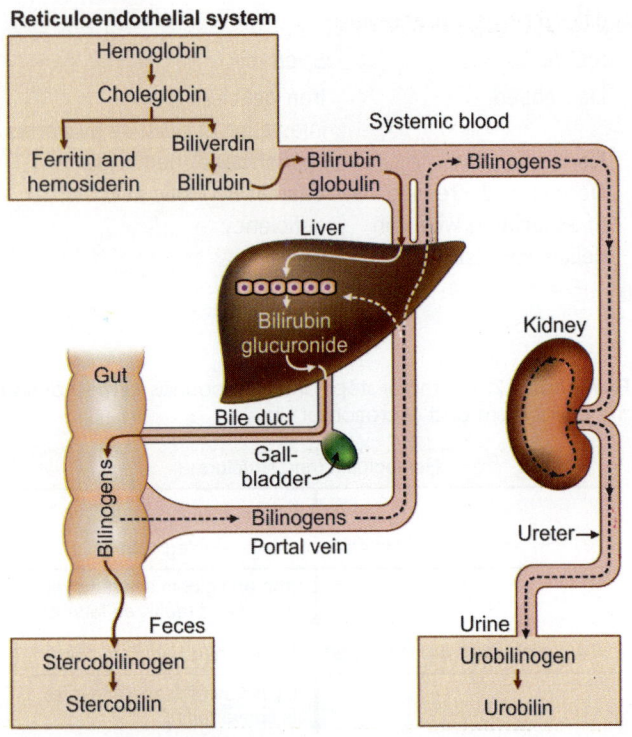

Fig. 1.8: Diagrammatic representation of major stages, compounds formed indicating the sites of formation and excretion of end products of Hb catabolism

- Normal serum bilirubin level is about 0.2–0.8 mg%.
- When it exceeds 2 mg% it results in clinical jaundice.

Depending on the cause, jaundice can be classified as:
a. Prehepatic (hemolytic), e.g. increased hemolysis for any reason, like in malaria, incompatible blood transfusion, sickle cell anemia.
b. Hepatic, e.g. viral hepatitis.
c. Posthepatic (obstructive), e.g. obstruction to the biliary tract.

The Table 1.4 gives some of the differences between the three types of jaundice.

Mostly conjugated hyperbilirubinemia:
a. Obstruction in biliary tract—stones and tumors.
b. Intrahepatic—hepatitis, drugs
c. Hepatocellular injury—acute or chronic

Mostly unconjugated hyperbilirubinemia:
a. Over production—hemolysis
b. Conjugation defects—neonatal, Gilbert's syndrome

Physiologic jaundice:
- Manifests approximately in about 72 hours after birth.
- Seen more commonly in premature births.
- Due to immaturity of the liver (less amount of glucuronyl transferase), liver is unable to cope with the demand and the unconjugated bilirubin accumulates in circulation.
- Treatment is to expose the infant to ultraviolet rays which quickens bilirubin metabolism.

Table 1.4: Certain important differences in various types of jaundice			
	Prehepatic	Hepatic	Post-hepatic
Urine			
1. Urobilinogen content	More	Less	Absent
2. Bilirubin	Absent	Present	Present
3. Bile salts	Absent	Present	Present
Stools			
1. Stercobilinogen	More	Less	Absent
2. Quantity and nature of stools	Normal	More, oily and foul smelling	More, oily and foul smelling
Vanden Bergh Reaction (with serum)	Indirect	Biphasic	Mainly direct
Liver function tests:			
1. Clotting time	Normal	Increased	Increased
2. Prothrombin time	Normal	Increased	May be increased
3. Plasma protein level	Normal	↓	↓
Change in blood			
Reticulocyte count	Increased	Normal	Normal

Table 1.5: Based on the staining with Leishman's stain, the characteristic features of the different types of white blood cells

Cell type	Size (microns)	Appearance of cytoplasm	Number of granules	Texture of granules	Nucleus	Chromatin
Neutrophil	10–14	Violet or pink	Plenty	Very fine	2–5 lobed	
Eosinophil	10–14	Red	Few compactly packed	Coarse	Usually bilobed	
Basophil	10–14	Blue	Very few	Coarse	Usually bilobed but nucleus will not be very conspicuous	
Small lymphocyte	8–10	Sky blue (thin rim at the periphery)			Large nucleus occupying almost the whole cell	Lumpy
Large lymphocyte	12–16	Sky blue			Centrally placed nucleus	Lumpy
Monocyte	16–21	Muddy gray			Horseshoe- or kidney-shaped nucleus	Reticular

A newborn infant, who is jaundiced at birth or develops jaundice within 24 hours after birth, is probably due to blood group incompatibility between mother and infant. This is probably due to Rh incompatibility or ABO grouping. This condition is known as erythroblastosis fetalis and details will be discussed with blood grouping.

Leukocytes (white blood cells)

- Lekocytes are the only nucleated cells in circulation.
- Size of the cell can range from as little as 8 μ to as much as 22 μ.
- Normal count in adult can be from 4 to 11 thousand cells per cu mm of blood. In children, it can be as much as 18 to 25 thousand cells per cu mm.
- The leukocytes can be classified as granulocytes or agranulocytes based on the presence or absence of granules in cytoplasm (when stained with Leishman stain) (Table 1.5 and Fig. 1.9).
- In the granulocyte group, the nucleus is lobed unlike in agranulocyte in which it is not lobed.
- Types of cells in the granulocyte group are neutrophils, basophils and eosinophils and in agranulocyte group are lymphocytes and monocytes (Table 1.5).

Granulocyte Group

Neutrophil (Fig. 1.10)
- Cell size 10–14 μ.

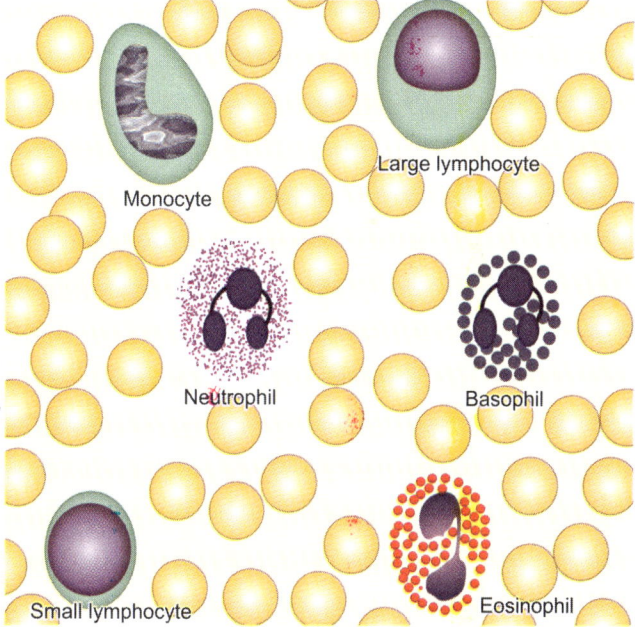

Fig. 1.9: Composite diagram of all types of white blood cells after treating with Leishman's stain

- Numerous fine granules in cytoplasm, which are violet or pink in color.
- Nucleus is lobed and the number of lobes may range from 2–7. Older cells will have more lobes.
- Lifespan may range from few hours to 2–5 days.

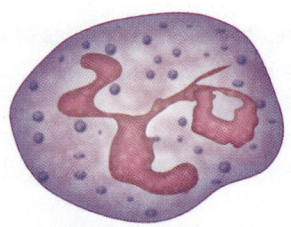

Fig. 1.10: Morphology of neutrophil

Eosinophil (Fig. 1.11)

- Cell size 10–14 µ.
- Coarse granules in cytoplasm, which are red in color and the number of granules is less.
- Nucleus is usually bilobed.
- Lifespan: 7–12 days.

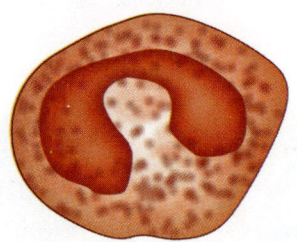

Fig. 1.11: Morphology of eosinophil

Basophil (Fig. 1.12)

- Cell size is 10–14 µ.
- Dark bluish coarse granules, which are very less in number.
- The affinity of granules for the stain is more. The nuclear material has least affinity for the stain and hence nucleus can't be seen distinctly. Usually the nucleus is bilobed.
- Lifespan is 12–15 days.

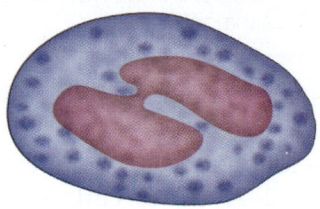

Fig. 1.12: Morphology of basophil

Agranulocyte Group

Lymphocytes can be divisible into small and large lymphocyte based on the size of the cell. They can also be classified into T and B lymphocytes based on the function. Lifespan of lymphocytes ranges from few days to few years.

Small Lymphocyte

- Cell size: 8–10 µ
- Nucleus occupies almost the whole of cell.
- Thin rim of sky blue cytoplasm is seen in one part of the cell.
- Lumpy distribution of chromatin material within the nucleus.

Large Lymphocyte (Fig. 1.13)

- Cell size: 10–14 µ.
- Large centrally placed nucleus.
- Contains more amount of cytoplasm.
- Sky blue cytoplasm surrounding the nucleus.
- Lumpy distribution of chromatin material within the nucleus

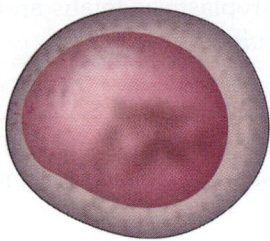

Fig. 1.13: Morphology of large lymphocyte

Monocyte (Fig. 1.14)

- Cell size: 16–22 µ.
- Horseshoe- or kidney-shaped nucleus and is eccentrically placed.

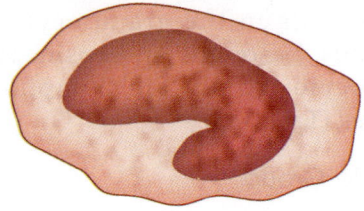

Fig. 1.14: Morphology of monocyte

- Muddy gray or frosted glass appearance of cytoplasm.
- Reticular distribution of chromatin material within the nucleus.

When leukocyte count is above the normal range, it is called as *leukocytosis*. This is seen in acute pyogenic (pus forming) infections like, appendicitis, tonsillitis, etc. Count is also increased in tuberculosis, following myocardial infarction. In leukemia, the increase in cell number will be very high and it may be as high as 80,000 to 1, 50,000. In addition to this, in leukemia, the cells present in peripheral circulation will be very immature.

When the count is less than the normal range it is called as leukopenia/leukocytopenia. This occurs in conditions, like malaria, typhoid, paratyphoid, and influenza.

When 100 white blood cells are counted and the percentage of different types of cells determined in that, it is known as differential leukocyte count (DLC). The normal percentage of different types of cells will be:

- *Neutrophil* is 40–70%. In children, it is less. Increase in the count above the range is called neutrophilia (in any acute pyogenic infections) and decrease is known as neutropenia (in typhoid, paratyphoid).
- *Eosinophil* is 2–4%. Increase in the count is known as eosinophilia (bronchial asthma, tropical eosinophilia, allergic conditions, hookworm infestation) and decrease is called eosinopenia (occurs in cortisol administration, typhoid fever).
- *Basophil* is 0–1%. Increase in the count is known as basophilia (myeloid leukemia, chickenpox).
- *Lymphocyte* percentage varies. In children, it is about 40% whereas in adult it is about 25–30%. Increase in the count is known as lymphocytosis (in most of the chronic conditions, like TB, viral infections) and decrease is known as lymphocytopenia (AIDS).
- *Monocyte* is 4–8%. When the count is above the normal range, it is known as monocytosis (syphilis).

Functions of Leukocytes

a. Phagocytic function—which is termed as non-specific/innate/passive immunity.
b. Specific/acquired/active immunity is provided by antibodies.
c. Role in allergic reactions and parasitic infections.
d. Anticoagulant function.

Phagocytosis

It is because of neutrophils (microphages) and monocytes (macrophages). The neutrophils are termed as first line of defense and monocytes are second line of defense. The neutrophils phagocytose less number (about 20) of bacteria when compared to monocytes (about 100). The monocytes of bone marrow are young and get matured in tissues. Both the types of cells indiscriminately phagocytose any type of bacteria and hence the immunity is known as non-specific.

Phagocytosis is brought about in the following steps:
- Margination
- Diapedesis
- Positive chemotaxis
- Phagocytosis proper
- Enzymatic digestion

Margination: At the site of infection, the velocity of blood flow decreases due to inflammatory exudates compressing the blood vessel. This leads to WBCs coming to the margin of the vessel wall from the central stream and this is termed as margination.

Diapedesis: The cells put forth pseudopodia-like processes and come out through the pores in the endothelial cell lining the capillaries to extravascular compartment.

Positive chemotaxis
- The chemical substances (toxins) liberated by the bacteria act as a chemoattractant and the leukocytes are attracted towards the bacteria. This is termed as positive chemotaxis.
- If the chemical substances liberated by bacteria are very strong (virulent), the leukocytes are repelled from the site of infection and is known as negative chemotaxis.

Phagocytosis proper
- The pseudopodia put forth by the WBCs engulf the bacteria completely.
- Now the bacteria would be ready for the chemical degradation by the enzymes released by the leukocytes.

Digestion
- The various enzymes, like lipolytic, proteolytic, lysozymes, hydrogen peroxide, superoxide, nitrous

Flow chart 1.3: The sites of sensitization and formation of different types of cells in cellular and humoral immunity

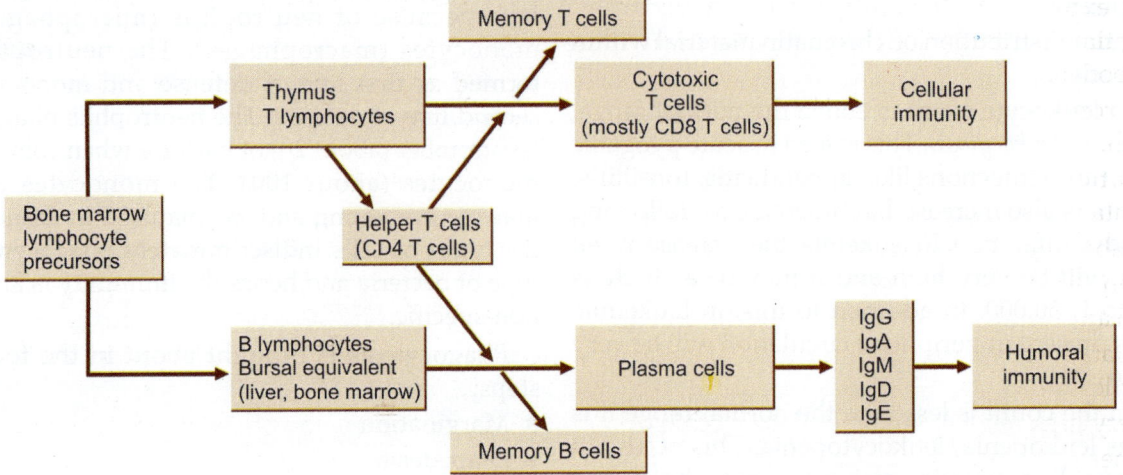

oxide, etc. act on the bacteria and bring about chemical degradation of the same.

- In the ensuing fight between the bacteria and neutrophils, not only the bacteria get killed, even the leukocytes and some of the neighboring cells also get destroyed. This leads to the formation of the pus.

Eosinophil Function

- Most of the allergens are proteins.
- Detoxify, disintegrate and remove foreign proteins.
- During allergic reaction, there will be production of histamine that is carried by eosinophils to the site of detoxification, which is the liver. They also have a parasiticidal function.

Basophil Function

- It is to transport substances, like histamine, heparin and serotonin.

- A large amount of heparin is secreted by the mast cells present in various tissues of the body as well.
- Heparin is the only naturally occurring anticoagulant and hence helps to maintenance of fluidity of blood.

Functions of Lymphocytes (specific or acquired or active immunity)

Functions of lymphocytes are depicted in Flow chart 1.3. Most of the circulating antibodies are IgG and IgM types. The memory cells will be present in the body for years and are responsible for prompt and immediate response for any subsequent infection by the same organism (antigen). The differences between cellular and humoral immunity have been indicated in Table 1.6.

Table 1.6: Differences between cellular and humoral immunity	
Cellular	*Humoral*
It is by T lymphocyte	It is by B lymphocyte
Cells are processed in thymus	Cells are processed in lymph nodes, liver and spleen.
Exposure to antigen produces helper, suppressor, memory and cytotoxic cells	Exposure to antigen produces memory and plasma cells
Lymphocytes bur holes in cells to be destroyed by releasing substances, like Interleukin, prostaglandin, etc.	Plasma cells synthesize and release free antibodies into circulation.
80% cells in peripheral circulation	20% cells in peripheral circulation
Has role in immune responses against bacteria, viruses, fungi and also against transplanted tissues.	Has role in immune response against bacteria only.

Importance of Sensitization

- First exposure to the antigen takes considerably long time (latent period) for the production of the antibody.
- The concentration of antibody produced is not much.
- Duration for which the higher antibody level maintained is also not much.

The above response is termed as primary response.

When there is subsequent exposure to the same antigen any time during the lifespan of the individual:

a. The latent period for the production of antibody is very less.

b. A very high level of antibody titer is achieved.

c. Higher concentration is maintained for prolonged duration.

This is termed as secondary response. Figure 1.15 indicates some of the salient aspects of primary and secondary responses in respect of latent period, concentration of antibodies and maintenance of antibody levels.

Basis for Immunization Program

Administration of attenuated antigens in small dose will bring about the sensitization (primary response) of the immune system. Attenuated antigens are those antigens which have lost their property to produce disease but have retained the capacity to induce the production of antibodies. When sensitization has occurred, the body can combat any subsequent infection by the same organism more vigorously and efficiently because of the secondary response. This prevents onset of many of the common diseases, like poliomyelitis, measles, mumps, rubella, viral hepatitis, smallpox, typhoid, etc.

Platelets (Thrombocytes)

- Third type of cell among the formed elements of blood.
- Is non-nucleated.
- Size is between 2 and 4 μ.
- May be circular- or oval-shaped.
- When treated with ammonium oxalate appears as shining bodies under the microscope.
- Normal count is about 2–4 hundred thousand cells/cu mm of blood.
- Lifespan is about 10 days.
- The cells are produced by the megakayocytes present in red bone marrow.
- Site of destruction is spleen, which contains reticuloendothelial system.

Physiological properties of platelets are:
- Adhesion.
- Aggregation.
- Agglutination.

Variations in Platelet Count

When the count is above the normal limit, it is known as thrombocytosis, which occurs in conditions, like:
- Surgical operation
- Fractures
- Accidents
- After parturition.
- After splenectomy.

When the count is below normal it is known as thrombocytopenia and is seen in conditions, like:
- Idiopathic thrombocytopenic purpura
- Depression of bone marrow due to radiation, drugs, etc.
- Viral fever
- Deficiency of vitamin B_{12}/folic acid.
- Hypersplenism

Functions of Platelets

- Hemostasis
- Blood coagulation

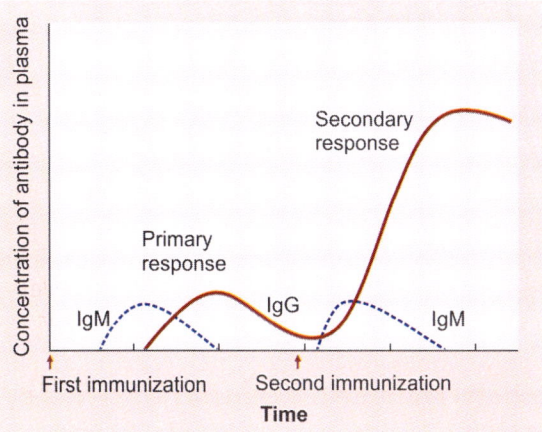

Fig. 1.15: Immune system response for the first and subsequent exposure to the same antigen in respect latent period, concentration of antibodies, etc.

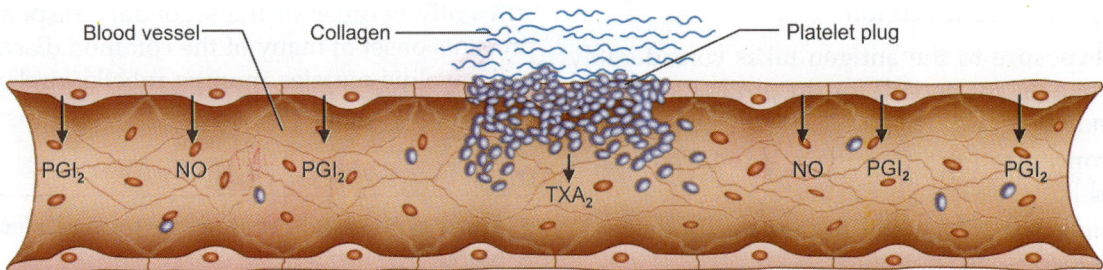

Fig. 1.16: Platelet plug formation at the site of injury to blood vessel, release of some of the substances, like NO, TXA$_2$, etc.

- Clot retraction
- Repair of capillary endothelium
- Transport of certain substances
- Phagocytosis.

1. **Hemostasis:** It is the spontaneous arrest of bleeding from small vessels, like capillaries and venules. This can be brought about by the following mechanisms:

   a. *Platelet plug formation* (Fig. 1.16):
      i. Breach of the blood vessel exposes sub-endothelial collagen.
      ii. Platelets start getting adhered to the sub-endothelial collagen.
      iii. Many platelets come together at the site of adhesion because of the property of aggregation and are aided by thrombxane A2 and ADP released by damaged platelets. This leads to platelet plug formation.
      iv. Site of injury is closed by this platelet plug and hence prevents loss of blood from the injured area.

   b. *Extravascular pressure factor:* Compressor pressure exerted by blood collected in the interstitial spaces over the capillaries.

   c. *Role of precapillary sphincter constriction in hemostasis:*
      i. Injury to the tissue leads to pain sensation.
      ii. This in turn brings about the reflex constriction of precapillary sphincter.
      iii. Flow of blood through the capillary is reduced.
      iv. Loss of blood is prevented.

   d. *By release of vasoconstrictor agent* like serotonin by the damaged platelets that bring about the constriction of the blood vessels and thereby reduce blood flow through the vessel and loss of blood from the injured area.

Determination of bleeding time:
- Prick the fingertip with aseptic precaution.
- Soon after pricking the time is noted.
- At the end of every 30 sec, the blood oozing out of the injured area is blotted on the filter paper.
- The procedure is continued till no stain of blood appears on the paper.
- The time is noted again.

The time interval from the onset of bleeding to the cessation of blood flow from the injured surface gives us the bleeding time.

Normal bleeding time is about 1 to 4 minutes. Increase in bleeding time occurs when there is thrombocytopenia.

Purpura
- It is a condition in which there are hemorrhagic spots beneath skin (cachetic state), mucous membrane.
- It is due to decrease in platelet count.
- Bleeding time is increased, but clotting time remains normal.
- Occurring due to decreased platelet count is called thrombocytopenic purpura and is also known as primary purpura.
- When it is due to some allergic reactions, infections, etc. it is known as symptomatic purpura.
- When it is thrombasthenic purpura, the platelet count will be normal but occurs due to defective platelet function.

The reason for idiopathic thrombocytopenic purpura is not known. The platelets help to repair the capillary endothelial cells whenever they are damaged.

2. **Coagulation of blood:** During the process of clotting, there is involvement of many of the substances and reactions. Platelets do contribute for

the proper clotting of blood by release of phospholipid that is required for the formation of prothrombin activator through the intrinsic mechanism.

3. *Clot retraction:*

- Freshly formed clot is big and soft.
- As time elapses, the size of the clot decreases and the texture of the clot changes. It becomes more firm. The fluid that squeezes out during clot retraction is serum.
- Size of clot decreases to about 40 to 60% of the original size in about an hour's time.
- Because of the clot retraction, the cut ends of the blood vessel come together which facilitate wound healing.
- When clot occurs within the blood vessels it is known as thrombosis. This obstructs the blood flow and this may cause damage to some of the vital organs, like heart, brain, etc.
- Clot retraction facilitates recanalization of the thrombosed veins and prevents thrombo-embolism.
- Clot retraction is due to involvement of protein present in platelets namely thrombasthenin (actomyosin-like complex).
- In thrombasthenia, the clot retraction suffers.

4. Certain substances, like serotonin, ADP, ATP, are present in the platelets.

5. Platelets are also involved in phagocytosis of non-living particles, like carbon, immune complexes.

HEMOSTASIS AND COAGULATION OR CLOTTING OF BLOOD

Blood that is in circulation is in fluid state. When fluid state of blood is converted to semisolid jelly-like mass, it is called as coagulation or clotting of blood. At the site of injury, clotting occurs over the platelet plug that has formed and hence it converts the temporary platelet plug into a permanent sealing of the injured area (Flow chart 1.4). This is very much essential as the platelet plug will not be very strong without superseded clot and will get washed away in course of time. This results in prolonged bleeding (as seen in hemophilia).

Blood coagulation involves mainly three steps:

1. Formation of prothrombin activator.

Flow chart 1.4: Steps in formation of temporary hemostate plug and later on sealing of injured area by definitive hemostate plug (clot)

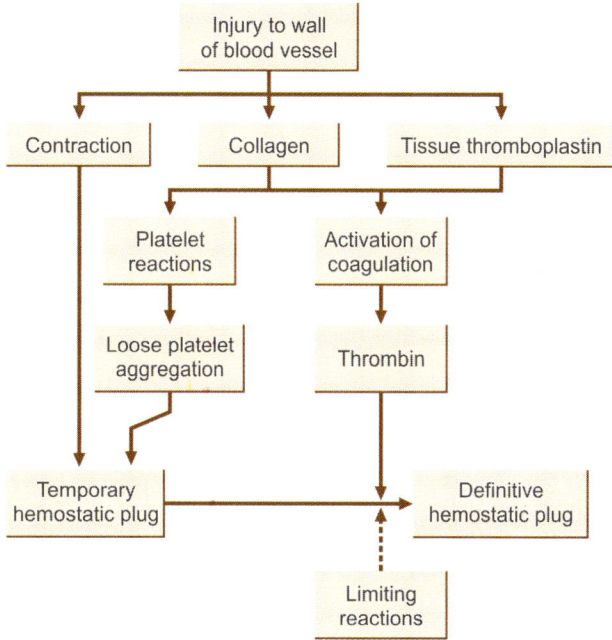

2. Conversion of prothrombin to thrombin by prothrombin activator.

3. Conversion of fibrinogen to fibrin by thrombin and clot formation.

Prothrombin activator can be formed by either intrinsic or extrinsic mechanism. In intrinsic system, the formation of prothrombin activator is by exposure of the collagen to platelets whereas in extrinsic system the substances released by damaged tissues are responsible. When clotting occurs in the body, it will involve both the intrinsic and extrinsic systems and these systems will complement each other.

Coagulation Factors

- The substances involved in coagulation are termed as clotting factors (Table 1.7).
- The factors are present in the inactive state in circulation.
- At the time of clotting, these substances are activated.
- They are designated with the Roman numerals.
- The number designated to any factor indicates the order of the discovery of the factor.
- Letter 'a' suffixed to the number indicates the active form of the factor.

Table 1.7: List of clotting factors

Factor no	Name
I	Fibrinogen
II	Prothrombin
III	Tissue thromboplastin (TF)
IV	Ca^{++}
V	Proaccelerin
VI	Absent
VII	Proconvertin
VIII	Antihemophilic factor
IX	Christmas factor
X	Stuart-Prower factor
XI	Plasma thromboplastin antecedent
XII	Hageman's factor
XIII	Fibrin stabilizing factor

Flow chart 1.5: Major steps involved during the process of coagulation of blood

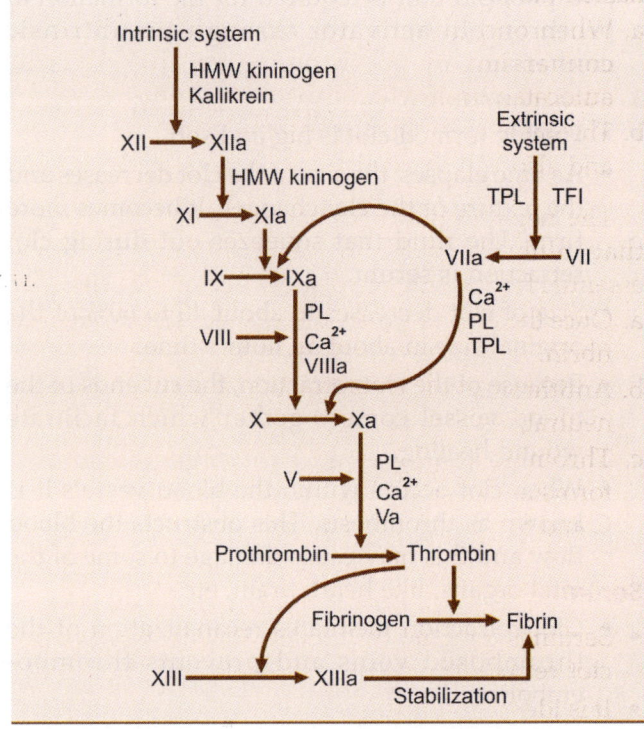

Xa along with phospholipids, Ca^{++}, Va acts as prothrombin activator. This converts prothrombin to thrombin. Thrombin later on converts fibrinogen to fibrin monomers by a process of proteolyis. This fibrin monomer is converted to fibrin polymer which is unstable. Unstable fibrin polymer will be acted upon by factor XIIIa, leads to the formation of stable fibrin threads. These threads entangle RBCs to form a stable clot (Fig. 1.17 and Flow chart 1.5).

Some of the important aspects of coagulation are:
- Up to the formation of prothrombin activator, the steps are different (it can be either by intrinsic or extrinsic system). Rest of the reactions involved is the same both for extrinsic and intrinsic mechanisms.
- There is enzyme substrate reaction.
- There is cascade of reaction.

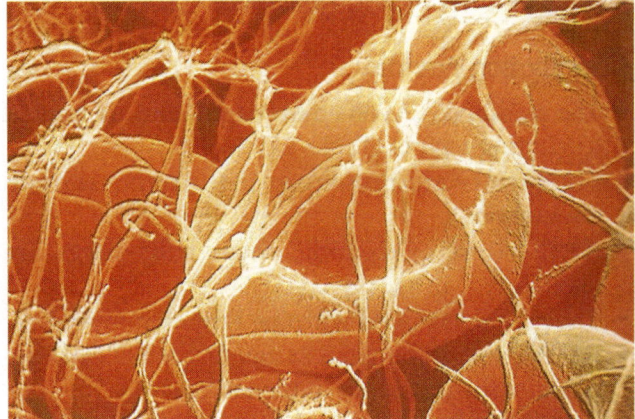

Fig. 1.17: RBCs entangled in fibrin threads to form stable clot

- Positive and negative feedback mechanisms are involved at various steps of coagulation.
- The whole set of reactions acts as a bioamplifier system.
- Calcium ions are necessary at various steps.

Enzyme substrate reaction is because of the active form of the factor acts as an enzyme and acts on another substrate (inactive factor) to activate it, e.g. XIIa acts as enzyme and converts the inactive factor XI (substrate) to XIa.

It is known as cascade reaction because as the reaction proceeds initial reaction require more time when compared to the final reactions that is each reaction accelerates the next step. The final few reactions (refer to prothrombin time) will occur in very few seconds, even though clotting time as a whole can be as much as 10 minutes.

Bioamplifier system because the factors involved in the earlier steps of reactions are present in very insignificant quantities in circulation and still have the ability to convert large amount of the next factor. In the final steps of reactions, some of the factors involved are to the extent of few hundred milligrams percent.

Positive feedback mechanism comes into play to hasten the process. They are:

a. When once thrombin is formed it brings about conversion of prothrombin to thrombin by autocatalytic reaction.

b. Thrombin also activates factors V, VIII, IX, X, XII and also XIII.

The negative feedback mechanisms also operate that inhibits the actions of thrombin and this is essential for limiting the process of clotting. They are:

a. Once the fibrin is formed it adsorbs thrombin on to fibrin.

b. Antithrombin III is present in the plasma, which neutralizes thrombin.

c. Thrombin combines with thrombomodulin and forms a complex. This complex activates proteins C and S which in turn inhibit factors V and VIII.

Serum

- Serum is the fluid part that is squeezed out during clot retraction.
- It is identical to plasma in almost all aspects except for the absence of factor number I, II, V, VIII and XIII. Hence it can't clot.
- It is used for many of the tests in the laboratory (e.g. estimation of Na$^+$ level).

Factors keeping blood in a fluid state are:

- Intact endothelial cell lining.
- A layer of glycocalyx (repel the clotting factors).
- Thrombomodulin and prothrombin complexes activate proteins C and S which in turn inactivate factors V and VIII.
- Small amounts of thrombin, if at all formed, get adsorbed to antithrombin III and fibrinogen.
- Presence of naturally occurring anticoagulant heparin.
- Velocity of blood flow.
- Fibrinolytic system brings about fibrinolyis.

Fibrinolysis is the process by which the clot is broken down (Flow chart 1.6a and b).

- It is essential to prevent clogging of the capillaries by the clot.
- After the clot is formed, the fibrinolytic system promptly comes into action and thereby tries to maintain the fluidity of the blood.

- Just like coagulation, even fibrinolysis involves many factors.
- These factors will also be in circulation in the inactive form.
- At the time of fibrinolysis, they get activated.
- The activation can be brought about by either the intrinsic or extrinsic system.
- Increased activity of the fibrinolytic system is dangerous. This occurs in prostatic/lung surgeries.

Anticoagulants: These are substances that prevent clotting of blood. They have important role to play in the normal functioning of the body. They can be classified into *in vivo* and *in vitro* anticoagulants.

In vivo anticoagulants are used to prevent coagulation of blood inside the body. *In vivo* anticoagulants are:

- Heparin
- Dicoumarol.

Heparin is produced by the mast cells and basophils. Mast cells are present in the lining of the blood vessels and lungs. Mechanism of action will be:

- Antithrombin action.
- Antithromboplastin action
- Prevent aggregation of platelets.

Therapeutically, heparin is used for preventing intravascular thrombosis, during dialysis, myocardial infarction, ischemic heart disease, etc.

Dicoumarol is not present in the body. Exogenous administration is essential.

- It can be taken orally.
- It acts as vitamin K antagonist.
- Vitamin K is essential for the synthesis of factors II, VII, IX and X by the liver.
- It binds to the receptors on the hepatocytes and prevents binding of vitamin K to these sites. Thereby dicoumarol acts as a competitive inhibitor.
- Hence the vitamin K dependent coagulation factors can't be synthesized.

In vitro anticoagulants are used to prevent coagulation of blood outside the body. They are:

- Heparin
- Sodium citrate (3.8%)
- Double oxalate (ammonium and potassium)
- EDTA (ethylenediaminetetraacetic acid).

Ionic calcium is necessary in many of the steps of coagulation. The inorganic salts will remove the ionic calcium.

Flow chart 1.6a and b: Process of fibrinolysis and factors affecting it

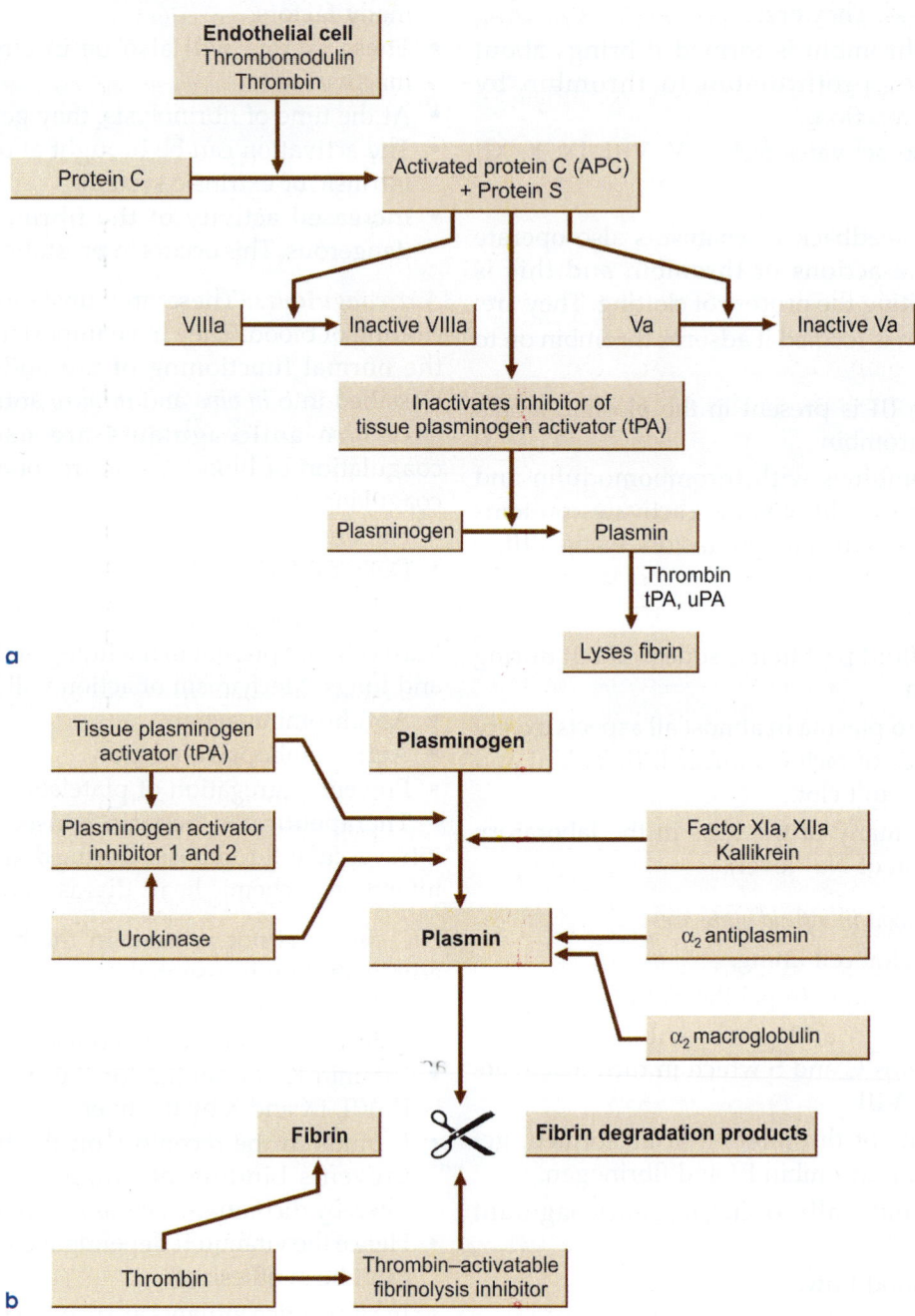

- By precipitating calcium ions as salts (sodium citrate, double oxalate)
- As chelating agent of calcium (EDTA).

Uses of anticoagulant outside the body are:
a. To store blood in blood bank. Anticoagulant used will be either acid citrate dextrose (ACD) or citrate phosphate dextrose (CPD).

b. To retain fluidity of blood to carry out certain tests (determination of PCV or ESR, for certain biochemical estimations) in the laboratory.

Clotting Time

- Clotting time is the time interval from the onset of bleeding till the appearance of fibrin threads.

- Normally it is about 4–10 minutes.
- Can be determined by capillary method or slide method.
- Increased in diseases, like hemophilia, Christmas disease, decrease in concentration of prothrombin or fibrinogen.

Prothrombin Time (Fig. 1.18)

- Prothrombin time is the time interval required to convert prothrombin to thrombin and final clot formation. There is inverse relationship between level of prothrombin and prothrombin time.
- Measures the extrinsic system involved in blood coagulation.
- Is normally about 12–16 sec.
- Increases in liver disease and forms one of the important liver function tests.
- Increases in vitamin K deficiency, as this vitamin is essential for the synthesis of prothrombin.
- Is used as a guide during anticoagulant therapy in any thrombotic condition. If the time exceeds more than 2½ times the control, the dosage of the anticoagulant drug must be reduced.

Disorders of Coagulation

Hemophilia (hemophilia A/ classical hemophilia)

- Hemophilia is a disorder of coagulation of blood.
- Is sex-linked inherited disease.

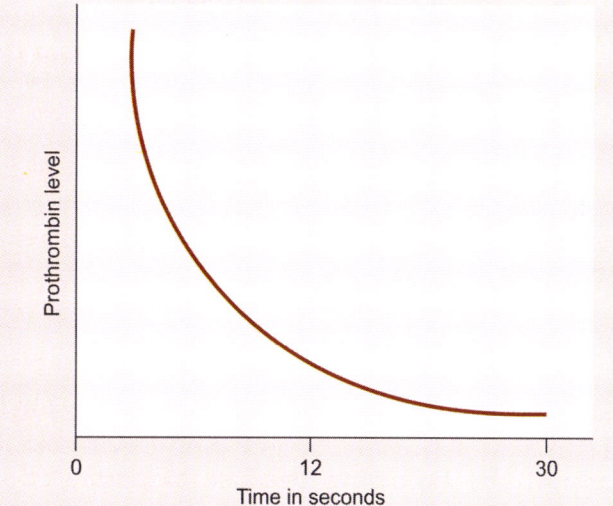

Fig. 1.18: Graph showing the inverse relationship between prothrombin level and prothrombin time

- Manifests only in males and hence they suffer and females are the carriers.
- The gene responsible is a recessive gene and is present on the X chromosome.
- In male, there is only one X chromosome and if the hemophilic gene is present on it, they suffer from the disease.
- Female has two X chromosomes. One of the X chromosomes will have the normal gene and if the other X chromosome carries the recessive gene, she doesn't suffer from the disease. Hence she becomes the carrier.
- Is because of deficiency of factor VIII.
- Is a characteristic disorder of the clotting and hence the clotting time is prolonged but bleeding time and prothrombin time will be normal. At times people continue to bleed for hours.
- Symptoms include painful swollen joints.
- Can be treated by administering fresh plasma or cryoprecipitate (concentrated form of deep frozen fresh plasma) or factor number VIII (anti-hemophilic globulin). Stored blood plasma cannot be given as factor VIII is destroyed during storing of blood.

Christmas disease (hemophilia B) is due to the deficiency of factor IX.

BLOOD GROUP

On the cell membrane of the RBCs, there may be presence of certain substances namely agglutinogen/antigen. The presence or absence of the group-specific agglutinogen on the RBC forms the basis for blood grouping. The chemical nature of these substances can be either glycoproteins or polysaccharides.

There are certain substances, which may be present in plasma and act against specific agglutinogen. These substances are termed as agglutinins/antibodies. The chemical nature of antibody is immunoglobulin/gamma globulin.

When a particular agglutinogen reacts with a corresponding agglutinin, the reaction is termed as agglutination. This reaction leads to agglutination (clumping) of the red blood cells.

Systems of Blood Grouping

The blood grouping of the human beings can be done under different systems based on certain criterion. The criterion is the presence or absence of group-specific agglutinogen on the red blood cells. Accordingly,

- A and B agglutinogens are considered in ABO system.
- D agglutinogen is considered in Rh system.
- M and N agglutinogens are considered in MN system.

The blood group specific agglutinogen can also be present in certain bodily secretions, like saliva, semen, and gastric juice. People in whom the group specific agglutinogen is present in the saliva, etc. are called as "secretors". About 85% of the people are secretors.

There are certain agglutinins/antibodies that are present in plasma. These agglutinins are called naturally occurring antibodies. The agglutinins are α (anti-A) and β (anti-B) with respect to ABO system of blood grouping.

Agglutinogen and agglutinin profile in ABO and Rh systems of blood grouping have been enumerated in Table 1.8. Based on the presence or absence of aforesaid agglutinogen and agglutinin (Table 1.8), Karl Landsteiner deduced the following law, which states that:

First part of the law: When a particular agglutinogen is present on the red blood cell the corresponding agglutinin will be absent in the plasma. The first part of the law is a logical outcome of the situation; otherwise there will be agglutination of the red blood cells. This part of the law holds good for all the systems of blood grouping.

Second part of the law: When a particular agglutinogen is absent on the red blood cell, the corresponding agglutinin will be present in the plasma. The second part of the law is applicable only to ABO system, as the agglutinins of ABO are naturally occurring one, unlike for Rh system. In Rh system, it is only when the Rh +ve cells are introduced into the body of Rh-ve individual, there will be production of anti-D agglutinin. Hence this agglutinin is not naturally occurring one. Because of this, Rh system will not obey the second part of the law.

Determination of Blood Grouping

Principle: A known agglutinin is made to react with red blood cells containing unknown agglutinogen. Agglutination or no agglutination in the reaction indicates the status of the agglutinogen presence or absence on the red blood cell.

ABO System

Procedure

- Prepare cell suspension (a drop of blood mixed with 1 ml of 0.9% NaCl solution)
- Mark slides anti-A and anti-B
- To the corresponding slides, add a drop of sera containing respective antibodies.
- Add a drop of cell suspension on to the slides and mix the same with serum.
- Wait for 10 minutes.
- Observe for the agglutination reaction first with naked eye, then under the microscope. Rule out possibility of pseudo agglutination, which gets disturbed on shaking the cell suspension on the slide, unlike true agglutination, which is an irreversible reaction.

Agglutination with anti-A serum	Blood group will be A
Agglutination with anti-B serum	Blood group will be B
No agglutination with both sera	Blood group will be O
Agglutination with both sera	Blood group will be AB

Rh grouping can also be done as above using anti-Rh antibody.

Since the antigens of ABO and Rh system are different, there is every possibility for them to co-exist. Because of this, the blood group of persons can be any of the following because of permutation combination:

A –ve, A +ve, AB +ve, AB –ve, B +ve, B –ve, O –ve, O +ve

Table 1.8: Agglutinogen and agglutinin normally present in various blood groups of different individuals

ABO system		
Agglutinogen on RBC	*Agglutinin in plasma*	*Blood group*
A present	Anti-B (β)	A
B present	Anti-A (α)	B
A and B present	Both absent	AB
A and B absent	Both present (α and β)	O
Rh system		
Agglutinogen on RBC	*Agglutinin in plasma*	*Blood group*
D present	Nil	Rh⁺
D absent	Nil	Rh⁻

Significance of blood grouping:

1. For transfusion of blood.
2. In certain medicolegal problems, like disputed paternity.
3. To understand the geographical distribution of the population for anthropological studies.

Types of blood transfusion and indication for transfusion:

a. Whole blood transfusion in hemorrhage.
b. Packed cells transfusion in anemia.
c. Fresh blood transfusion in hemophilia.
d. Plasma transfusion in burns.
e. Exchange transfusion when the newborn infant is suffering from erythroblastosis fetalis.
f. Platelets and white blood cell components also can be separated and transfused depending on the situation.

Before any transfusion is done, it should be ascertained whether the donor and recipient's blood are matching. To assess the compatibility, the following tests have to be performed:

a. Major cross-matching wherein the donor's cell suspension is made to react with recipient's plasma.
b. Minor cross-matching wherein the donor's plasma is made to react with recipient's cell suspension.

If there is agglutination in any of the tests, then the two groups are said to be incompatible.

Note:

a. O blood can be donated to any recipient provided the agglutinin titer is low and hence O –ve with low agglutinin titer is termed as universal donor.
b. AB +ve person can receive blood from any group and hence called as universal recipient (Table 1.9 and Fig. 1.19).

Table 1.9: Intergroup compatibility chart of ABO system blood types

Donor	Recipient			
	A	B	AB	O
A	–	+	–	+
B	+	–	–	+
AB	+	+	–	+
O	–	–	–	–

– sign denotes compatibility (matching)
+ sign incompatibility (not matching)

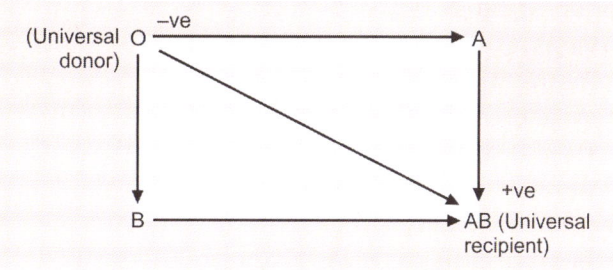

Fig. 1.19: Simple line diagrammatic representation of compatibility in ABO system

Dangers of Blood Transfusion

Dangers Pertaining to Compatible Blood

a. Transmission of diseases, like AIDS, viral hepatitis, syphilis, and malaria.
b. Over loading of the heart, if the volume of blood transfused is more than what is required. This happens in massive transfusion.
c. Ionic imbalances leading to hypokalemia, and hypocalcemia. This affects the excitability of nerve and muscle.
d. Reactions of transfusion, like fever, and shivering.

Dangers associated with Incompatible Blood

a. *Minor reaction:* In-apparent hemolyis because the donor's red blood cells react with recipient's plasma and hence the red blood cells will get hemolyzed. Consequent to hemolysis, there is release of hemoglobin from the hemolyzed cells.
b. *Moderate reaction:* After about a day or two, the serum bilirubin level rises. This is because of the hemolysis of red blood cells and production of more amount of bilirubin. Due to an increase in the bilirubin level, the person develops jaundice. Since the jaundice is consequent to transfusion, it is called as post-transfusion jaundice.
c. *Severe reaction:* The agglutinated mass, which is in circulation, blocks the circulation in the capillaries. Because of this, the blood flow through the organs and tissues suffers. This results in compression in chest, pain at the back and may also lead to the failure of organs, like kidney and brain. The renal failure can also be due to filtration of hemoglobin into the renal tubules and affecting the functioning of the kidneys. The loss of kidney function leads to oliguria or anuria. This leads to uremia, hyperkalemia or hypokalemia.

Inheritance of Blood Group

a. The genes responsible for blood group are dominant genes.

b. They are present on autosomes.

c. Even if the dominant gene is present on any one of the chromosomes of the pair, the particular blood group is manifested.

d. Because of this, e.g. if the blood group of a father is A, the probable genotype is AA or AO. The former genotype is known as homozygous and the latter heterozygous. Likewise, if the blood group of mother is B, the probable genotype could be BB or BO.

e. During the gametogenesis, each of the parents passes on one gene to the gamete.

f. The fertilization of the egg by the spermatozoa will result in the zygote having two genes, one from the father and another from mother.

g. Supposing the parents' blood group is A and B and if genes are in homozygous state, the offspring's genotype has to be AB. This results in the offspring having blood group of AB.

h. However, if blood group of the one of the parents is A with genotype AO and others blood group is B with genotype BO, the gamete may get A/O or B/O gene. The zygote formation from such gametes results in the genotype of the offspring AB/AO/BO/OO. Hence the blood group of the offspring can be A/B/AB/O (Fig. 1.20).

Erythroblastosis Fetalis

- It occurs due to blood group incompatibility between mother and fetus.

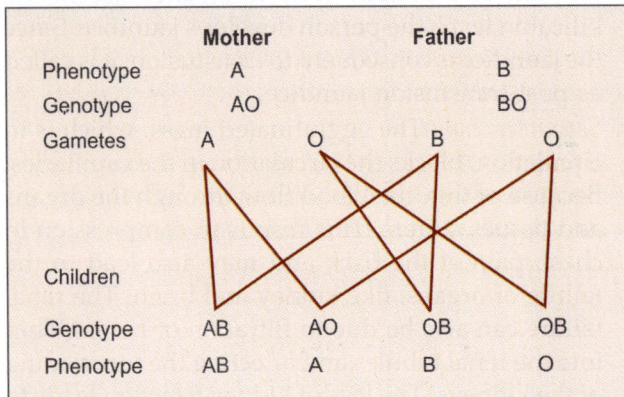

Fig. 1.20: Schematic representation of inheritance of blood group by the offspring when parents are in heterozygous state

- Fetal blood group will be Rh+ve and that of mother's will be Rh–ve.
- Usually in the first pregnancy, there will not be any problem for the fetus unless the mother had received Rh+ve blood transfusion earlier.
- During delivery, some of the erythrocytes of fetus enter the maternal circulation and sensitize the immune system of mother and bring about the production of Rh antibodies.
- In the subsequent pregnancy, supposing the fetus happens to be Rh+ve, and even if a small number of fetal erythrocytes enter maternal circulation due to any breach in the placenta, the mother's body is able to produce large number of anti-Rh antibodies (secondary response) because of previous sensitization.
- These antibodies belong to IgG type and hence have the ability to cross placental barrier to reach fetal circulation.
- On reaching fetus, they bring about the agglutination of the red blood cells of fetus resulting in hemolysis.
- This results in serious type of hemolytic jaundice.

How to Prevent Erythroblastosis Fetalis?

a. Never give Rh+ve blood transfusion to any female who is Rh–ve till her child-bearing period is over.

b. Immediately after delivery of an Rh+ve infant, the mother has to be injected with anti-D antibodies.

c. These antibodies agglutinate fetal red blood cells having Rh+ve antigen.

d. This prevents the sensitization (primary response) of the immune system of mother.

e. Since very small quantity of antibodies is injected, neither the quantity nor longevity of the antibody will be sufficient enough for any problem in subsequent pregnancies.

f. Another way to prevent is by spacing of pregnancies.

How to make out whether the Newborn Infant is Suffering from Erythroblastosis Fetalis?

Clinical features of newborn that is suffering from erythroblastosis fetalis are:

a. Anemic (may or may not be).

b. Jaundiced at birth or within 24 hours of birth.

c. Presence of large number of immature nucleated erythrocytes (erythroblasts) in peripheral circulation.

d. Very high reticulocyte counts in blood (50–60%).

e. Increase in the concentration of bilirubin in circulation due to excessive hemolysis and hence causes jaundice. Bilirubin may get deposited on the basal ganglia nuclei in brain due to incomplete development of blood–brain barrier. This condition is known as kernicterus.

f. Marked enlargement of liver and spleen (hepatosplenomegaly)

Treatment of newborn infant suffering from erythroblastosis fetalis:

- An exchange transfusion with Rh–ve blood.
- A known volume of blood is transfused and an equal volume is withdrawn. This procedure has to be continued till the newborn is out of danger.
- The reason for this type of transfusion is to maintain the blood volume and also to reduce the concentration of antibody in the neonate's circulation to prevent any more agglutination. In the course of time, the newly formed Rh+ve cells of the neonate will not be agglutinated.
- There is no agglutination of the transfused red blood cells as the transfused cells belong to O–ve group.

Advantages of exchange transfusion:

1. Respiratory functions of the blood are taken care off as transfused RBCs are not agglutinated.
2. Anti-D titer is reduced since they have come from maternal circulation.
3. Decreased bilirubin level reduces the intensity of jaundice and chances of kernicterus are prevented.

BLOOD VOLUME

- Normally is about 5 liters in adult male weighing 70 kg.
- In relation to body weight is about 70 ml/kg in adults and 90 ml/kg in children.

Blood volume determination can be done in different ways, namely:

a. Direct method, which needs the sacrificing of the animal and hence cannot be employed on human beings.

b. Indirect method that is based on dilution principle. In this method, either the plasma or RBC volume only will be determined and by applying certain formula the final blood volume can be calculated.

Principle of Dilution

- A known quantity of substance is dissolved in certain volume of fluid.
- This solution will be injected into the body of person whose blood volume has to be determined.
- After complete and proper dilution, the concentration of the substance is measured per ml and the total volume of the fluid is calculated.

While determining blood volume, the substances used may either get attached to plasma proteins or the concentration of the marker RBCs (RBCs tagged with radioactive material) injected get decreased due to dilution in circulation. The substances, which get attached to plasma proteins will be T_{1824} dye (Evan's blue), RIHSA, etc. Radioactive iron, chromium, etc. bind to the RBCs only.

Procedure when T_{1824} dye used will be:

- Obtain a sample of blood of the person and estimate *PCV* (Assume it to be 40%).
- Dissolve known quantity of dye (e.g. 3 mg in 1 ml) and inject.
- Wait for about 20 min for the dye to get diluted in the plasma volume.
- Take a sample of plasma and estimate the concentration of dye in it (e.g. 0.001 mg/ml).

Plasma volume can be calculated as follows:

Step 1

- Total quantity of dye injected—3 mg.
- 0.001 mg of dye is present in 1 ml of plasma after the dye has got uniformly diluted in plasma.
- In order to get the above dilution, what should be volume of total plasma (X).

$$\text{Calculation will be } 3 \times 1 = 0.001 \times (X)$$

$$\text{So } (X) = \frac{3 \times 1}{0.001} = 3000 \text{ ml}$$

Step 2

Assume *PCV* as 40%. So the blood volume will be

$$\text{Blood volume} = \frac{\text{Total plasma volume} \times 1}{(1 - PCV)}$$

$$= \frac{3000 \times 1}{(1 - 0.40)} = 5000 \text{ ml}$$

Some of the criteria the substance used must possess are:
The substance should

- Get distributed evenly in the plasma.
- Not to leave the circulatory system.
- Not to alter the blood volume.
- Be non-toxic.
- Not get metabolized in the body and concentration can be estimated easily.

Above principle can be used to measure the total body water content and ECF volume as well. Total body water content can be determined by using heavy water (Deuterium). ECF volume can be determined using Na^+, Cl^-, inulin, etc.

Blood volume is increased in conditions, like pregnancy (20 to 30% increases), anemia, administration of steroid, hyperaldosteronism, etc.

Blood volume gets decreased in burns, hemoconcentration (severe vomiting, diarrhea), hemorrhage, etc.

Regulation of Blood Volume

1. *Capillary fluid shift mechanism is most sensitive.* Even when there is loss of few ml the mechanism gets activated to restore the blood volume. The mechanism starts acting within few seconds of decrease in the volume of blood.

   - When there is decrease in blood volume, there will be reflex precapillary sphincter constriction due to stimulation of sympathetic nerves.
   - This leads to less amount of blood flow through the capillary.
   - The hydrostatic pressure (out driving force) in the capillary is decreased. Because of this hydrostatic pressure will be less than the colloidal osmotic pressure (in driving force) throughout the length of the capillary.
   - Due to in driving force (colloidal osmotic pressure) being more than the out driving force, fluid is drawn into the intravascular compartment from the tissue spaces throughout the length of capillary.
   - This increases the blood volume (Fig. 1.21).

2. *Secretion of hormones* like aldosterone, ADH and atrial natriuretic peptide or factor (ANP/ANF) will also help in the regulation of blood volume.

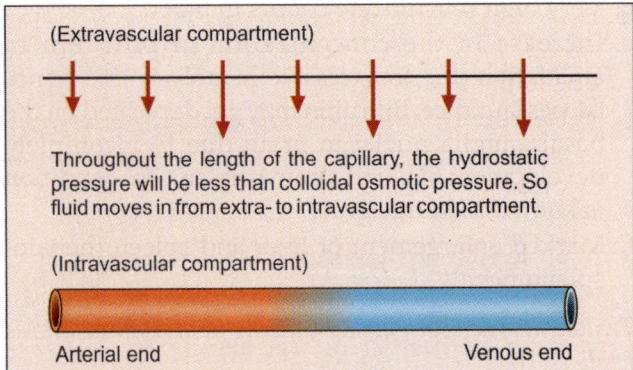

Fig. 1.21: Shift of fluid from extravascular region to intravascular region when there is loss of blood

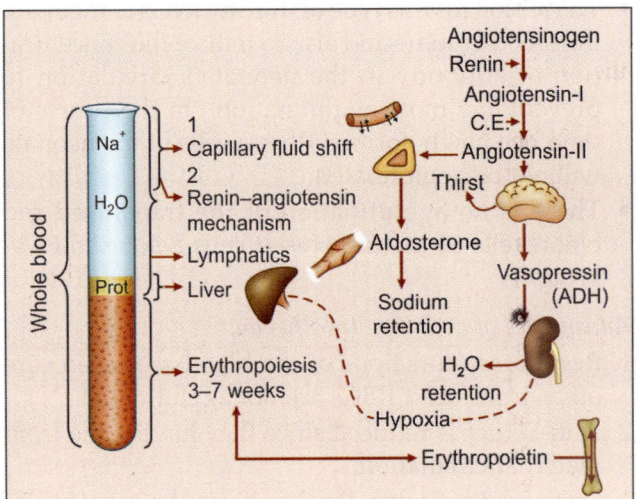

Fig. 1.22: The role of renin-angiotensin-aldosterone mechanism in the restoration of blood volume

i. *The role of aldosterone will be as follows* (Fig. 1.22):
   a. Aldosterone increases sodium reabsorption in kidney and hence increased water reabsorption leading to increased blood volume.
   b. Aldosterone is secreted from adrenal cortex
   c. Decreased blood flow to kidney in hypovolemia leads to the activation of the renin angiotensin system. More amount of renin secretion will also be due to increased sympathetic stimulation.
   d. Angiotensin II in turn acts on adrenal cortex to increase the secretion of aldosterone.
   e. Angiotensin II also stimulates thirst center and the person drinks more water.

ii. *ADH increases water reabsorption in the kidney to restore blood volume.* Increased secretion of ADH is due to the following:

- Decreased blood volume leads to decreased stimulation of volume/low pressure receptors present in the walls of great veins, right atrium etc.
- So less inhibitory impulses along the afferent vagus nerve to supraoptic nucleus in hypothalamus.
- Activity of the supraoptic nucleus increased.
- More impulses along the hypothalamo-hypophysial tract to posterior pituitary gland.
- This increases ADH release into circulation. This in turn increases water reabsorption in the collecting tubules and hence blood volume is increased.

iii. *Atrial natriuretic peptide is secreted from the wall of the atrium.*

- When there is increase in blood volume, there will be increased distension of the walls of the atria.
- This increases the secretion of ANP.
- ANP acts on the kidney and decreases the reabsorption of sodium and water.
- This leads to decrease of blood volume.

When hypovolemia is because of loss of water alone, the above first two mechanisms come into action and may restore the blood volume. But if the decrease in blood volume is due to hemorrhage, plasma and formed elements are also lost. So the restoration of the plasma proteins may occur in a week's time and formed elements number (especially of RBCs) in about few months time.

LYMPH

Lymph is nothing but the interstitial fluid which has entered the lymphatic vessels. It is almost identical to plasma except for proteins concentration which is far less than in plasma.

Formation of lymph can be explained on capillary dynamics or Starling's hypothesis.

- At the level of capillaries, hydrostatic pressure is about 35 mm Hg at the arterial end, tries to drive out fluid into interstitial spaces.
- This is countered by the colloidal osmotic pressure, which is about 25 mm Hg.

- However, since the hydrostatic pressure is higher than the colloidal osmotic pressure, some amount of fluid goes out to the tissue spaces.
- Whereas, at the venous end of the capillary, the colloidal osmotic pressure continues to be same, but the hydrostatic pressure will have fallen down to only about 16 mm Hg.
- Due to this some amount of fluid from the tissue spaces returns to the vascular compartment.
- However, a small volume of fluid left behind in the tissue spaces is brought back to circulation by lymphatic vessels.

Functions of Lymph

- Return of tissue fluid and lost proteins into circulation and maintains blood volume.
- Transport of lymphocytes from the lymph nodes into circulation.
- Transport of fats absorbed from the intestine into circulation.
- Transport of microorganisms to lymph nodes for initiation of immune responses.

Lymph Nodes

Lymph nodes (Fig. 1.23) are present at strategic positions in the body along the flow of lymph. They

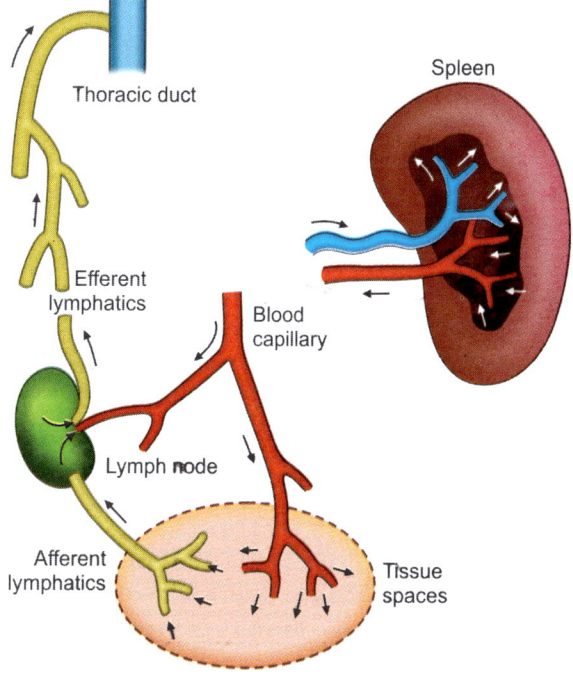

Fig. 1.23: Lymphatics and the course of lymph flow

are concentrated in neck, axilla, inguinal region, tonsils, appendix, etc. Hence inflammation of the lymph nodes in any of these regions will definitely indicate infections in the body.

Functions of the lymph nodes are:
- Production of lymphocytes.
- Production of antibodies (immunoglobulins/ gamma globulins)
- Act as filters for bacteria and thereby prevent the spread of infection to different parts of body (so the infection is localized).

Spleen

Spleen is one of the biggest lymphoid organs. Despite this, spleen is not an essential organ as person can survive even after removal of spleen (splenectomy). Spleen has many functions.

Some of the important functions of the spleen are:
- Production of RBCs in fetal life.
- Destruction of senile RBCs throughout the lifespan.
- Production of lymphocytes and antibodies.
- May have control over production of WBCs and platelets.
- In lower animals, acts as a storage organ for blood.

In hypersplenism (Banti's syndrome), the person most often suffers from anemia, thrombocytopenia and leukocytopenia.

BODY FLUID pH REGULATION

The regulation of H+ is very essential for the maintenance of normal pH of body fluid. The intracellular pH varies from region to region, the lowest being found in the canaliculi of parietal cells of gastric glands (here it can be as low as 1). The pH of blood should be maintained around a value of 7.4 ±0.04 for the functioning of tissues to go on smooth. A minute variation of pH above or below the normal range affects the chemical reactions in the tissues. The hydrogen ion concentration can be ascertained by measuring the pH, as pH has inverse relationship with hydrogen ion concentration (Fig. 1.24).

Hydrogen ions are constantly produced in the body due to various metabolic activities, like:

1. Oxidation of carbon compounds to produce carbon dioxide

$$CO_2 + H_2O \leftrightarrow H_2CO_3 \leftrightarrow +H^+$$

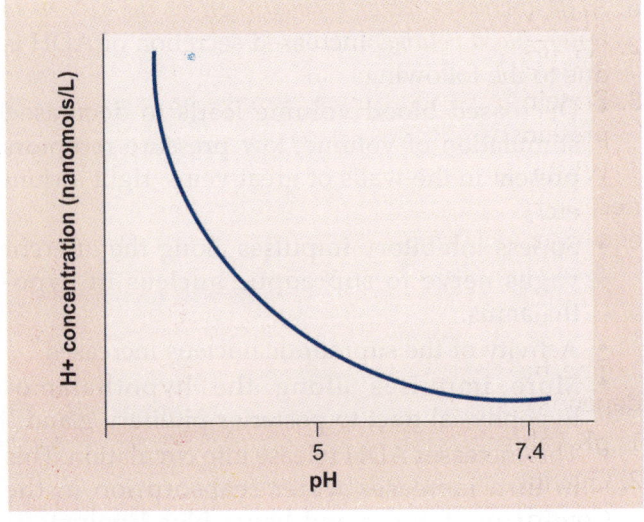

Fig. 1.24: Graph showing the relationship between H+ concentration and pH

2. Conversion of neutral foodstuff into organic acids
   Neutral carbohydrates—fats + proteins→
   intermediary metabolites → $CO_2 + H_2O$

3. Oxidation of sulfur in organic compounds
   Methionine + $O_2 \rightarrow H_2SO_4$ + Urea + $H_2O + CO_2$

4. Medication—ammonium salts (NH_4Cl), organic acids.

When these H+ are produced and added, the following mechanism comes into play to maintain its concentration.

a. Blood buffers and intracellular buffers act immediately to neutralize the H+. The respiratory system—in the regulation of body fluid pH and its efficiency is only to the extent of 75%.

b. The renal system—it takes a little longer time to act, but when once it starts acting, its capability is almost 100%, e.g. if the pH of body fluid is reduced to 7 (acidosis) with respiratory system alone it is corrected only to about 7.3. But with kidney it is corrected to 7.4. Respiratory system and kidney play a very vital role in the H+ homeostasis.

Blood Buffers

There are 3 important buffer systems operating in blood to maintain the pH of blood around 7.4. They are:

1. $\dfrac{(HCO_3^-)}{(H_2CO_3)}$ Bicarbonate buffer pair

2. $\dfrac{(HCO_4^-)}{(H_2PO_4)}$ Phosphate buffer pair

3. Protein buffer (includes hemoglobin and plasma proteins)

While discussing the regulation of pH, it is necessary to understand Henderson-Hasselbalch equation, which states that

$$pH = pK + \log \dfrac{Base}{Acid}$$

The buffering capacity of a buffer substance depends on its:

1. pK value

2. Quantity of the buffer substance.

Considering the above two, Table 1.10 depicts the details of all the three buffer systems of blood.

Table 1.10: The relative capability of different buffer systems

Buffers	pK value	Quantity	Buffering capacity
HCO_3/H_2CO_3	6.1	+++	++
HPO_4/H_2PO_4	6.8	+	+
Proteins	7.4	+++++	+++++

+ve denotes the relative concentration and buffering capability.

Since large amount of proteins are available in blood and the pK value of protein buffer system is nearer to the pH of blood, and as blood buffer it is the most efficient one. However, as for the entire body is concerned, it is the HCO_3 buffer which is more important, because the concentration of buffer pair HCO_3/H_2CO_3 is more easily maintained by the respiratory system (H_2CO_3) and by the kidney (HCO_3). As long as the proportion between the buffer pair is maintained, the pH is also maintained.

For the bicarbonate buffer system, the normal ratio will be:

$$\dfrac{HCO_3^-}{H_2CO_3} = \dfrac{24\ mEq/L}{1.2\ mEq/L}$$

And finally the ratio will be 20:1

So the pH $= 6.1 + \log \dfrac{20}{1} = 6.1 + 1.3 = 7.4$

Reactions involved with the bicarbonate buffer system:
When an H^+ or OH^- is added, $NaHCO_3 + HCl \rightarrow H_2CO_3 + NaCl$

Powerful acid (HCl) is converted into a weak acid H_2CO_3.

When OH^- is added
$NaOH + H_2CO_3 \rightarrow NaHCO_3 + H_2O$

A powerful base (NaOH) is converted to a weak base $NaHCO_3$.

Protein buffers:

Phosphate buffer system:
When an acid is added
$NaHPO_4 + HCl \rightarrow NaH_2PO_4 + NaCl$

Strong acid HCl is converted to weak acid NaH_2PO_4.

When an alkali is added
$NaH_2PO_4 + NaOH \rightarrow Na_2HPO_4 + H_2O$

A strong alkali is converted to a weak base.

Phosphate buffers play an important role in the renal tubules. They buffer the H^+ secreted into the tubular fluid and maintain the tubular fluid pH above 4.2.

Isohydric principle: Whenever the body fluid pH changes, all the buffers react simultaneously to rectify the pH and this is known as isohydric principle. *The four major types of acid-base disturbance include:*

1. *Respiratory acidosis* occurs in acute pulmonary edema, bronchial asthma, and depression of respiratory center due to poisoning or bulbar polio. In all these conditions, carbon dioxide is not washed-out properly and is retained as carbonic acid (H_2CO_3). This alters the ratio between HCO_3/H_2CO_3 and pH falls towards the acidic side. Kidney corrects this by excreting more of H^+ in urine.

2. *Respiratory alkalosis* will be due to excessive stimulation of respiratory centers. This leads to more amount of CO_2 getting washed-out from the body and as a result H_2CO_3 concentration

decreases. This also creates an imbalance in HCO_3/H_2CO_3 ratio and hence leads to increase of pH and alkalosis. This occurs in conditions like hypoxic hypoxia in high altitudes, hysteria, salicylate poisoning. Kidney helps to restore the pH back to normal by excreting more amount of HCO_3. Kidney also decreases the excretion of H^+ in the urine.

3. *Metabolic acidosis* occurs in diabetes mellitus (ketone bodies), lactic acidosis and in severe diarrhea (excessive loss of bases). This decreases the HCO_3 concentration. The pH is restored back to normal by respiration by eliminating more CO_2 from the body and hence the H_2CO_3 content decreases. The kidney also increases the excretion of H^+ ions and reabsorption of HCO_3.

4. *Metabolic alkalosis* occurs in severe vomiting (loss of HCl), ingestion of excessive amount of $NaHCO_3$. The elevated pH depresses the respiratory center and hence washout of CO_2 from the body is decreases. So H_2CO_3 concentration gets increased. In addition to this, kidneys retain H^+ and excrete more HCO_3 in the urine. The complementary efforts of the respiratory and renal systems try to **restore** the ratio between HCO_3/H_2CO_3 and the pH as **well**.

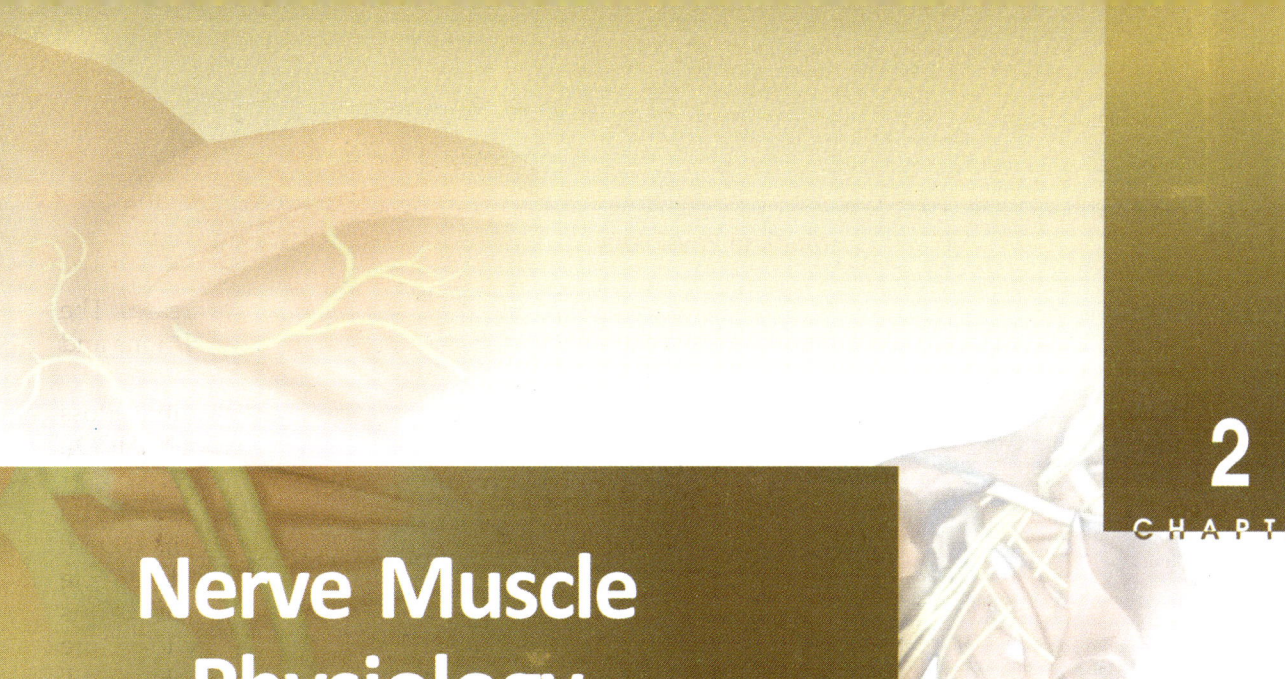

Nerve Muscle Physiology

2
CHAPTER

This system deals with the structure and function of both neuron and muscles in the body in general. For the sake of convenience, in this chapter neuron and muscle part will be dealt separately.

NEURON

- Neuron is the structural and functional unit of nervous system.
- There are about 100 billion neurons in central nervous system (CNS).
- Apart from this, neurons and nerves are also present in the peripheral nervous system and this is outside the CNS.
- The neurons of peripheral nervous system help to establish contact between CNS and the structures present in different parts of body.
- Function of nervous system is to receive, integrate and transmit the information required to bring about the intended actions.

Some of the important definitions that need to be understood are:

1. *Neuron:* Is the structural and functional unit of nervous system.
2. *Nerve/nerve trunk:* Is the collection of nerve fibers outside the CNS.
3. *Ganglion:* Is the collection of nerve cell bodies outside CNS.
4. *Nucleus:* Is the collection of nerve cell bodies inside the CNS.

5. *Synapse:* Is the functional junction between parts of two different neurons.
6. *Tract:* Is collection of nerve fibers in CNS having common origin, course, termination and function.
7. *Excitability:* Is the ability of the tissues to respond to a stimulus.
8. *Stimulus:* Is the sudden change in the external or internal environment, to which a tissue responds.
9. *Threshold stimulus:* Is the minimum strength of stimulus that is required to elicit a response.
10. *Action potential or impulse:* Is an electrical change brought about by movement of charged ions across the cell membrane, which is self-regenerating one and is conducted in a decrimentless fashion along the whole length of the nerve fiber.

The structural and the functional unit of the nervous system is a neuron. They are present in both central and peripheral nervous system. Each nerve cell possesses a cell body, an axon and many dendrites. The nerve cells are classified into:

1. *Unipolar:* The dendrite and the axon arise from a common stem and divide into two, one forming the axon and the other forms the dendrite. This type of cell is seen in the posterior nerve root ganglion cells.
2. *Bipolar cells:* The axon and the dendrite are located on either poles of the neuron. They are typically seen in the bipolar cell layer of the retina and the vestibulocochlear ganglion of the eighth cranial nerve.
3. *Multipolar cells* (Fig. 2.1): This type of nerve cells will have a single axon and a number of dendrites

33

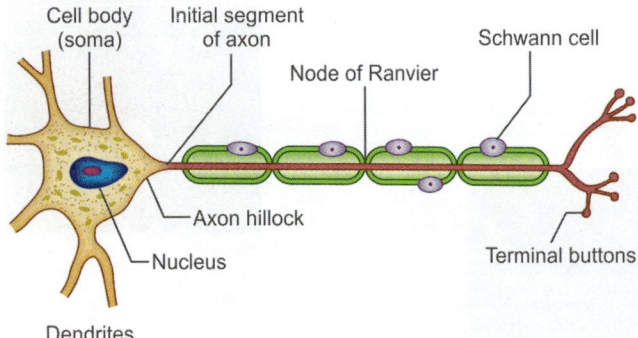

Fig. 2.1: A multipolar neuron

and the dendrites repeatedly branch to form a network. These cells are seen in the cerebral cortex, in the cerebellar cortex and in the anterior horn cells of the spinal cord.

Nerve cells can also be classified as motor and sensory based on their function. Motor neurons are present in the cerebral cortex, subcortical regions, as well as in the anterior horn of the spinal cord. Sensory nerve cells are present in the posterior horn of the spinal cord, thalamus and in the sensory cortex of the brain. The nerve cell body contains neurofibrils, fine thread like structures which course through the cell body.

The cell body also contains Nissl granules, rough endoplasmic reticulum, Golgi apparatus and mitochondria. Nissl granules disintegrate when there is injury to the axon, and this is known as chromatolysis.

Dendrites are the extensions of the cell body. They repeatedly branch forming arborizations.

There is only one axon for a neuron and it takes its origin from the axon hillock. It lacks rough endoplasmic reticulum, free ribosome and Golgi apparatus. Therefore, the axon degenerates when it is disconnected from the cell body.

Neuroglial cells form a supporting framework of the central nervous system. In the central nervous system, the glial cells present are astrocytes, oligodendroglial cells, microglial cells and ependymal cells.

Astrocytes buffer the external environment with respect to their chemical environment.

Oligodendroglial cells ensheath the axons of the central nervous system.

Microglial cells are phagocytic in nature. They remove the products of cellular damage.

Ependymal cells separate the central nervous system from the cerebrospinal fluid. Specialized ependymal cells are responsible for the secretion of cerebrospinal fluid.

Nerve Fiber or Axon

Axon is the part of the neuron, which conducts impulse/action potential along the whole length. Thereby it helps for establishing the communication between nervous system and any part of the body.

Classification of Nerve Fibers

Based on the presence or absence of myelin sheath, they are classified into myelinated or non-myelinated nerve fibers. In the peripheral nervous system, the Schwann cells are responsible for the formation of the myelin sheath. In the central nervous system, the oligodendroglial cells are responsible for the formation of the myelin sheath. This sheath is broken at regular intervals known as the nodes of Ranvier. Here only the neurilemmal membrane will separate the interior and exterior of the nerve fiber.

Nerve fibers can be classified based on different criteria:
1. Histologically, as myelinated or non-myelinated (Fig. 2.2).
2. Functionally, as afferent (sensory) or efferent (motor).
3. Based on diameter and conduction velocity which is known as Gasser and Erlanger's classification.
4. Based on the type of neurotransmitter released from their terminals as adrenergic, cholinergic, dopaminergic, etc.

In myelinated nerve fiber, the wrapping of the axon by the myelin sheath provided Schwann cell occurs. Whereas in non-myelinated nerve fiber, the Schwann cell just covers the nerve fiber without wrapping. In myelinated nerve fibers, at certain places the myelin

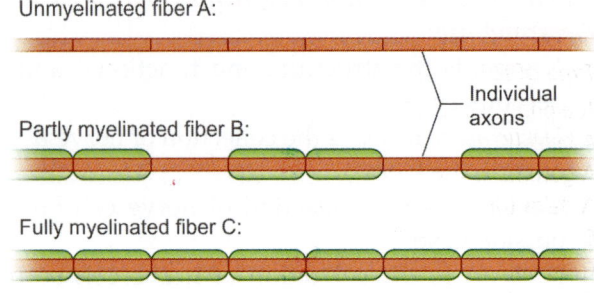

Fig. 2.2: A typical non-myelinated and myelinated nerve fiber

sheath is absent. These areas are called as nodes of Ranvier. The protoplasm present in the axon region is known as axoplasm. The transport of materials within the axoplasm can occur in either direction (from the cell body towards the axon and vice versa). When the substance is transported from the cell body towards the axon terminals, it is known as anterograde transport (fastest—400 mm/day). This type of movement of axoplasm helps for transport of neurotransmitter, proteins, etc. from the cell body to the end of the nerve terminals. When the transport of substance occurs in opposite direction (that is from the nerve terminals towards the cell body), it is known as retrograde transport (slowest—200 mm/day). Many of the viruses (rabies virus, polio), bacteria (tetanus), etc. reach the cell bodies in the nervous system because of the retrograde transport.

Myelinogenesis

Myelinogenesis is the process by which myelination of the nerve fiber takes place. In the peripheral nervous system, the myelinogenesis is contributed by the Schwann cells whereas in the CNS it is being contributed by the oligodendroglial cells. The sheath of Schwann cell wraps the axon by about 80–100 times. The cell membrane lipids form the myelin sheath.

Functions of the Myelin Sheath

1. In myelinated nerve fibers, the velocity of impulse transmission is faster because the process of depolarization occurs only at the nodes of Ranveir and, therefore, it appears as if the impulses are jumping from one node to the successive node (Fig. 2.3). This type of impulse transmission is known as saltatory or leaping type of conduction. Because of this type of impulse transmission, the energy required for conduction is markedly reduced.

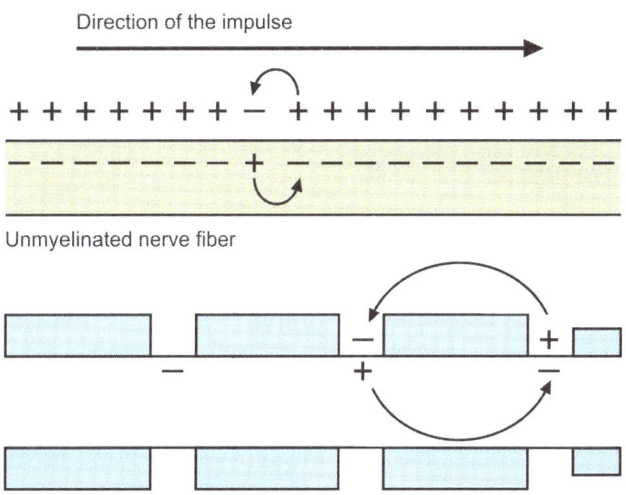

Direction of the impulse

Unmyelinated nerve fiber

Myelinated nerve fiber

Fig. 2.3: The process of impulse conduction in unmyelinated and myelinated nerve fibers. In myelinated nerve fiber, the impulse jumps from one node of Ranvier to the next

2. It acts as a protective sheath minimizing injury to the nerve fiber.
3. It acts as an insulator and prevents cross transmission of impulses from one fiber to the other in a mixed nerve.

Based on the diameter and velocity of impulse conduction, the nerve fibers are also classified into A, B and C types. And A is further divided in to A alpha, A beta, A gamma and A delta fibers. This classification is known as Erlanger and Gasser classification. Diameter and conduction velocity have direction relationship.

A and B group fibers are myelinated whereas C group fibers are non-myelinated (Table 2.1).

Properties of Nerve Fibers

Excitability is the most important property of a nerve fiber. They are highly excitable when compared to any other tissues. They have the least chronaxie. Nerve

Table 2.1: Indicating diameter, conduction velocity and function of nerve fibers			
Type of fiber	Diameter (microns)	Velocity (m/sec)	Function
A alpha (α)	12–20	70–120	Somatic motor, proprioception
A beta (β)	5–12	30–70	Touch, pressure
A gamma (γ)	3–6	15–30	Motor to muscle spindle
A delta (δ)	2–5	12–30	Pain and temperature
B	<3	3–15	Preganglionic autonomic
C dorsal root	0.4–1.2	0.5–2	Pain and temperature
C sympathetic	0.3–1.3	0.7–2.3	Postganglionic sympathetic

Table 2.2: Susceptibility of fibers to various factors

	Highly	Moderate	Least
Local anesthetics	C	B	A
Pressure	A	B	C
Hypoxia	B	A	C

fibers respond to electrical, mechanical, chemical and thermal stimuli.

Among the different stimuli, electrical is the best to stimulate a tissue for the following reasons:

1. The current strength used can be easily measured and regulated.
2. It produces the least mechanical damage to the tissue.
3. The events that occur in the tissue are of the electrical in nature that is the depolarization and repolarization.

Property of conductivity: This is the most important function of the nerve fiber. Myelinated nerve fibers conduct at a much faster rate than the non-myelinated nerve fibers. The maximum velocity of impulse transmission in a myelinated nerve fiber in human being is about 70 to 120 meters per second. In a sensory nerve fiber, the impulses are transmitted from the periphery towards the center known as orthodromic transmission. If the transmission is in the opposite direction that is from the center towards the periphery in a sensory fiber, it is known as antidromic transmission.

Factors affecting the velocity of impulse conduction are:

1. Diameter of the nerve fiber and myelination.
2. Ideal space between nodes of Ranvier (about 1 mm apart).
3. Temperature.
4. Pressure (Table 2.2).
5. Hypoxia (decreased oxygen supply) (Table 2.2).
6. Actions of hormones like thyroxin.
7. Diseases (multiple sclerosis, diabetes mellitus) etc.

Strength Duration Curve (Fig. 2.4 and Table 2.3)

Chronaxie is the minimum time required to elicit a response from the tissue with double the rheobasic current. The excitability of any tissue has inverse relationship with chronaxie.

Rheobase is the minimum current required to stimulate a tissue without considering the time factor.

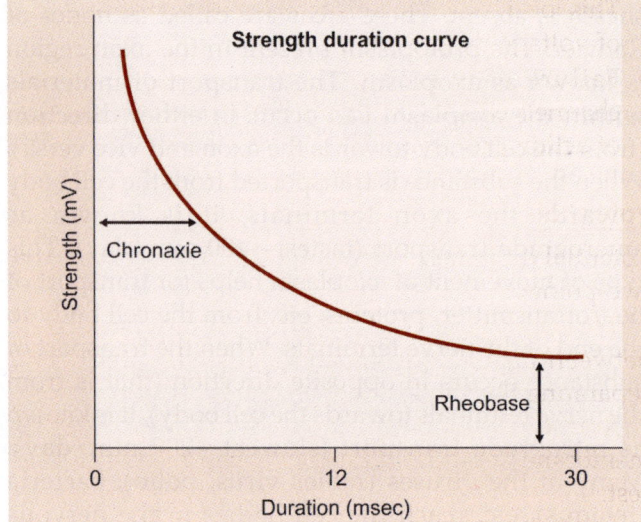

Fig. 2.4: Graph shows the relationship between the strength of stimulation and the duration to respond

Table 2.3: Excitability of different types of nerve fibers

Tissue	Chronaxie (msec)
Large myelinated nerve fiber	0.01
Small unmyelinated nerve fiber	0.1
Skeletal muscle	0.03
Cardiac muscle	1–3
Smooth muscle	30–100

Importance of chronaxie

1. Studies involving nerve degeneration and regeneration.
2. Principle of diathermy wherein in surgeries, short duration high frequency stimuli are applied which would be less than the chronaxie durations. This brings about increase of local temperature which facilitates early coagulation of blood and hence loss of blood is reduced (thermocautery).

Some of the other factors, which affect excitability, are:

a. Ionic composition.
b. Temperature.
c. Local anesthetics, etc.

Mechanism of action of local anesthetics in blocking impulse conduction will be as follows:

- These substances block voltage-gated sodium channels.
- So, when stimulus is applied, there is development of local potential.

- This local potential fails to bring about the opening of voltage-gated sodium channels.
- Failure of opening of voltage-gated sodium channels will not be able to bring about production of action potential.

Potentials

Potential difference is the voltage difference between two points.

Transmembrane potential is the voltage difference between inside and outside (across the membrane separating ECF and ICF).

Resting membrane potential is the steady transmembrane potential difference when the tissue is at rest.

Equilibrium potential is the voltage difference at which the net flux of ions between ECF and ICF is zero (influx = efflux).

Graded potential is potential change of variable amplitude and duration, which can't get conducted over long distance and time. Examples of local potentials are excitatory post-synaptic potential (EPSP), inhibitory post-synaptic potential (IPSP), receptor potential and end plate potential (EPP).

Action potential is the brief depolarization (all or none in nature) of the membrane that occurs on application of threshold stimulus or above the threshold strength and gets conducted over long distance without any variation in the amplitude.

Resting Membrane Potential

- It is the potential difference between ECF and ICF when the tissue is at rest.
- The ICF is normally negative when compared to ECF.
- It is due to inequality in the distribution of charged ions in ECF and ICF, and difference in the permeability of the membrane for the movement of charged ions (Table 2.4).
- The cell membrane is freely permeable to K^+ and is less permeable to Na^+.

Table 2.4: Distributions of inorganic ions (mEq/L water) in ECF and ICF

Ions	ECF	ICF
Na^+	150	15
K^+	5	150
Cl^-	110	10

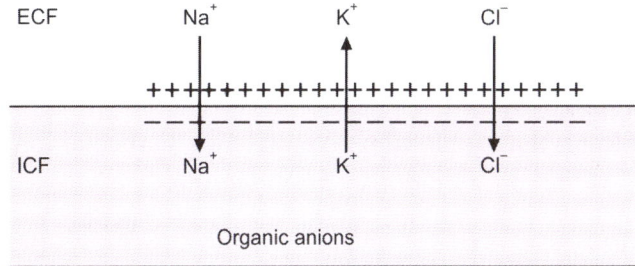

Fig. 2.5: Distribution of the charged ions across the cell membrane and the tendency of the ions to move across the cell membrane

- Na^+ moves in along the electrical and concentration gradient, K^+ tries to move out along the concentration gradient. Chloride doesn't move much. The cell membrane is not permeable to organic anions (Fig. 2.5).
- Na^+–K^+ pump keeps up the electrical gradient. This pump is known as electrogenic pump.
- For every 3 Na^+ that are pumped out into the ECF, 2 K^+ will be brought back into ICF from the ECF.
- RMP of nerve is usually around –70 mV. That for skeletal and cardiac muscle is around –90 mV.

Major reasons for negative charge inside the cell will be:

a. More K^+ efflux because of concentration gradient and more permeability.

b. Cell membrane impermeability for organic anions like proteins.

c. Decreased Na^+ permeability at rest.

d. Operation of the Na^+–K^+ pumps which keeps up the gradient. Though K^+ is diffusing out, major part is brought back because of more permeability of cell membrane for K^+.

The magnitude of the RMP depends on two factors:

1. Difference in ion concentration across the membrane.

2. Difference in the membrane permeability for the ion.

The equilibrium potential for one ion can be different in magnitude and direction from those for other. In the ECF and ICF, concentration gradient for different ions varies and the direction of movement of the ions also.

If concentration gradient is known for any ion, based on Nerst equation, equilibrium potential can be calculated.

According to Nernst equation

$$E\, ion = \frac{60}{Z}\log\frac{(C_o)}{(C_i)}$$

$E\, ion$ is the equilibrium potential for a particular ion.

C_i is the concentration of the ion inside.

C_o is the concentration of the substance outside.

Z is the valence of the ion.

60 is constant (gas constant, temperature and Faraday electric constant)

Based on the above, the equilibrium potential for
a. Potassium ion will be –89 mV.
b. Sodium ion will be +60 mV.

Since in the body, apart from positively charged ions, even negatively charged ion (chloride) is also involved in the development of membrane potential. The following equation helps us to derive the net equilibrium potential when all the three different ions are considered. In this equation, not only the ionic concentration is considered, but also the permeability of the membrane for different ions. This equation is known as Goldman equation (which is the expanded form of Nernst equation).

$$V_m = 60\log\frac{P_{Na}(Na_o) + P_K(K_o) + P_{Cl}(Cl_i)}{P_{Na}(Na_i) + P_K(K_i) + P_{Cl}(Cl_o)}$$

For chloride, the position is reversed in the equation because, chloride is a negatively charged ion and its movement has opposite effect.

When one calculates the equilibrium potential taking all the above three ions into consideration, it comes to about –70 mV which is nearer to equilibrium potential of potassium. It is not more negative (–89 mV) because, there are some leaky channels in the membrane through which some amount of sodium ions diffuse from ECF to ICF.

When any threshold or above strength of stimulus is applied, the RMP is altered. This will give rise to generation of action potential.

When the strength of stimulus is less than threshold (that is subthreshold), there will not be production of action potential. But still, there will be some amount of potential change occurring locally and this is termed as local potential. There are subtle differences between local potential and actions potentials (Table 2.5).

Table 2.5: Comparing local potential and action potential

	Local potential	*Action potential*
Size	Graded	All or none
Conduction	Not well (decrementing type)	Decrimentless
Summation Polarity	Possible depolarizing or hyperpolarizing type	Not possible always depolarizing type
Intensity of stimulus	Not fixed	Threshold and above
Refractory period	Nil	Present
Function served	Signal over short distances	Signal over long distances

Action Potential

Action potential is a brief or temporary propagation of the depolarization (physicochemical change) brought about by a threshold stimulus or above. It is a self-regenerating one, and gets conducted in a decrimentless fashion.

Types of action potential:
1. Monophasic (Figs 2.6 and 2.7)
2. Biphasic/diphasic
3. Compound.

Of the three, the first two can be recorded from a single nerve fiber whereas the compound action potential can be recorded from a nerve trunk (group of nerve fibers).

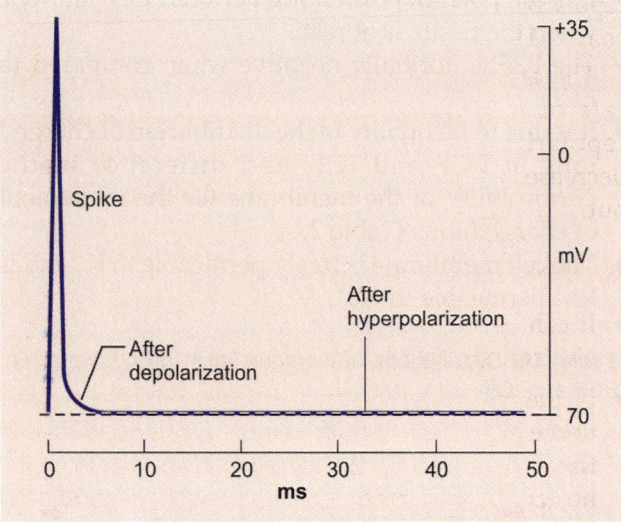

Fig. 2.6: Monophasic action potential—actual recording

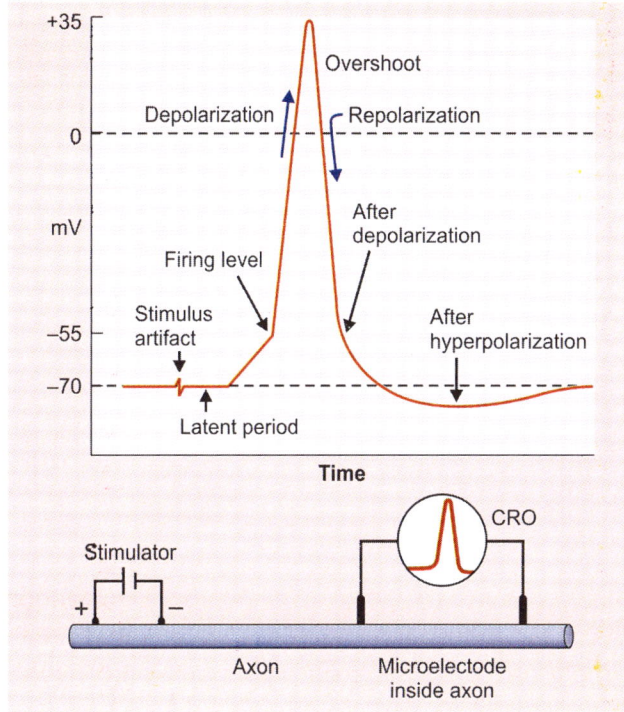

Fig. 2.7: Monophasic action potential—schematic drawing

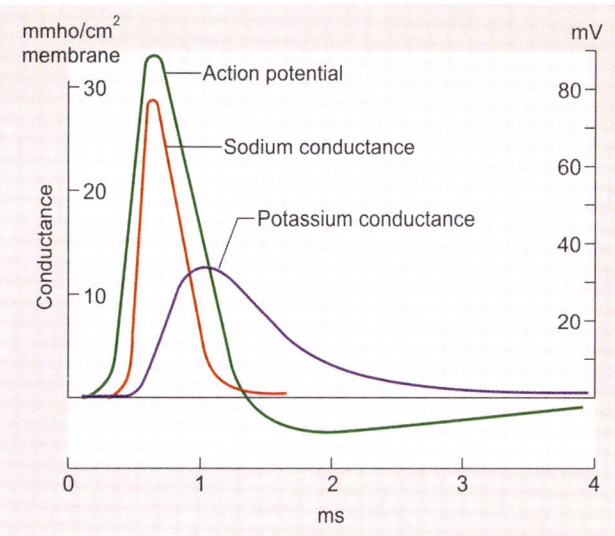

Fig. 2.8: Ions responsible for the process of depolarization and repolarization

Flow chart 2.1: The influx of Na+ ions responsible for the process of depolarization

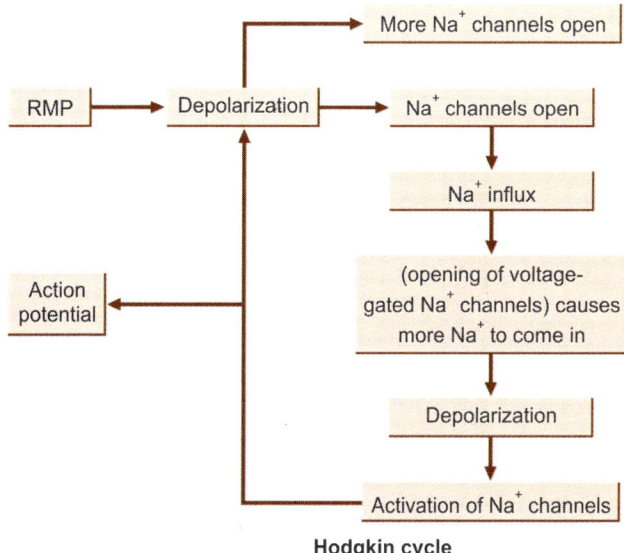

Monophasic Action Potential

To record a monophasic action potential, one of the recording electrodes should be in ECF and the other in ICF. For biphasic action potential recording, both the recording electrodes can be placed either in ECF or ICF.

The depolarization is because of influx of Na^+ and repolarization is because of efflux of K^+ (Fig. 2.8) (Flow chart 2.1).

The after depolarization is because of decreased rate of movement of K^+ out of cell, as during repolarization phase, the efflux of K^+ gradually decreases the concentration gradient for K^+ to move out.

Biphasic Action Potential

- It can be recorded by placing both the recording electrodes either in the ECF or ICF.
- In the Y axis when there is no stimulation of the nerve fiber, there is no potential difference between the two recording electrodes and hence the horizontal line recorded is known as isopotential line.
- The recording will have two peaks and one will be the mirror image of the other (Fig. 2.9).
- The isopotential duration between the mirror images will depend on the distance between the two recording electrodes and is directly related.
- The ionic basis of the potential recorded will be same as far monophasic action potential.

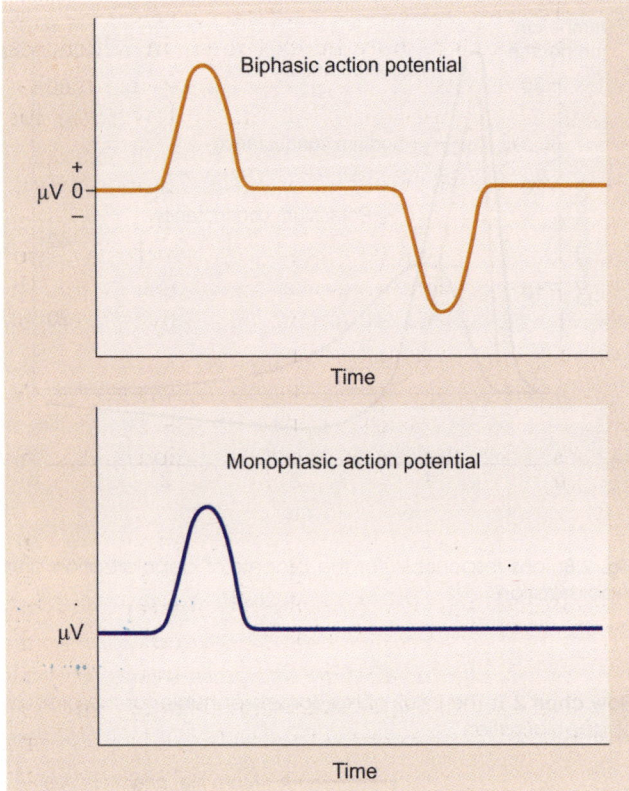

Fig. 2.9: Configuration of monophasic and biphasic action potentials

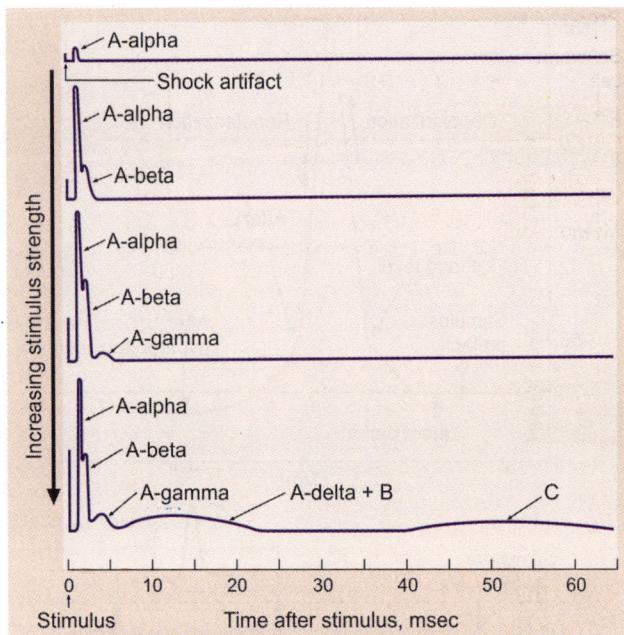

Fig. 2.10: Peak appearing at different intervals when a mixed nerve is stimulated

Compound Action Potential

- It can be recorded from a mixed nerve.
- A mixed nerve may be either the nerve having both the afferent and efferent fibers and fibers belonging to different groups as per Gasser and Erlanger classification.
- The peaks appear at different intervals because of the difference in the conduction velocities (Fig. 2.10).
- The relative amplitude of the peaks, depends on the number of nerve fibers of a particular group present in the mixed nerve.

Nerve Injuries

Whenever a nerve is damaged, depending on the type of injury and intensity of the damage, there will be certain structural and functional changes. The details of the same will be discussed under degeneration and regeneration.

Types of Nerve Injuries

1. *Neurapraxia* is physiological paralysis wherein the conduction of impulses in the intact nerve fibers will be lost temporarily. It may be due to stretch / distortion without any rupture. There is no physical damage to the nerve fibers and hence there will not be any degenerative changes. The recovery will be complete in this type of nerve injury.
2. *Axonotmesis* is intrathecal rupture of nerve fibers with an intact sheath. Degenerative changes occur in the nerve fibers and recovery from such injury will be complete.
3. *Neurontmesis:* In this type, there will be partial or complete damage to both the sheath and nerve fibers. Following this type of an injury, only about 80% of the functional recovery is observed.

Effect of sectioning the axon Wallerian degeneration:
- Changes are seen distal to the site of injury.
- Changes are seen proximal to the site of injury.
- Changes are seen in the cell body.

a. ***Changes seen distal to the site of injury can be described under four headings:***
1. *Histological changes* (Fig. 2.11): The myelin sheath is broken down into fragments and the lipid material into oily droplets while the axis cylinder remains intact. This is followed by proliferation of Schwann cells and macrophages. Macrophages act as scavengers and remove the cell debris. Schwann

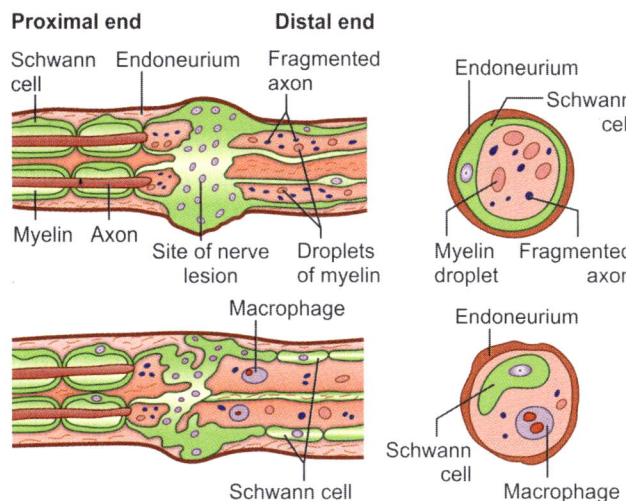

Fig. 2.11: Histological degenerative changes in nerve fiber

cells help in the guiding the regenerative sprouts into the distal tube during the process of regeneration.

2. *Biochemical changes:* Synthesis of acetylcholine becomes defective; acetylcholine estrase activity is markedly reduced. If the cut ends of the nerve fibers are not separated, the nerve fiber may be able to transmit impulses for about two to three days. At the end of this period, impulse transmission is completely stopped.

3. *Functional changes:* If the nerve fibers are sensory one, the sensations are lost over the area of the skin supplied by this nerve. If it is a motor nerve, there will be paralysis of the muscle-nerve supplied by this nerve.

4. *Electrical changes:* This change is known as the reaction of degeneration, an altered response to galvanic and faradic shocks by a muscle when its motor nerve supply is cut and has undergone degeneration. When a denervated muscle is directly stimulated it will not respond to faradic shocks and for galvanic shocks it responds very slowly and sluggishly.

b. *Similar changes are also seen proximal to the site of injury until the first node of Ranvier.*

c. *In case the injury is severe, the cell body also demonstrates certain degenerative changes.* They are:
   a. Nissl substances start disintegrating.
   b. The cell body gets swollen up by imbibing water from the ECF.

c. The nucleus may be pushed to a side. At times the nucleus may be extruded, in which case regeneration of nerve fiber cannot take place.

d. Staining property of the cell will be lost gradually.

e. Neurofibrils will also undergo fragmentation.

The entire process of degeneration in nerve fibers takes about 8 to 32 days at the end of which the neuron may recover. The regeneration is possible in the peripheral nervous system but generally not possible in the central nervous system.

One of the important differences between the CNS and PNS is as far as degeneration is concerned it occurs at both the places, but regeneration occurs only in PNS.

Regeneration (Fig. 2.12): Many neurofibrils get sprouted at the proximal end of the nerve fiber. These sprouts begin to grow from the proximal end towards the distal end. One of these is attracted towards the empty neurilemmal tube and continues to grow further. The rest of the fibers start disintegrating and this has to occur in order to avoid certain problems. The full diameter of the nerve fiber previous to injury may not be achieved. The functional recovery may be about 80%. In the meantime, the myelination also occurs by the proliferated Schwann cells. The complete regeneration takes about 20 to 80 days. Nissl granules reappear when the cell recovers.

If the growing sprouts fail to enter the distal tube, they get entangled to form a small tumor-like swelling

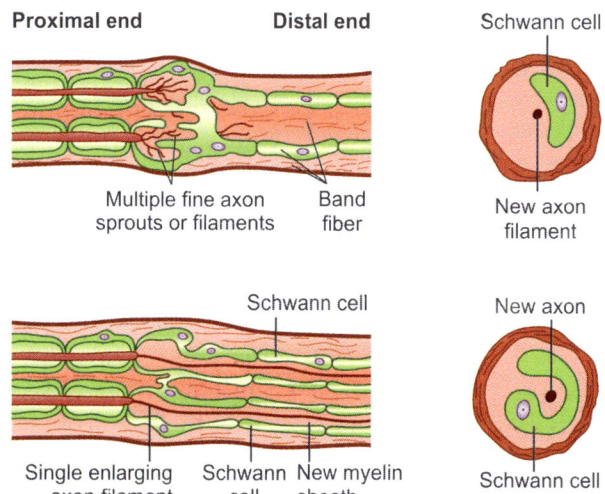

Fig. 2.12: Regenerative changes occurring in a damaged nerve fiber

called the neuroma. Neuroma associated with the sensory nerves is very painful.

Factors affecting regeneration:

1. The gap between the cut ends of the fiber should not be more than 3 mm. If it is more than 3 mm, regeneration will not occur. To facilitate regeneration, if the gap is more, suturing is done to minimize the gap to facilitate regeneration.

2. Some other tissue or fluid or foreign body should not fill up the gap. Cleaning of the injured area tries to clear these particles, if any.

3. Infection and inflammation should not be there at the site of injury. This can be avoided by maintaining the injured area as much hygienic as possible.

4. If the damaged nerve is a mixed type, regeneration may not be very effective.

5. A good protein diet facilitates regeneration.

6. If the injury is closer to the cell body, regeneration may not occur.

7. In young people, regeneration is better than in aged people.

Properties of Nerve Fibers

1. *Excitability:* When a stimulus is applied, the nerve fiber demonstrates a change in its electrical activity from its resting state.

2. *Conductivity:* It is the ability of the nerve fiber to transmit impulses all along the whole length of axon without any change in the amplitude of the action potential. This type of conduction is termed as decrimentless conduction.

3. *Refractory period* (Fig. 2.13): It is the duration after an effective stimulus, when a second stimulus is applied, there will be no response for the second stimulus.

   a. From the time of the application of the stimulus till the initial one-third of the repolarization phase, the nerve fiber excitability will be zero and is completely refractory for the second stimulus. This duration is known as absolute refractory period.

   b. Relative refractory period is the duration after an effective stimulus, when a second stimulus, which is slightly above threshold, is applied there will be response for the second stimulus as well.

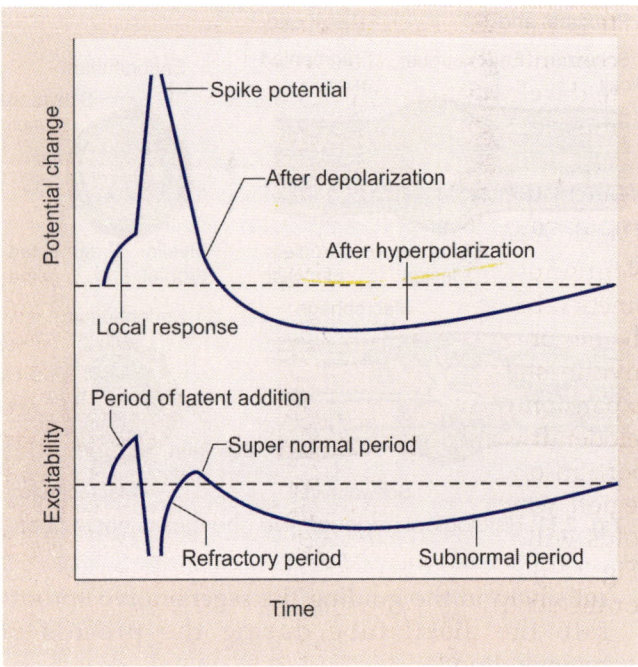

Fig. 2.13: Excitability of the nerve fiber during absolute and relative refractory periods

4. *All or none law:* It states that, when the tissue is stimulated with threshold or more than threshold strength, the amplitude of response will remain the same but for a stimulus of less than threshold strength, there will not be any response. All or none is obeyed by:

   a. A single nerve fiber.

   b. A single skeletal muscle fiber.

   c. A motor unit.

   d. Whole of cardiac muscle.

   e. A single fiber of multi-unit smooth muscle.

   f. Whole of visceral smooth muscle.

Role of Calcium in Nerve Function

Unlike sodium and potassium ions of ECF, which are directly involved in the development of action potential, the calcium's role is an indirect one. It does affect the excitability of the tissue but in an indirect way. The details are:

- At rest, calcium ions keep sodium channels closed. So when calcium ion in ECF is low, the number of sodium channels remaining in the closed state will be less.

- This leads to more sodium entry from ECF to ICF.

- This increases the excitability of the tissues.

• It is for this reason, when the ECF calcium ion concentration is reduced, the person has tendency to develop tetany (sustained state of contraction of muscle).

Neuromuscular Junction and Transmission of Impulses across this Junction

Neuromuscular junction (Fig. 2.14) is a functional junction between a nerve fiber and a muscle fiber. As the motor nerve approaches this junction, it loses the myelin sheath and the bare nerve expands. This expansion is known as the sole foot region or axon telodendria or terminal boutons. The corresponding portion on the muscle membrane is the end plate region, which is thrown into a number of folds. These folds will have the receptor sites for acetylcholine (Fig. 2.15). The folds increase the surface area available for the action of acetylcholine.

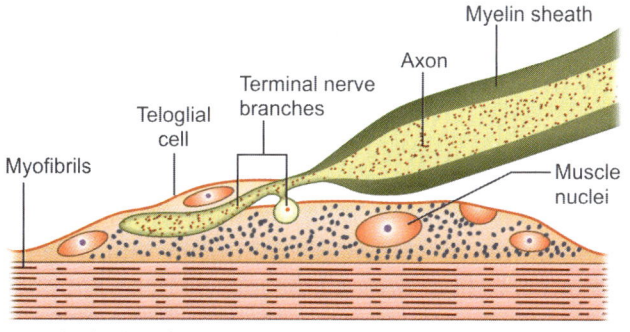

Longitudinal section through the end-plate-neuromuscular junction

Fig. 2.14: Overview of NMJ

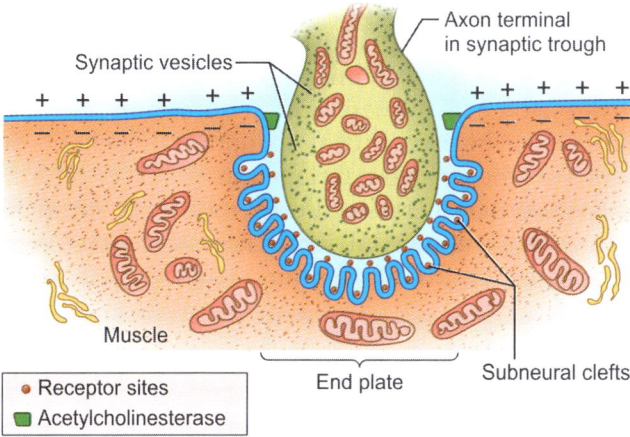

Electron micrographic appearance of one junction

Fig. 2.15: Details of terminal bouton, end plate with receptor sites

Neuromuscular transmission: It is the process by which the nerve action potential is converted into a muscle action potential. Events involved in the neuromuscular transmission are:

• Action potential reaching the motor neuron terminal.
• Depolarization of motor neuron terminal.
• Calcium ion influx into the terminals of the neuron.
• Synaptic vesicles binding to the pre-junctional membrane.
• Release of neurotransmitter (acetylcholine—ACh) by exocytosis.
• Diffusion of ACh through the synaptic clefts.
• Binding of ACh to the receptors present on the post-junctional membrane.
• Opening of ligand-gated sodium channels at the end plate region of the post-junctional membrane.
• Slow influx of sodium ions.
• Development of end plate potential.
• When end plate potential reaches sufficient value (firing level), there will be opening of the voltage-gated sodium channels at the extra-junctional region of the muscle.
• Sudden rush of sodium ions from ECF into ICF.
• Development of action potential in the muscle fiber.
• Removal of ACh by diffusion and degradation by cholinesterase enzyme present on the post-junctional membrane.

For all practical purposes, end plate potential is also a local potential and hence it has all the characteristic features of local potential. Even at rest, there will be very small amount of release of ACh at NMJ and this brings about the development of minute amount of potentials namely miniature end plate potentials. Since they will be very weak, they die off without producing any effect.

The structural difference between neuromuscular junction and synapse is, at synapses the post-junctional region is contributed by part of some other neuron and not by muscle.

Neuromuscular blockers: Blocking of neuromuscular transmission can be done by different ways. Some of the substances used to block the transmission by acting at the pre-junctional region and some at the post-junctional region. Blocking the transmisson leads relaxation of the muscle.

Prejunctional blockers: Botulinum toxin (from *Clostridium botulinum*) prevents the synthesis and release of ACh.

Clinically, the neuromuscular blockers are used extensively. The mechanism of action of the different blockers varies.

1. *Competitive inhibitors* (e.g. tubocurarine). They bind to the receptors available on the post-junctional membrane. Hence these receptors will not be available for ACh to bind when ACh gets liberated from the prejunctional regions. Because of this, there will not be opening of ligand-gated sodium channels and hence no development of end plate potential. Consequently, muscle action potential cannot get developed. Unlike ACh, which gets metabolized fast, curare group of drugs metabolism is slow, and hence action continues for prolonged duration.

2. *Depolarizing blockers:* (e.g. succinylcholine). They also bind to the ACh receptors present on the post-junctional membrane and bring about the depolarization of the post-junctional membrane much like ACh. However, since the metabolism of this substance cannot be brought about by cholinesterase, there will be a persistent end plate potential at the post-junctional membrane. Because of this, the post-junctional membrane cannot get stimulated again.

3. *Anticholinesterases* (e.g. neostigmine, physo-stigmine, nerve gas (di-isopropyl fluorophosphate). All these substances antagonize/inactivate the enzyme cholinesterase. Hence ACh cannot get metabolized. This will also bring about the persistent depolarization of the post-junctional membrane. When the muscle is not in the resting state, the production of action potential cannot occur. And hence block the transmission.

Muscle relaxants are used:
1. During surgeries.
2. During electroconvulsive therapy.

Myesthenia Gravis—Disease of Neuromuscular Junction

- It is an autoimmune disease.
- Antibodies are produced against the ACh receptors present on the post-junctional membrane.
- So the receptors get destroyed.

- ACh liberated during neuromuscular transmission fails to find adequate number of receptors for its action.
- The amplitude of end plate potential is minimized.
- This leads to no development of action potential in the muscle.
- Features are easy fatigability, weakness.
- If the condition is severe, it can lead to respiratory paralysis and death.
- Treatment will be administration of anticholin-esterase to prolong the action of acetylcholine. Some of the other ways of treatment are:
  a. Thymectomy to reduce antibody production
  b. Administration of immunosuppressants to minimize the production of antibody.

Motor Nerve Fibers and Motor Units

Motor nerve fibers supply the skeletal muscle fibers. They take their origin from the anterior horn cells or the corresponding cranial nerve motor neurons. Any time the motor fibers are damaged the muscle fibers undergo paralysis.

A motor unit is an anterior horn cell or corresponding cranial nerve motor neuron with its axon and the number of muscle fibers supplied by it. A motor unit is a functional contractile unit. When a motor nerve fiber fires, all the muscle fibers supplied by this fiber contract synchronously. The number of motor unit which are present in a muscle fibers varies.

Small motor units are seen in the rectus muscle of the eye. A motor nerve fiber supplies only a small number of muscle fibers. This helps to control the movement of the eye precisely. In contrast, the motor units supplying the postural muscles are large, that is each nerve fiber supplies a large number of muscle fibers. Hence movements are not too precise. Increasing the number of motor units coming into play can alter the tension developed in a muscle and this can be done by increasing the strength of the stimulus. The type of summation, which is produced this way, is known as quantal summation or multi-fiber summation.

MUSCLES

Muscles are essential to the body to provide stability and mobility. They are present in almost all the parts of the body and the type of muscle that is present in a particular part of the body is functionally very well suited for that region. Like neurons, even muscles are excitable tissues.

The classification of muscle can be done based on various criteria.
- Functionally, they can be classified into voluntary and involuntary.
- Histologically into striated and non-striated.

The three groups of muscles present in the body are:
a. Skeletal
b. Cardiac (explained late in Cardiovascular System)
c. Smooth

Skeletal Muscles

- They are striated.
- Voluntary in function.
- Attached to the skeleton through tendon.
- Composed of many muscle fibers, which are parallel to each other in arrangement.
- Each of the muscle fiber in turn is made of many sarcomeres, which are also arranged serially.
- For the muscle to act, the impulse has to come from CNS (brain or spinal cord).

Sarcomere (Fig. 2.16)

- Band A is present in the center is made up of myosin proteins. In the center of the A band, there is narrow gap that is known as H band. In the center of the H band is the M line. A band (anisotropic band) is so-called because light cannot pass through this band.

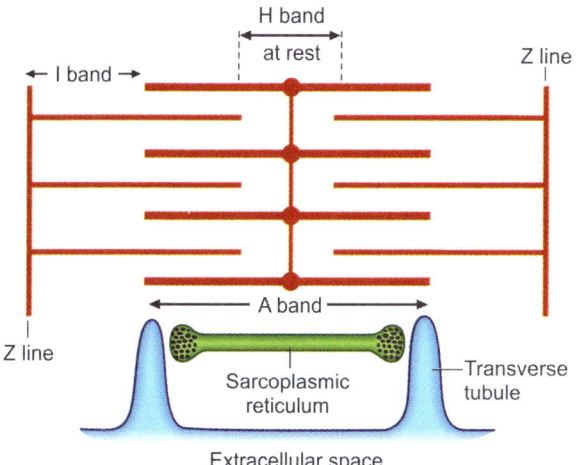

Fig. 2.16: Sarcomere showing the details, the various bands with sarcotubular system

- Extending from the Z line on either side of the A band is I band. This is called I band (isotropic band) because light can pass through this band.
- I band is composed of actin proteins. In addition to this, in I band there will be presence of troponin and tropomyosin proteins.
- Under resting conditions though there is some amount of overlap between bands A and I, there is some gap in the center and this is H band.
- During contraction, I band slides over the A band and bring about the shortening of the muscle fiber.
- Myosin and actin proteins are the contractile proteins in a sarcomere.
- In addition to these proteins, the other proteins present are troponin and tropomyosin. These are called as regulatory proteins.
- The protoplasmic membrane namely the sarcolemmal membrane covers the muscle fiber. This membrane shows dipping in at specific parts that is at the junction of bands A and I. This part of the sarcolemmal membrane is known as T tubule (transverse tubule).
- Sarcoplasmic reticulum is placed horizontally and between the two consecutive T tubules. These are known as L tubules (longitudinal tubules). The ends of the L tubules are dilated and are known as lateral cisterns.
- The function of the T tubule is to conduct the impulse through the muscle fiber and that of L tubules (terminal cisterns of this) is to store and release of calcium ions during the process of contraction.
- Two T tubules and one L tubule together constitute sarcoplasmic triad.

Microscopic examination also shows two other important structures in the muscle. The sarcolemmal sheath covering the muscle dips into the muscle forming the T tubules. The action potentials produced at the neuromuscular junction travel along the sarcolemmal membrane enter the interior of the muscle fiber along the T tubules.

The other structure is the longitudinal tubules (L tubules) with their expanded ends as the lateral cisterns. They closely surround the myofibrils. These form the sarcoplasmic reticulum. The expanded portion (terminal cistern) stores ionic calcium, which plays important role in excitation–contraction coupling of muscle.

Excitation-Contraction Coupling

Events during Excitation-Contraction Coupling

A muscle action potential reaches the T tubule by traveling along the sarcolemmal membrane. This triggers the release of the calcium ions from the cisterns of the longitudinal tubules. The calcium ions occupy the C part of the troponin molecule. This in turn brings about a conformational change in the tropomyosin molecule. This change is responsible for exposing the active site on the actin filaments. The head of the myosin filament gets attached to the active sites and stepwise it gets attached and detached to the active sites. In this process, the actin filament is drawn inwards towards the center of the sarcomere. This requires energy and it is supplied by the breakdown of ATP. Myosin head itself acts as ATPase (actin myosin ATPase) and ATP is broken down to ADP and high energy PO_4 is released. The number of crossbridges occupied depends on the amount of ionic calcium available. Greater the amount of ionic calcium, greater will be the number of binding between actin and myosin and, therefore, greater will be the force or tension developed. During this process, the width of the H band decreases and hence the width of the sarcomere decreases (Figs 2.17a to c). The width of the A band remains unchanged. There may be overlapping of the actin filaments at the center of the sarcomere. This is known as the sliding filament theory of muscle contraction. Immediately following this, the calcium ions are actively pumped back into the L tubules by means of calcium pump. The pumping of calcium into cisterns also requires expenditure of energy. Thus ATP has two important roles in the muscle: (1) it is necessary for muscle contraction and (2) also necessary for muscle relaxation (Figs 2.18 and 2.19). This action of ATP is known as the plasticizer action of ATP.

Four important changes occur in the muscle when it is stimulated to contract.

1. Electrical—in the form of muscle action potential
2. Mechanical—in the form of muscle contraction.
3. Chemical—in the form of breakdown of ATP and creatnine phosphate
4. Thermal—in the form of heat production.

Mechanical changes: When a muscle is made to contract, two types of contractions may be noted.

1. Isotonic contraction
2. Isometric contraction

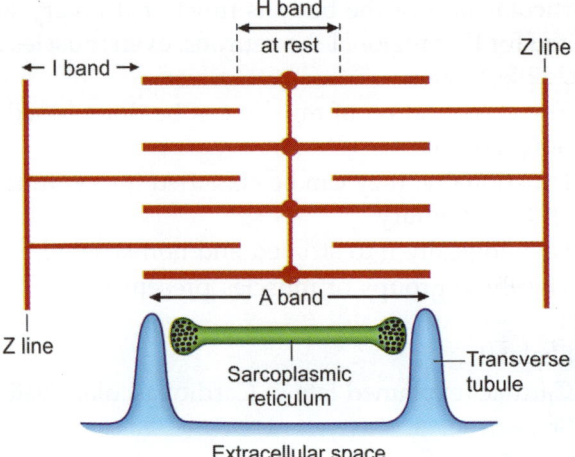

Fig. 2.17a: Sarcomere in resting state

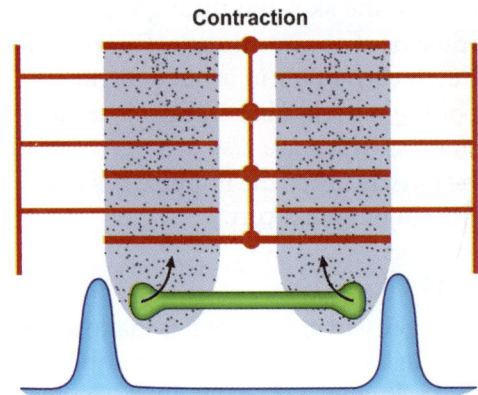

Fig. 2.17b: Sarcomere in contracting state

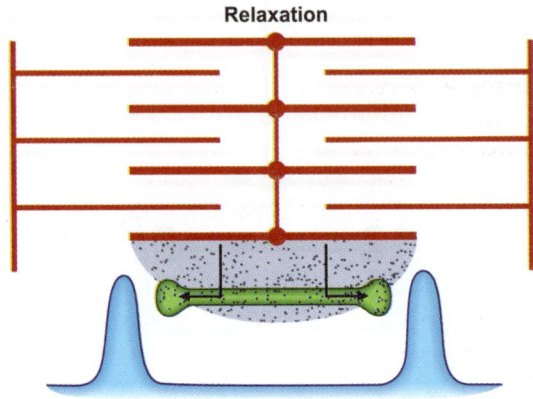

Fig. 2.17c: Sarcomere in relaxed state

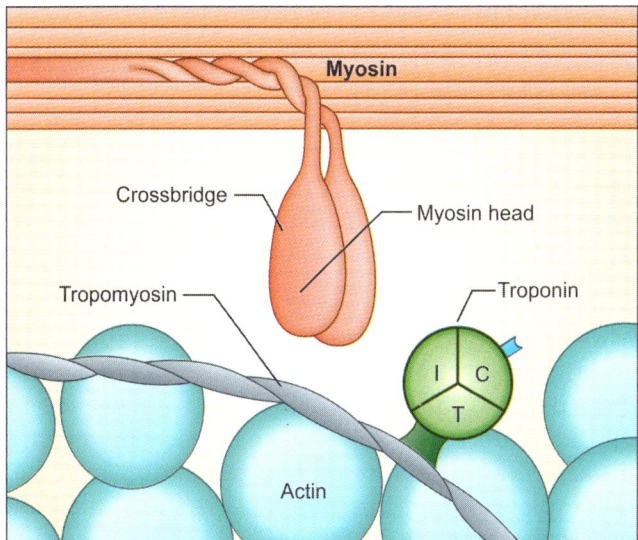

Fig. 2.18: Head of myosin is not attached to actin in resting state

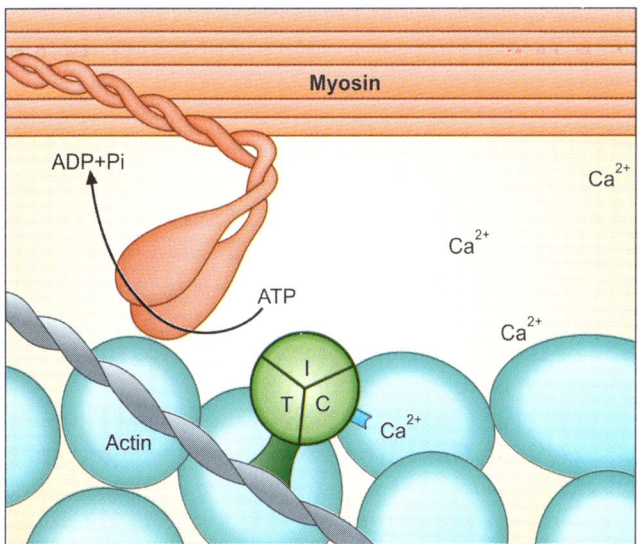

Fig. 2.19: Head of myosin movement over actin during contraction

During an isotonic type of muscle contraction, the length of the muscle fiber decreases but the tension in the muscle fiber remains the same. When a weight is lifted leads to certain amount of external work is done, and this is an example for isotonic contaction.

In isometric type of muscle contraction, the length of the muscle fiber remains the same but the tension developed in the muscle is increased. Example for isometric contraction is pushing against a wall. Walking is a good example for both isometric and isotonic type of contraction. The muscles of the limb which is on the ground contract isometrically to support the body weight and the muscles in limb which is lifted up to move contract isotonically.

Chemical changes that occur in the muscle during muscular contraction: The immediate source of energy supply for muscle contraction is by the breakdown of adenosine triphosphate (ATP). During muscular contraction, it is found out that the ATP content of the muscle is not markedly decreased. This shows that ATP is not only broken down but it is also getting synthesized. The PO_4 (high energy phosphate), required for the resynthesis of ATP from ADP, is obtained from the breakdown of creatine phosphate. During repeated contraction of the muscle, the required energy can also come from the breakdown of glucose or glycogen. Free fatty acids can also provide energy for muscular contraction.

Thermal changes: A certain amount of heat is released even when the muscle is at rest. This is known as the resting heat. When the muscle is made to contract, some amount of heat is generated known as the heat of shortening. During relaxation of the muscle, the heat that is produced is known as the heat of relaxation. These can be measured by using thermocouples.

A gastrocnemius-sciatic (GS) nerve preparation is used to study the properties of skeletal muscle contraction. When a threshold stimulus is applied to the sciatic nerve, the muscle responds by contraction, which can be recorded on a moving drum. The recording is known as a simple muscle twitch. There is a short time lag between the application of the stimulus and the onset of contraction. This duration is known as the latent period.

Causes for the latent period are:
1. The time taken for the nerve action potential to reach the neuromuscular junction.
2. The time taken for the release of ACh.
3. Time taken for the production of the muscle action potential, etc.

Following this, the muscle starts contracting and the contraction reaches its maximum. This duration from the onset of contraction until the peak of contraction is known as the contraction period. After the contraction peak, the muscle fibers start relaxing. The duration from the peak of contraction until the complete relaxation is called relaxation period. The total time required for the twitch period (from the moment of application of stimulus to the relaxation of muscle is complete), will be approximately about 100 milliseconds.

The latent period is approximately 10 milliseconds. The first half of the latent period is absolute refractory period. After the first stimulus, whatever is the intensity of the second stimulus applied during this period, it will not have any effect on the muscle.

Following the absolute refractory period, during the contraction phase, if a second stimulus is applied, a bigger contraction is obtained. This effect is known as wave summation. The effect of two stimuli is added together resulting in a bigger contraction.

If a second stimulus is applied during the relaxation period of the first response, a second contraction is obtained; the second stimulus will not allow the muscle to relax completely before another contraction starts. The response is termed as superposition.

If a second stimulus of the same strength is applied after the complete relaxation period for the first response, the curve obtained is bigger than the first response. This is known as the beneficial effect. The beneficial effect is due to:

1. Increase in the ionic calcium available at the actin and myosin level.
2. Slight decrease in the viscosity of the muscle proteins.
3. Slight increase in the temperature due to the previous contraction.
4. Slight fall in pH in muscle.

Instead of a second stimulus after the relaxation has started, if a number of stimuli are applied one following the other at very short intervals during the contractile phase, the responses for the different stimuli get added up. This results in a sustained contraction called as tetanus (tetanic type of a response). This type of a response can be produced in the skeletal muscle fibers. Since the cardiac muscle fiber has a long absolute refractory period, it cannot be tetanized.

Starling's law: It is applicable to all the types of muscle fibers. The law states that force of contraction in the muscle is directly proportionate to the initial length of the muscle fiber within physiological limits. Greater the initial length, greater will be the force of contraction. This can be demonstrated by performing experiments on a gastrocnemius-sciatic preparation.

Muscle contractions are recorded when the muscle is preloaded or when it is after-loaded state. It is observed that the height of the contraction obtained is much larger when the muscle is preloaded than when it is after-loaded. Preloading a muscle will increase its initial length unlike when it is after-loaded wherein the load starts acting on the muscle only after muscle starts contracting. This will not alter the initial length of the muscle fiber.

Muscle fatigue: When a muscle is repeatedly stimulated, the amplitude of the response gradually gets decreased. The work done by the muscle gradually decreases and a stage is reached when the muscle fails to respond. The relaxation becomes incomplete. When this happens, it shows that the muscle has undergone fatigue.

Which is the seat of fatigue?

In an isolated GS preparation, the seat of fatigue is the neuromuscular junction. It is due to exhaustion of acetylcholine. This can be proved by directly stimulating the muscle after the GS preparation has failed to produce a response when stimulated through the nerve. When the muscle is stimulated directly, the muscle responds again. The motor nerve is not the seat of fatigue. Recording action potentials from the nerve of a GS preparation which has demonstrated fatigue can prove this. The muscle might have undergone complete fatigue but action potentials can still be recorded from the nerve fiber. This shows that the nerve is not the seat of fatigue.

In the case of human beings, the seat of fatigue is muscle itself. This can be proved by finger ergography. Blood pressure cuff is tied over the upper arm and the sling of the ergometer is hooked to the index finger. The person is asked to repeatedly lift the weight attached to the instrument till the muscles get tired. This performance can be recorded and the duration for which the exercise was carried out can be noted. During the exercise, the blood flow to the exercising muscle gets increased and this washes away the metabolic products that are produced. Next the whole procedure is repeated by inflating the blood pressure cuff so that the venous return is prevented. Inflation of cuff prevents the metabolic waste getting washed away. Hence they get accumulated at the muscle itself. The duration at the end of which fatigue sets in is noted and compared. The fatigue sets in early when the cuff is in inflated state suggests that the seat of

Table 2.6: Some of the important differences between visceral and multi-unit smooth muscles

Criteria	Visceral smooth muscle	Multi-unit smooth muscle
Structure	Sheet or bundles	Made up of individual muscle fibers
Innervation	Both the divisions of ANS supply (sympathetic and parasympathetic divisions). Only few fibers are supplied by nerves but not all.	Either sympathetic or parasympathetic. Each muscle fiber has nerve supply
Propagation of action potential	From cell to cell	No cell to cell propagation
Generation of action potential	Is spontaneous	No spontaneous activity
Nature of activity	Nerve regulated	Nerve operated
Plasticity property	Demonstrates this property	No plasticity property
All or none law	The whole of the muscle obeys this law	Each fiber obeys all or none law
Contractions	Non-graded	Graded

fatigue is the muscle itself and it is due to accumulation of the metabolic waste. Muscular contraction is associated with production of lactic acid. As more lactic acid accumulates at the actin and myosin site, it prevents the sliding mechanism. The site of fatigue in the CNS is the synapse.

Fatigue can be postponed in the human body. During exercise, adrenaline is secreted. This in turn increases the blood glucose and free fatty acid levels in the circulation. These supply the necessary fuel for muscular contraction. It also increases the blood flow to the muscle tissue by bringing about vasodilatation. Thus adrenaline postpones fatigue and this action of adrenaline is called Orbelli's effect.

Smooth Muscle

- This is another type of muscle present in the body.
- It is non-striated that is there are no definite cross-striations in the muscle fibers.
- Thick and thin filaments are present with no regular arrangement of the filaments.
- It is supplied by nerve fiber belonging to autonomic nervous system.
- Hence the function of these muscles is not under voluntary control.

Types of Smooth Muscle (Table 2.6)

There are two types of smooth muscle namely visceral/single unit/unitary smooth muscle and multi-unit smooth muscle.

Visceral Smooth Muscle

- In this type of muscle, the propagation of action potential is from cell to cell. That is the whole of the muscle acts as a single unit (structural syncitium).
- It shows spontaneous development of action potential.
- Present in the walls of GI tract, uterus, urinary bladder, etc.

Multi-unit Smooth Muscle

- Each fiber is almost similar to the skeletal muscle fiber but there are no definite cross-striations.
- There is no cell to cell propagation of impulse just like what is seen in skeletal muscle fiber.
- There is no spontaneous activity in the muscle fiber.
- Present in iris, and other examples are ciliaris muscle, erector pilorum muscle, etc.

The activity of the visceral smooth muscle is influenced by:

1. Impulses coming along the autonomic nervous system.
2. Stretch of the smooth muscle.
3. Hormones adrenaline, thyroxine, etc. acting on it.
4. Local factors like hypoxia, hypercapnia, acidosis, and other inorganic ions, like potassium, sodium, etc.
5. Apart from, ICF calcium, even ECF calcium has role to play in the process of contractions.

3

C H A P T E R

Cardiovascular System

Cardiovascular system deals with study of heart and blood vessels. The human heart is made up 4 chambers namely; 2 atria and 2 ventricles. Atria are thin-walled chambers. Right atrium receives venous blood from peripheral parts of body. The venous blood is brought to right atrium by superior and inferior vena cavae. Left atrium receives oxygenated blood from lungs. This blood is brought to left atrium by pulmonary veins. The two atria also act as weak pumps and blood is pumped from right and left atria into right and left ventricles, respectively (Fig. 3.1).

Comparatively, ventricular walls are thicker than the atrial walls. Right ventricle is less thick-walled than the left ventricle. The ventricles act as primary pumps. From the right ventricle, blood is pumped into pulmonary circulation and from the left ventricle blood is pumped into systemic circulation (Fig. 3.2). Volume of blood pumped out by the right or the left ventricle every minute is the cardiac output. Normal cardiac output is about 5 liters per minute.

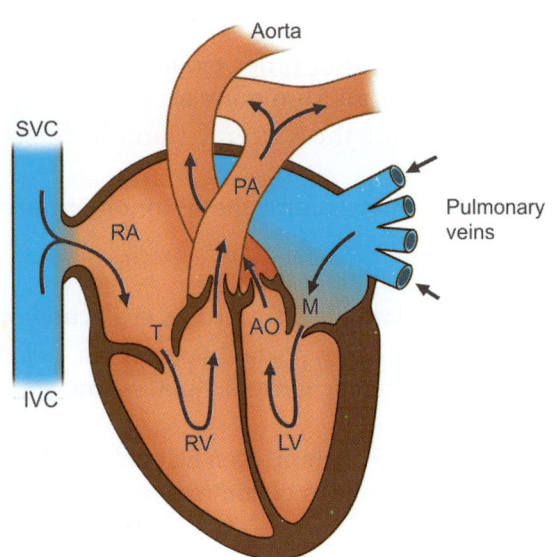

Fig. 3.1: Chambers of heart with valves and blood vessels and direction of flow of blood through chambers and blood vessels

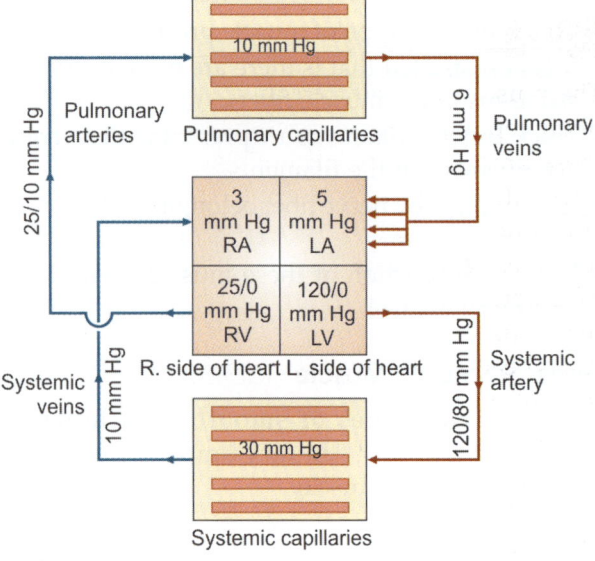

Fig. 3.2: Vessels and chambers of heart involved in systemic and pulmonary circulations and the pressure

50

Blood Vessels

The systemic circulation starts with aorta. Aorta acts as a damping vessel. Aortic wall contains plenty of collagen and elastic fibers. Collagen fibers prevent rupture of the vessel. The elastic fibers are stretched when blood enters aorta from left ventricle during ventricular systole (contraction of ventricle). Blood that enters aorta during ventricular systole is accommodated due to the stretching of elastic fibers. During ventricular diastole (relaxation of ventricle), the accommodated blood in aorta is made to flow towards periphery due to the recoiling of the elastic fibers. It is because of this, aorta acts as a secondary pump.

Blood that enters systemic circulation supplies oxygen and nutrients to the tissues and at the same time it removes carbon dioxide and metabolic wastes from tissues. Systemic circulation is a high pressure area. The pressure will be around 120/80 mm Hg.

Venous blood that has entered right ventricle is pumped into pulmonary artery. This blood takes part in exchange of gases at lungs. Because of this, oxygen from lung diffuses into blood and at the same time carbon dioxide is diffuses from blood into alveolar air. The oxygenated blood is returned to left side of heart by pulmonary vein. The pulmonary circulation is a low pressure area and the pressure will be around 25/10 mm Hg.

CARDIAC MUSCLE

The muscle is involuntary and striated. The muscle fibers repeatedly branch and interdigitate. Wherever these branches come in contact an intercalated disk present, it will maintain continuity with the surrounding fibers through gap junctions. These are the areas which offer least resistance for the passage of electrical current. Therefore, the process of depolarization, wherever it is produced in the heart, can spread all over (conductivity) the heart causing it to contract as a single unit. Because of this, heart muscle acts like a functional syncitium.

Once the cardiac muscle is depolarized, calcium ions (Ca^{++}) enter into the ICF. This triggers the release of calcium ions from the cisterns of the L tubules. This inturn will bring about excitation contraction coupling of the cardiac muscle.

Properties of the Cardiac Muscle

1. Excitability
2. Autorhythmicity
3. Conductivity
4. Contractility
5. Distensibility
6. All or none phenomenon
7. Absolute and relative refractory period

Excitability: Cardiac Muscle Responds to All Types of Stimuli

The resting membrane potential of the ventricular muscle fiber is –90 mV. When a threshold stimulus is applied, it initiates the depolarization of the fiber (phase–0). The interior becomes +20 mV. Depolarization is due to influx of sodium ions through sodium channels. When once the interior becomes +20 mV, further influx of Na^+ is prevented. Now there will be opening up of K^+ channels and, therefore, K^+ efflux (K^+ going out from ICF to ECF) is responsible for the initial repolarization (Phase I). This phase is a very short-lived phase, because during this time there is opening of Ca^{++} channel. Ca^{++} influx occurs. Further process of repolarization is slowed, giving rise to a plateau (Phase II) phase of action potential. At the end of this phase, further repolarization becomes faster. This is again due to K^+ efflux (Phase III) which is followed by phase IV, during which the resting membrane potential is restored back to normal. The total duration of the action potential is about 200–300 milliseconds. The duration of the action potential is dependent on heart rate.

Factors Influencing the Excitability of the Cardiac Muscle

1. The ionic composition of the ECF like Na^+, K^+, Ca^{++}
2. Presence or absence of sympathetic/parasympathetic stimulation
3. Temperature
4. Drugs like digitalis, adrenaline/noradrenaline.

Action Potentials from Pacemaker Region

The resting membrane potential of the pacemaker region is about –60 mV and is not stable. Gradually, it becomes less and less negative. And when this slope reaches the firing level and action potential is automatically produced. This slope is known as the pre-potential/pacemaker potential. It is due to Ca^{++} influx along the T channels (T for transients). The rest of the action potential (the upstroke) is due to Ca^{++} influx along the L (long-lasting) channels.

The time taken for the prepotential to reach the firing level can be decreased by increasing the temperature or sympathetic stimulation. This inturn produces more number of action potentials in given time and, therefore, increases the heart rate. The opposite effect is brought about by decreasing the temperature (cold on SA node) or by vagal stimulation. This is how the vagal stimulation (parasympathetic) decreases/stops the heart. Even under resting condition, vagus exerts some amount of inhibitory influence and this is known as vagal tone.

Autorhythmicity

Heart is capable of producing its own impulses at regular intervals. The area concerned with the generation of impulse on its own is known as the pacemaker of heart.

Sinus venosus is the pacemaker of the frog's heart. This can be proved by Stannius ligature experiments or by applying warm and cold saline on sinus venosus.

The pacemaker of the human heart is the SA node (sinoatrial node). The SA node is located at the junction of the superior vena cava with the right atrium as it opens into the right atrium.

Contractility of the Myocardium

The contractile mechanism is somewhat similar to the contractile mechanism involved in the contraction of the skeletal muscles. The calcium that is necessary for the excitation–contraction coupling comes from the ECF. This inturn triggers the Ca^{++} release from the lateral cisterns. Factors influencing the force of contraction of the cardiac muscle fibers are:

- The initial length of the fiber depends on the end diastolic volume which in turn depends upon the venous return.
- Starling law is applicable to the cardiac muscle fibers also. It states that the force of contraction is directly proportionate to the initial length of the muscle fiber within physiological limits. As the venous return is increased, the ventricle is filled to a greater extent, the initial length of the muscle fiber is increased, resulting in an increase in the force of contraction. This is reflected by an increase in the stroke volume.

Factors Influencing Myocardial Contractility

1. *Sympathetic stimulation:* Increases the force of contraction. This is not due to a change in the initial length but sympathetic stimulation increases the Ca^{++} influx. And this increases the intracellular calcium and increases the excitation–contraction coupling. Hence stroke volume is increased without any increase in end diastolic volume.

2. Parasympathetic stimulation brings about the opposite effect.

3. *Effect of electrolytes:* A decrease in Na^+ concentration decreases the force of myocardial contraction.

4. An increase in ECF potassium stops the heart completely.

5. Increase in ionic calcium increases the force of contraction. If the ionic calcium level is further increased, the cardiac muscle fiber contracts even more and remains in a state of contraction. This is known as calcium rigor.

6. Temperature also affects the force of contraction. Increased temperature increases the force of contraction.

7. *Drugs:* Adrenaline, noradrenaline, digitalis bring about an increase in the force of contraction (positive inotropic effect).

Distensibility

Distensibility of the cardiac muscle fibers is limited because of the pericardium. This fibrous sheath covers the entire heart. Distensibility of the cardiac chambers is further decreased, if fluid/blood accumulates in the pericardial cavity.

Absolute and Relative Refractory Periods of Cardiac Muscle

Heart muscle has long absolute refractory period. It extends throughout the duration of ventricular systole (Fig. 3.3). Due to its long absolute refractory period, cardiac muscle fiber cannot be tetanized. During the relative refractory period, cardiac muscle responds to a second stimulus, provided the second stimulus is of a higher intensity. The response obtained is known as an extra-systole or premature contraction and this is followed by a compensatory pause. Following which the rhythm is brought back to normal.

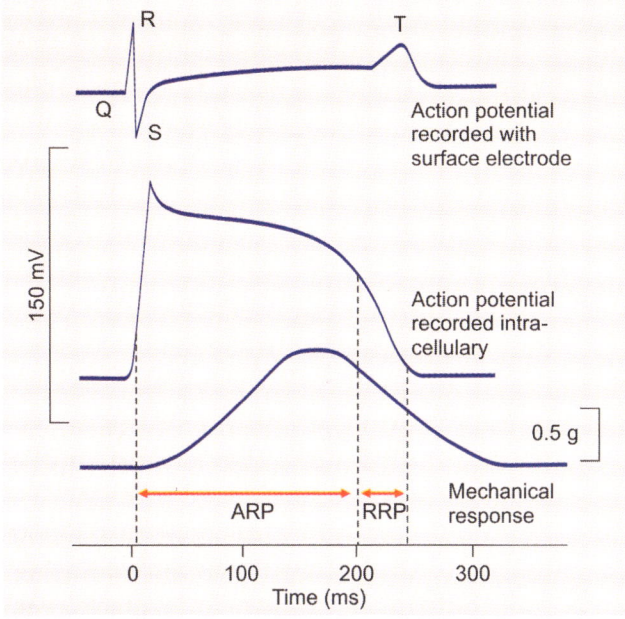

Fig. 3.3: Duration of absolute and relative refractory periods during the mechanical phase of ventricular muscle comparing with that of ECG recorded

All or None Law

The entire heart (all the cardiac muscles) obeys this law. If the stimulus strength is of threshold value, the entire heart responds maximally. A further increase in the strength of stimulus will not alter the response of the cardiac muscle. If the stimulus strength is not adequate, it does not respond at all.

Properties of Cardiac Muscle in Nutshell

1. Excitability is affected by ionic concentration, like K^+, Ca^{++}, Na^+, sympathetic and parasympathetic nerve stimulation and drugs
2. Autorhythmicity
3. Conductivity
4. Contractility
5. Absolute and relative refractory periods
6. Distensibility

Conducting System of Human Heart

Cardiac function does not require intact innervations. Frog's heart removed from the body, and in human beings who have transplanted heart, the heart continues to function. The perfusion of the isolated heart in the laboratory will also continue to beat at regular intervals.

In a frog's heart when the chambers are separated, each of the chambers shows regular contractions on its own. The rate of contraction per minute varies. In the case of frog's heart, the sinus venosus shows maximal rate of contractions when compared to any other chamber of heart.

This can also be proved by applying first and second Stannius ligature or effect of temperature on sinus venosus. It proves that sinus venosus is pacemaker of the frog's heart.

Mammalian Heart/Human Heart

The SA node or sinoatrial node is the pacemaker. Automaticity and rhythmicity are the properties responsible for this. Action potentials from the various chambers (regions) of human heart have been shown in Fig. 3.4.

SA Node

- It is about 8 mm long, 2 mm wide.
- Lies posteriorly in the groove at the junction between the superior vena cava and right atrium.
- Contains two types of cells namely small round cells (pacemaker cells)—P cells, and slender, elongated cells responsible for conducting impulses within the cells.

Action Potential from the Pacemaker Cells of SA Node

- The membrane potential of SA node is not stable. Hence there is nothing as resting membrane

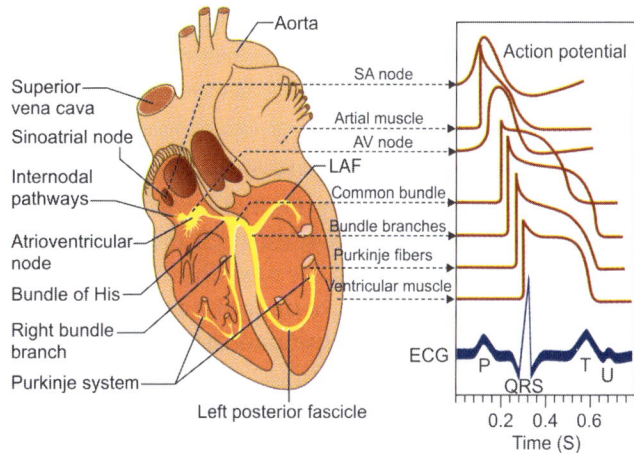

Fig. 3.4: The action potentials from the different parts of conducting system and ventricular muscle with ECG correlation

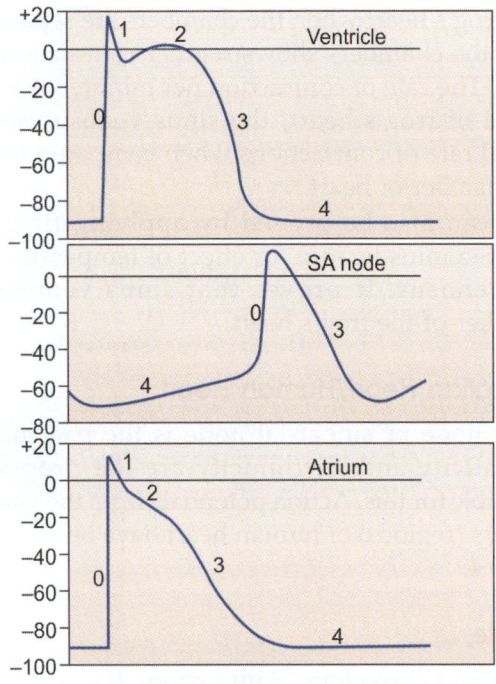

Fig. 3.5: Action potential of SA node correlated with ventricular and atrial muscle action potential

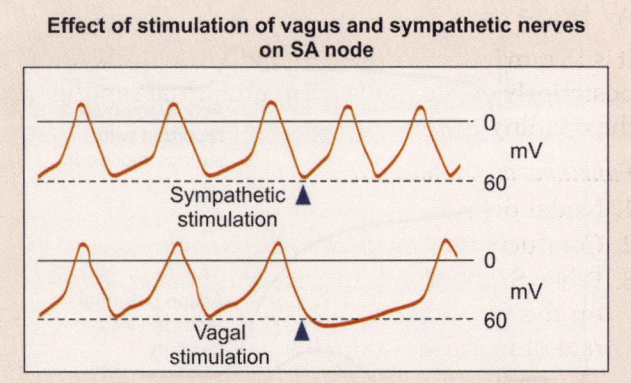

Fig. 3.6: Variation in the gradation of prepotential when sympathetic and parasympathetic nerve stimulated

potential. Before the impulse generation from the SA node occurs, the membrane potential at SA node is about –60 mV.

- During the process of depolarization, the polarity of the interior gets reversed and it becomes positive. In the recording, the upstroke is called as depolarization and this part is less steep.
- After the depolarization, there will be reestablishment of the polarized state of the tissue. The down stroke (re-establishment of polarity) is known as repolarization and this phase is steeper. Figure 3.5 shows the action potential recording from ventricle, SA node and atrium.

Ionic Basis

Tetradotoxin, which blocks the sodium channels, has no influence on the action potential recorded from the pacemaker region. This suggests that the upstroke of the action potential is not due to sodium influx. Effect of stimulation of sympathetic and parasympathetic nerves on the activity of the pacemaker is shown in Fig. 3.6.

Adrenergic transmitter—increases all the currents whereas acetylcholine increases hyperpolarization by increasing K^+ efflux, though acetylcholine regulates potassium channels.

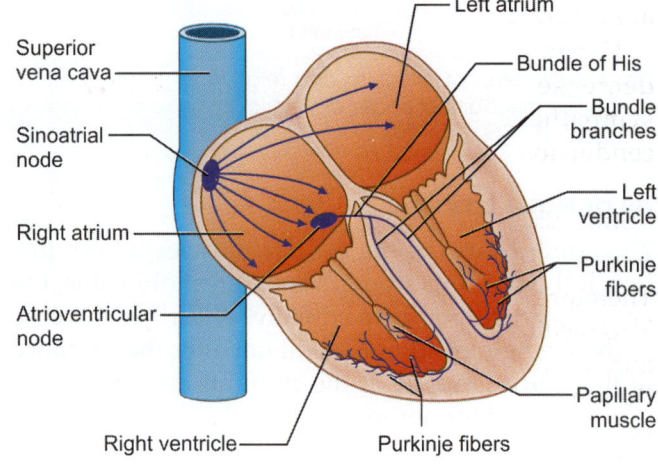

Fig. 3.7: The different parts of conducting system (shown in blue color) in human heart

The different parts of conducting system in human heart are (Fig. 3.7):
- SA node (sinoatrial node)
- Internodal fibers
- AV node (atrioventricular node)
- Bundle of His and its branches
- Purkinje fibers

The velocity of conduction of the impulse in the different parts of human heart is:
- SA and AV nodes—0.05 m/sec
- Atrial and ventricular muscles—1.0 m/sec
- Internodal fibers, Bundle of His and its branches—1.0 m/sec
- Purkinje fibers—4.0 m/sec

AV Node

It is 15 mm long, 10 mm wide and 3 mm thick. Located posteriorly on the right side of interatrial septum near the opening of coronary sinus.

Functions of AV node are:

1. Nodal delay
2. Conduction of the impulse to bundle of His
3. When SA node fails to act as pacemaker, it can take up the function of pacemaker, but at a decreased rate of impulse production.

The nodal delay does not permit the impulse that has reached the AV node from SA node to get conducted immediately. The normal delay in the AV node is about 0.1 sec. This facilitates proper filling of the ventricular chambers and also prevents the ventricles from contracting simultaneously when atria are contracting.

Vagal stimulation, calcium channel blockers, decrease the velocity of conduction, whereas sympathetic stimulation increases the velocity of conduction at the nodes.

Ventricular Conduction

Purkinje fibers: Purkinje fibers are 70–80 microns. Therefore, conduction velocity is as much as 4 m/sec. This facilitates simultaneous contraction of both right and left ventricles. Like ventricular muscle fibers, the Purkinje fibers also have a long absolute refractory period.

Right vagus nerve predominantly supplies the SA node whereas the left vagus nerve influences the activities of the AV node.

When vagus nerve is stimulated, acetylcholine is liberated, and it inhibits the activity.

The last portion to be depolarized is the posterior basal part of the ventricles, pulmonary conus and upper most part of the septum.

Arrhythmia refers to irregularity in the beating of heart.

Heart rate varies depending on the phase of respiration. This is known as sinus arrhythmia. This occurs even in normal human beings and hence it is quite physiological one.

- When the pacemaker is located in the SA node and heart beats accordingly, it is known as *sinus rhythm.*
- If AV node acts as pacemaker, it is known as *nodal rhythm.*

- If ventricular muscle fibers act as pacemaker, it is known as *idioventricular rhythm.*

Ectopic beats occurs when regions other than the SA node produces the impulses.

In complete heart block, there will be delayed conduction or no conduction of impulse to ventricular muscle fibers from the SA node. Heart blocks are:

1. *First degree block* wherein there will be delayed conduction of impulse from the SA node.
2. *Second degree block* in which some impulses from SA node only get conducted to the ventricles.
3. *Third degree block* is also known as complete heart block in which the impulses generated from the SA node will not get conducted to ventricular muscle fibers. The ventricle starts contracting on its own. There is complete dissociation between atria and ventricular contractions.

Vasovagal attack/syncope occurs due to intense stimulation of vagal fibers.

Sick sinus syndrome—ectopic foci producing 100–150 impulses per min. Normal SA node activity is inhibited by the ectopic foci. Before the SA node starts producing impulses, there is delay during which cardiac output falls to almost zero. Hence the person loses consciousness.

Cardiac Muscle Action Potential

Cardiac muscle is also an excitable tissue. Accordingly, the membrane potential of cardiac muscle will also be in the polarized state at resting condition. This is known as resting membrane potential.

While discussing the electrical activity of cardiac muscle, the representative part of the muscle that is considered will be taken from the ventricular region. The atrial, ventricular and Purkinje fibers demonstrate a fast response. In myocardial infarction, the fast response becomes a slow response.

In slow response, the action potential gets conducted more slowly than the fast response. The conduction is more likely to get blocked compared to fast response.

- Under normal resting conditions, the resting membrane potential of the cardiac muscle fiber will be around –90 mV.
- The action potential recorded from the single cardiac muscle fiber differs from the one that is recorded from a bulk of the cardiac muscle.

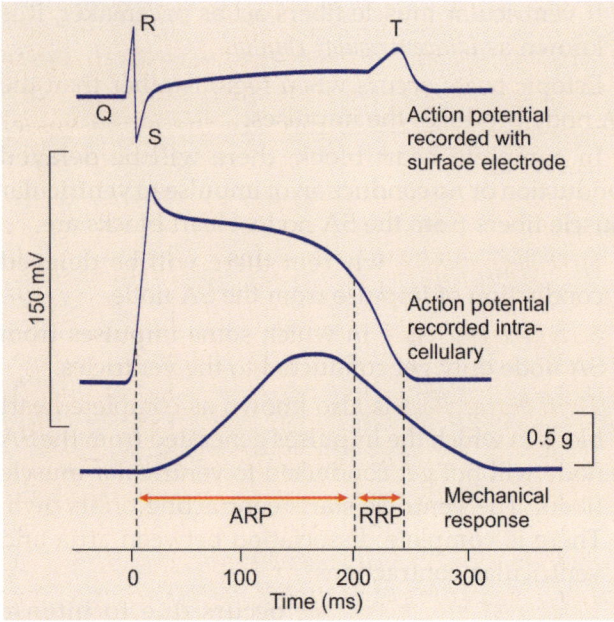

Fig. 3.8: Ventricular muscle action potential correlated with ECG and mechanical response

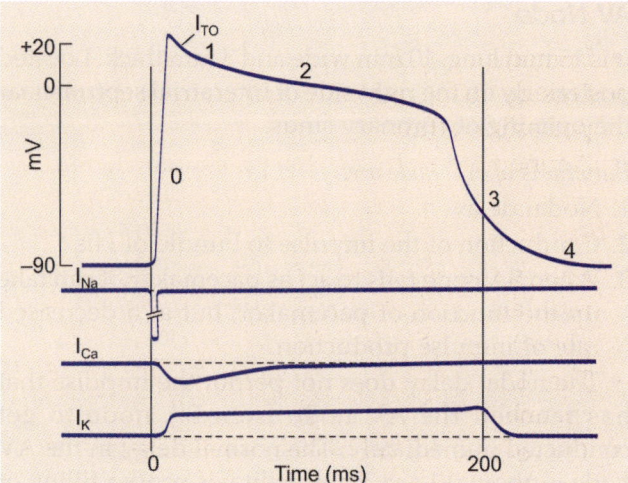

Fig. 3.9: Ventricular muscle action potential phases and the ions involved in various phases

- The configuration of the single fiber recording will be entirely different from the one that is recorded from the whole of cardiac muscle.
- The whole of the cardiac muscle recording is a summated recording and is known as electrocardiogram (ECG).
- The configuration and ionic basis of cardiac muscle fiber action potential is different from the action potential recorded from either the single skeletal muscle fiber or a nerve fiber.
- There is lot of correlation between the cardiac muscle action potential duration with that of the contractile process that is occurring in the ventricular muscle fibers (Fig. 3.8).

The action potential has 5 phases, numbered from 0 to 4 (Fig. 3.9).

   a. Fast depolarization phase is 0.

   b. The slight falling phase is 1 (early repolarization).

   c. The plateau phase of depolarization is 2

   d. The steep repolarization which follows phase 2 is phase 3.

   e. Restoration of the resting membrane potential is phase 4.

- RMP is –90 mV.
- On application of the effective stimulus, there will be production of propagated action potential.

- Net amount of ionic diffusion depends on the permeability of the membrane for a given ion, transmembrane concentration difference, and transmembrane potential difference.

Ionic Basis of the Action Potential (Fig. 3.10)

Phase 0

- It is almost due to an increase in permeability to sodium ions.
- There will be sudden increase of sodium influx.
- Sodium enters through fast sodium channels (this channel can be blocked by tetradotoxin).

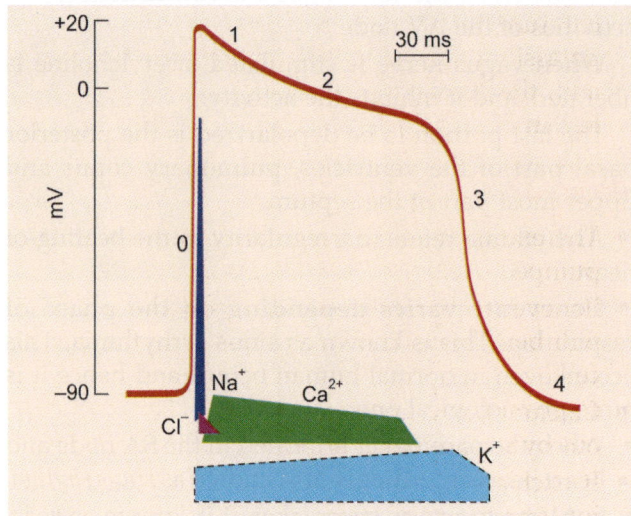

Fig. 3.10: Ionic basis of ventricular muscle action potential

Phase 1

- Immediate repolarization.
- Due to transient outward current carried by potassium efflux.
- Aminopyridine blocks the potassium channels.

Phase 2

- Following phase 1, the further process of repolarization becomes much slower (plateau phase).
- The "L" channels refer to the long-lasting calcium channels.
- There will be increased permeability of the membrane throughout the duration of this phase for calcium ions from ECF to ICF.
- Therefore, there will be calcium influx.
- Calcium also takes part in excitation–contraction coupling.
- Calcium conduction is increased by catecholamine, isoproterenol and is decreased by acetylcholine.
- Calcium channel antagonists, like verapamil, diltiazem, etc., decrease calcium conductance.
- Increased calcium conductance increases the force of contraction of the muscle.

Final Repolarization

- Starts when the efflux of potassium becomes more than the calcium influx.
- The duration of the plateau is less in atrial muscle because at phase 2, potassium efflux is greater than calcium influx. In addition to this, outward potassium current is also greater in atrial muscle and, therefore, the duration of action potential is less in atrial muscle fiber.

Phase 4

- The excess of sodium that has entered the cell is pumped out by sodium–potassium ATPase.
- For every three sodium ions transported out, there will be transport of two potassium ions into the cell.
- Calcium that has entered will also be transported out by sodium–calcium exchanger.
- It exchanges three sodium ions for one calcium ion transported out by an ATP-driven calcium pump.

Biophysical Aspects of Circulation

Blood vessels are a closed system of conduits that carry blood from the heart to the tissues and back to the heart. Blood flows through the blood vessels primarily because of the forward motion imparted to it by pumping ability of the heart, although in the case of systemic circulation diastolic recoil of the walls of the arteries, compression of veins by skeletal muscles during exercise and negative intrapleural pressure also move blood towards the heart. The resistance to flow is affected by many factors but one of the most important being the diameter of the blood vessels. The resistance offered by the blood vessels to flow of blood is predominantly provided by the arterioles.

The blood flow to each organ or tissue is regulated by local, neural and humoral mechanisms. These factors either dilate or constrict the vessels to adjust the flow according to the needs of the concerned part of body. In pulmonary circulation, all the blood flows to lungs, whereas in systemic circulation, it is made up of numerous different circuits. The arrangement permits wide variation in regional blood flow without changing the total systemic flow.

The design of the various parts of the vascular system is in conformity to the dynamics of circulation. The intraluminal diameter, the wall thickness, the histological structure of the walls are designed in such a way that the circulation in the overall parts of the body is smooth with specific basic functions to be complied with.

The wall of arteries are made up of three layers, namely:
- The outer most connective tissue layer, the tunica adventitia
- The middle layer is made up smooth muscle, the tunica media
- And the innermost layer is made up of endothelial cell, the tunica intima.

The walls of the aorta and other large diameter arteries contain relative large amount of elastic tissue (Fig. 3.11) that permit distensibility and collagen fibers. Collagen prevents overstretching; elastic fibers recoil and act as secondary pump in facilitating blood flow during ventricular diastole. They are stretched during ventricular systole and recoil during ventricular diastole. The smooth muscles present in the blood vessels are innervated by sympathetic noradrenergic fibers, which bring about the constriction of the blood

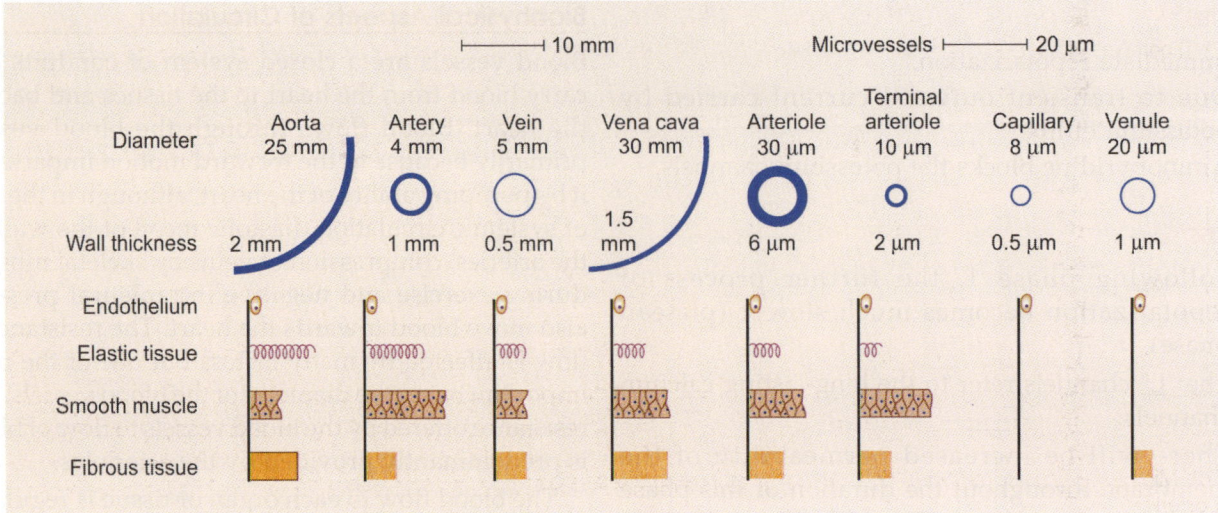

Fig. 3.11: Different tissues contribution in the walls of aorta, artery, capillary and veins

vessels. The parasympathetic innervations to the smooth muscle are almost insignificant. The arterioles are the major site of resistance to the blood flow.

Blood always flows from areas of higher pressure to areas of lower pressure except in certain situations when momentum transiently sustains flow (forward flow of blood in aorta during protodiastole phase of ventricular diastole. In this phase, in spite of semilunar valves being in the open state and the pressure being more in the aorta than in left ventricle, there will not be back flow of blood into the ventricle from the aorta).

Shear Stress

- Flowing blood creates a force on the endothelium that is parallel to the long axis of the vessel.
- This shear stress is proportionate to the viscosity (η) times the shear rate.
- Shear rate is the rate at which the axial velocity increases from the vessel wall towards the lumen.

Average Velocity

- It is important to distinguish between velocity and flow.
- Velocity is rate of displacement per unit time, whereas flow is rate of volume flow per unit time.
- Velocity is proportionate to

$$V = \frac{Q}{A}$$

V = velocity; Q = flow; A = area of the conduit
Hence $Q = A \times V$

The average velocity of blood is inversely proportional to the total cross-sectional area. Therefore, the average velocity of blood flow is high in aorta, decreases gradually in the arterial compartment and is least at the level of capillaries (the cross-sectional area of capillaries will be few thousands of times to that of the aorta). The average velocity of blood again increases slight in the veins.

Viscosity and Resistance

- The resistance to flow is determined not only by the radius of blood vessels but also by viscosity of blood.
- Blood is about 5–6 times more viscous to that of water.
- In large vessels, increase in hematocrit causes appreciable increase in viscosity.
- In small vessels, the change in hematocrit does not affect the viscosity much. This is because of change in the type of blood flow.
- That is why changes in hematocrit will have relatively no effect in the change of viscosity.
- Apart from hematocrit, the other factors of blood which contribute for viscosity are fibrinogen and immunoglobulin in plasma. Hence, any increase in fibrinogen and immunoglobulin levels in circulation affects viscosity.

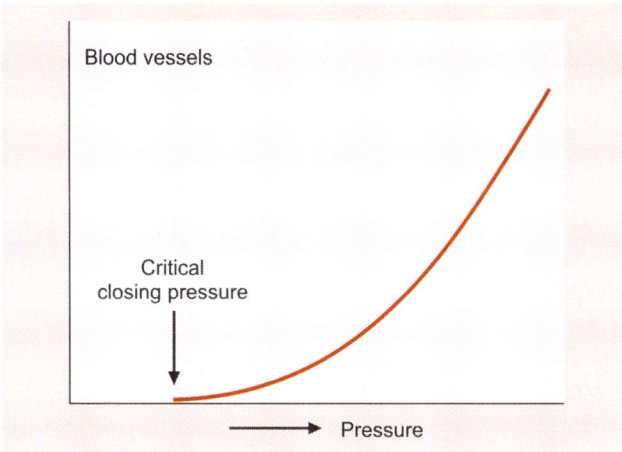

Fig. 3.12: Minimum pressure required to maintain the patency of the arteries

Critical Closing Pressure or Critical Opening Pressure (Fig. 3.12)

- Critical closing pressure is the minimum pressure that should be exerted by blood in order to maintain the patency of vessels in the arterial compartment.
- Normally, it is around 20 mm Hg.
- Since blood vessels are collapsible, when the blood pressure is less than 20 mm Hg, the walls of the blood vessels get collapsed and there will be no flow of blood through the blood vessel.

Peripheral Resistance

- It is the resistance offered by vessel wall for flow of blood.
- The unit used to measure resistance (pressure divided by flow) is dynes/cm. In other words, resistance in cardiovascular system is generally expressed as R units (Reynold's number), which is obtained by dividing the pressure in mm Hg by flow in ml/sec. For example, if the mean arterial pressure is 90 mm Hg and the left ventricular output is 90 ml/sec, the total peripheral resistance is

$$\frac{90 \text{ mm Hg}}{90 \text{ ml/sec}} = 1 \text{ R unit}$$

In general, the resistance offered by the vessel wall is influenced by:

$$R = \frac{8 \, \eta, \, l}{\pi r^4}$$

Wherein

8 is the integer of velocity of flow

η is viscosity of blood

l is length of blood vessel

r is the radius of blood vessel (4th power of radius)

The length and viscosity of the blood vessel do not vary much easily. Hence varying the radius of the blood vessel can bring about a lot of moment-to-moment alterations of peripheral resistance. This can be easily altered by sympathetic nerve fibers and chemical factors.

Role of Arterioles in Maintenance of Peripheral Resistance

- Peripheral resistance is maximum at the level of arterioles.
- Hence arterioles are known as seat of peripheral resistance.
- It is maximum at arterioles because in the walls of the arterioles, there are plenty of smooth muscle fibers.
- The contractility of the smooth muscle is constantly under the influence of vasoconstrictor impulses coming from the lateral horn cells of spinal cord reaching the arterioles along the sympathetic fibers.
- Apart from the neural influence that can affect the contractility of the smooth muscle, there are local and hormonal factors, which can alter the contractile state of vascular smooth muscle.
- Some have constrictor influence and some other substances have dilator effect.
- Therefore, peripheral resistance is controlled by neural and chemical mechanisms.

Neural Mechanism

- The role of vasomotor center present in the brainstem is very important.
- The vasomotor center exerts its influence through the sympathetic nerves on the smooth muscle of the arterioles (Fig. 3.13).
- Sympathetic tone or arteriolar tone refers to constant excitatory influence by sympathetic nerves on smooth muscles of arterioles. About 1–3 impulses per second reach the arterioles. These impulses come from the lateral horn cells of spinal cord. The frequency of impulses can be increased up to 10/second.

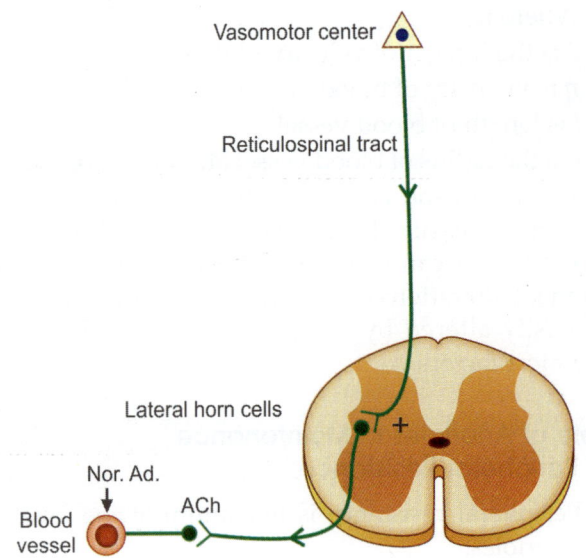

Fig. 3.13: Vasomotor center influence over blood vessels through sympathetic nerves

- Intervention to the vasomotor–sympathetic pathway affects peripheral resistance and concomitant changes in the blood pressure.
- Sympathetic constrictor influence is not only to the smooth muscles present in the walls of the arterioles, but also on the smooth muscles present at the beginning of the capillaries (pre-capillary sphincters), post-capillary sphincters and on the walls of the veins.

Hormonal Mechanism (Table 3.1)

- Norepinephrine exerts a powerful vasoconstrictor effect.
- However, adrenaline in certain areas has vaso-constrictor effect and in certain other areas has vasodilator effect. In the skeletal region, the vasodilator effect is brought about by the action through beta receptors whereas in most of the other

Table 3.1: Chemicals acting on vascular smooth muscle

Vasoconstrictors	Vasodilators
1. Noradrenaline	Bradykinin
2. Adrenaline	Histamine
3. 5 HT	Adrenaline
4. Vasopressin	Adrenosine
5. Angiotensin II	Hypoxia ($\downarrow$ pO_2)
	Hypercapnea ($\uparrow$ pCO_2)
	Lactic acid
	Adenosine

parts of body, the vasoconstrictor effect will be mediated through the alpha receptor activity. Vasoconstrictor effect of adrenaline is used clinically in the treatment of epistaxis.

- The role of these hormones secreted from adrenal medulla is of much importance in physiological conditions, like muscular exercise, etc. But they have vital role to play in certain pathological conditions, like cardiovascular shocks.
- Apart from adrenaline, and noradrenaline, the other blood-borne factors which have role in altering peripheral resistance are serotonin (5HT), angiotensin II, vasopressin, histamine, etc. In addition to blood-borne factors, there are certain other local factors like adenosine, bradykinin, etc., which also have the ability to alter peripheral resistance.

EXTRINSIC CONTROL OF PERIPHERAL BLOOD FLOW

The relationship between the mean pressures, mean velocity and cross-sectional area is designed in different parts of the circulatory system to suit the demands of the parts of the body (Figs 3.14, 3.15 and Table 3.2).

Flow which is nothing but the blood flow is equal to effective perfusion pressure in that part of body divided by the resistance. The effective perfusion pressure is the mean transluminal pressure at the arterial end minus the mean pressure at the venous end. The units of resistance (pressure divided by flow) are dynes/cm. In other words, resistance in cardio-vascular system is generally expressed as R units (Reynold's number), which are obtained by dividing the pressure in mm Hg by flow in ml/sec. For example, if the mean arterial pressure is 90 mm Hg

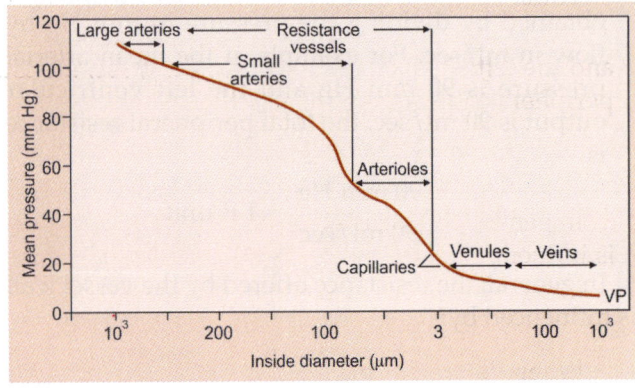

Fig. 3.14: Pressure profile in vascular tree

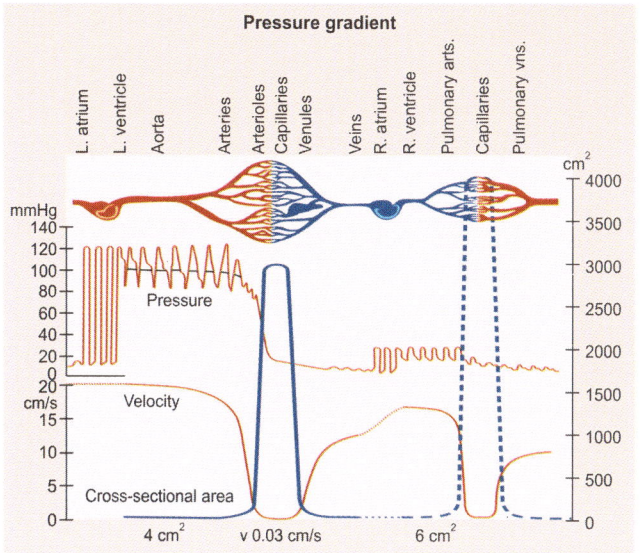

Fig. 3.15: Pressure profile throughout cardiovascular regions correlated with velocity and cross-sectional area

Table 3.2: Comparing diameter, mean velocity and mean pressure in vascular tree

	Diameter (mm)	Mean vel (cm.s^{-1})	Mean pressure (mm Hg)
Aorta	20–25	20	100
Medium-sized		10–15	95
Very small arteries		2	70–80
Arterioles	0.06–0.02	0.2–0.3	35–70
Capillaries			
Arterial end			30–35
Middle	0.006 }	0.03	20–25
Venous end			15–20
Very small veins		0.5–1.0	10–15
Small to medium veins		1–5 }	
Large veins	5–15	5–10 }	10 or less
V. cavae	30–35	10–16 }	

and the left ventricular output is 90 ml/sec, the total peripheral resistance is

$$\frac{90 \text{ mm Hg}}{90 \text{ ml/sec}} = 1 \text{ R unit}$$

In general, the resistance offered by the vessel wall is influenced by

$$R = \frac{8\,\eta,\,l}{\pi r^4}$$

Where in
8 is the integer of velocity of flow

η is viscosity of blood

l is length of blood vessel

r is the radius of blood vessel (4th power of radius)

The length and viscosity of the blood vessel do not vary much easily. Hence varying the radius of the blood vessel can bring about a lot of moment-to-moment alterations of peripheral resistance. This can be easily altered by sympathetic nerve fibers and chemical factors.

Poiseuille-Hagen Formula

The formula explains relationship between the blood flow to that of pressure gradient that is available and the total peripheral resistance in the body. According to the formula,

$$F = \frac{(P_1 - P_2)\,\pi r^4}{8\,\eta l}$$

Wherein

F = flow

$(P_1 - P_2)$ is the pressure difference between the two ends of the blood vessel

r^4 = fourth power of radius

8 is the integer of velocity of flow

η is viscosity of blood

l is length of blood vessel

The flow is directly proportional to the pressure difference between the two ends of blood vessel that is in considerations. P_1 is mostly the pressure that gets reflected in the down steam of blood vessel from the left ventricle. Hence a change in P_1 is not all that easy and not practical one either to regulate the blood flow in a particular part of body. P_2 is the pressure at the venous end of the capillaries. If P_2 is increased, the hydrostatic pressures in the capillaries are increased and this can give rise to accumulation of fluid in the interstitial spaces and edema.

The flow is inversely proportional to the fourth power of radius. Supposing the radius of blood vessel changes from one to two, the rate of change of flow that is observed will be about 16 times. In the body, when flow of the blood has to be adjusted in a particular tissue or organ, it is the radius of the blood vessel, which gets altered in the concerned part of body to suit the required volume of blood flow.

- The activity of the pre-capillary sphincter is altered in state of cardiovascular shocks, injury to any part of the body. These events will try to maintain the cardiovascular dynamics and reduce the volume of blood lost from the injured area respectively.

- There is venomotor tone, but compared to arteriolar tone this is much less.
- Capacitance vessels would not show much of alterations in the lumen diameter and since they are larger and very little smooth muscle is present in their walls; they do not contribute for regulation of peripheral resistance. Blood gets mobilized from these capacitance vessels to peripheral circulation in conditions, like hypovolemia thereby try to restore the normal cardiovascular dynamics.
- The influence of parasympathetic nerves to vascular smooth muscle is not much. There is some amount of parasympathetic innervation to the vascular smooth muscles present in head, viscera and genitalia.

Sympathectomy and Blood Flow

In certain cases, the sympathetic innervation to the blood vessels may have to be abolished permanently. In such a case, following sympathectomy, in the initial periods there will be increase of blood flow due to loss of arteriolar tone. However, in course of time, the flow of blood gets decreased markedly. This is because of denervation hypersensitivity or denervation supersensitivity. As long as the post-ganglionic sympathetic innervations to the vascular smooth muscles are intact, the responsiveness of the vascular smooth muscle is restricted to circulating chemical substances. However, after sometime following denervations, the vascular smooth muscle becomes hyper-responsive to circulating chemical substances. This results in increased vascular tone and causes the blood flow to decrease.

VENOUS RETURN

Continuous return of blood to the atria from respective circulations is called venous return. Generally, venous return refers to returning of deoxygenated blood from peripheral parts of body to the right side of heart. The return of blood to the right side of the heart will be due to the pressure gradient from the peripheral parts of body towards the right atrium. Either a positive pressure from the peripheral parts may keep propelling blood into the right atrium or there is creation of negative pressure (suction force)

Table 3.3: Factors influencing venous return

1. Pressure gradient
2. Varieties of pumps
   - Skeletal muscle pump
   - Abdominal pump
   - Thoracic pump
3. *Vis-a-tergo*
4. *Vis-a-fronte*
5. Venomotor tone
6. Extent to which the venous compartment is already filled
7. Drugs—veneconstrictor, noradrenaline
8. Presence of valves
9. Gravity and posture

in the right atrium to draw blood from the venous compartment to the right atrium. The venous return is affected by many factors. Factors affecting venous return are (Table 3.3):

i. Pressure gradient
ii. Varieties of pumps
   - Skeletal muscle pump
   - Abdominal pump
   - Thoracic pump
iii. *Vis-a-tergo*
iv. *Vis-a-fronte*
v. Venomotor tone
vi. Extent to which venous compartment is already filled.
vii. Drugs—veneconstrictor, noradrenaline
viii. Posture and gravity
ix. Presence of valves

1. Pressure Gradient

The pressure in the right atria (central venous pressure) into which the superior and inferior vena cavae open is around 0 mm Hg. In the peripheral veins, the pressure is around 8 mm Hg and the pressure in the veins nearer to the heart goes on decreasing. In the right atrium, the pressure (central venous pressure) is almost 0 mm Hg. So the pressure gradient along the veins towards the right side of the heart is responsible for the flow of blood into right atrium. When central venous pressure becomes positive as seen in pulmonary hypertension, the gradient is reduced. Hence there will be decreased venous return (Fig. 3.16).

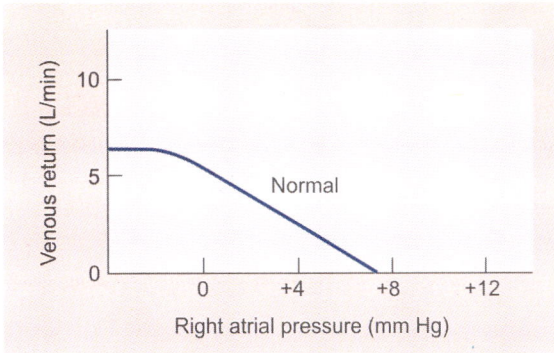

Fig. 3.16: Right atrial pressure influence over venous return

2. Vis-a-Tergo (force acting from behind)

The contraction of the left ventricle creates a pressure that pushes blood from behind all along the vascular tree throughout the body. This pressure from the left side of heart which is ultimately responsible for pushing of blood from behind towards the right side of heart is called vis-a-tergo. This is proved by stimulating the vagus. The heart stops contracting and venous return is reduced.

3. Vis-a-Fronte (force acting from front)

As stated earlier, the pressure in the right atrium is normally around 0 mm Hg. During ventricular contraction, the atrioventricular ring is pulled down. As a result of this, the atria get expanded. This creates a negative pressure in right atrium and the negative pressure is also created during sudden rush of blood from atria to ventricle. This negative pressure exerts suction effect on the great veins and draws blood into the atrium. This is known as vis-a-fronte.

4. Skeletal Muscle Pump

The veins are arranged in between the skeletal muscle fibers and are arranged parallel to skeletal muscle fibers. So when the muscle contracts the veins get squeezed. Due to the compressor effect of the muscle fibers on the vein, blood is made to flow through them. However, blood is made to flow in the direction of heart due to the presence of valves in veins, which prevent back flow. If the skeletal muscles do not contract, there will be pooling of blood especially in the lower parts of body in the erect posture. This is because of two reasons, namely
a. No activity of muscle pumps.

b. The gravitational force acts as counter-force for venous return and try to retain as much blood in the dependent parts of body.

In soldiers, prolonged standing at attention, venous return is decreased and in some of the cases it may fall to zero. This decreases cardiac output and hence the person may collapse.

5. Thoracic Pump

During inspiration, the intrapleural pressure becomes more negative. A simultaneous increase of pressure in the abdomen and a more negative pressure in thorax, increase the pressure gradient for flow of blood towards the heart from the abdomen. Hence venous return is more during inspiratory phase when compared to expiratory phase during which the intrapleural pressure is less negative.

6. Abdominal Pump

Normally, veins present in the splanchnic region act as reservoir for blood. When the abdominal muscles contract, there will be increase of intra-abdominal pressure and hence compression of veins occurs in the abdominal region. This increases venous return by increasing the gradient towards the thoracic cavity (heart).

7. Venomotor Tone

The constant excitatory influence by sympathetic nerves on the smooth muscle of veins is called venomotor tone. Because of this, the walls of the veins remain in a partially contracted state even under resting condition. When the venomotor tone is increased, the capacity of veins decreases. This increases the venous return.

8. Posture and Gravity

As such the pressure in the veins is very less. When gravitational force acts on the lower parts of body especially in the erect posture, it will decrease the venous return from the lower limbs. The gravitational force tries to pull down blood from the dependent parts of the body. This keeps on increasing the pressure in veins in the dependent parts of body. In addition to this, pulling down of blood in the arterial compartment due to gravitational force, increases the hydrostatic pressure in the capillaries. The overall effect will be more fluid transudation from the intra-vascular compartment to interstitial spaces. This will give rise to edema. This may be one of the reasons for swelling of legs in long-distance flights; wherein prolonged erect posture in the absence of muscular contractions will lead to swelling of legs. The stasis of blood in the venous compartment, at times may lead to intravascular clotting and this is known as deep vein thrombosis.

When a person is in recumbent posture, the gravitational force acts equally on all the parts of body. This is going to facilitate venous return. People who have been standing almost stationary for prolonged time, have tendency to fall unconscious is because of decreased venous return. This decreases the cardiac output and hence reduces blood flow to brain. The falling down of such people in fact is a natural defense mechanism to facilitate venous return and restoration of blood flow to brain.

ELECTROCARDIOGRAM (ECG/EKG)

Pacemaker of the heart automatically and rhythmically gets depolarized and repolarized. This inturn depolarizes and repolarizes both atrial and ventricular muscle fibers. The potential changes produced can be recorded by placing pair of electrodes over the myocardium itself or suitable points on the body surface. The points that are commonly selected are the right arm, the left arm and the left leg. When these points are connected to each other it forms an equilateral triangle, the heart is said to lie in the center of the triangle. The electrical potentials generated by the heart spread towards these points by the volume conduction principle. Placing a pair of electrodes and connecting these electrodes to a galvanometer or to a cathode ray oscilloscope can record the potential changes. The summated potential recorded this way is known as an ECG recording. The recordings are made on a standard, calibrated paper. Along the horizontal axis is the time scale, the smallest division is equal to 0.04 seconds. And along the vertical scale the amplitude-voltage is recorded in millivolt (mV)— one small division is equal to 0.1 mV.

Spread of potential through conducting system to muscle mass in different parts in heart has been shown in Fig. 3.17.

Lead System

A lead is nothing but a pair of electrodes placed in a definite position on the body surface, connected to

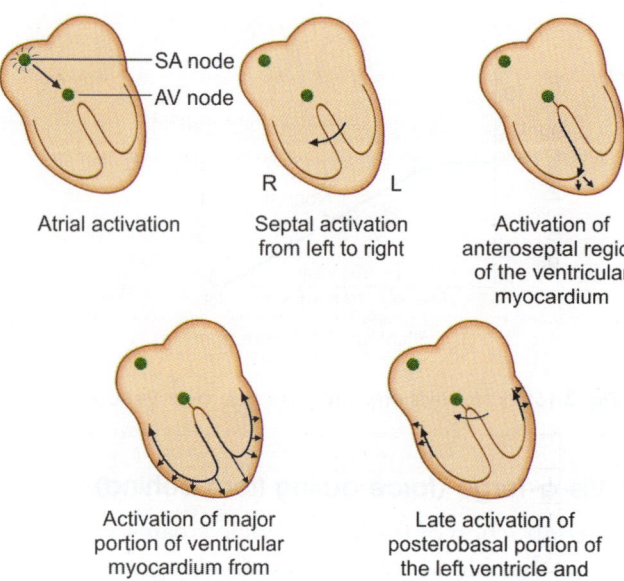

Fig. 3.17: The sequential spread of action potential from the pacemaker region to ventricular muscle

the negative and to the positive terminals of an oscilloscope.

Standard Bipolar Limb Lead System (Fig. 3.18)

Records the potential difference between the two electrodes. Accordingly, there are three leads namely lead one (L I), lead two (L II), and lead three (L III).

In L I, the right arm is connected to negative and the left arm to positive terminals.

In L II, the right arm is connected to negative and the left leg to positive terminals.

In L III, the left arm is negative and the left leg to positive terminals.

It has been mathematically shown that the potential recorded in lead two (L II) is usually the biggest and potential at lead two is always equal to the sum of the potentials recorded at lead I and lead III (Fig. 3.19). This is because, when the electrical axis of the heart is parallel to the axis of a lead, maximum recording will be obtained. On the other hand, if the electrical axis of the heart is perpendicular to the axis of a lead the recording will be the smallest.

Unipolar Lead System

It has been shown by Einthoven that when the three points on the body surface are connected to a common terminal by means of resistance wires of 5000 ohms,

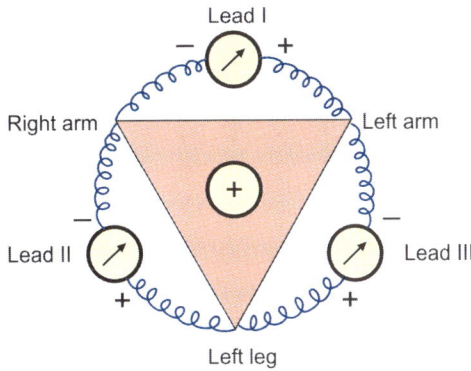

Standard bipolar limb leads

	Rt. arm	Left arm	Left leg
Lead I	(−)	(+)	
Lead II	(−)		(+)
Lead III		(−)	(+)

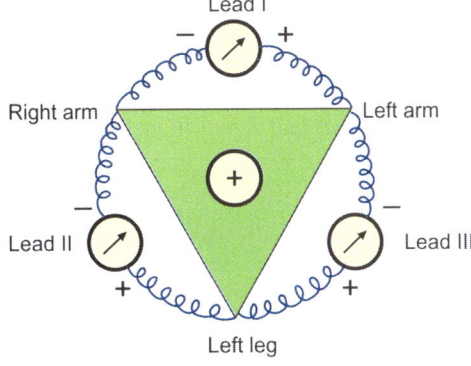

Einthoven's triangle

Fig. 3.18: The terminals to which the different leads are connected for standard bipolar limb lead ECG recording

Einthoven's law

It states that if the electrical potentials of any two of the three bipolar limb leads are known at any given instant, the third one can be determined mathematically from the first two by simply summing the first two (but note that the positive and negative signs of the different leads must be observed when making this summation)

since lead II potential is equal to lead I + III potentials, a zero potential is recorded. This is used as an indifferent electrode, and connected to the negative terminal of the recording device. The other electrode is used as an active electrode and connected to the positive terminal of the recording device. Unlike the bipolar recording, the unipolar recording gives us the potential that exists over a particular area on the body surface. Under the unipolar lead system (Fig. 3.20):

1. VR VL and VF
2. aVR, aVL and aVF
3. Chest leads V_1 to V_6 to V_9

To interpret the details of an ECG recording, the standard bipolar limb lead II recording is usually considered.

Normal Recording
(in the limb lead II recording) (Fig. 3.21)

- The recording shows three positive deflections and two negative deflections.
- P, R and T are the positive deflections and Q and S are the negative deflections.

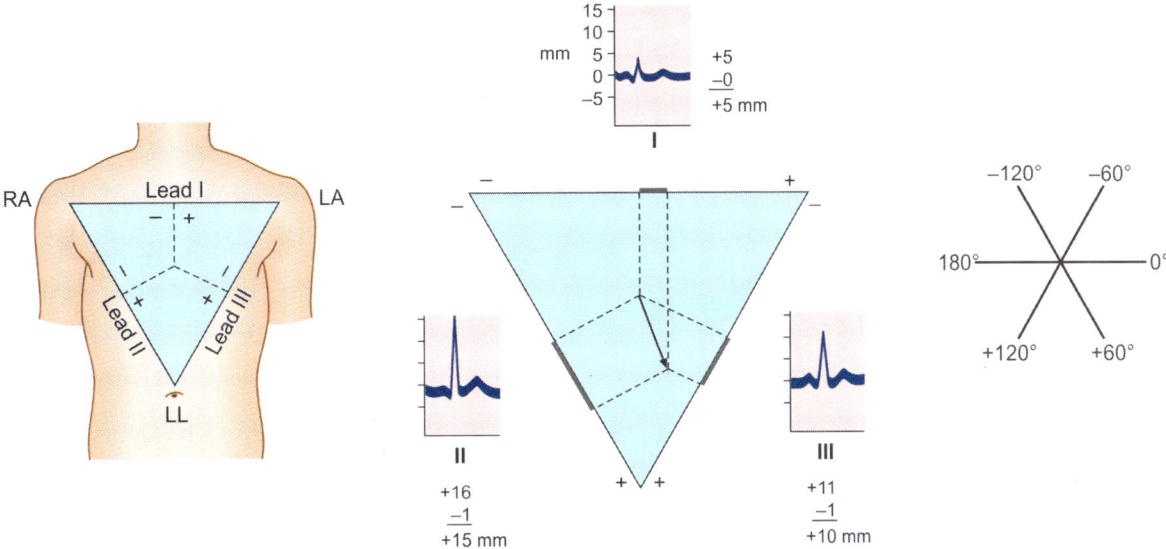

Fig. 3.19: The ECG recording from the standard bipolar limb leads correlated with the electrical axis

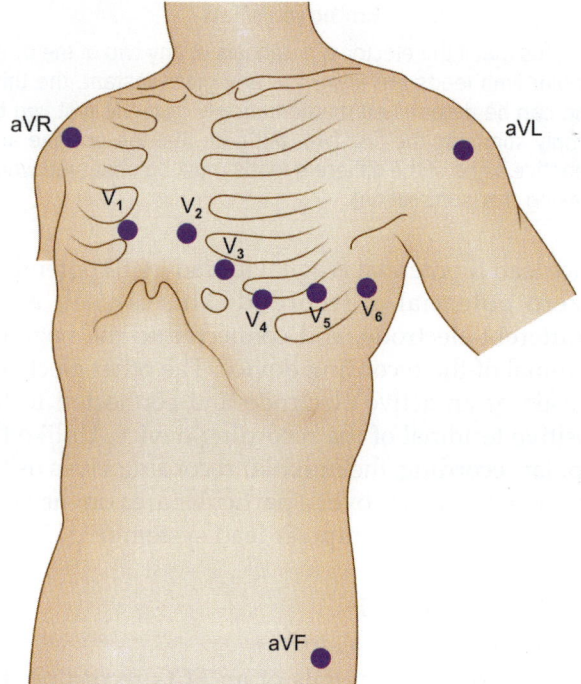

Fig. 3.20: Position of precardial chest leads and augmented limb leads

- PQ and ST are the segments.
- PQ or PR, QT, PP, RR are the intervals.
- Rarely following a T wave a U wave may be seen.

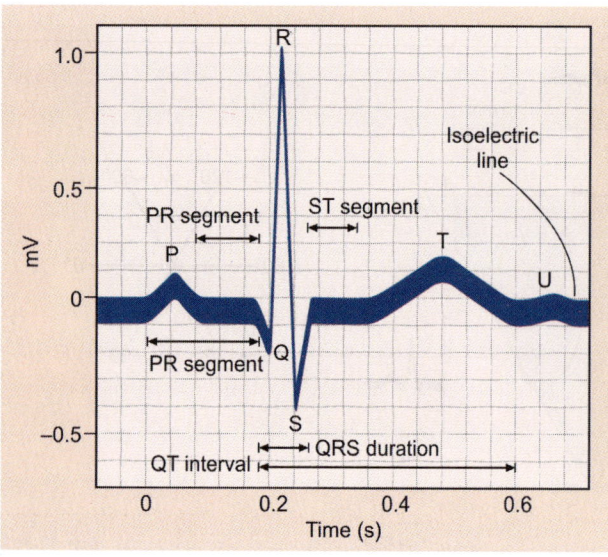

Fig. 3.21: ECG recorded from standard bipolar limb lead

Cause for the Various Waves (standard bipolar limb lead II is considered for explanation)

P Wave

- P wave is due to atrial depolarization.
- It is an upward deflection.
- The duration of the P wave is 0.08 seconds and the amplitude is 0.1 to 0.3 mV.
- Clinical importance: Increase in the amplitude is suggestive of atrial hypertrophy, as it can occur in mitral or tricuspid stenosis. It may be absent in atrial fibrillation and being replaced by fibrillatory waves. The configuration of the wave is also altered in mitral stenosis, due to hypertrophy of the left atrium.

QRS Complex

- Represents the depolarization of the inter-ventricular septum and the ventricles.
- In lead II, the normal value is 0.08 to 0.1 sec.
- Normal height of the R wave is 1.2 to 1.3 mV.
- If the height of the R wave is more than 2.5 mV, it is suggestive of ventricular hypertrophy.
- The normal duration should not exceed 0.1 seconds.

T Wave

- It is due to ventricular repolarization.
- The amplitude of the wave is 0.1 to 0.3 mV.

P-Q/R Interval

- Denotes the time taken for the impulse to spread from the SA node to the Purkinje fibers.
- Normal duration is 0.12 to 0.16 seconds.
- Measured from the beginning of P wave to the beginning of Q/R wave.
- If it exceeds 0.2 seconds, it is suggestive of a first degree heart block.
- If it is less than normal, it is suggestive of an ectopic foci situated nearer to the AV node, acting as the pacemaker.

Q-T Interval

- It is the time interval between the beginning of the Q wave and to the end of the T wave.
- It includes depolarization and repolarization of the ventricular muscle.
- The normal duration is 0.37 to 0.43 seconds.

P-P or R-R interval denotes the time taken for one cardiac cycle.

The electrical axis of the heart: The normal axis is plus 59 degrees. The normal range is from minus 30 to plus 110 degrees. If it is more negative, it is known as left axis deviation as seen in left ventricular hypertrophy, and left bundle branch block. If it is more positive, it is known as right axis deviation which occurs in right ventricular hypertrophy and right bundle branch block.

Clinical Significance of ECG (Table 3.4)

1. Anatomical orientation of the heart, could be vertical or horizontal (Fig. 3.22). Left or right axis deviation of heart could be made out.
2. Detect different types of arrhythmias (conduction blocks, fibrillations, flutters, varieties of tachycardias)
3. Hypertrophy of various chambers
4. Detection of myocardial infarction
5. Electrolyte imbalances particularly of K^+, Na^+, and Ca^{++}
6. Monitoring administration of digoxin group of drugs
7. Hyperkalemia (plasma K^+ ±7 mEq/L), there is tall slender T wave.
8. Hyperkalemia (plasma K^+ ±8.5 mEq/L) P wave is absent; QRS complex is broad and slurred. The T wave remains tall and slender.
9. Hypokalemia (plasma K^+ ±3.5 mEq/L) PR interval is almost 0.2 sec, prominent U wave.
10. Hypokalemia (plasma K^+ ±2.5 mEq/L) PR interval is very much prolonged, ST segment

Table 3.4: Uses of ECG in nutshell
1. To note the anatomical orientation of the heart a. Horizontal heart b. Vertical heart
2. To find out the relative size of the cardiac chambers
3. Abnormality in rhythm [arrhythmia and conduction (conduction block)]
4. Detection of myocardial ischemia/infarction—location, extent, duration and progress
5. ECG electrolyte imbalance with respect of ECF—K^+ and Ca^{++}
6. Action of certain drugs—digitalis
7. To monitor moment to moment status of patient in post-operative wards

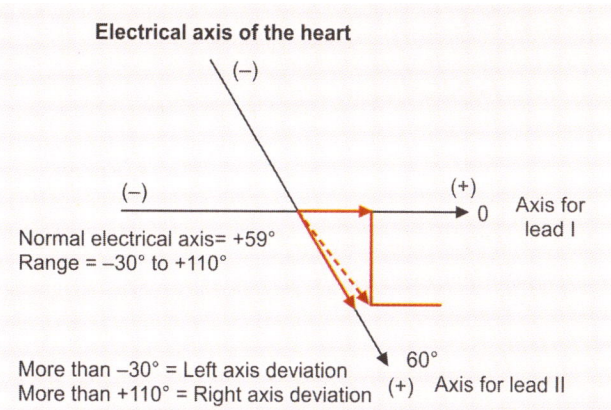

Fig. 3.22: The normal electrical axis

depressed and T wave is inverted, prominent U wave.
11. Some of the normal ECG recordings have been shown in Fig. 3.23.

CARDIAC CYCLE

SA node, the pacemaker has the property of automaticity and rhythmicity. Because of this, it produces action potentials, which spread all along the atrial and ventricular muscle fibers. This in turn brings about depolarization and repolarization. Following this, various changes occur in the heart, which is repeated from beat to beat. These events are known as the events of the cardiac cycle. The events are (Fig. 3.24):

• Mechanical changes in the form of contraction (systole) and relaxation (diastole) in atria and ventricles.
• Hemodynamic changes that is pressure and volume changes in atria and ventricles.
• Acoustic changes that is the production of heart sounds.

Duration of cardiac cycle depends on the heart rate per minute. For example, if the heart rate is 60 per minute, the cardiac cycle duration will be 1 sec. There is an inverse relationship between the duration of cardiac cycle and heart rate. Hence when the heart rate is increased to 120 beats per minute, the cardiac cycle duration will be about 0.5 sec.

Duration of atrial and ventricular systole and diastole will be as follows: when the heart rate is about 75 times per minute the duration of systole and diastole in different chambers will be (Table 3.5):

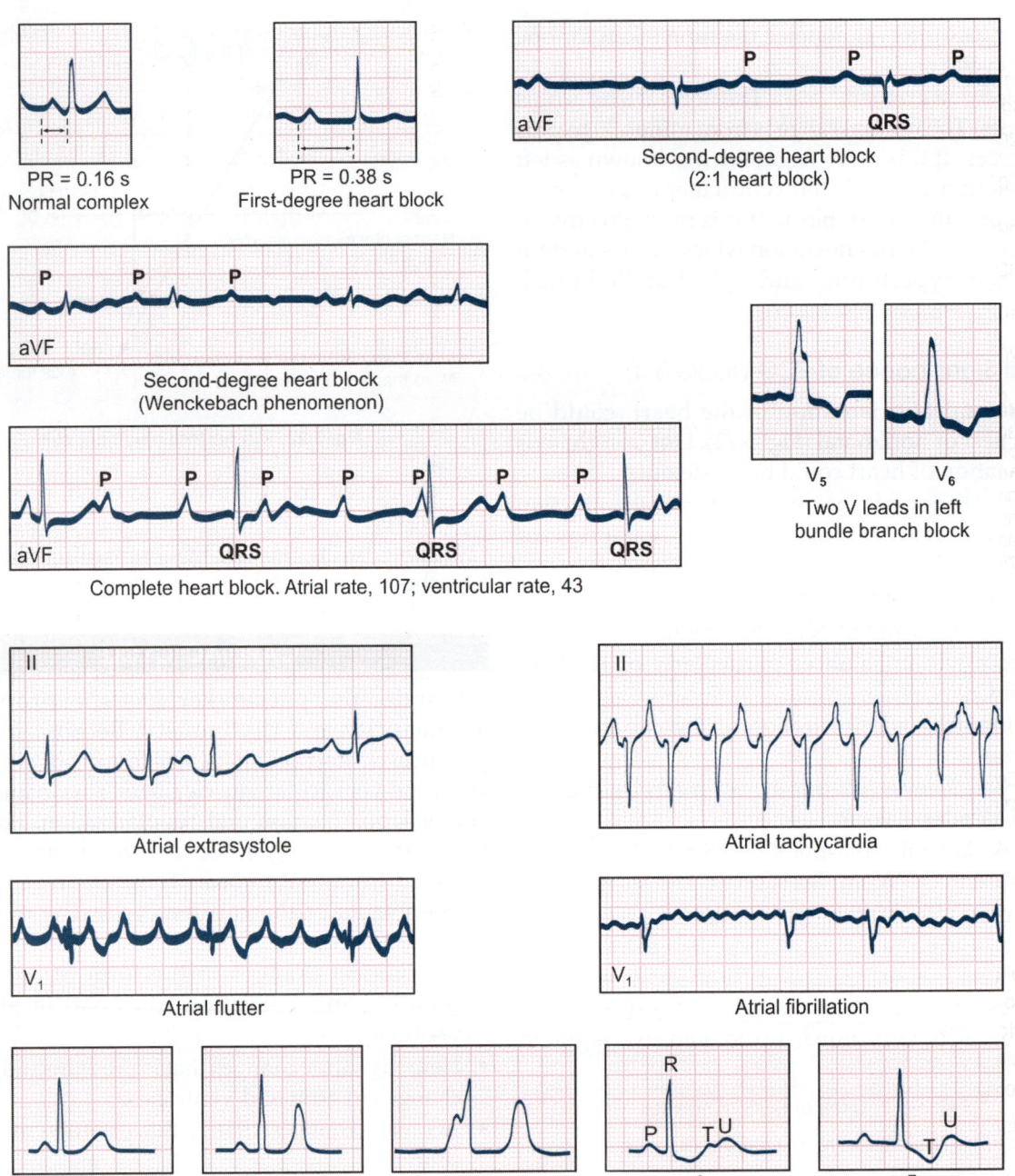

Fig. 3.23: Examples of some abnormal ECG recordings

- *Atria:*

  a. Systole is about 0.1 sec.

  b. Diastole is about 0.7 sec.

- *Ventricular:*

  a. Systole is about 0.3 sec.

  b. Diastole is about 0.5 sec.

From the above, it is obvious that the systole of atrial chambers will be followed by the systole of ventricular chambers. The ventricular and atrial systole will never coincide. Part of ventricular diastole and atrial diastole occur simultaneously. That is part of atrial diastole will occur when the ventricles are also in diastolic phase.

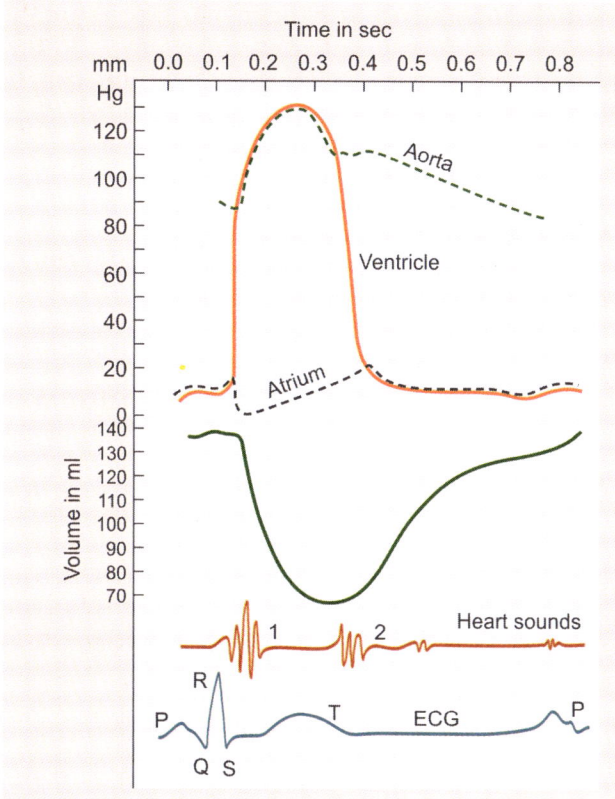

Fig. 3.24: Electrical, pressure, volume and acoustic changes during a cardiac cycle

Table 3.5: Events during cardiac cycle

Cardiac cycle (0.8 sec)
a. Atrial cycle
   Systole 0.1 sec
   Diastole 0.7 sec
b. Ventricular cycle
   Systole 0.3 sec
   Diastole 0.5 sec

Mechanical events
a. Atrial
   Systole   Volume change
                              Pressure change

b. Ventricular
   Systole   Volume change
                              Pressure change
   Diastole   Volume change
                              Pressure change

The further events of the cardiac cycle occurring in the ventricular chambers are discussed on the basis of intraventricular pressure changes. The pressure

recording and the volume changes in the ventricular chambers can be made out with the help of cardiac catheterization (Fig. 3.25).

At the end of the atrial systole, the ventricular systole starts. The ventricular chamber is filled with blood. The left intraventricular pressure is about 5–8 mm Hg. As the chamber begins to contract, the intra ventricular pressure begins to rise. Blood in the ventricle tries to go back into the atrium. This is prevented by the closure of atrioventricular valves and this is responsible for the production of the 1st heart sound. The semilunar valves, which are present at the beginning of aorta, are yet to open, as the aortic pressure is around 80 mm Hg. Hence the ventricle now contracts isometrically as a closed chamber. Because of this, the intraventricular pressure rises sharply. So, the phase of ventricular systole during which both the AV and SL valves are in closed state, and which gives raise to sharp increase of intra ventricular pressure is known as isovolumetric contraction/isovolumetric ventricular contraction. The duration of this phase is about 0.05 sec. The ventricular pressure rapidly rises from about 5 mm Hg to about 80 mm Hg. When the intraventricular pressure rises beyond 80 mm Hg, the SL valves are forced open and this leads the next sub-phase of ventricular systole, which is known as maximum ejection phase.

Maximum Ejection Phase

• Duration of this phase is about 0.11 sec.

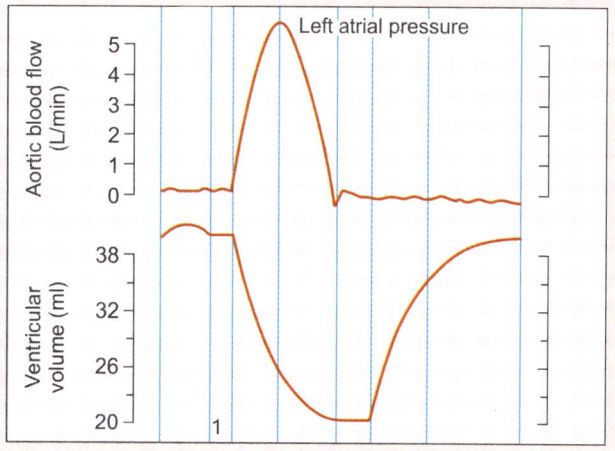

Fig. 3.25: Pressure in aorta and left ventricular volume change during a cardiac cycle

- The ventricular fibers contract isotonically.
- The pressure in the chamber increases gradually to about 120 mm Hg.
- Approximately, 70% of the stroke volume is pumped out from the ventricle into the aorta during this phase.

Reduced Ejection Phase

- Duration is about 0.14 sec.
- Some of the ventricular muscle fibers have already started relaxing.
- About 30% of the stroke volume is pumped out into the aorta during this phase.
- The intraventricular pressure slowly starts decreasing.

Protodiastole Phase

- Duration is about 0.04 sec.
- This is the time interval from the end of ventricular systole to the closure of the SL valves.
- When once the intraventricular pressure falls below the aortic pressure, blood from the aorta tends to flow back into the ventricle.
- This is prevented by the sudden closure of aortic valves.
- The closure of aortic valves is responsible for the production of the 2nd heart sound.

The time interval between the 1st and 2nd heart sounds is known as clinical systole.

Isovolumetric Relaxation Phase

- Duration is about 0.08 sec.
- AV valves which were closed at the beginning of ventricular systole are still in the closed state and the SL valves have also got closed.
- Now the ventricular muscle starts relaxing, and the ventricle relaxes as a closed chamber. Therefore, the pressure in the ventricle falls sharply without any alterations in the volume of blood in the ventricle
- The pressure falls rapidly to as low as zero mm Hg.

Right from the moment the closure of AV valves, the blood that is returning to the heart from the venous compartment keeps getting accumulated in the atria. This is responsible for slow raise of pressure in the atrium. The increase of pressure in the atrium continues until the AV vales open which occurs at the end of isovolumetric ventricular relaxation and this will lead to the next phase namely the initial rapid filling phase.

Initial Rapid Filling Phase

- Duration is about 0.09 sec.
- During this phase, there is pressure gradient between the atrium and the ventricle.
- Due to this, blood starts flowing from the atrium to ventricle.
- The sudden rush of blood from the atrium to ventricle is responsible for the production of the 3rd heart sound.
- About 70% of ventricular filling occurs during this phase.
- Since no active contraction of the muscle is involved for ventricular filling, only a pressure gradient facilitates this, the ventricular filling occurs by a passive process.

Clinical significance: Conditions like atrial fibrillations wherein atrial muscles stop contracting. Due to the passive process of filling of ventricle, cardiac output does not fall considerably.

Diastasis (slow filling phase)

- Duration is about 0.19 sec.
- As blood flows from the atrium to ventricle, the pressure falls in the atrium.
- Rushing of blood from the atrium into the ventricle, blood accumulates in the ventricle and increases the intraventricular pressure.
- Due to this, the pressure gradient between the atrium and ventricle gradually decreases. This stops the further blood flow from the atrium to the ventricle during this phase.

Though there is no blood flow, this phase has lot of practical significance, when there is increase or decrease of heart rate, cardiac cycle duration will also change. Normally, the duration of the ventricular systole does not get altered much when compared to the duration of the ventricular diastole. Even in the ventricular diastole, it is the duration of the diastasis that is affected. When there is an increase of heart rate, the duration of the diastasis is compromised. Therefore, in spite of an increase in the heart rate, ventricular filling remains fairly normal.

Final Rapid Filling Phase

- Duration is about 0.1 sec.
- This corresponds to the phase of atrial systole.
- Now the active contraction of atrial muscle pumps blood from atrium to ventricle.
- About 25% of ventricular filling occurs during this phase.
- Blood flow into the ventricle causes the production of 4th heart sound.

Phonocardiogram: Refers to graphical recording of heart sounds.

Heat sounds can be heard using a stethoscope at specified areas on the precardial region. Almost any one who is trained better, can hear the 1st and 2nd heart sounds and sometimes the 3rd sound also. But the 4th sound can only be graphically recorded. The heart sounds are affected in conditions like stenosis of valves, incompetence of valves, etc.

At times, in very rare cases, the 1st heart sound may split due to asynchronous closure of mitral and tricuspid valves.

The 2nd heart sound is replaced or followed by murmur in aortic incompetence.

Some of the important features of 1st and 2nd heart sounds have been shown in Table 3.6.

Jugular Venous Pulse (Fig. 3.26)

- Pressure change in jugular pulse is almost similar to pressure changes in right atrium.
- 'a' wave is due to atrial systole.
- 'a-x' is due to relaxation of atrial muscle.
- 'c' wave indicates slight increase in pressure due to bulging of tricuspid valves into right atrium at the beginning of ventricular systole.
- 'c-x' is due to the atrioventricular ring being pulled down towards the apex of the heart during ventricular systole leading to drop in pressure.

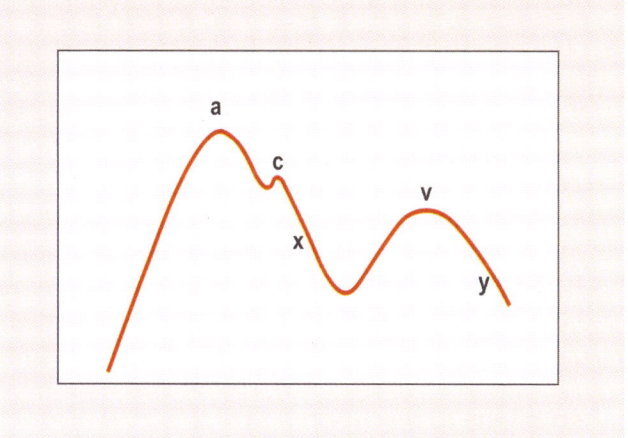

Fig. 3.26: Jugular venous pulse recording

- 'x1-v' gradual filling of atria throughout the ventricular systole and till the end of isovolumetric ventricular relaxation.
- 'v-y' is due to blood flowing from atrium into the ventricle during initial rapid filling phase.

HEART RATE AND ITS REGULATION

Normal heart rate is about 60–90 beats per minute. On an average, the rate at which the heart beats is about 75 per minute. It depends on the balanced activity between the sympathetic and parasympathetic nerve influence that are acting on it. Heart rate can be increased because of either an increased activity of sympathetic nerve fibers or a decreased activity of parasympathetic nerve fibers and vice versa for a decrease in heart rate.

In a newborn infant, the heart rate is about 120 beats per minute. The rate at which the heart beats is proportionate to the metabolic rate of the body. In canary birds, it can be as much as 1000 beats per minute.

Table 3.6: Differences between 1st and 2nd heart sounds

	1st heart sound	*2nd heart sound*
Produced due to	Closure of AV valves	Closure of SL valves
Duration (sec)	0.12–0.16	0.1–0.14
Frequency (cycles/sec)	Less than 40	More than 40
Pitch	Low	High
Heard better in	Mitral and tricuspid areas	Aortic and pulmonary areas
Indicates	Beginning of ventricular systole	Beginning of ventricular diastole
Carotid pulse relationship	Corresponds to carotid pulse	Follows carotid pulse

An increase in heart rate is known as tachycardia and a decrease is known as bradycardia.

Factors Influencing Heart Rate

Tachycardia	*Bradycardia*
Exercise	Athletes
Sympathetic stimulation	Conduction blocks
Anger, anxiety	Grief
Arrhythmias	Sleep
Thyrotoxicosis	Hypothyroidism
Fever	

Innervations to the Heart (Fig. 3.27)

- The efferent nerve supply to the heart is from both sympathetic and parasympathetic nerves.
- The parasympathetic nerve supplying the heart comes along the vagus whereas sympathetic is from the lateral horn cells of T1–T5 segments of spinal cord. The sympathetic fibers reach heart as superior, middle and inferior cardiac nerves.
- Vagus nerve takes origin from the cardioinhibitory center present in the reticular formation of the brainstem. The preganglionic fibers synapse in the ganglion cells present in the walls of the atria. From these the short postganglionic fibers supply almost all parts of heart except the apex. The neurotransmitter liberated both at the pre- and postganglionic regions will be acetylcholine. The receptors through which acetylcholine acts at the preganglionic region are termed as nicotinic receptor and at the postganglionic region are muscarinic receptor. The right vagus predominantly supplies the SA node whereas the left vagus predominantly supplies the AV node.
- Even under normal resting conditions, there is some amount of constant activity of the vagus on heart. This is termed as vagal tone. Because of this, the normal heart rate is maintained around 75 beats per minute. If there is bilateral vagotomy (cutting of vagi on either side), even at rest the heart rate may increase to about 140–180 beats per minute.
- The sympathetic fibers take origin from the lateral horn cells of the upper five thoracic segments. The preganglionic fibers that have emerged out of the spinal cord ascend up and synapse in the superior, middle and inferior cervical ganglia. From these ganglia, the postganglionic fibers take origin and supply the heart. The neurotransmitter liberated

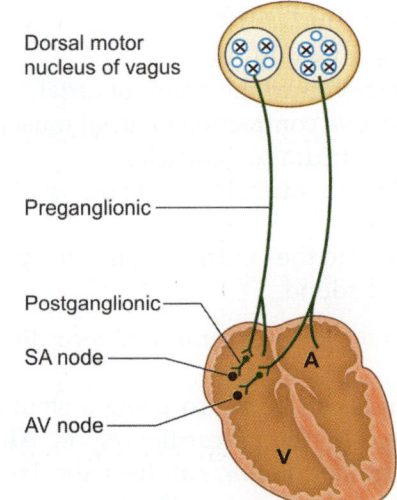

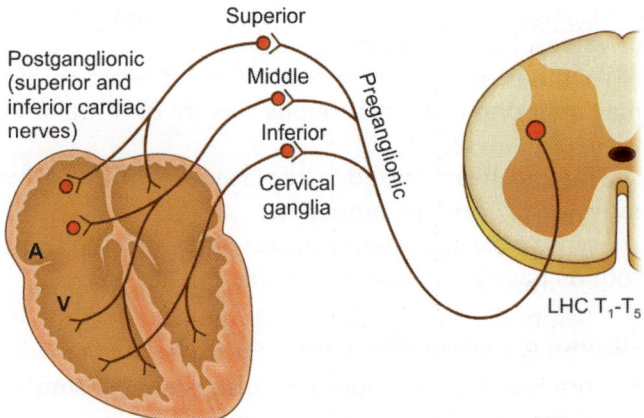

Fig. 3.27: Motor innervations to heart by parasympathetic and sympathetic nerves (above diagram is of parasympathetic and below is sympathetic)

by the preganglionic fibers is acetylcholine and the postganglionic fibers release noradrenaline.

The influences of parasympathetic and sympathetic nerve stimulation on various activities of the heart have been indicated in Table 3.7.

Phases of Respiration and Heart Rate

Sinus arrhythmia: During inspiration, the heart rate is increased and during expiration, it is decreased.

Mechanism

a. During inspiration, there will be irradiation of the impulses from the inspiratory center to the cardioinhibitory center which is present nearby in the reticular formation of the brainstem. These

Table 3.7: The effects of sympathetic and parasympathetic nerve stimulation on heart

Parasympathetic stimulation	Cardiac activity	Sympathetic stimulation	Tropic effect
↓	Heart rate	↑	Chronotropic
↓	Force of contraction	↑	Inotropic
↓	Conduction velocity of impulse	↑	Dromotropic
↓	Excitability	↑	Bathmotropic

impulses from the respiratory center will inhibit the activity of the cardioinhibitory center and this in turn decreases the activity of vagus nerve and hence vagal tone. Consequently, heart rate gets increased.

b. During inspiration as air enters the alveoli, the stretch receptors present in the walls of the alveoli get stimulated. The impulses are carried to the brainstem through afferent vagal fibers. These afferent impulses not only inhibit the inspiratory center but also the cardioinhibitory center. Hence vagal tone is decreased and heart rate increases.

Regulation of Heart Rate

Baroreceptor Mechanism

- There are specialized receptors namely the baroreceptors in the walls of carotid sinus and arch of aorta. The carotid sinus is located at the beginning of the internal carotid artery.
- The baroreceptors are stretch receptors present in the walls of the above blood vessels. Whenever there is an increase in blood pressure, the receptors get stimulated. They respond better when the blood flow in the above vessels is pulsatile.
- The afferent impulses from the carotid sinus are carried by sinus nerve a branch of glassopharyngeal nerve and from arch of aorta by aortic nerve a branch of vagus.
- The afferent impulses will stimulate the cardio inhibitory center present in the brainstem. This will increase the number of efferent impulses along the vagus to heart. The end result will be a decrease in heart rate (Fig. 3.28). The vagal tone depends on the impulses coming from the baroreceptors. When the baroreceptors are denervated vagal tone is lost completely.
- There is an inverse relationship between blood pressure and heart rate. Heart rate is inversely proportional to blood pressure and this is termed as Marey's law. Accordingly, when blood pressure increases the heart rate is decreased. In certain

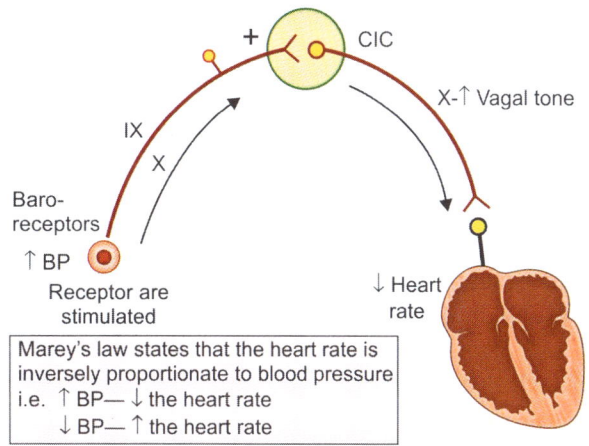

Marey's law states that the heart rate is inversely proportionate to blood pressure i.e. ↑ BP— ↓ the heart rate ↓ BP— ↑ the heart rate

Fig. 3.28: The reflex pathway involved in Marey's reflex

conditions, like muscular exercise, anxiety, etc., there is increase of both blood pressure and heart rate (exception to Marey's law).

Nerves: From baroreceptors (BR) to CIC—IX and X cranial nerves.

Chemoreceptor Mechanism

- These receptors are called as carotid and aortic bodies.
- The carotid body is present at the bifurcation of the common carotid artery (at the commencement of occipital artery) and aortic bodies are present at the arch of aorta.
- The afferent nerve that carries impulses from these receptors will be sinus nerve and aortic nerve respectively.
- They respond for chemical changes in blood namely, decrease in pO_2, increase of pCO_2 and increase in hydrogen ion concentration.
- When chemoreceptor get stimulated by any of the above factors, the afferent impulses from these receptors are carried by sinus and aortic nerves.
- The end result will be an increase in heart rate.

Bainbridge Reflex (Fig. 3.29)

- In the walls of great veins, there are stretch receptors present. They are termed as low pressure or volume receptors.
- Distension of the great veins leads to stimulation of these receptors.
- Afferent impulses from these receptors will be carried by vagus nerve.
- The afferent impulses inhibit the activity of cardio-inhibitory center and thereby leading to increase in heart rate.
- The afferent impulses along the vagus will also stimulate the neurons present in the brainstem which can increase the activity of sympathetic nerves. This leads to increased sympathetic activity on heart and heart rate increases.

The other factors which can influence the heart rate are (Table 3.8):

1. Pain receptor stimulation will have differential effect. When pain is from superficial parts of body (cutaneous pain), it brings about an increase in heart rate and if pain is visceral in origin, it leads to decrease in heart rate.
2. Joint receptors that are present in and around the joint will get stimulated during muscular exercise and increase the heart rate during exercise.
3. Increased intracranial tension: When there is an increased intracranial tension (e.g. in improper drainage of CSF), this will bring about a reflex bradycardia.
4. Oculocardiac reflex: When pressure is applied on the eyeball, it will bring about a decrease in heart rate.

Table 3.8: Factors regulating heart rate
1. Higher centre activity
2. Baroreceptors
3. Bainbridge reflex
4. Chemoreceptors
5. Joint receptors
6. Pain receptors
7. Circulating chemical substance, like adrenaline

5. Increase of body temperature will bring about an increase of heart rate.
6. Effect of adrenaline and noradrenaline: In an intact heart, adrenaline increases the heart rate while noradrenaline decreases the same. The decrease of heart rate by noradrenaline is brought about by reflex mechanism acting through baroreceptors since noradrenaline brings about an increase of mean arterial blood pressure.
7. Impulses coming from higher parts of the CNS, like limbic system, hypothalamus will also influence the heart rate, e.g. anger, fear, worry excitement, etc.

CARDIAC OUTPUT

Cardiac output is defined as volume of blood pumped out per ventricle per minute (Table 3.9). Right ventricle pumps blood into pulmonary circulation and during the same time an identical volume of blood is also pumped out from the left ventricle into systemic circulation.

Right ventricular = Left ventricular output = 5L/min output

- The normal cardiac output is about 5 liters/ventricle/minute
- Cardiac output is a product of stroke volume and heart rate.
- Stroke volume (SV) is volume of blood pumped out per ventricle per beat, which is normally about 70 ml.
- The normal heart rate (HR) can be considered as about 70 per minute. In which case

Cardiac output = HR × SV
                = 70 × 70 = 4900 ml

Cardiac output has direct relationship with body surface area. Hence expression of the absolute value of cardiac output is not very appropriate. It is better to express as cardiac index.

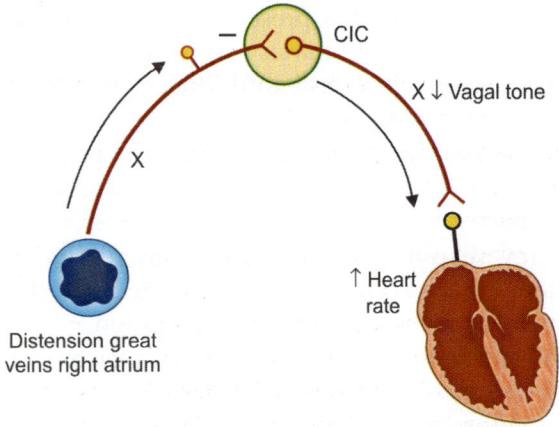

Fig. 3.29: The pathway involved in Bainbridge reflex

Table 3.9: Definition of cardiac output

It is the volume of blood pumped out per ventricle per minute

RL ventricle output = Lt. ventricle output = 5 L/min.

Stroke volume is volume of blood pumped out per ventricle per beat

Cardiac Index

- Expression of cardiac output in relation to body surface area
- Normally, it is expressed as L/Sq m Body surface area (BSA)/min
- To calculate cardiac index, cardiac output must be divided by body surface area.

$$\text{Cardiac index} = \frac{\text{Cardiac output (L/min)}}{\text{BSA (m}^2)}$$

Assuming that cardiac output is 5 L/min, BSA is 1.7 m^2

Cardiac index will be $\dfrac{5}{1.7}$ = about 3 L/min/m^{2}BSA

Determination of Cardiac Output

It can be done by many methods. Some of the common methods employed are (Table 3.10):

1. Using Fick's principle.
2. Dye method.
3. Thermodilution method.

Fick's Principle

It states that the quantity of a substance taken up by an organ or given out by an organ is equal to concentration difference of the substance in arterial and venous blood multiplied by blood flow through the organ per minute. Hence, Fick's principle can also be used for determination of blood flow through organs, like brain, coronary, renal, etc.

According to this principle:

$$Q = \frac{(C_a - C_v)}{\text{Blood flow through the organ}} / \text{min}$$

Q is quantity of substance taken up or given out by the organ per minute

Table 3.10: List of methods to determine cardiac output

1. By using Fick's principle
2. Dye technique Evan's blue/T$_{1824}$
3. Thermodilution

C_a concentration of the substance in arterial blood

C_v concentration of the substance in venous blood.

While determining cardiac output by this method, the quantity of substance taken up or given out by the organ per minute and arteriovenous concentration of the substance must be known. Hence, the volume of blood flow through the ventricle per minute (which is nothing but cardiac output) has to be calculated.

So the formula has to be rewritten:

$$\frac{(C_a - C_v)}{\text{Blood flow through the organ } (CO)} / \text{min} = Q$$

So cardiac output will be:

$$CO = \frac{Q}{(C_a - C_v)} / \text{min}$$

For determination of cardiac output by applying this principle, either oxygen or carbon dioxide content of blood can be used. More often, it is the oxygen content of blood that is used.

While determining cardiac output by using oxygen, the following data are required:

1. Volume of oxygen used up by the body per minute (Q). This can be estimated by making the person to breathe from a bag containing 100% oxygen.
2. The arterial oxygen content can be estimated by taking a sample of arterial blood (C_a).
3. The venous blood oxygen is estimated by taking a sample of mixed venous blood. Mixed venous blood sample can be obtained from pulmonary artery by cardiac catheterization (C_v).

Assuming the data as follows:

1. $Q = 250$ ml /min
2. $C_a = 20$ ml/100 ml
3. $C_v = 15$ ml/100 ml

$$\text{So cardiac output} = \frac{Q}{(C_a - C_v)} = \frac{250}{5} \times 100$$

$$= 5000 \text{ ml/min}$$

Dye Method

The dye that is normally used is T$_{1824}$, which is also known as Evan's blue. Any dye which is used should possess the following criteria:

- Should get diluted properly in plasma.
- Should be non-toxic.
- Should not alter hemodynamics.
- Should not alter blood volume.
- Concentration of the dye can be easily estimated.

Procedure

- Dye has to be dissolved in an isotonic fluid.
- A known quantity of dye has to be injected into a peripheral vein.
- A series of blood samples have to be collected from an artery at regular intervals (may be every 3 sec).
- Concentration of the dye in the sample of blood is determined.
- The data has to be plotted on a semi-log paper (Fig. 3.30).
- In the graph, there will be a gradual increase in the concentration of dye till it reaches maximum. After this, the concentration of dye goes on decreasing till a point wherein there will be again a slight increase in concentration of dye. The slight increase in the concentration of dye is because of recirculation of blood.
- Wherever the concentration of dye starts increasing for the second time, the rising point will be taken as mean concentration of dye.
- From the lowest concentration point, line is extrapolated to cut the X axis. This will indicate the time required for one circulation.
- Calculation of cardiac output has to be done based on the above available data. For example:
  1. Quantity of dye injected is 3 mg in 1 ml of isotonic fluid.
  2. Concentration of dye in it is about 1.5 mg/ml
  3. Time for one circulation is 30 sec.

$$Cardiac\ output = \frac{Quantity\ of\ dye\ injected}{Mean\ concentration\ of\ dye} \times \frac{Time\ in\ seconds}{Time\ for\ one\ circulation}$$

$$= \frac{3}{1.5} \times \frac{60}{30} = 4\ liters\ per\ minute$$

Thermodilution Method

- Equipment used is thermister.
- A double lumen catheter is introduced into the heart.
- Through one of the lumens of the catheter, cold saline of known temperature and volume is introduced into right atrium.
- This saline from right atrium enters right ventricle from where it is pumped into pulmonary artery. The change in the temperature of the saline that was introduced is measured by the devise in the pulmonary artery.
- The extent to which a change in the temperature has taken place depends on the right ventricular output.
- This is said to be more advantageous because:
  a. Since the indicator used is cold saline, in cases where cardiac output has to be determined repeatedly it can be done easily.
  b. Since blood is pumped out into systemic circulation, whatever changes that have occurred with respect to temperature can be minimized further by the tissues as blood flows through the tissues. Because of this, the temperature of venous blood will not be altered much.

There are many conditions in which cardiac output is altered. Some of the conditions in which cardiac output will be more than normal are:

1. Muscular exercise in which it can be as much as 35 L/min that is about 7-fold increase.
2. Sympathetic stimulations, like anxiety, anger, fear, etc., will also increase cardiac output.
3. In pregnancy, anemia, hyperthyroidism also
4. More in the recumbent posture when compared to erect posture

Conditions in which cardiac output decreases will be:

1. Hemorrhage
2. Arrhythmias

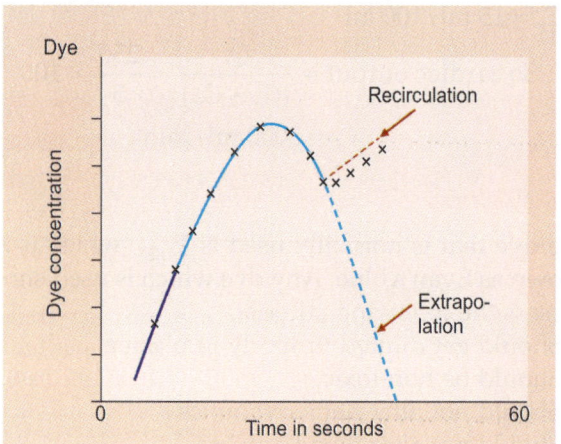

Fig. 3.30: Changes in concentration of dye against time factor

3. Left ventricular failure
4. Sleep
5. Hypothyroidism

Regulation of Cardiac Output

- Determinants of cardiac output are heart rate and stroke volume.
- Hence any factor, which affects either the heart rate, or stroke volume, or both will alter the cardiac output.
- Peripheral resistance also affects cardiac output by altering the stroke volume. This is brought about because of after-load effect.
- In addition to this, some of the other factors, which try to regulate cardiac output, will be distensability of cardiac chambers.

Hence regulation of the cardiac output can be discussed under the following headings (Fig. 3.31 and Table 3.11):
1. Factors which are going to affect the heart rate
2. Factors that are going to affect the stroke volume

Heart rate alterations can be brought about by:
1. Neural mechanism
2. Hormonal mechanism

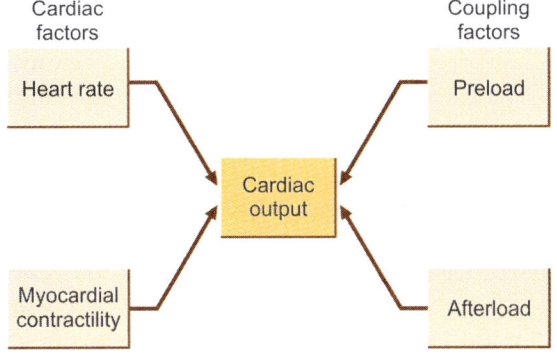

Fig. 3.31: Factors affecting cardiac output

Table 3.11: Factors regulating cardiac output
1. Venous return
2. Heart rate
3. Force of contraction
4. Peripheral resistance
5. Distensibility of the cardiac chambers

Neural Mechanism

Stimulation of parasympathetic nerve (vagus) is going to have negative chronotropic effect. Hence it is going to decrease the heart rate and decreases cardiac output. But a moderate decrease of heart rate is not going to alter the cardiac output for the reason that when there is decrease of heart rate, the ventricular filling time is increased and thereby the end diastolic volume increases, increases stroke volume based on Starling's law and hence the stroke volume will increase.

Stimulation of sympathetic nerve will increase the heart rate by exerting positive chronotropic effect and hence increases the heart rate and cardiac output. An increase in the heart rate up to a certain extent increases the cardiac output. But on further increase in the heart rate, the cardiac output starts decreasing. When the heart rate increases beyond a certain range, the ventricular filling time decreases. This decreases the end diastolic volume, stroke volume and, therefore, cardiac output.

Hormonal Mechanism

- Thyroxin is going to increase the sensitivity of beta-receptors in the heart for catecholamine action. In addition, it also increases the number of beta-receptors in cardiac muscle. Because of this, in hyperthyroidism, there will be increase of heart rate and cardiac output.
- Catecholamines (adrenaline and noradrenaline) due to their action on the cardiac muscle through beta-receptors will also increase the heart rate. This action is similar to the action that is brought about the sympathetic stimulation. Sympathetic stimulation increases not only the heart rate but also the force of contraction. This brings about a marked increase in cardiac output.

Stroke volume is altered by many of the factors. Stroke volume is difference between end diastolic volume (EDV) and end systolic volume (ESV).
- End diastolic volume is volume of blood present in the ventricle at the end of diastole, which is normally about 140 ml.
- End systolic volume is volume of blood present in the ventricle at the end of systole, which is normally about 70 ml.
- Ejection fraction (SV/EDV): It is the fraction of EDV that has been ejected out during ventricular systole, which in this case will be about 0.5 or 50%.

- Either by altering the EDV or ejection fraction, stroke volume can be affected.
- There are many factors, which can alter either the EDV or ejection fraction. They are:
  a. Preload effect (venous return)
  b. After-load effect (peripheral resistance)
  c. Myocardial contractility

Preload Effect

- Preload means load acting on the muscle before it starts contracting.
- In the case of cardiac muscle, preload is exerted by the extent of venous return. Therefore, the end diastolic volume and preload effect have direct relationship.
- When venous return increases, more blood is brought to ventricle.
- This brings about distension of the chambers.
- Stretching of the ventricular muscle fibers.
- Hence as per Starling's law, force of contraction gets increased (Starling's law states that force of contraction is directly proportional to initial length of muscle fibers within physiological limits).
- Hence any factor which affects venous return will alter stroke volume and cardiac output.

After-load Effect

- After-load means it is load acting on the muscle after the muscle has started contracting.
- In the case of ventricle, for blood to get pumped out, there should be opening of the semilunar valves present at the origin of aorta.
- The semilunar valves normally open at a particular pressure (when the ventricular pressure exceeds that of the diastolic blood pressure).
- So the ventricles are able to experience the resistance offered by the semilunar valves only after the ventricle has started contracting and because of this, it is termed as after-load effect.
- When the after-load effect is more, the volume of blood pumped out by the ventricle decreases because lot of the exertion of the ventricle will be spent to overcome the resistance offered by the semilunar valves.
- It is for this reason, in condition of severe hypertension especially that of diastolic hypertension person may tend to go into left ventricular failure.

- In hypertension, since the ejection fraction decreases and the end systolic volume increase. In the mean time, the volume of blood (venous return) returning to the heart will continue to be as usual. This will increase the further distension of the ventricles. So abnormal stretching of the ventricle may occur beyond a limit and the ventricle may fail to contract.
- It is for this reason, whenever a patient is suffering from diastolic hypertension, due attention has to be paid to reduce the blood pressure in order to reduce the stress on the left ventricle exerted because of the after-load effect and prevent consequent cardiac failure.

Myocardial Contractility

Keeping the preload and after-load effects constant, there are many factors which can just affect the myocardial contractility and hence the stroke volume and cardiac output. Myocardial contractility is affected by factors, like (Fig. 3.32):

1. Effect of sympathetic and parasympathetic stimulation because of their inotropic effects. The increase in the force of contraction when sympathetic nerve is stimulated will increase the stroke volume at the expense of end systolic volume. Normally, the end systolic volume will be about 70 ml. When there is sympathetic nerve stimulation, for the same end diastolic volume, the force of contraction gets increased because of positive inotropic effect. This increases the ejection fraction.
2. Hypoxia, hypercapnia and acidosis of myocardium, which occurs when there is decrease in blood flow through coronary vessels. When the coronary blood flow decreases, due to the above changes, there will be decrease in force of contraction of the ventricle.
3. Death of myocardium as it occurs in myocardial infarction will decrease the muscle mass and hence decreases the stroke volume.
4. Functional depression of myocardium will reduce the force of contraction.
5. Inotropic agents action: Positive inotropic agents, like digitalis, facilitate the force of contraction, whereas verapamil, diltiazem, etc., by reducing the calcium conductance into ICF, will decrease the force of contraction.
6. Catecholamines are going to imitate the sympathetic stimulation action and hence bring

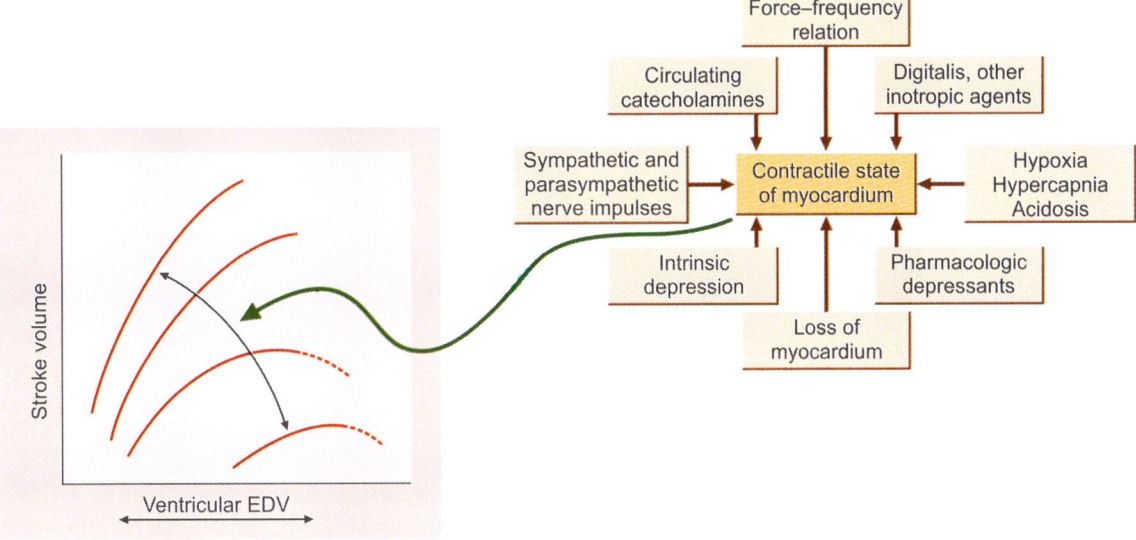

Fig. 3.32: Relationship between EDV and SV and factors influencing myocardial contractility

about a positive inotropic effect and increase the force of contraction.

Distensability of the cardiac muscle is decreased in pericardial effusion, hemopericardium and when the patient has recovered from myocardial infarction. When distensability is decreased the stroke volume and cardiac output also decreases.

The influence of various factors in the regulation of cardiac output can be studied with the help of heart-lung preparation.

Cardiac Catheterization

Cardiac catheterization is an invasive technique in which a thin tube is (catheter) is introduced into the peripheral blood vessel and guided to reach the different parts of heart. It was first performed by Frossmann in the year 1929. Later on he won the Nobel prize for this path breaking technique which he had first performed on himself.

To reach the right side of heart, the catheter has to be introduced into a peripheral vein. This type of catheterization is called as anterograde catheterization.

To reach the left side of heart, the catheter has to be introduced into a peripheral artery. This type of catheterization is known as retrograde catheterization.

Advantages of cardiac catheterization
- Measure pressure changes in different chambers of heart.

- Measure volume changes in ventricles (EDV and ESV).
- Obtain a sample of mixed venous blood.
- Study septal defects.
- Introduce drugs directly into heart.
- Stimulate pacemaker region.
- ECG can be recorded directly from heart.

Disadvantage of cardiac catheterization: Catheterization may induce fibrillations in ventricular muscle.

BLOOD PRESSURE

Blood pressure is defined as the lateral pressure exerted on the vessel wall by column of flowing blood or it is also termed as end arterial pressure.

Systolic blood pressure is defined as maximum pressure that can be recorded in arteries during ventricular systole. In a normal adult of 20 years it ranges from 100 to 140 mm Hg and the mean pressure is 120 mm Hg.

Diastolic blood pressure is the minimum pressure that can be recorded in arteries during ventricular diastole. In a normal adult of 20 years, it ranges from 60 to 90 mm Hg and the mean will be 80 mm Hg.

Mean arterial pressure is the mean pressure in the arteries during a cardiac cycle. It is diastolic pressure plus one-third of pulse pressure. So it will be 80 + 40/ 3 = about 94 mm Hg.

Pulse pressure is the difference between systolic and diastolic pressure. So it is 120 – 80 = 40 mm Hg.

Factors influencing blood pressure are:
1. Age
2. Sex
3. Body build
4. Posture
5. Exercise
6. Emotional aspects

Factors that maintain the normal blood pressure are:
1. Cardiac output
2. Peripheral resistance
3. Blood volume
4. Viscosity of the blood
5. Elasticity of the blood vessel

Cardiac output: Systolic blood pressure depends entirely on the cardiac output. An increase in the cardiac output increases the systolic pressure and a decrease in the output will have the opposite effect.

Peripheral resistance affects the diastolic pressure and has a direct relationship. The seat of resistance is the arterioles. Arterioles contain large number of smooth muscle fibers that are supplied by sympathetic vasoconstrictor fibers. Vasoconstriction increases the resistance offered to blood flow and, therefore, the diastolic blood pressure is increased.

Blood volume: If blood volume is reduced, it decreases the blood pressure. Decreased blood volume decreases the systemic filling pressure. This in turn will decrease the venous pressure, decrease the

---

Blood pressure

- Later pressure
- End arterial pressure
- Normal BP $\dfrac{120}{80}$ mm Hg

  120 mm Hg—systolic BP
  80 mm Hg—diastolic BP

Pulse pressure = Systolic–Diastolic
= 120–80
= 40 mm Hg

Mean arterial BP = Diastolic + rd of pulse pressure
= 80 + (13 or 14)
= 94 mm Hg

Measurement of BP

1. *Direct:* Inserting a needle into an artery
2. *Indirect:*
   - Sphygmomanometer
     - Palpatory method
     - Auscultatory method

---

venous return and cardiac out put and, therefore, the blood pressure.

Viscosity of the blood: Increased viscosity offers increased resistance to blood flows and, therefore, increases the blood pressure. This is usually seen in cases of polycythemia vera.

Elasticity of the blood vessels: As age advances, the amount of elastic fiber decreases in the vessel wall. The blood vessel becomes more rigid tubes, the distensibility of the blood vessel is reduced. As a result, the systolic blood pressure is increased and the diastolic pressure is decreased. However, in practice, what is seen is an increase in the diastolic pressure. This is because of atherosclerotic changes, the tube (blood vessel) diameter decreases and, therefore, offers greater resistance to blood flow.

Measurement of blood pressure can be done both by direct and indirect methods. But the direct method is not done during routine measurement of blood pressure as the technique is invasive and needs insertion of needle into an artery to determine blood pressure. Hence the indirect method is preferred. Indirect methods are:
1. By palpatory method
2. By auscultatory method.

By palpatory method, only the approximate systolic pressure can be measured. Diastolic blood pressure cannot be measured by this method.

Auscultatory method is the most accurate method of measuring the blood pressure. Both systolic and diastolic pressures can be measured by this method. Instrument used to measure blood pressure is known as sphygmomanometer.

In palpatory method, an approximate systolic pressure is obtained whereas in auscultatory method an accurate systolic and diastolic pressure can be obtained.

While determining blood pressure by auscultatory method, the sounds heard using stethoscope is known as Korotkoff sound. Korotkoff sounds are produced due to turbulence created by flow of blood through the partially obstructed blood vessel. In the normal course, the blood flow through the blood vessel is laminar or silent as there is no obstruction. In laminar flow, the central most layer of blood will be flowing at maximal velocity and the velocity of flow of the layer of blood nearer to the wall of vessel will be least.

In a completely occluded vessel, there is no flow beyond the area of occlusion. When the vessel is partially opened (occlusion is removed partially), now blood has to pass through the narrow area. This creates turbulence beyond the area of partial obstruction. This turbulence is responsible for production of Korotkoff sound. When the occlusion is completely removed, the turbulent flow is replaced by laminar flow. Hence there will be no more sound production.

Regulation of Blood Pressure

This can be discussed as under:
1. Local mechanisms
2. Spinal cord in the regulation
3. Medulla oblongata in the regulation
4. Higher centers in the regulation
   Or
1. Immediate mechanisms
2. Intermediate mechanisms
3. Long-term mechanisms

Local mechanisms include the production of vasodilator or vasoconstrictor substances. The vasoconstrictor substances are noradrenaline, angiotensin II, 5-hydroxytryptamine and others. The vasodilator substances are bradykinin, histamine, and adrenaline in certain regions. Hypoxia, hypercapnea, warmth, acidosis, etc. also bring about vasodilatation. These substances mainly alter the peripheral resistance and, therefore, the diastolic blood pressure.

Spinal Cord in the Regulation of Blood Pressure (Fig. 3.33)

Complete transverse section of the spinal cord (at the level of T1 segment) is followed by a marked fall in blood pressure. During the recovery phase, the lateral horn cells recover, send vasoconstrictor impulses to the blood vessels, blood vessels constrict, the blood pressure improves though it may not come back to normal. During the state of spinal shock, carbon

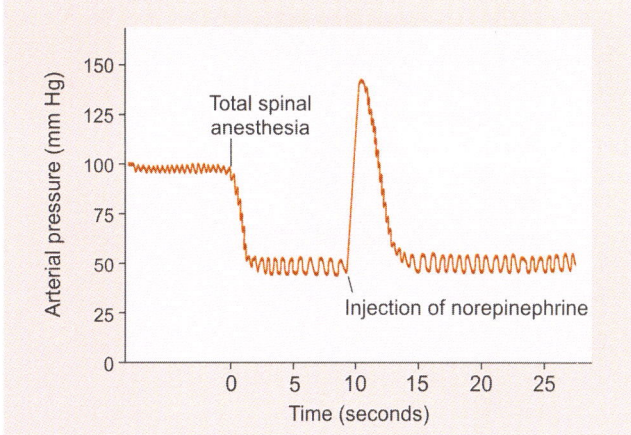

Fig. 3.33: Role of sympathetic nerve activity in the maintenance of normal blood pressure

dioxide breathing will stimulate the lateral horn cells directly and increases the blood pressure. Influence of VMC is mediated through the lateral horn cells and the impulses from VMC on the lateral horn cells are always excitatory.

Role of Medulla Oblongata in the Regulation of Blood Pressure

Medulla oblongata is the most important region of the central nervous system that is involved in the regulation of blood pressure. Collectively, these neurons are called as the vasomotor center (VMC). Stimulation of these neurons will give rise to vasoconstriction, which increases the peripheral resistance and increases the blood pressure. On the other hand, when this neuronal activity is decreased it leads to vasodilation and, therefore, decreases the peripheral resistance and hence decreases the blood pressure.

Factors controlling the activity of the vasomotor center are (Fig. 3.34):
1. Impulses coming from the baroreceptors
2. Impulses from the chemoreceptors
3. Impulses from the higher centers.
4. Impulses from the pain receptors and from joint receptors
5. Impulses from the visceral receptors.

Baroreceptor Mechanism in the Regulation of Blood Pressure

- Baroreceptor mechanism is the most important mechanism in the regulation of blood pressure.

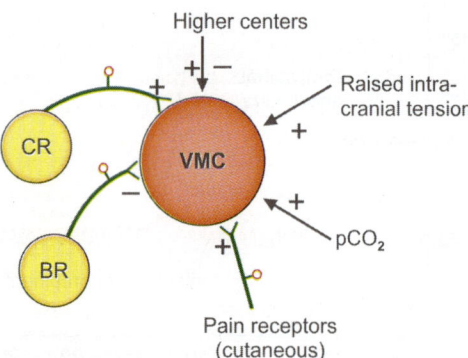

Fig. 3.34: Various factors influencing activity of vasomotor center present in the brainstem

- Carotid sinus and arch of aorta contain the baroreceptors (Fig. 3.35).
- Carotid sinus is located at the bifurcation of the carotid artery and at the commencement of the internal carotid artery.
- Aortic arch receptors are located in the arch of the aorta.
- A branch of the glassopharyngeal nerve supplies carotid sinus and the aortic nerve a branch from the vagus nerve supplies the aortic arch (Fig. 3.36).
- These receptors are stretch receptors. An increase in the blood pressure further stretches the receptors area resulting in production more number of impulses (Fig. 3.37).
- More number of impulses are produced and these impulses reach the following centers (Fig. 3.37):
  a. Vasomotor center
  b. Cardioinhibitory center
  c. Respiratory center

Role of Vasomotor Center (Fig. 3.38)

i. Impulses going to the vasomotor center from the baroreceptors are inhibitory in nature and therefore, the activity of the vasomotor center is inhibited. This in turn decreases the number of impulses going to the lateral horn cells in the spinal cord. The activity of the lateral horn cells is decreased. Vasoconstrictor impulses going to the arterioles are reduced, leading to vasodilatation, decreased peripheral resistance and a decrease in diastolic blood pressure.

ii. Inhibition of vasomotor center also decreases the venomotor tone; blood gets pooled in the venous compartment. This decreases the venous return, decreases the cardiac output and, therefore, the blood pressure.

iii. Inhibition of vasomotor center decreases the amount of catecholamine secretion from the adrenal medulla which in turn decreases the peripheral resistance and cardiac output.

iv. Due to decreased sympathetic activity, the heart rate and force of contraction of the heart are also reduced, reducing the systolic blood pressure.

The loss of function of baroreceptor (Fig. 3.39, when baroreceptor area is denervated or when baroreceptor area is not prefused—Figs 3.40 and 3.41) on BP variations has been depicted.

Role of Cardioinhibitory Center

Impulses coming from the baroreceptors are excitatory to the cardioinhibitory center. Stimulation of cardioinhibitory center increases the vagal tone, which in turn decreases the heart rate and force of

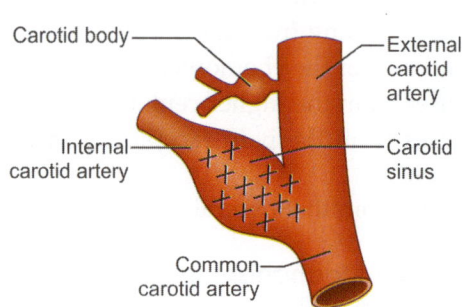

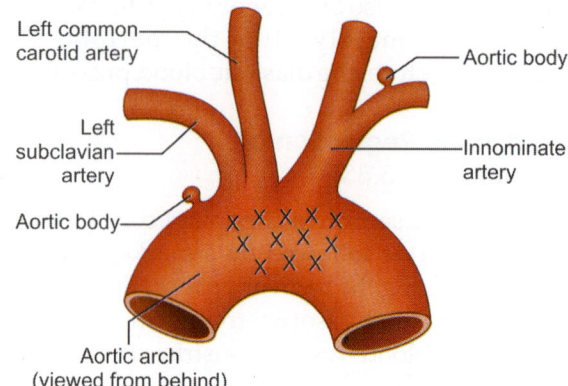

Fig. 3.35: Location of baroreceptors and chemoreceptors

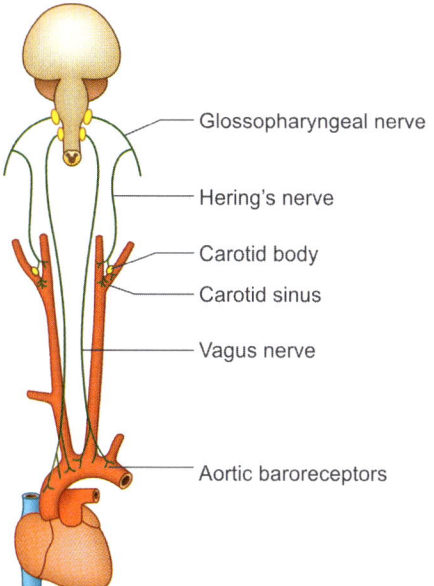

Fig. 3.36: Afferent nerves carrying impulses from baroreceptors

- Glossopharyngeal nerve
- Hering's nerve
- Carotid body
- Carotid sinus
- Vagus nerve
- Aortic baroreceptors

contraction of the heart. This will lead to decreased cardiac output.

Marey's law states that heart rate is inversely proportionate to blood pressure. Whenever the blood pressure is increased, acting through the cardio-inhibitory center, it reflexly lowers the heart rate and blood pressure.

Role of Respiratory Center

Impulses coming from the baroreceptors are inhibitory to the respiratory center. This in turn decreases the rate and depth of respiration. Because of this, the changes in the intrapleural pressure become less. This will lead to decreased venous return. Decreased venous return decreases the cardiac output and, therefore, blood pressure.

Chemoreceptor Mechanism

- Chemoreceptors are the carotid bodies and aortic bodies.
- Decreased blood pressure decreases the blood flow through the chemoreceptors decreasing the oxygen supply.
- Hypoxia, hypercapnia and acidosis stimulate these chemoreceptors.

The impulses from the chemoreceptors in general are going to stimulate the vasomotor center, respiratory center and inhibit the cardioinhibitory center during the course of regulation of blood pressure. Stimulation of VMC increases the peripheral resistance and hence the blood pressure.

CNS Ischemic Response

If the blood pressure falls to a greater extent, the blood flow to the brain is markedly reduced, metabolic waste products accumulate, the resulting hypercapnea and acidosis stimulate the vasomotor center directly and

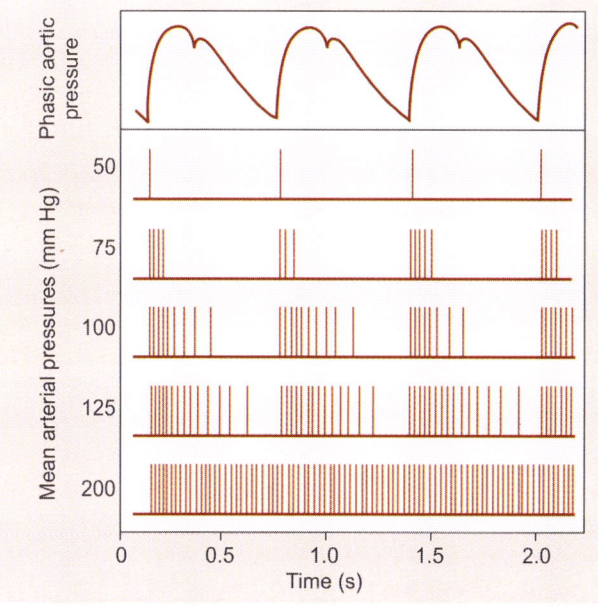

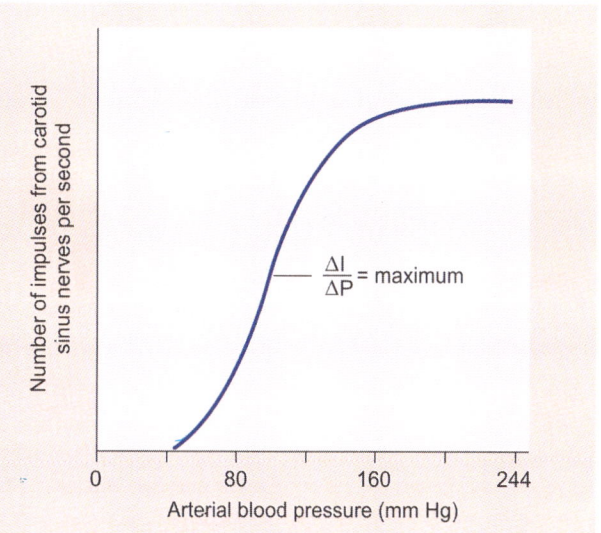

$\dfrac{\Delta I}{\Delta P}$ = maximum

Fig. 3.37: The relationship between mean arterial pressure and frequency of impulse discharge in the sinus nerve

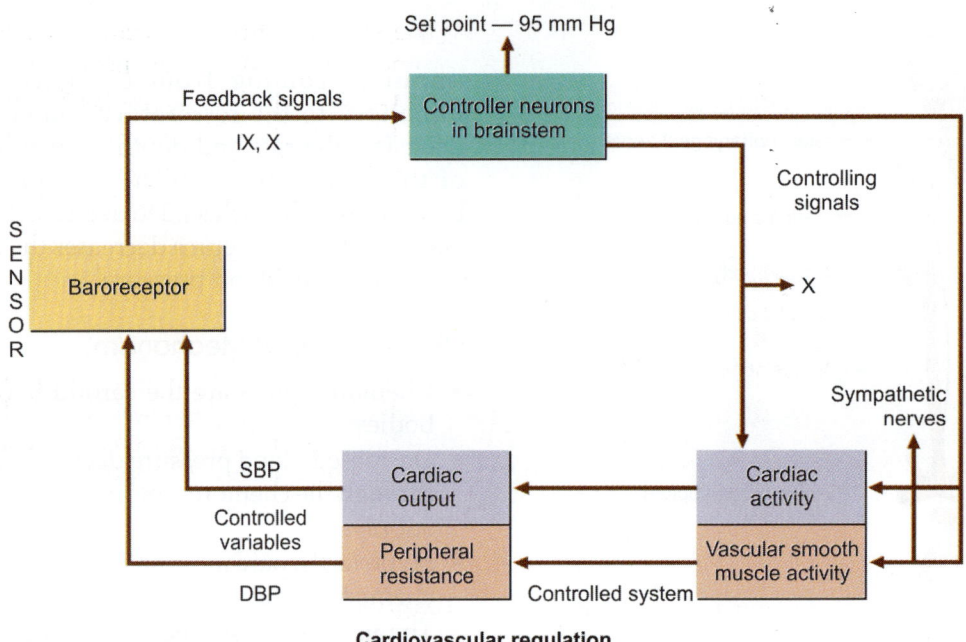

Cardiovascular regulation

Fig. 3.38: Feedback circuit indicating the role of baroreceptors in the regulation of BP by altering the cardiac output and peripheral resistance

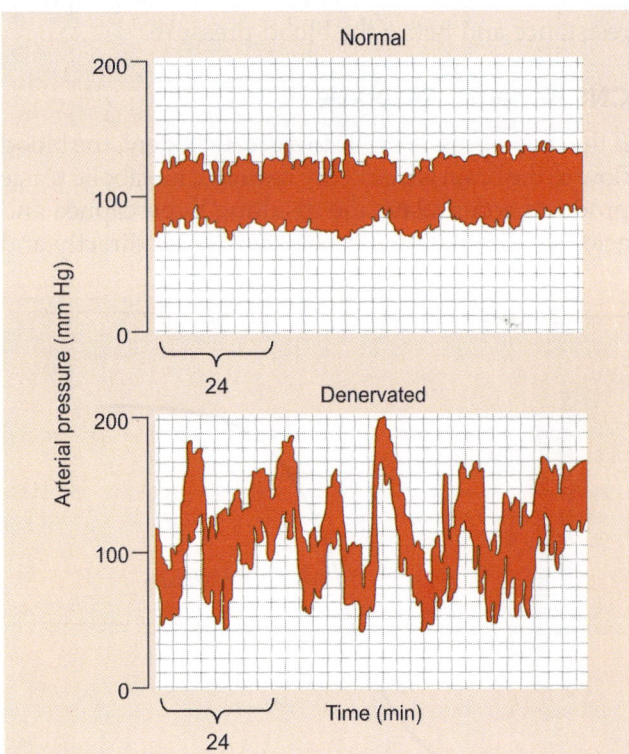

Fig. 3.39: Variation in blood pressure even under resting conditions when the carotid sinus baroreceptor area is denervated when compared to the normally innervated carotid sinus baroreceptor area

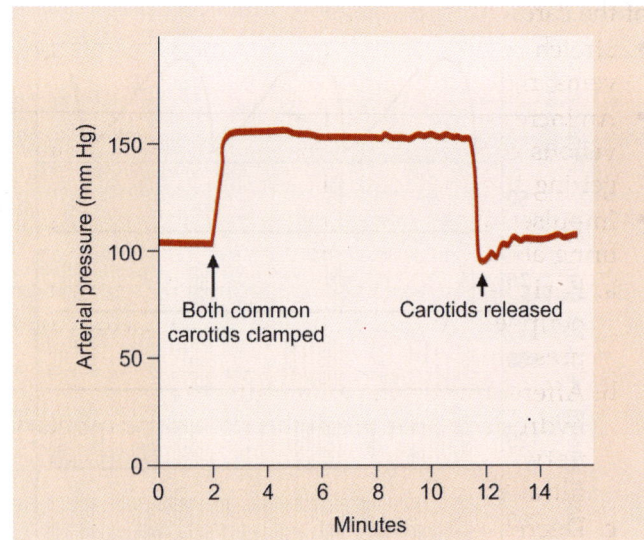

Fig. 3.40: Increase in blood pressure when the common carotids of both the sides are occluded thereby preventing blood flow through the carotid sinus and consequent non-stimulation of carotid sinus baroreceptors

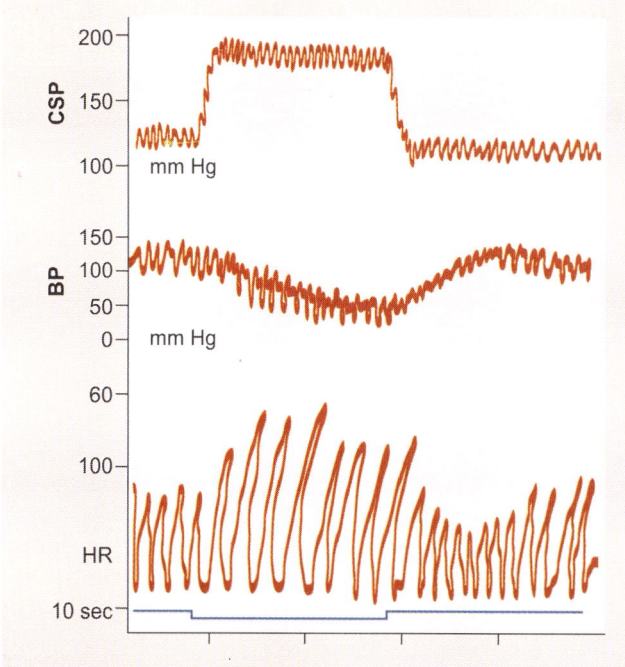

Fig. 3.41: Decrease in blood pressure and decrease in heart rate when the blood pressure in the carotid sinus region is increased

more powerfully. Peripheral blood vessels under go marked vasoconstriction and increases the blood pressure to a greater extent.

Stretch receptors present in the low pressure areas of the cardiovascular system:

- Stretch receptors are present in the walls of great veins, right atrium.
- An increase in the blood volume, distension of the venous compartment. This leads to the receptors getting stretched and stimulated.
- Impulses travel to the higher centers and reflexly bring about the following changes:
  a. Peripheral arteriolar dilation, decreased peripheral resistance, therefore, a fall in the blood pressure.
  b. Afferent arteriolar dilation leads to increased hydrostatic pressure in the glomerular capillary network leading to increased glomerular filtration rate and increase the fluid loss.
  c. Decreased release of ADH will increase the urinary output. This in turn decreases the blood volume and blood pressure.

Atrial natriuretic factor: A chemical substance released from the atrial muscle fibers due to distension

of the atrium. This can occur whenever the blood volume is increased or whenever the venous return is increased. Any time this hormone is released it brings about peripheral vasodilation, increased excretion of water and salt. This in turn decreases the blood pressure.

Factors Regulating Blood Pressure— Intermediate Mechanisms

Fluid shift mechanism: Any time the blood pressure falls, the pre-capillary sphincter contracts, this decreases the hydrostatic pressure in the capillaries. All along the capillaries, the colloidal osmotic pressure remains high and, therefore, the fluid shifts from the extravascular compartment to the intravascular compartment. This increases the blood volume and blood pressure.

Renin–angiotensin mechanism (Fig. 3.42): Decreased blood flow to the kidney due to a fall in the blood pressure will bring about the release of renin from the juxtaglomerular cells. This converts angiotensinogen to angiotensin I which is converted to angiotensin II. This is a powerful vasoconstrictor substance which brings about constriction of the arterioles, increasing the peripheral resistance and blood pressure. This mechanism also increases the production of aldosterone. This hormone acts on the renal tubules, increasing the reabsorption of salt and

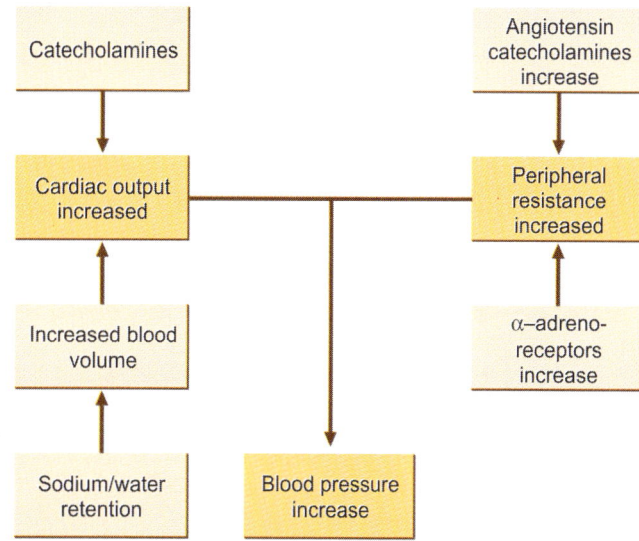

Fig. 3.42: Role of catecholamines and angiotensin in the regulation of blood pressure

water, increasing the blood volume and blood pressure.

ADH mechanism: Any time when the blood volume is increased, the blood pressure is increased. The volume receptors are stimulated. Impulses arising from these receptors reach the hypothalamus and inhibit the secretion of ADH. More amount of water is lost from the kidneys, lowering the blood volume and blood pressure.

Long-term Regulation of Blood Pressure

Kidneys play a very important role in the long-term regulation of blood pressure. Thus the fluid volume is maintained and, therefore, the blood volume and blood pressure is maintained.

Increased blood pressure in person with normal kidney excretes more of salt and water known as pressure natriuresis and pressure diuresis. The efficiency of the kidney in this respect is infinite (Fig. 3.43).

Baroreceptors of carotid sinus and aortic arch show the property of adaptation. Sustained increase in blood pressure occurs in essential hypertension. Sustained increase of blood pressure will lead to resetting of the baroreceptors due to the property of adaptation. Therefore, the baroreceptors fail to lower the blood pressure.

Regional Circulations

Cerebral Circulation

• Two internal carotid arteries
• Two vertebral arteries, which join to form basilar artery.
• Human brain weighs 1400 gm
• Blood flow to the brain = 750 ml/min.
• Venous drainage is through the internal jugular vein.
• The total volume of blood in the cranial region remains same all the time. If any part of the brain is more active, there will be redistribution of blood from less active region to more active regions (Fig. 3.44).
• Autoregulation of blood flow is well developed with respect to the cerebral circulation. Because of this, in spite of variation of blood pressure, the volume flow remains constant between a pressure range of 60 and 160 mm Hg.

Nerves supply to these blood vessels are the sympathetic postganglionic fibers. They have vasoconstrictor influence on cerebral blood vessels.

There is well-developed blood–brain barrier because of which certain substances present in the

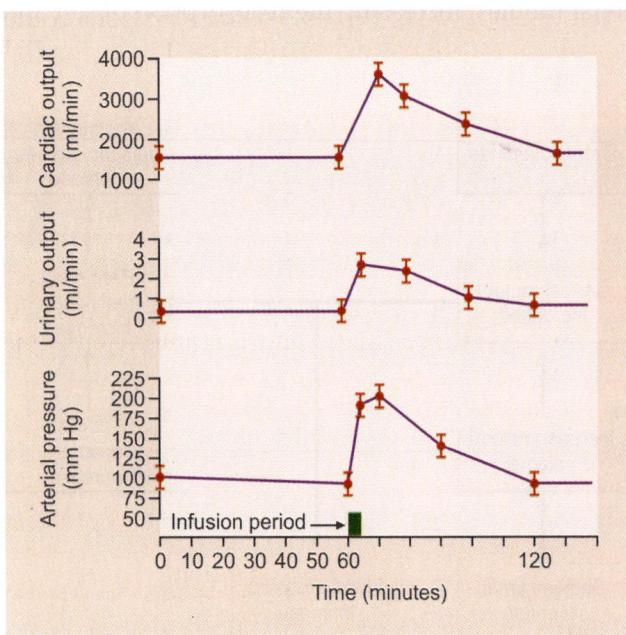

Fig. 3.43: Role of kidney in the regulation of blood pressure in long-term

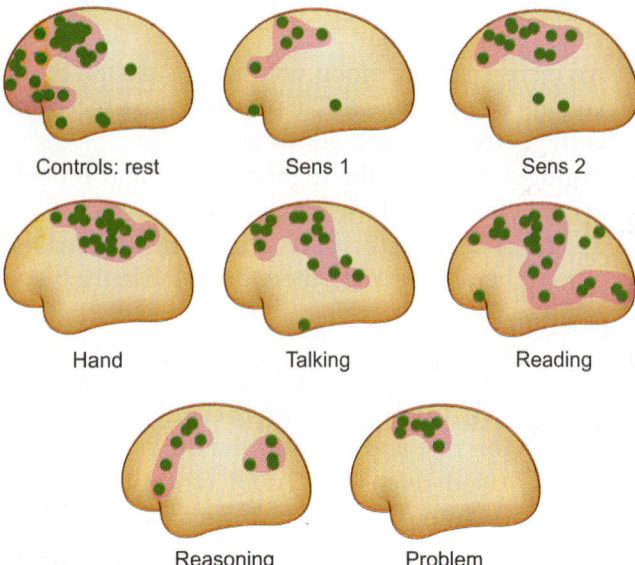

Fig. 3.44: Variation in the regional blood flow depending on the activity of certain part of brain

blood cannot reach brain and water, oxygen and carbon dioxide, etc., enter the brain with ease from the blood.

Factors influencing the substance penetrating the blood–brain (CSF) barrier:

1. Inversely related to the molecular weight of the substance
2. Directly related to the lipid solubility. Greater the lipid solubility greater is the penetration.

Determination of Blood Flow to the Brain (CBF)

1. By Kety's method
2. Fick's principle is employed

Substance of choice N_2O (nitrous oxide)

$$CBF \text{ (cerebral blood flow)} = \frac{Q}{A_C - V_C} \text{ ml/minute}$$

Wherein

Q is the quantity of nitrous oxide taken up by brain tissue.

A_C is the concentration of the substance in arterial blood.

V_C is the concentration of substance in venous blood.

Regulation of Blood Flow

1. Increased carbon dioxide tension (increased pCO_2) is the most important factor.
   - CO_2 is a power full vasodilator of the cerebral blood vessels. Increasing the CO_2 content of the inspired air (3–5%) almost doubles the blood flow to the brain. Voluntary hyperventilation decreases the pCO_2, and brings about vasoconstriction and decreases the cerebral blood flow. This gives rise to dizziness.
2. Increased H^+ concentration of the CSF increases the cerebral blood flow.
3. Hypoxia (decreased pO_2) also increases the cerebral blood flow.
4. A rise in the intracranial tension compresses the blood vessels supplying the brain. This decreases the cerebral blood flow (Monro-Kellie doctrine).
5. Stimulation of sympathetic/parasympathetic never fibers has very little effect on cerebral blood flow.

Monro-Kellie doctrine: Since the three compartments are placed in rigid box (cranium) expansion of any one of the compartment can occur only at the expense of compromise of the other two compartments. When the CSF compartment expands (due to increased accumulation of CSF) the vascular compartment is pressed upon. This decreases cerebral blood flow.

Coronary Blood Flow

- Blood flow through the coronaries supplies the heart muscle (myocardium).
- The right and the left coronary arteries take their origin from the root of the aorta.
- Normal coronary arterial blood flow is about 250 ml/minute.
- Arteriovenous oxygen difference is highest even under resting conditions. It is about 14 ml (20–6 ml)/100 ml.
- Therefore, whenever there is an increased demand for oxygen by the heart muscle it is met with only by increasing the coronary blood flow.
- The venous blood from the myocardium is drained into the coronary sinus and the anterior cardiac veins.
- There is variation in blood flow during cardiac cycle. More blood flows through the coronary vessels during ventricular diastole than during systole. This is more so with respect to left coronary artery (Fig. 3.45).
- The volume flow variation is more phasic in the endocardial region when compared to epicardial region.

Determination of Coronary Blood Flow

- By applying Fick's principle.
- Nitrous oxide is the substance of choice. Radioisotope thalium (Tl-201) can also be used.
- The venous blood from the myocardium is drained into the coronary sinus and the anterior cardiac veins.

$$CBF \text{ (coronary blood flow)} = \frac{Q}{A_C - V_C} \text{ ml/minute}$$

Wherein

Q is the quantity of nitrous oxide taken up by brain tissue.

A_C is the concentration of the substance in arterial blood.

V_C is the concentration of substance in venous blood.

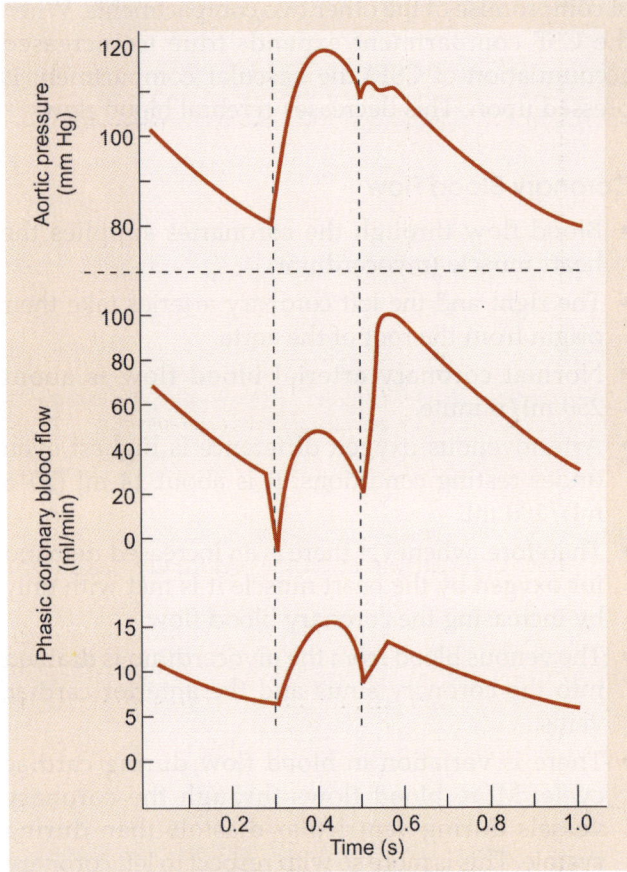

Fig. 3.45: Phases of cardiac cycle and blood flow through the right and left coronary arteries

Factors Influencing the Blood Flow

1. Coronary blood flow is subjected to an auto-regulation.
2. The pressure head (aortic pressure minus coronary sinus pressure)
3. Phasic blood flow
4. Chemical factors (blood gases), the most important one being the oxygen supply (hypoxia) and decreasing in oxygen tension (fall in pO_2). Any hypoxic situation will be promptly followed by an increase in blood flow.
5. Sympathetic stimulation

Left Coronary Flow

- During isometric contraction phase as the intraventricular pressure is suddenly increasing, the blood vessels are compressed upon and, therefore, the blood flow decreases.

- During maximum and reduced ejection phase, the cardiac muscle fibers contract and the intra-ventricular pressure increases to 120 mm Hg. The endocardial blood vessels are compressed and hence blood flow decreases.
- During the same time epicardial blood vessels are not compressed to a great extent. The total blood flow remains low (about 40 ml/minute)
- During diastole, as the intraventricular pressure rapidly falls, the compressor force on the blood vessels decreases and this leads to an increase in blood flow.

Right coronary arterial blood flow remains high both during ventricular systole and diastole, because the blood vessels supplying the right heart are not subjected to greater compression. This is because the pressure changes in the right ventricle during a cardiac cycle remains low (10–25 mm Hg).

Chemical Factors

Mechanism involved:

1. Hypoxia produced leads to production of adenosine an end product of anaerobic metabolism and adenosine is a powerful vasodilator substance to the coronary blood vessels. The effect of hypoxia is not direct one but it is through the production of adenosine.
2. An increase in pCO_2 or an increase in H^+ will also bring about coronary vasodilatation, and increase in the blood flow.

Sympathetic Stimulation (Fig. 3.46)

Coronary arteries contain both and receptors. Stimulation of receptors will bring about coronary

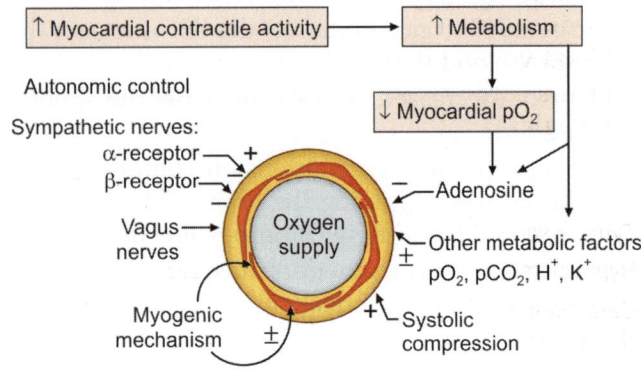

Fig. 3.46: Factors affecting the lumen diameter of coronary vessels

vasoconstriction. Stimulation of receptor results in coronary vasodilatation. However, stimulation of sympathetic fibers to the heart is associated with coronary vasodilatation. Sympathetic fiber stimulation to the heart increases the force of contraction and, therefore, metabolism of the cardiac musculature. Metabolic end products bring about coronary vasodilatation. Therefore, the net effect of sympathetic stimulation is coronary vasodilatation and increase in blood flow.

Acetylcholine (ACh): Parasympathetic (ACh is the neurotransmitter liberated by these nerve terminals) nerve stimulation is associated with coronary vasodilatation and increase in the blood flow. Other coronary vasodilators include:

• Potassium
• Lactate
• Prostaglandin
• And NO (nitric oxide), nitroglycerin, nitrates are used clinically as coronary vasodilators.

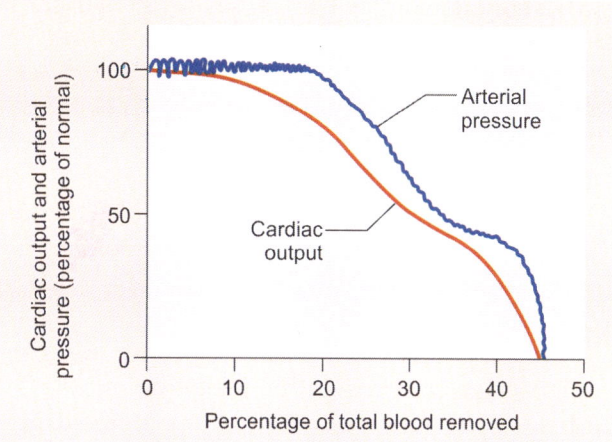

Fig. 3.47: Fall in cardiac output and blood pressure consequent to experimental decrease in blood volume

CARDIOVASCULAR SHOCK

Shock is defined as lack of tissue perfusion which occurs when there is an imbalance between the volume of blood present in the circulatory system and the capacity of the circulatory system itself.

Types of Shock (Table 3.12)

1. *Hypovolemic (hemorrhagic shock)* is due to loss of blood or body fluids, the remaining volume of the blood are not sufficient to fill the system and supply oxygen to the tissues (Fig. 3.47).
2. *Neurogenic shock* is loss of sympathetic tone resulting in vasodilatation. The volume of the cardiovascular system is increased. However, the blood volume remains normal, since the capacity of the cardio vascular system is increased even though the blood volume remains normal it is not

sufficient to fill the system completely, therefore, the blood pressure falls.

3. *Cardiogenic shock* is due to sudden failure of the left ventricle, which is unable to pump the blood into systemic circulation. This occurs usually in myocardial infarction or ventricular fibrillation.
4. *Anaphylactic shock* is a very severe type shock often occurs during allergic reaction. The antigen antibody reaction brings about release of histamine, which is a very powerful vasodilator substance. This results in vasodilatation of the all the blood vessels, decreased peripheral resistance and, therefore, a profound fall in the blood pressure.
5. *Septic shock* is due to the release of the endotoxins from gram-negative bacteria. Endotoxins are very powerful vasodilator substance resulting in fall in blood pressure. This is usually associated with very high body temperature (fever).

Signs and Symptoms of Shock

In hypovolemic shock, the patient is apprehensive, stuporous, and highly talkative; reticular formation is inhibited due to accumulation of metabolites (lactic

Table 3.12: Pathophysiology of shocks and the clinical conditions when occur		
Type of shock	*Pathophysiology*	*Clinical examples*
Hypovolemic	Decreased blood volume	Hemorrhage, vomiting, burns, diarrhea, dehydration
Cardiogenic	*Pump failure*	*MI, arrhythmia*
Neurogenic	Loss of Symp. NS activity	Trauma involving spinal cord, brainstem
Septicemic	*Bacterial infection*	*Gram-negative bacteria*
Anaphylactic	Histamine release	Type I hypersensitivity

acid) or stimulated due to increased catecholamine in the blood.

1. Skin—cold and clammy due to peripheral vasoconstriction and sweating
2. Pulse—rapid and thready
3. Respiration—shallow and hurried
4. Blood pressure is usually decreased or it may remain normal, if compensatory mechanism has already set in.
5. Tongue becomes dry, eyes sunken.
6. There may not be any visible bleeding (bleeding might have occurred within the body).
7. Muscle tone is reduced, feeling of extreme degree of fatigue or weakness.
8. Patient repeatedly asks for water (thirsty).
9. Urinary output may be markedly decreased (oliguria) or not at all (anuria).

Stages of Shock

a. Non-progressive or reversible or compensatory shock
b. Progressive or irreversible or non-compensatory shock.

Compensatory Shock

Signs and symptoms of shock are seen but given time the compensatory mechanisms come into play and blood pressure returns to normal and the person recovers. Compensatory mechanisms try to restore the blood volume and the blood pressure.

Compensatory mechanisms to restore the blood pressure include:

1. Baroreceptor mechanism
2. Chemoreceptor mechanism
3. CNS ischemic response
4. Secretion of various hormones, like ADH, renin, angiotensin, aldosterone, adrenaline, noradrenaline, etc.
5. The sympathetic system is very powerfully stimulated. All these mechanisms are geared to restore the blood pressure rather than to restore the cardiac output (this can be made out from the above diagram) (Fig. 3.48).

The blood volume is restored back to normal relatively slowly. Components of the blood (RBCs, WBCs and platelets) are restored within a few weeks. If the volume of blood lost is too much, the

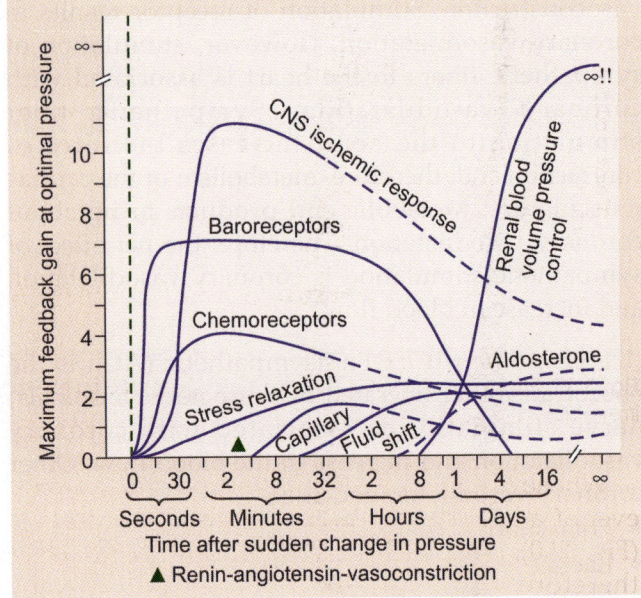

Fig. 3.48: Composite graph showing various mechanisms involved in the maintenance of blood pressure depending on the time factor

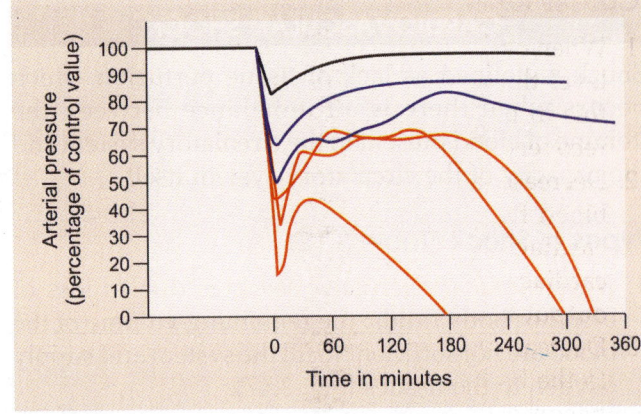

Fig. 3.49: Extent of fall of blood pressure following decrease in the blood volume

compensatory mechanisms fail to restore the blood pressure. Hence the shock becomes progressive and may become irreversible (Fig. 3.49).

In the first three sets of dogs, the fall in blood volume and blood pressure is progressively increased. However, given time all the three sets of animals recover. In the IV, V and VI sets, the fall in the blood volume and blood pressure is comparatively much greater. The compensatory mechanisms try to restore the blood pressure. In spite of this, due to a much greater fall in blood pressure, tissues deterioration has occurred to such an extent that the animals ultimately die.

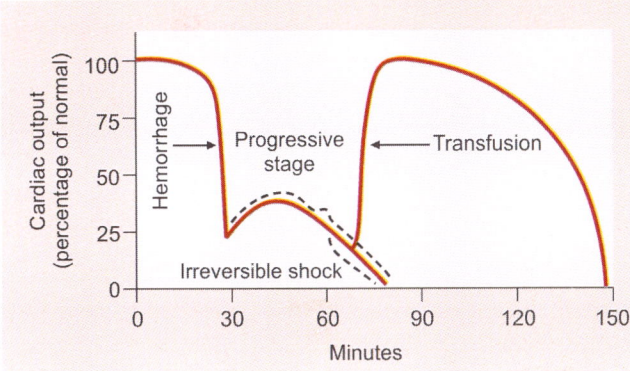

Fig. 3.50: Effect of transfusion when the animal has gone into irreversible stage of shock

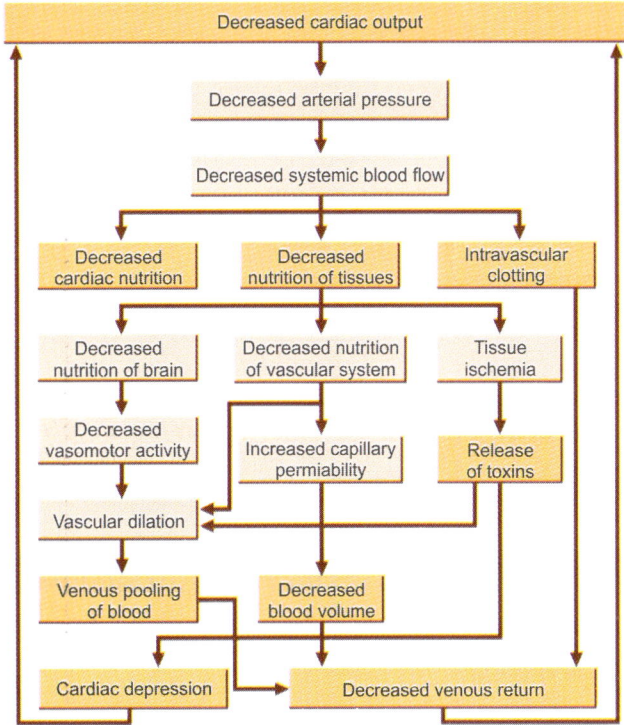

Fig. 3.51: The events occurring in irreversible stage of shock

Whenever the progressive stage of shock sets in, even if a blood transfusion is done after a time lag (Fig. 3.50), it fails to restore the blood pressure. And, therefore, the animal dies. Hence the dictum is whenever shock is diagnosed; the treatment must be started without any further wastage of time.

Causes for Irreversibility (Fig. 3.51)

1. When once the blood pressure falls below a critical level the positive feedback mechanisms develop, this in turn decreases the blood pressure further, recovery becomes impossible.
2. Decrease in cardiac output decreases the coronary blood flow. Because of this, oxygen supply to the cardiac muscle suffers. This in turn makes the cardiac contraction weaker decreasing the cardiac output further.
3. Decreased blood pressure decreases the blood flow to the brain resulting in hypoxia of the brain and vasomotor center. Vasomotor center function deteriorates resulting in peripheral vasodilatation giving rise to a further fall in blood pressure. This fall in blood pressure further decreases the blood flow to brain.
4. Nutrition and oxygen supply to the capillary endothelial lining cells is decreased resulting in damage to these cells. Fluid from the capillary leaves to the extravascular compartment, decreasing the blood volume and decreasing the blood pressure.
5. Metabolic waste like lactic acid accumulates in the tissues. This acts on the heart, depressing the myocardial contraction.
6. Inhibition of sodium–potassium pump leads to altered cell membrane permeability.
7. Endotoxins from the gastrointestinal tract enter the circulation. These are powerful vasodilators and they also are toxic to the myocardium.

When once irreversibility sets in, any amount of treatment may be in the form of blood transfusion becomes useless. Therefore, treatment should be commenced at the earliest.

Treatment of Shock

If the cause is blood loss, blood transfusion is must. If the blood is not available then plasma expanders must be used.

In hypovolemic shock, noradrenaline administration is not beneficial because the sympathetic system is already maximally stimulated releasing lot of noradrenaline. In fact, it may do more harm than good because if the blood vessels remain contracted for long time, nutrition of the endothelial cells becomes defective and they suffer.

Vasoconstriction decreases the renal perfusion pressure leading to decreased formation of urine. Toxic materials will accumulate of which urea is the most important. This substance has deleterious effect on the brain.

Dopamine is more beneficial because it brings about renal vasodilatation; it has a positive inotropic effect on the heart. Oxygen may be useful in some cases.

Raising the foot end of the cot is beneficial. It facilitates the blood flow to the brain.

The following things are not to be done:

1. Trying to keep the patient warm by covering the patient with woolen blankets because this will induce peripheral vasodilatation, increase the blood flow to skin and decrease the blood flow to vital organs.

2. Hanging the patient or hold the patient feet end up trying to improve the blood flow to the brain. The diaphragm will not be in a position to contract properly and this will decrease pulmonary ventilation.

AUTOREGULATION OF BLOOD FLOW

Mean arterial pressure determines the blood flow through the vascular region. At the level of organ or tissue, it is the perfusion pressure, which is nothing but pressure difference between the beginning of the flow (P_1, arterial end pressure) and at the end of flow (P_2, venous pressure). There is a direct relationship between this perfusion pressure ($P_1 - P_2$) and the blood flow. In most of the tissues or organs, the pressure difference ($P_1 - P_2$) will be around 70 mm Hg.

Organs and tissues in which autoregulation of blood flow occurs are:

1. Coronary flow (blood flow through the myocardium)
2. Cerebral flow (blood flow through brain)
3. Renal flow (blood flow through kidney)
4. Skeletal blood flow, etc.

The above organs have well-developed autoregulatory mechanism to maintain the flow constant within a particular range of pressure. This is termed as autoregulation of blood flow.

By definition, autoregulation of blood flow states that it is the ability of an organ or tissue to regulate its own blood flow despite a change in blood pressure.

Critical Closing Pressure/
Critical Opening pressure (Fig. 3.52)

Critical closing pressure is the minimum mean arterial pressure that is essential to keep the arteries in a distended state. If the pressure in the vessel is below the minimal value, the blood vessels collapse. Normally, the critical closing pressure is around 20 mm Hg. Below this pressure, since the blood vessels

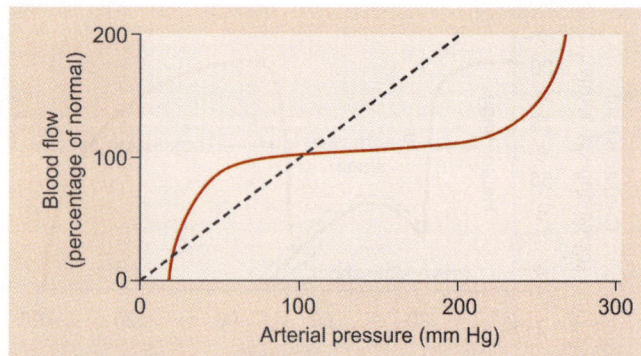

Fig. 3.52: Flow of blood in a rigid tube (hatched lines) and flow of blood through blood vessel (solid line)

collapse, the blood flow through the organ stops completely.

As the pressure increases above the critical closing pressure, the volume of blood flow also increases proportionately till a limit. So they will have a direct relationship. However, when once the pressure exceeds a particular value, in spite of an increase in pressure, there will not be any further increase in blood flow. This is termed as autoregulatory ability of the organ to regulate the blood flow.

Most of the organs have the ability to autoregulate their flow between a pressure range of 60 and 180 mm Hg. Beyond 180 mm Hg, the autoregulatory mechanisms fail and hence there would be further increase of blood flow proportionate to the increase in pressure. Autoregulation of blood flow is seen even in a denervated isolated organ. This suggests that the nerve supply is not responsible for autoregulation mechanism.

There are many theories which try to explain the mechanism of autoregulation. They are:

1. Myogenic theory
2. Tissue metabolite theory
3. Tissue fluid pressure theory
4. Renin–angiotensin theory, etc. (this theory is applicable only in kidneys)

Myogenic Theory (Fig. 3.53)

According to this theory:

- When there is an increase in pressure, initially there will be an increase of blood flow.
- When blood flow increases, the smooth muscles present in the walls of the blood vessels get stretched.
- The stretching of the muscle will act as a stimulus (mechanical stimulus) to the muscle.

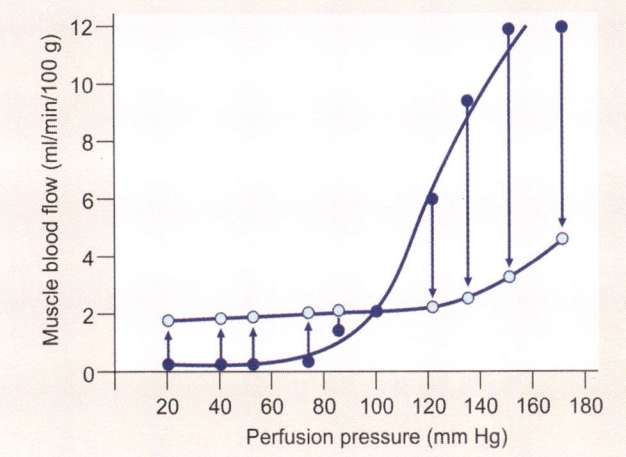

Fig. 3.53: Autoregulation of blood flow based on myogenic theory

- The muscle starts responding to the stimulus by contracting.
- Contraction results in the narrowing of the lumen diameter. Decreased lumen diameter increases the resistance to the flow (decrease in the radius of the lumen) and restricts the increase in the flow.
- Greater is the stretch; greater is the contraction of the smooth muscle fibers. Therefore, the total blood flow remains the same.

The role of myogenic theory in regulation of blood flow can be experimentally proved. When papavarine is injected, papavarine brings about the paralysis of smooth muscles. Hence, after injection of papavarine, when the perfusion pressure is increased, there will be increase of blood flow without any autoregulation. It proves the role of smooth muscle fibers of blood vessels in the auto regulatory mechanism. This theory holds good for almost all organs.

Tissue Metabolite Theory

- At any given time, there will be some amount of metabolites in the tissues, e.g. the pCO_2 in the tissues will be generally around 45 mm Hg.
- These metabolites exert vasodilator effect. Hence some amount of vasodilatation is maintained by these metabolites.
- When there is increase in perfusion pressure, to start with, there will be slight increase of blood flow.
- This brings about increased washout of metabolites from the tissues.
- So the concentration of metabolites in the tissue is reduced.

- This reduces the vasodilator effect and leads to a little more vasoconstriction.
- Decreased lumen diameter will regulate the blood flow.

This theory holds good for all organs.

Tissue Fluid Pressure Theory

- There will be constant movement of fluids between blood and tissues at the level of capillaries.
- Exchange of fluid occurs at the level of capillaries because of the capillary dynamics.
- When there is increase of perfusion pressure, initially there will be increase of blood flow.
- This increases the hydrostatic pressure both at the arterial and venous end of capillaries.
- Because of this, more fluid goes out at the arterial end of the capillary and less fluid returns at the venous end of the capillaries.
- This leads to increased accumulation of fluid in the tissue spaces.
- This in turn leads to compression of blood vessels.
- So blood flow is regulated.

This theory is applicable in the case of encapsulated organs, like kidney, liver, etc.

Renin–Angiotensin Theory

- When there is increase in perfusion pressure, there will be increase of blood flow to the kidney.
- This increases the filtration pressure in the nephrons.
- So the volume of filtrate is more in the nephrons.
- Because of this, more sodium will reach the distal convoluted tubules in the nephrons.
- The amount of sodium reaching the distal convoluted tubules will be sensed by the macula densa of distal convoluted tubules.
- This leads to more renin getting released from juxta-glomerular cells.
- Renin acts on angiotensinogen present locally and brings about formation of angiotensin I.
- This angiotensin I is converted to angiotensin II (by converting enzyme present in the endothelial cell lining the blood vessels).
- Increased angiotensin II brings about the constriction of the arterioles (especially the afferent arteriole) in the kidneys.
- This decreases the lumen diameter and the blood flow to the kidney is regulated.

This theory is applicable only to the kidneys.

4

Respiratory System

Introduction

The respiratory system is concerned with delivery of oxygen from the atmosphere to tissues and excretion of carbon dioxide from the tissues to atmosphere. Oxygen diffuses into blood from the alveoli and at the same time carbon dioxide is evolved out of blood into lungs. Exchange of gases at the level of lungs is known as external respiration.

At the level of tissues, the reversal occurs. Oxygen diffuses into tissues from blood and at the same time carbon dioxide diffuses into blood from the tissues. This is known as internal respiration (Fig. 4.1).

Respiratory Tract

Parts of respiratory system starting from the nasal apertures, extends through pharynx, larynx, trachea, bronchi, bronchioles and into alveoli. Alveolus is the structural and functional unit of respiratory system. The part extending from the nasal apertures up to terminal bronchioles forms the respiratory tract and is known as conducting zone. This region is also known as anatomical dead space (Fig. 4.2).

The concept of dead space is part of respiratory system in which in spite of air being present, it does not take part in exchange of respiratory gases. The normal anatomical dead space volume (DSV) is about 150 ml.

Functions of Upper Respiratory Tract (Fig. 4.2)

1. Warming up of air, as the temperature of air reaching the alveoli should be brought to body temperature, for better diffusion of gas.
2. The epithelial cells lining the respiratory tract add on water molecules to the air getting into the alveoli. This is known as humidifying of air.
3. Filtration of air is essential before the air reaches alveoli. Partial filtration of dust particles will be taking place due to the presence of hairs in the nose

Fig. 4.1: The areas of external and internal respiration

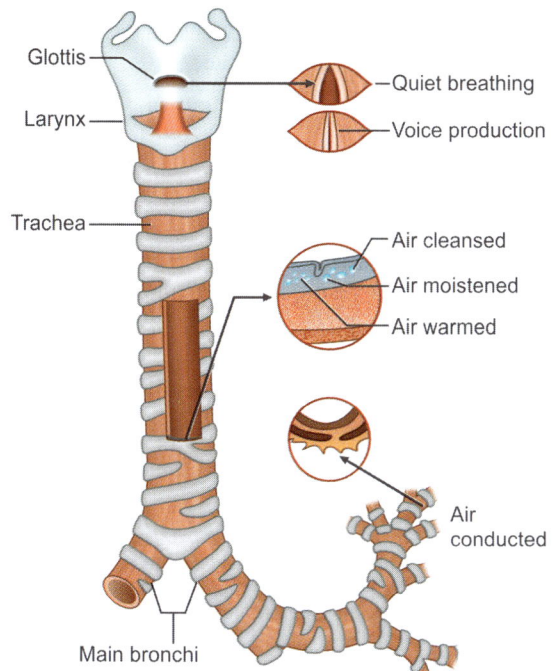

Fig. 4.2: Parts of respiratory tract (that is a dead space region) showing various functions of the tract while air is passing through

Glottis

Larynx

Trachea

Quiet breathing

Voice production

Air cleansed

Air moistened

Air warmed

Air conducted

Main bronchi

and also because of the ciliated cells on which a layer of mucus is present.

All the aforesaid aspects in general are known as air conditioning. In addition to this, the passage of air through the larynx is responsible for production of sound.

Functions of respiratory system can be broadly classified into:

a. Respiratory

b. Non-respiratory.

Respiratory Function

It is to provide adequate volume of oxygen to the tissues. Normal person at rest needs about 250 ml of oxygen per minute. Atmospheric air enters the lungs during inspiration. Oxygen from the air diffuses through the alveoli into pulmonary capillary blood. The oxygenated blood reaches the left ventricle and from there it gets pumped to reach all parts of the body.

About 200 ml of carbon dioxide is produced in the body every minute because of tissue metabolism. From the tissues, carbon dioxide enters the blood to reach the lungs for the process of excretion. When deoxygenated blood reaches the lungs, carbon dioxide

gets diffused from the pulmonary capillaries into the alveoli. The air from the alveoli is expelled out from the lungs by the process of expiration.

Non-respiratory Functions

1. Regulation of acid-base (pH) balance.
2. Mast cells present in the lungs produce heparin, which acts as an anticoagulant.
3. Macrophages in the alveoli have phagocytic function.
4. Converting enzyme present in the lungs play a role in converting angiotensin I to angiotensin II, which is a powerful vasoconstrictor.
5. The passage of the air through the larynx is essential for vocalization and has role in communication by speech.
6. Plays a minor role in body temperature regulation.

Parts of Respiratory System

Nose

a. Hairs are present in the nasal cavity. These hairs serve to filter the air that is entering the respiratory system. Any particle whose size is more than 6 μ gets filtered in the nose.

b. The mucous membrane of the nose is highly vascular. As the air passes through the nose, it gets:

 i. Warmed up to the body temperature,

 ii. Its water vapor content is also increased. This is essential because if dry air passes through the trachea, it may lead to drying up of the trachea and it can produce a cough reflex.

Trachea

a. It is made up of a number of incomplete cartilaginous rings, which prevent the trachea from kinking when the neck is rotated. The posterior 1/6th of the trachea is free from cartilage and is made up of fibrous tissue, which permits certain amount of expansion of trachea during inspiration.

b. The trachea is lined by ciliated columnar epithelium. Underneath this lining, lot of goblet cells are present. These goblet cells secrete certain amount of mucus. The particles which escape filtration at nose, get trapped in the mucus present here and swept towards the nose by the movements of the cilia. These particles are get rid off from the body by the process of coughing. Some of the finest

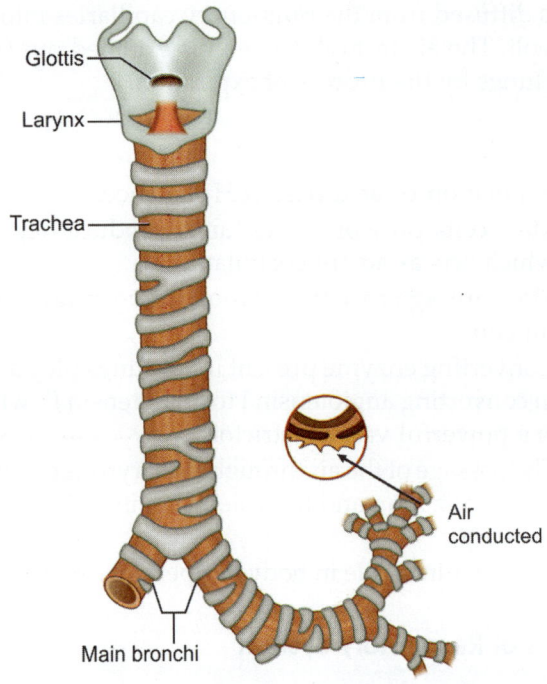

Fig. 4.3: The branching of bronchi from the trachea

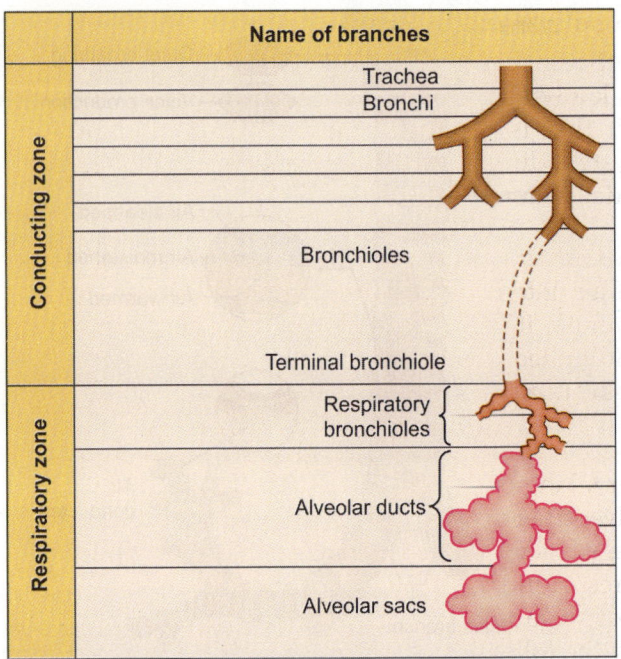

Fig. 4.4: Branching of airways until the alveoli

particles may escape from getting filtered here and reach alveoli. They are removed by the macrophages lining of the alveoli or the parenchyma of the lungs.

The trachea divides into right and left bronchi (Fig. 4.3). The branching of the trachea is the most sensitive part of the tracheobronchial tree. The right bronchus is larger than the left and the angle at which it originates from the trachea is also less acute. Because of this reason, any foreign body entering the trachea is found more commonly in the right lung than in the left.

Bronchi

The bronchi, which are the branches of the trachea, divide further. These branches are called as lobar bronchi that again divide into segmental bronchi. As the branching proceeds, the amount of cartilage present in the walls goes on decreasing. They also acquire a coat of smooth muscle fibers. These smooth muscle fibers are supplied by both sympathetic and parasympathetic nerve fibers. Sympathetic nerve stimulation or administration of sympathomimetic drugs (adrenaline) brings about relaxation of smooth muscle and hence bronchodilation. This leads to decrease of the airway resistance. This knowledge is useful in the treatment of bronchial asthma. Parasympathetic nerve stimulation brings about bronchoconstriction.

The bronchi divide to form bronchioles. These bronchioles further divide to form terminal and respiratory bronchioles. The respiratory bronchioles lead to alveolar duct and finally into the alveoli (Fig. 4.4).

Changes that occur as the branching proceeds from trachea to bronchioles:

1. The cross-sectional area goes on increasing. The branching decreases the resistance offered to the flow of airflow (particularly during inspiration).
2. The amount of cartilaginous tissue also goes on decreasing to be replaced by smooth muscle fibers.
3. The mucous membrane which is lined by columnar ciliated epithelium is changed to flattened nonciliated at the level of alveoli.

Flattened epithelial cells line the alveoli. Alveolus is approximately 70–300 µ in diameter. The total surface area of all the alveoli together will be approximately 70 m^2. At any given time approximately 60–80 ml of blood will be present in the capillaries surrounding the alveoli. Therefore, any given time about 1 ml of blood is spread over 1 m^2. This facilitates rapid exchange of gases between air in alveoli and blood in pulmonary capillaries.

Normal respiratory rate is about 12–16/min and is known as rate of respiration (RR). The volume of air that is taken in or expired out of respiratory system during a normal quiet breathing is known as tidal volume and is about 500 ml.

Pulmonary ventilation: It is defined as the volume of air entering or leaving the respiratory system per minute. It is the product of rate of respiration (RR) multiplied by tidal volume (TV), which is about 6 L/min (12 × 500 = 6000 ml/min).

Alveolar ventilation: It is defined as the volume of air taking part in the exchange of gases at the level of alveoli per minute. As stated already, the alveolar area region is where the exchange of gas occurs but the air present in the conducting zone does not take part in exchange of gases (dead space air). It can be calculated by the following formula:

$$\text{Alveolar ventilation} = RR \times (TV - DSV)$$
$$= 12 \times (500 - 150)$$
$$= 4200 \text{ ml/min}$$

RR—rate of respiration
TV—tidal volume
DSV—dead space volume

Covering of the Lungs

The lungs are covered by pleura that are closely adherent to the surface of the lung tissue. This layer of pleura is known as visceral pleura. Another layer of pleura adheres to the inner surface of the wall of the thorax. This layer is known as parietal pleura. A thin film of fluid is present between the two layers of pleura in the potential space known as pleural space. This fluid keeps the pleural layers adherent to each other. The two layers cannot be separated but can slide over one on the other. In animals, introduction of needle into the pleural space allows us to record the pressure in the intrapleural space. In the case of human beings, it can be measured from the lower one-third of esophagus by balloon technique. Normally intrapleural pressure is always negative (less than the atmospheric pressure). Sometime the pleural space may get filled with fluid/air giving rise to pleural effusion and pneumothorax, respectively.

Mechanics of Respiration

Respiration has two phases namely inspiration and expiration. During normal quiet inspiration due to contraction of muscles of inspiration, the chest and lungs expand. The pressure inside the alveoli (intra-alveolar pressure) falls below the atmospheric pressure. Due to the pressure gradient developed in the direction of the alveolus, air moves from the atmosphere into the lungs. Because inspiration is brought about by the contraction of the muscles, the process of inspiration is an active one.

However, the process of expiration is normally a passive process. The relaxation of the muscles of inspiration and the recoiling of the elastic fibers present in the lungs is more than enough to bring about the expiration. During expiration, since the alveoli are trying to recoil, the intra-alveolar pressure becomes more than the atmospheric pressure and hence air can be driven out of the lungs into the atmosphere. In forced expiratory states, expiration needs the active contraction of certain muscles. Hence in such states even expiration becomes an active process.

Muscles of inspiration: Diaphragm and external intercostals are the muscles of inspiration during a normal quiet breathing. However, during forced inspiration, contraction of sternocleidomastoid, scalene, serratus anterior and platysma muscles is very much required. These muscles are known as accessory muscles of inspiration.

Muscles of expiration: The normal quiet expiration is a passive process. However, in forced expiration, even this phase becomes an active process and requires active contraction of certain muscles. The muscles that are involved in forced expiration are known as accessory muscles of expiration and they are internal intercostals and muscles of the anterior abdominal wall.

Thorax is separated from the abdominal cavity by the diaphragm, a dome-shaped muscle. The thorax has three different diameters namely vertical, transverse and anteroposterior. During inspiration, the thoracic volume gets increased because of increase in the diameters of chest. The increase in the thoracic volume decreases the intra-alveolar pressure.

The most important muscle of inspiration is diaphragm supplied by the phrenic nerve. This is responsible for about 70% increase in the thoracic volume and the rest volume increase in thorax is contributed by the contraction of external intercostals supplied by the intercostal nerves. This type of respiration is called as abdominothoracic type. In case the external intercostals play a major role in expansion of thorax, the type of respiration is known as thoraco-abdominal type.

Contraction of the diaphragm alters the vertical diameter whereas the contraction of the external intercostals increases the anteroposterior and transverse diameters of the thoracic cavity.

Intrapleural and Intra-alveolar Pressure (Fig. 4.5)

Intrapleural Pressure

- It is the pressure that is prevalent in the pleural space.
- It is always sub-atmospheric (less than 760 mm Hg).
- At the beginning of inspiration, it is minus 3 mm Hg (3 mm Hg less than the atmospheric pressure).
- As the inspiration proceeds, it becomes more negative and in normal quiet inspiration, it reaches a value of about minus 6 mm Hg at the end of inspiration.

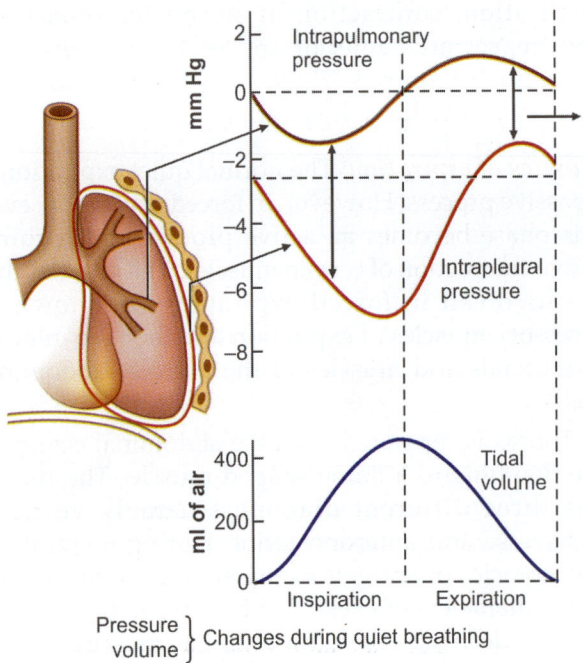

Fig. 4.5: Graph of intrapleural and intra-alveolar (intrapulmonary) pressures tidal volume during a normal quiet respiration

- During expiration, it becomes less negative as the expiration proceeds. And reaches minus 3 mm Hg at the end of expiration.
- During forced inspiration, it becomes much more negative and can be as low as minus 60 mm Hg.
- When there is forced expiration against closed glottis (as occurs in coughing, sneezing, etc.), the pressure can become positive and can be as high as plus 40 mm Hg.
- During inspiration, as the chest wall expands, the two layers of pleura have a tendency to recoil in the opposing directions. The visceral pleura along with the lungs tend to recoil in the direction of the hilum of the lungs and the parietal pleura towards the chest wall. This makes the intrapleural pressure to become more negative. When the inspiration becomes deeper, the recoiling tendency becomes greater because of further increase in the expansion of the alveoli. The intrapleural pressure becomes more negative in forced inspiration.
- The intrapleural pressure can be measured in animals by introduction of needle into the pleural space and connecting it to a manometer. In the case of human beings, it can be recorded by introduction of balloon into the lower one-third of esophagus.

Significance or Functions of Negative Intrapleural Pressure

1. Facilitates the venous return from dependent parts of the body into the heart.
2. Maintains the patency of bronchioles both during inspiration and expiration and decreases airway resistance during inspiration.
3. This decreases the intra-alveolar pressure, which facilitates air entry into the alveoli.
4. Prevents the collapsing tendency of the alveoli.
5. Facilitates lymph flow.

Pressure Changes in the Alveoli during Respiration

- Alveoli are connected to the atmosphere outside the body through the respiratory tract. The entry or exit of air through this tract is always in the direction of the pressure gradient (along a pressure gradient).
- The pressure recorded from the alveoli is known as intra-alveolar pressure.

- At the beginning of inspiration, the pressure is 0 mm Hg. As the inspiration proceeds, it becomes negative. It can be as little as minus 1 or 2 mm Hg by mid-inspiration. During the later part of inspiration, it starts becoming less negative and at the end of inspiration, it will be 0 mm Hg once again.
- The pressure gradient during inspiration facilitates the entry of air from atmosphere into the alveoli.
- The accumulation of air in the alveoli, gradually makes the pressure to become less negative and at the end of inspiration it becomes 0 mm Hg. This puts an end to the pressure gradient and hence air entry into the alveoli ceases.
- The recoiling tendency of the alveoli during expiration brings about the compression of air present in the alveoli. This increases the intra-alveolar pressure and becomes positive (more than the atmospheric pressure), and it can be as much as plus 1 or 2 mm Hg by mid-expiration. This forces air from the alveoli into the atmosphere. As the air moves out of the alveoli, the pressure inside decreases and at the end of expiration the pressure returns to 0 mm Hg. Pressure gradient ceases and hence expiration comes to an end.

Lung Compliance (Fig. 4.6)

- It is the change in the volume of lungs per unit change in transpulmonary pressure (pressure difference between intrapleural and intra-alveolar compartments).
- The unit being cm H_2O for pressure and ml for the volume.
- It is about 130 ml per cm H_2O pressure (for lungs and chest wall put together).
- It is about 200 ml per cm H_2O for lungs alone.
- When it is plotted in the form of graph for inspiratory and expiratory phases, the curves will not overlap but bring about the formation of hysteresis loop. It is due to a change in the elastic property of the lungs and chest walls.

Factors influencing the compliance of the lungs are:
a. Presence or absence of surfactant
b. Initial lung volume
c. Posture

Compliance of lung decreases in conditions, namely:
1. Pulmonary edema.

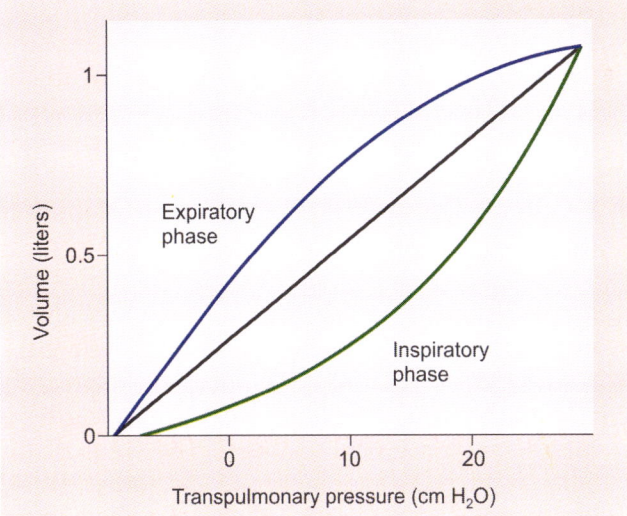

Fig. 4.6: Compliance of lungs during inspiration and expiration phases

2. Fibrosis.
3. Atelectasis.
4. In the lying down posture, due to accumulation of blood in the lungs (increase in pulmonary blood volume).

Compliance can be measured by making the person to inspire 50 ml of air at a time and a short time is allowed for pressure equilibration to occur. Then the pressure measurements are made. This is continued till the person breathes 500 ml of air (tidal inspiration). Procedure is repeated by expiring 50 ml of air at a time and recording of the pressure. The result is plotted on the graph paper. With the help of this, the airway resistance and non-elastic tissue resistance can also be measured. This measures the static lung compliance. If pressure measurements are made as the air is entering into or coming out of lungs, this is known as dynamic lung compliance.

Collapsing Tendency of the Lungs

- It is because of the presence of layer of water molecules in the alveoli, which exert surface tension (get attracted towards each other). This is responsible for about two-thirds of the collapsing tendency.
- The lungs contain large amount of elastic fibers that have a tendency to recoil. This is responsible for the remaining one-third of the collapsing tendency.

Factors preventing collapsing tendency of lungs/alveoli:
- A layer of surfactant opposes the collapsing tendency of the lungs, which is present in the alveoli. The surfactant covers the layer of water molecule present in the alveoli. Hence, prevents the air–water molecular interface.
- Recoiling tendency of the chest walls in the opposite direction.
- The negative intrapleural pressure also contributes for preventing the collapsing tendency of the alveoli by maintaining a distension force on the lungs.
- Another factor that also has a role in preventing the collapsing tendency of the alveoli is interdependence of the alveoli. The walls of the adjacent alveoli are adhering to each other. When one alveolus tries to recoil, the elastic fibers in the surrounding alveoli gets stretched. As a result of which they try to recoil in the opposite direction.

Blood flowing through the collapsed alveoli is unable to take part in diffusion of gases and hence this blood remains as deoxygenated blood. When this blood mixes with oxygenated blood coming from other alveoli, it can lead to some amount of shunting (Fig. 4.7). This type of shunting is detrimental to body functioning.

Surfactant

- It is a chemical substance namely dipalmitoyl-phosphatidylcholine (DPPC).

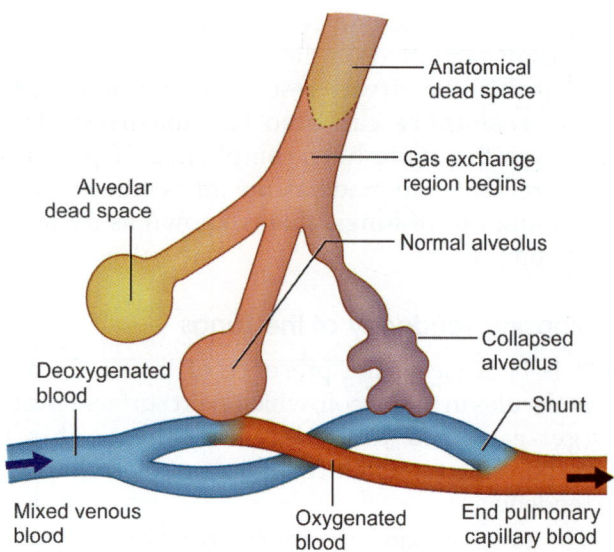

Fig. 4.7: Collapsed alveoli thereby contributing for shunting of blood

- It is secreted by type II pneumocytes (alveolar epithelial cells)
- Covers the thin layer of water molecules present in the alveoli and instead of air–water interface, there will be air-surfactant interface. This decreases the surface tension exerted by the water molecules by about 10–14 times.
- Two-thirds of collapsing tendency of the lungs is prevented by this.
- The secretion of surfactant starts from the 7th month of intrauterine life. The secretion is affected by the hormones thyroxine and cortisol.
- In the premature newborn infant when surfactant is deficient, the lungs remain collapsed. This leads to respiratory distress syndrome or hyaline membrane disease. In this condition, fluid is retained in lungs.
- Steroids or injection of surfactant may help these patients.
- In adult when surfactant is deficient, it leads to adult respiratory distress syndrome (ARDS). In smokers, the production of surfactant is decreased and may lead to ARDS.

Spirogram

Spirometry is a technique by which recording of the different lung volumes and capacities can be done.

Spirogram is the graphical recording of the lung volumes (Fig. 4.8) and capacities.

- *Tidal volume* (TV) is the volume of air inspired or expired during a normal quiet respiration and it is about 500 ml.
- *Inspiratory reserve volume* (IRV) is the volume of air inspired forcibly over and above a tidal inspiration—3000 ml.
- *Expiratory reserve volume* (ERV) is the volume of air expired forcibly after tidal expiration—1100 ml.
- *Residual volume* (RV) is the volume of air still remaining in the lungs even after a forced expiration—1200 ml.

A capacity is sum of two or more different lung volumes.

- *Functional residual capacity* (FRC) is the volume of air remaining in the lungs after a normal expiration (RV + ERV) and is about 2300 ml. This air is responsible for making the exchange of respiratory gases a continuous process. Because of this, the partial pressure of the gases in artery gets maintained constant.

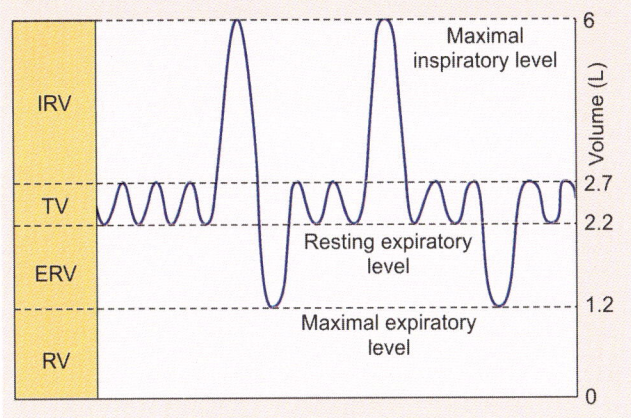

Fig. 4.8: Spirogram showing different lung volumes

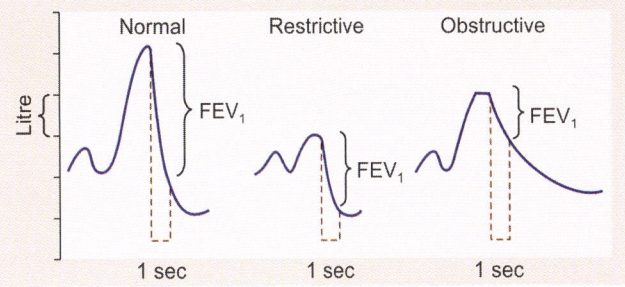

Fig. 4.9: Timed vital capacity and vital capacity in different types of lung diseases when compared to normal

- *Total lung capacity* is the maximum volume of air present in the lungs at the end of forced inspiration. It is sum of IRV, TV, ERV and RV, which is around 5800 ml.
- *Vital capacity* (VC) is the volume of air expired forcibly after a maximal inspiration. It includes TV, ERV and IRV. Normally in a male, it is about 4600 ml.
  a. In relation to body surface area, vital capacity is about 2.8 l/mts^2 in males and 2.3 l/mts^2 in females.
  b. Vital capacity determination forms one of the important lung function tests. It is normal in obstructive type of lung diseases and decreased in restrictive type of lung diseases.
  c. Vital capacity is also dependent on the age, sex, posture and build of the individual.
  d. Vital capacity decreases in fibrosis of lungs, paralysis of respiratory muscles, pleural effusion, poorly developed respiratory muscles, restricted movement of diaphragm (due to increased intra-abdominal pressure).

Timed vital capacity is the percentage volume of vital capacity expired at the end of successive seconds. Usually it is denoted as FEV$_1$, FEV$_2$ and FEV$_3$ wherein FEV refers to the forced expiratory volume and the number suffixed refers to the end of a particular second. To calculate timed vital capacity at the end of first second, the following formula is applied

$$FEV_1 = \frac{\text{Volume of air expired at the end of first second}}{\text{Vital capacity}} \times 100$$

Normal value:
- FEV$_1$ is 75–80%
- FEV$_2$ is 85–90%
- FEV$_3$ is about 97%

Timed vital capacity decreases in obstructive type of lung diseases (bronchial asthma) even though vital capacity remains normal. Vital capacity is decreased in restrictive type of lung diseases but the timed vital capacity remains normal (Fig. 4.9; Table 4.1).

Ventilation Perfusion Ratio

- It is the ratio between the volumes of air taking part in the exchange of gases at the alveoli to the volume of blood flow through the lungs per minute.

$$\text{V-P ratio} = \frac{\text{Ventilation (alveolar ventilation l/min)}}{\text{Perfusion (pulmonary blood flow l/min)}}$$

- Normal value is 0.8 because, alveolar ventilation is about 4 liters and pulmonary blood flow is 5 liters per minute, respectively.
- This value is mean for the lungs assuming that all the parts of the lungs have proportionate ventilation and perfusion.

Table 4.1: Differences between obstructive and restrictive type of lung diseases

Type of lung disease	Vital capacity	Timed vital capacity	Occurs in conditions
Obstructive type	Almost normal	Decreases	Bronchial asthma, emphysema
Restrictive type	Decreases	Normal	Paralysis of respiratory muscles, pleural effusion, lobectomy, hydrothorax

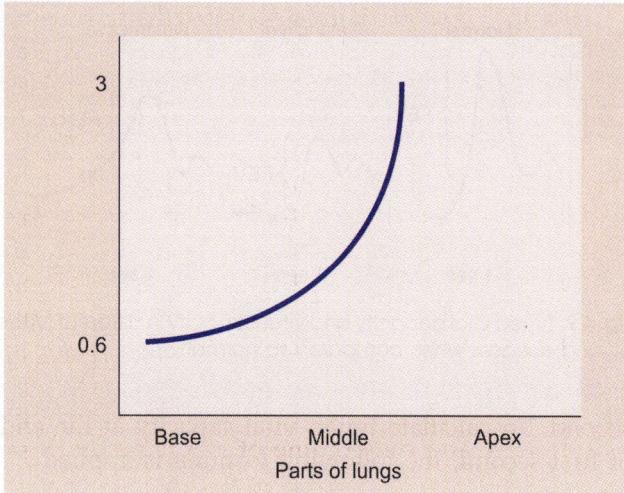

Fig. 4.10: Graph showing the difference in V-P ratio in different parts of lungs

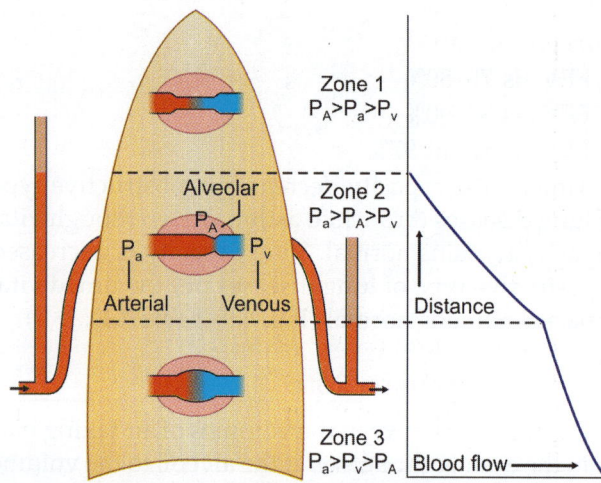

Fig. 4.11: Model tries to explain variation in the blood flow in different parts of lungs based on the pressure in artery, vein and alveoli (P_a–pressure in artery, P_v–pressure in vein, P_A–pressure in alveoli)

- In the sitting posture, it is slightly different between the apical, middle and basal parts of the lungs. In erect posture, the perfusion of blood to the apical parts will be low as against a high perfusion to the basal parts. Hence at the apical parts, the V:P ratio will be more than 0.8 and at base it will be less than 0.8 (Figs 4.10 and 4.11). It is the middle part, which has V:P ratio of almost 0.8.

- A higher value (>0.8) indicates wastage of ventilation (physiologic dead space) and low value (<0.8) indicates wastage of blood flow (blood is not getting oxygenated adequately).

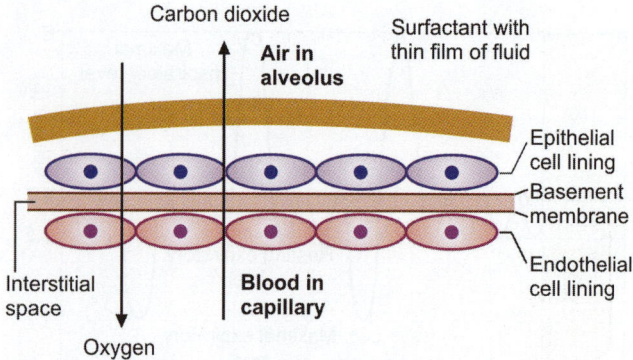

Fig. 4.12: Diagram of respiratory membrane

Respiratory Membrane (Fig. 4.12) and Exchange of Gases

- It is also known as alveolocapillary membrane or blood–gas barrier.
- The average thickness of the membrane is about 0.5 μ.
- The average surface area available for gas exchange will be about 60–80 sq mts.
- The membrane is made up of different layers.
- On one of the sides of the membrane will be air and on the other side will be blood. Hence the name blood–gas barrier.

Factors affecting diffusion of gas across the membrane: The volume of gases diffusion across the membrane can be explained based on the Fick's law of diffusion. According to this law,

D–volume of gas diffused.
A–surface area available for diffusion
T–thickness of respiratory membrane.
S–solubility of the gas

Square root of molecular weight of the gas and solubility of the gas are constant. So, the alterations in any of the other factors affect gas diffusion across the respiratory membrane, the three factors namely pressure gradient for the gas, surface area available for diffusion and thickness of respiratory membrane affect the volume of gas diffused.

Pressure Gradients (Fig. 4.13)

In the alveolar air, the pO_2 is around 104 mm Hg and pCO_2 is 40 mm Hg, whereas, in the pulmonary capillary blood pO_2 is 40 mm Hg and pCO_2 is 46 mm

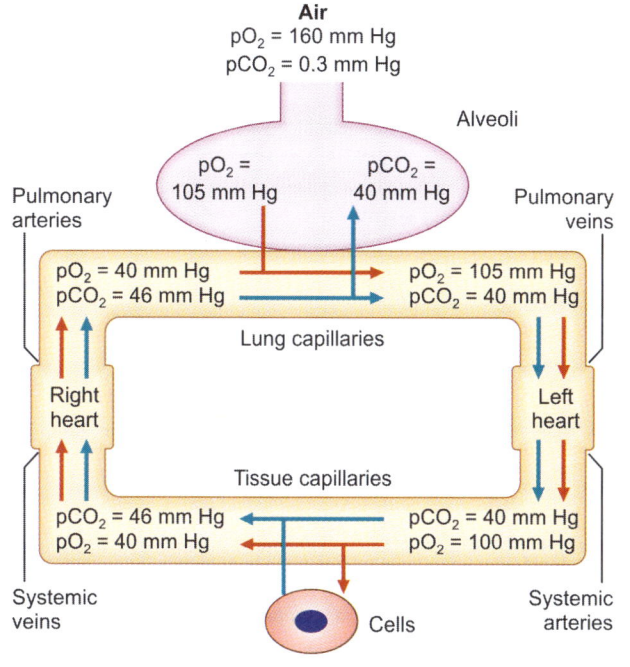

Fig. 4.13: Partial pressure of gases at different regions in the body

Hg. For O$_2$ to diffuse into blood from the alveolar air, the pressure gradient available will be about 64 mm Hg. And for CO$_2$ to diffuse out from pulmonary blood into the alveolar air, it is about 6 mm Hg. Though the pressure gradient available for CO$_2$ diffusion is only 6 mm Hg (10 times less than for oxygen) when compared to 64 mm Hg available for O$_2$, still CO$_2$ can diffuse easily because the rate of diffusion ratio between CO$_2$ and O$_2$ is 20:1. CO$_2$ has a high diffusion coefficient. Because of this, in respiratory disorders where the respiratory membrane is affected (pulmonary edema), the patient will have more of signs and symptoms of hypoxia (decreased oxygen supply to tissues) and not of hypercapnia (increased pCO$_2$ in circulation).

Diffusion coefficient of a gas: Can be defined as the volume of gas that is diffused per unit area (cm^2) area of respiratory membrane for a pressure gradient of 1 mm Hg per unit time.

Diffusing capacity is the volume of gas diffusing across the respiratory membrane per minute per mm Hg pressure gradient. For oxygen, it is about 21 ml/ mm Hg/minute.

When the gases start diffusing across the membrane the equilibration point (the partial pressure of the gas on either side of the respiratory membrane when gets equaled) is achieved when blood has traversed only about one-third of the distance and time available in the capillary. So the pulmonary capillary blood pO$_2$ will have got increased to 104 from 40 mm Hg and pCO$_2$ will have got decreased to 40 from 46 mm Hg. Rest of the distance along the capillary, the blood flows without there being any net diffusion of gas. This distance and time will act as a safety factor in certain demanding situations like in muscular exercise during which the velocity of blood flow increases considerably and the volume of gas has to diffuse will also be more than normal in unit time.

Pressure gradient gets decreased in conditions, like:
• Hypoventilation of alveoli (bronchial asthma, paralysis of respiratory muscles)
• Hyperventilation of alveoli (at high altitudes)
  Surface area availability is normally around 60–80 sq mts.

Decrease in surface area occurs in:
• Emphysema
• Collapse of the lungs
• Pneumonia
• Collapse of lung lobes (atelectasis) due to pleural effusion, pneumothorax, etc.
  Thickness of the respiratory membrane is only 0.5– 1 micron. It is increased in conditions, like pulmonary edema.

Muscular exercise: During muscular exercise, the oxygen demand by the body is increased and the volume of carbon dioxide produced will also be more. So, certain respiratory adjustments have to be brought about by which the rate of diffusion of gas can be

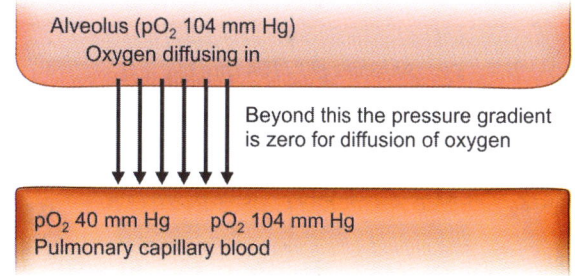

Fig. 4.14: Diffusion of gas across the respiratory membrane (that is between alveolar air and pulmonary, capillary blood)

enhanced. The respiratory adjustments that are brought about to meet the increased demands are:

- Increase in rate and depth of respiration.
- Further distension of the alveoli.
- The almost dormant alveoli are opened up for diffusion of gases.
- Opening of new capillaries

Oxygen Transport

Oxygen transport from the atmospheric air to the tissues is "down the hill" transport along a pressure gradient.

Along a pressure gradient (Fig. 4.15), oxygen diffuses from the alveolar air into the pulmonary capillary blood. The diffusion takes hardly 0.3 sec though blood remains in the pulmonary capillary for about 0.8 sec. Within this short duration (Fig. 4.16), the pO_2 of the pulmonary capillary blood gets increased from 40 to 104 mm Hg and thereby equilibration is achieved. To start with, during diffusion of oxygen there will be a pressure gradient of 64 mm Hg.

By the time oxygenated blood is pumped out from the left ventricle, the pO_2 is reduced to about 95 mm Hg. This is due to admixture of venous blood (physiologic shunt). The reasons for the physiologic shunt are:

- A small volume of venous blood from bronchial veins gets directly mixed with the oxygenated blood present in the pulmonary veins (Fig. 4.17).
- A small volume of venous blood from the coronary circulation supplying the myocardium gets drained

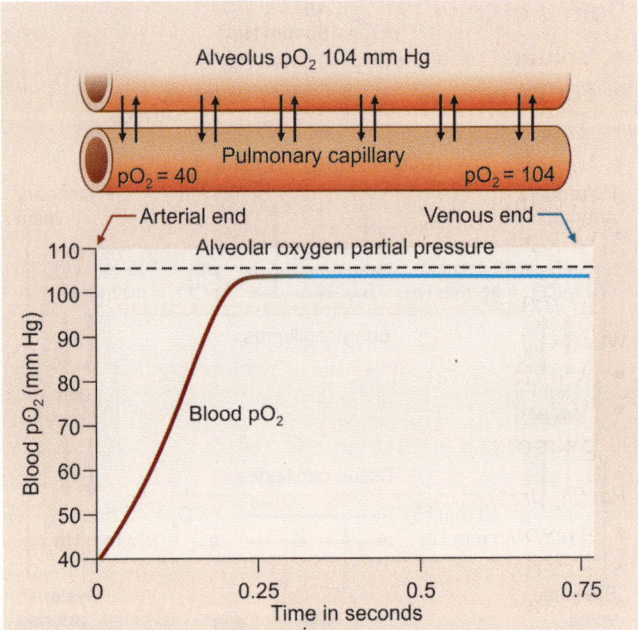

Fig. 4.16: Length and time in which the oxygen equilibration of pressure is achieved with that of alveolar air in capillary blood

directly into the chamber of the left ventricle that contains oxygenated blood.

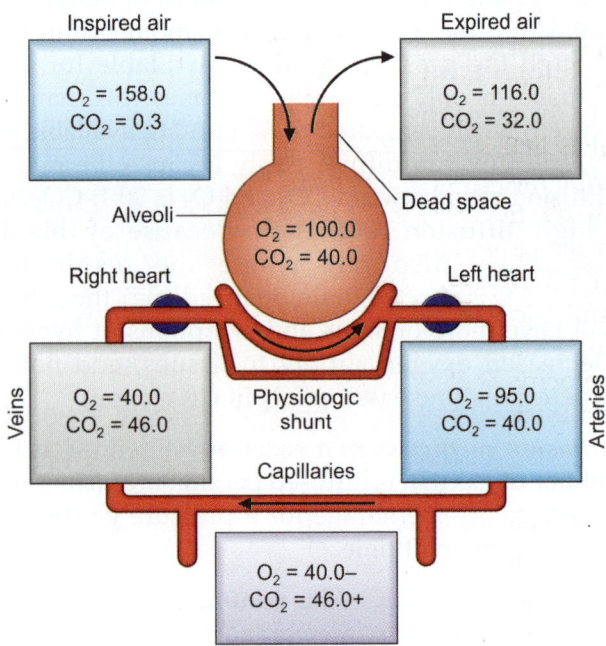

Fig. 4.17: pO_2 and pCO_2 in different regions and the vessels contributing for physiologic shunt

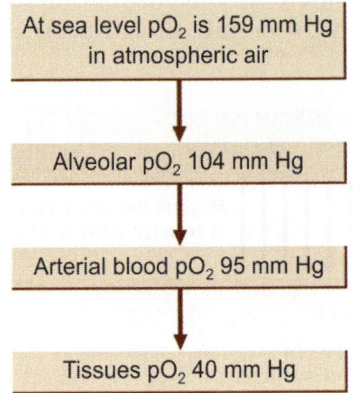

Fig. 4.15: The pressure profile from atmosphere until the tissues

Details of Oxygen Transport

- Volume present in 100 ml of blood
- Partial pressure at different regions
- Forms of transport
- Importance of dissolved form
- In combination with hemoglobin
- Oxygen hemoglobin dissociation curve and factors influencing

In 100 ml of blood, the volume of oxygen present will be:

- Arterial blood about 20 ml
- Venous blood about 15 ml (mixed venous blood in pulmonary artery).

Partial pressure at different regions will be:
- Alveoli—104 mm Hg at sea level.
- Arterial blood—95 mm Hg.
- Tissues—<40 mm Hg.
- Venous blood—40 mm Hg (mixed venous blood in pulmonary artery)

	Arterial blood	Venous blood (mixed venous blood)
pO$_2$ (mm Hg)	95	40
% saturation of Hb	95–97	70–75
Content (ml/100 ml)	20	15

So when pulmonary arterial blood, which contains mixed venous blood, flows through the lungs, to start with there will be a pressure gradient of about 64 mm Hg for the diffusion of oxygen into blood from the alveoli. Because of this, oxygen starts getting diffused from the alveolar air into pulmonary capillary blood. By the time blood has traversed about one-third the distance along the pulmonary capillary, the pressure equilibration is brought about between alveolar air and blood. This acts as safety factor for better oxygenation during muscular exercise wherein the velocity of flow of blood through the pulmonary circulation will be very fast (Fig. 4.16).

Forms of Transport

- Dissolved form
- In combination with hemoglobin.

In the dissolved form, it is about 0.3 ml/100 ml in the arterial blood and 0.1 ml/100 ml in the venous blood. But still this particular form of transport is very essential as this form of gas alone can exert partial pressure that is necessary for diffusion of any gas. Oxygen gets dissolved in water available both in plasma and red blood cells. The volume of oxygen that is getting into the dissolved form in blood is directly proportional to the partial pressure.

As the pO$_2$ is increased, the volume of oxygen getting dissolved will also increase (Fig. 4.18). At pO$_2$ of 104 mm Hg, it is about 0.3 ml of oxygen goes into the solution form. At pO$_2$ of 1000 mm Hg, it is about 3 ml. In cases of severe anemia, oxygen in the dissolved form alone can cope up with the demands of oxygen supply to the tissues. This can be achieved by allowing the patient to breathe oxygen under high pressure (pO$_2$ 1000–2000 mm Hg) intermittent hyperbaric oxygen administration.

Oxygen is transported mainly by hemoglobin. Volume of oxygen transported by hemoglobin in the arterial blood is about 19.5 ml/100 ml and in venous blood it is about 14.5 ml/100 ml. Presence of Hb increases the oxygen carrying capacity of blood by about 65 times.

$$Hb + O_2 \rightleftharpoons HbO_2$$

The percentage saturation of hemoglobin is about:
- 97% in arterial blood (oxygenated blood)
- 70% in the venous blood (deoxygenated blood)

One gram of hemoglobin can maximally carry about 1.34 ml of oxygen on full saturation.

Even though about 20 ml of oxygen is available in arterial blood for utilization by the tissues, the tissues normally use only about 5 ml of oxygen when 100 ml of blood flows through them in one minute. In other

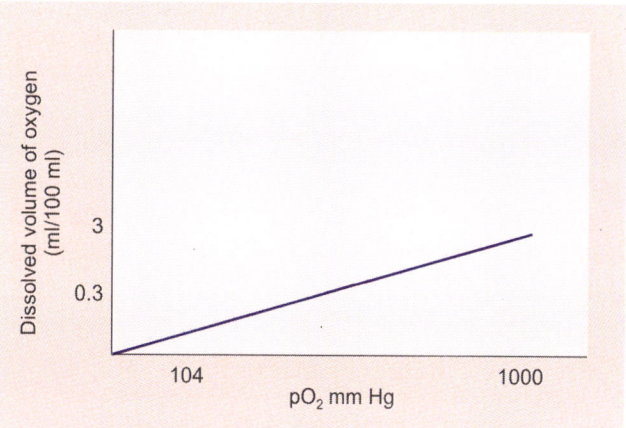

Fig. 4.18: Graph showing relationship between dissolved form of oxygen and partial pressure (note the direct relatioship between the volume of O$_2$ present in dissolved form when there is increase in pO$_2$)

words, only a part of oxygen available to them will be utilized. This is known as utilization coefficient. The ratio between the volume of oxygen used to the volume of oxygen available for utilization by the tissues is known as utilization coefficient. The utilization coefficient of oxygen is normally about 25%. In severe muscular exercise, it can go up to about 75%.

Oxygen binds to the heme part of hemoglobin. The reaction is a physical one. The reaction will be oxygenation and not oxidation, as the ferrous form of iron in hemoglobin does not get oxidsed to ferric form. Each molecule of hemoglobin with 4 atoms of iron can carry 4 molecules of oxygen. The reactions occur in stepwise fashion and it is known as heme-heme interaction. This type of binding of oxygen facilitates the rate of binding of oxygen to hemoglobin.

Details of heme—heme interaction steps:

$$Hb_4 + O_2 \longleftrightarrow Hb_4O_2$$
$$Hb_4O_2 + O_2 \longleftrightarrow Hb_4O_4$$
$$Hb_4O_4 + O_2 \longleftrightarrow Hb_4O_6$$
$$Hb_4O_6 + O_2 \longleftrightarrow Hb_4O_8$$

Reaction between oxygen and hemoglobin can be studied by plotting an oxygen dissociation curve.

- A series of (at least 10) tonometers are used. These are conical-shaped glass tubes of 5 ml capacity.
- In each one of these tonometers, 1 ml of blood is taken.
- These blood samples are exposed to different partial pressure of oxygen starting from 10 to 110 mm Hg, sealed and centrifuged.
- Oxygen combines with Hb and Hb gets saturated to different extents depending on the pO_2 to which it is exposed.
- The oxygen content of each of the tonometer is determined.
- Then one sample of blood is also exposed to 760 mm Hg pO_2 to fully saturate the Hb. This will give us the oxygen combining capacity of Hb.
- The amount of oxygen after full saturation is found out.
- From these figures available, the % saturation of Hb is calculated.

Percentage saturation of hemoglobin is ratio between volume of oxygen carried by hemoglobin to the maximum oxygen carrying capacity of hemoglobin times hundred.

$$\% \text{ Saturation of Hb} = \frac{O_2 \text{ carried (content)}}{O_2 \text{ carrying ability (capacity)}} \times 100$$

Oxygen dissociation curve: It is the graphical representation of % saturation of hemoglobin in relation to partial pressure of oxygen (Fig. 4.19). For adult Hb, it is sigmoid in shape whereas for fetal Hb, it has different configuration. Fetal Hb has greater affinity for oxygen as has been depicted in the graph. It is for this reason, fetal Hb dissociation curve when plotted is to the left of the adult Hb dissociation curve.

pO_2 mm Hg	% Saturation of HbA	% Saturation of HbF
20	35	70
40	70	95
104	97	

Factors affecting dissociation are:
1. Partial pressure of carbon dioxide.
2. H^+ in blood (decrease pH).
3. Temperature.
4. Conc. of 2–3 DPG.

Increase in all above factors shift the oxygen dissociation curve to the right. Converse happens (shift to left) when there is decrease in any of the above mentioned factors. Increase in pCO_2 or decrease in pH, which shifts the curve to right, is known as Bohr's effect. The extra oxygen requirement by the tissues during exercise is, therefore, met with by the above factors and hence the utilization coefficient is increased from 25 to about 75%. Therefore, oxygen

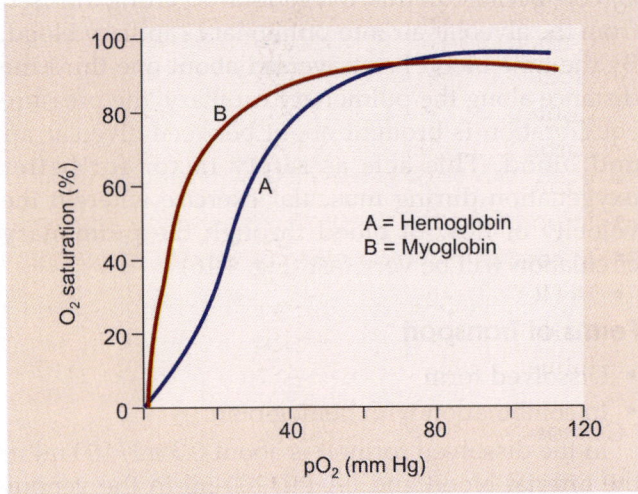

Fig. 4.19: Graph comparing oxygen-Hb dissociation curve with that of myoglobin

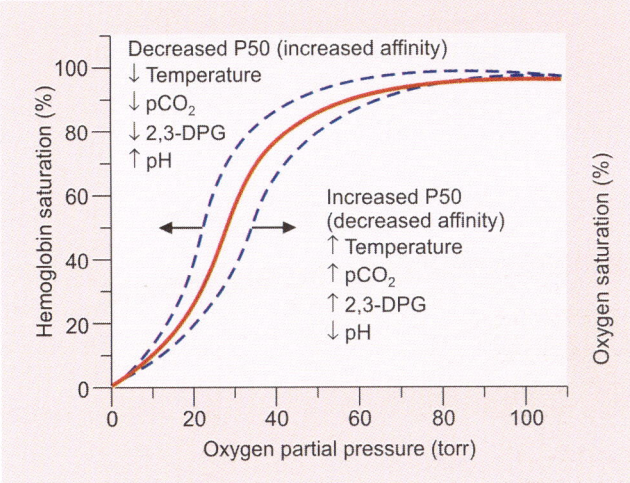

Fig. 4.20: Variation in P50 depending on various factors influencing the O₂ dissociation curve

supply to the tissues during exercise can be increased from 250 to 750 ml/min by the above mechanism only. Another 5–7-fold increase in the supply of oxygen can be achieved by increasing the cardiac output to about 25–35 l/min.

P50 is the partial pressure of oxygen at which hemoglobin is saturated to 50%. At sea level, P50 is about 28 mm Hg (Fig. 4.20).

Carbon Dioxide Transport

Carbon dioxide is the end product of oxidative tissue metabolism. When arterial blood flows through the tissues, because of pressure gradient, carbon dioxide diffuses from tissues into blood.

Carbon dioxide transport will be discussed under the following headings:

- Content
- Partial pressure at different levels
- Forms of transport
- Importance of dissolved form
- In combination with hemoglobin/plasma protein
- In HCO₃ form
- Carbon dioxide dissociation curve and factors influencing the same.

Content

In the arterial blood, it is about 48 ml/100 ml and in the venous blood (mixed) is about 52 ml/100 ml. Partial pressure at different regions:

a. In arterial blood is 40 mm Hg.
b. In tissues is about 46 mm Hg.
c. In venous blood, it is 46 mm Hg (mixed venous blood)
d. In alveoli, around 40 mm Hg.

	Arterial blood	Venous blood
pCO₂ (mm Hg)	40	46
Content (ml/100 ml)	48	52

Forms of Transport (Fig. 4.21)

1. As dissolved form 10%
2. As bicarbonate 68%
3. As carbamino compound 22%

Dissolved form: In arterial blood, it is about 2.5 ml and in venous blood it is about 2.8 ml per 100 ml of blood. It is this form of gas which exerts partial pressure. It gets dissolved in water available in plasma and in red blood cells. The volume of carbon dioxide getting transported in the dissolved form is directly proportional to partial pressure of the gas (Fig. 4.22).

As carbamino compound form: When hemoglobin reacts with hydrogen ion, the hemoglobin now is called reduced hemoglobin. The reduced hemoglobin reacts with carbon dioxide to form carbamino hemoglobin, which is also one of the forms of carbon dioxide transport. Unlike oxygen that binds to the heme part, carbon dioxide is attached to the globin part of hemoglobin.

Carbon dioxide is transported as bicarbonate both in red blood cells and plasma. But the formation of bicarbonate occurs mostly in erythrocytes because of the presence of the enzyme carbonic anhydrase. Bicarbonate thus formed inside the red blood cells, diffuse into the plasma along the concentration gradient.

At the tissue level, carbon dioxide diffuses from tissues into blood. This carbon dioxide apart from getting dissolved in water presents in the plasma, some amount also gets diffused into the red blood cells. In the erythrocytes also, some amount is transported in the dissolved form. However, the presence of carbonic anhydrase enzyme in red blood cell facilitates the reaction between carbon dioxide and water and there will be formation of carbonic acid. This acid is an unstable weak acid. Immediately, it dissociates to form bicarbonate and hydrogen ion.

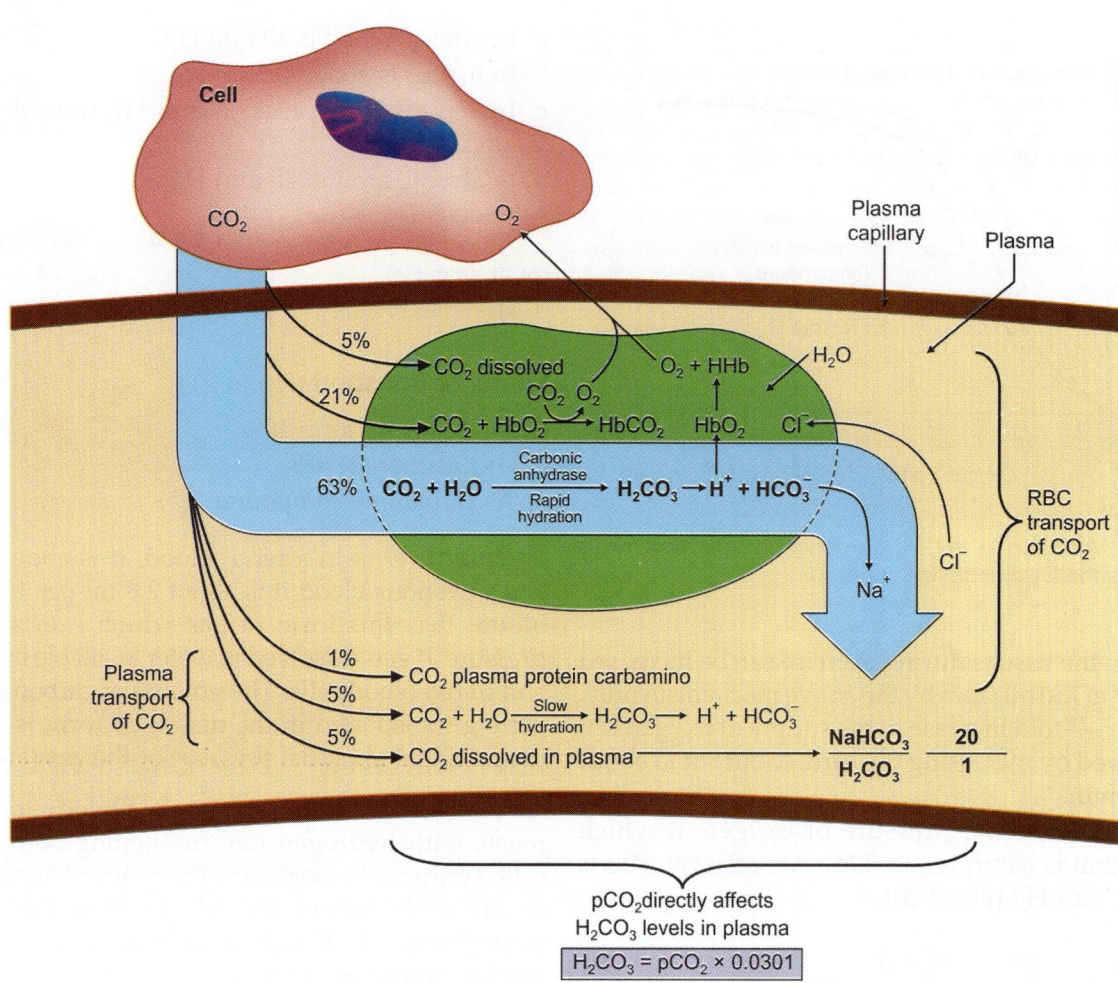

Fig. 4.21: Details of CO_2 transport in RBCs and plasma

Hemoglobin present in RBCs buffers the hydrogen ion that is formed during the reaction between carbon dioxide and water (Fig. 4.23).

Bicarbonate thus formed inside the red blood cell diffuses into plasma along the concentration gradient. Electrical activity of both red blood cells and plasma gets affected since bicarbonate is a charged ion. In order to maintain electrical neutrality, when bicarbonate diffuses out of cells, chloride ion diffuses into red blood cells from the plasma. This is known as *chloride shift* or *Hamburger's phenomenon*. This will be followed by diffusion of water into the red blood cells to maintain the tonicity. This increases the volume of RBCs. Hence PCV of venous blood will be slightly more than the arterial blood.

The whole set of reactions get reversed at the level of lungs during the process of diffusion of gas and thereby leads to the removal of carbon dioxide from the blood.

Carbon Dioxide Dissociation Curve (Fig. 4.24)

Graphical relation between partial pressure of carbon dioxide and the volume of carbon dioxide present in 100 ml of blood.

Haldane's effect: When venous blood flows through the pulmonary capillaries carbon dioxide diffuses out from blood into alveoli. Because of this, the pCO_2 of blood falls to 40 mm Hg from 46 mm Hg. If diffusion of carbon dioxide alone were to happen in the alveoli, what will happen to the volume of carbon dioxide at 40 mm Hg? When carbon dioxide dissociation curve is plotted for venous blood (pO_2–40 mm Hg), it is seen that when pCO_2 has fallen from 46 to 40 mm Hg, the

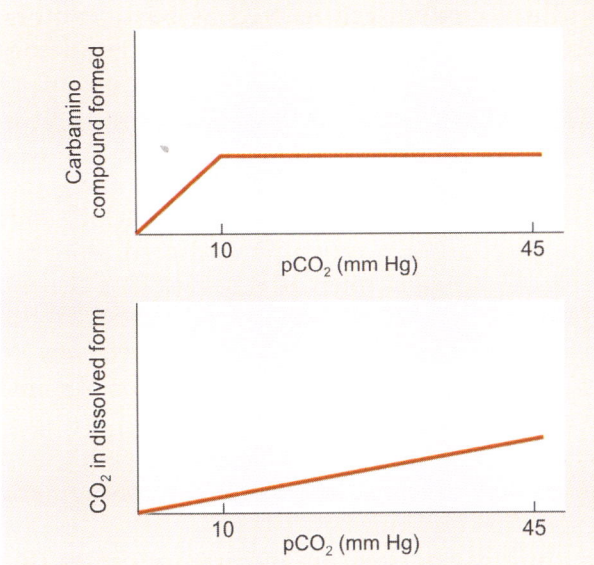

Fig. 4.22: Relationship between volume of CO_2 in dissolved form, carbamino compound form and partial pressure of CO_2

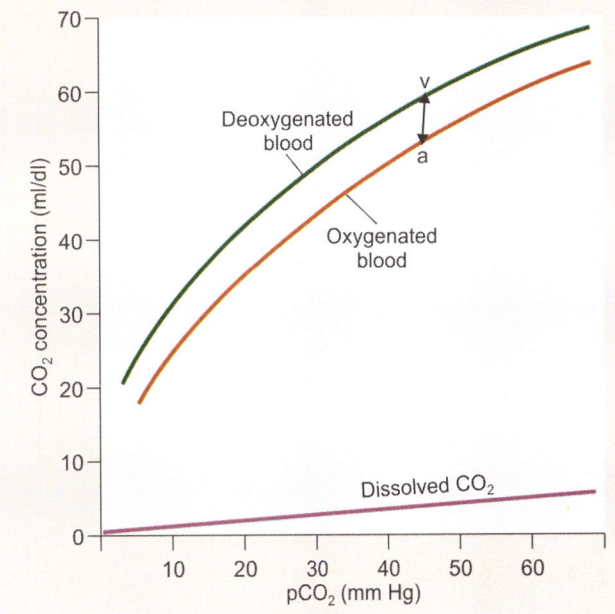

Fig. 4.24: Carbon dioxide dissociation curve

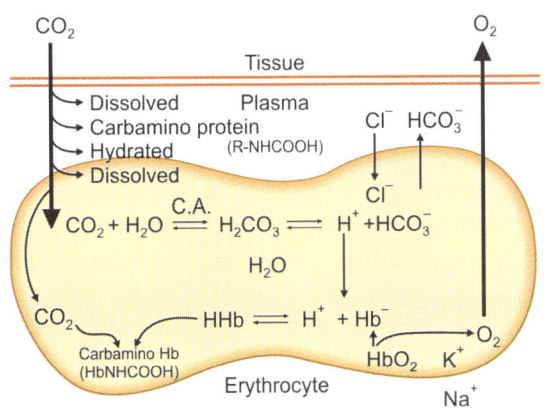

Fig. 4.23: Reactions within RBCs during carbon dioxide transport

carbon dioxide content gets reduced from 52 to 50 ml (point a in graph) only and not to 48 ml. For every 100 ml of blood flowing through the pulmonary capillaries only about 2 ml of carbon dioxide is removed.

But the important aspect to be remembered here is that at the lungs when carbon dioxide is diffusing out, there will be simultaneous oxygenation of capillary blood. This will increase the pO_2 of blood from 40 to 104 mm Hg. The increase in pO_2 shifts carbon dioxide dissociation curve to the right, so that point B on the dissociation curve gets shifted to point C. This

facilitates an additional 2 ml of carbon dioxide being removed from blood. Because of this, when pCO_2 falls from 46 to 40 mm Hg due to simultaneous increase of pO_2, the content of carbon dioxide in blood falls from 52 to 48 ml/100 ml. This enables the removal of 4 ml of carbon dioxide from every 100 ml of blood flowing through the pulmonary capillaries. This is made possible because when oxygen enters blood, it combines with Hb to form oxyhemoglobin. This compound has a much lower affinity for carbon dioxide. Exactly the opposite happens when blood flows through the tissue capillaries.

In the lungs, when carbon dioxide is diffusing out, there is simultaneous diffusion of oxygen into blood. The increase in pO_2 (formation of oxy Hb) facilitates the release of more amount of carbon dioxide. Increase of pO_2, which shifts CO_2 dissociation curve to right, is known as Haldane's effect. Haldane's effect will help both the uptake (at tissue level) as well as giving out of carbon dioxide (at lungs).

Regulation of Respiration

Oxygen requirement by the body differs depending on the activity. It is lowest at rest and increases during routine activity and further increases in muscular exercise. Similarly production of carbon dioxide also is dependent on the rate of metabolic activity in the

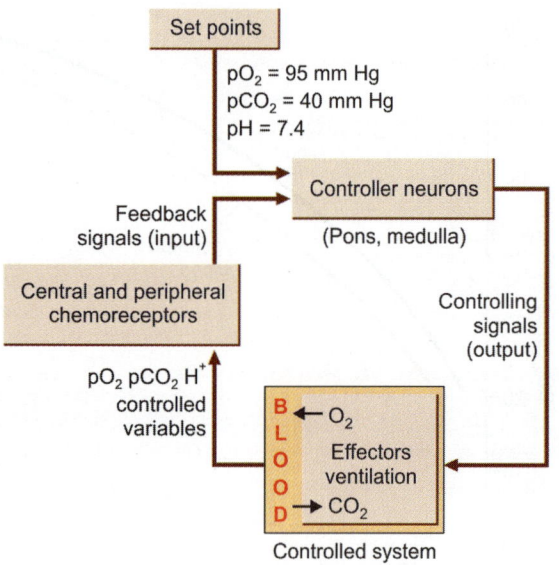

Fig. 4.25: Feedback circuit involved in the regulation of respiration

body. Respiratory system has the responsibility of meeting needs of the body by altering the rate and depth of respiration in order to keep the pO_2 and pCO_2 at normal levels.

The regulation of respiration can be brought about by:

1. Neural mechanism.
2. Chemical influence.
3. Non-chemical influence.

The chemical and non-chemical influence has to act through the neural mechanism only (Fig. 4.25).

Neural Mechanism

Centers are present in brainstem. The brainstem centers are required for rhythmic respiration whether during asleep or awake. The cerebral cortical center is required for voluntary alterations in respiration.

Brainstem centers are present in the reticular formation of pons and medulla oblongata. In the pons, the centers present are:

- Pneumotaxic
- Apneustic

In medulla oblongata, the centers present are:

- Inspiratory (dorsomedial group of neurons)
- Expiratory (ventrolateral group of neurons)

There is a lot of interconnection between the various centers. The interplay of the different centers is essential for a proper regulation of respiration. The

medullary centers are termed as basic centers, whereas the pontine centers are called regulatory centers. The pontine centers act through the medullary centers and bring about smooth rhythmic respiration.

From the medullary centers, which are also spontaneously active, the impulses are sent to spinal cord through the reticulospinal pathway, which ends on the anterior horn cells in spinal cord. Both the phrenic (C3–C5) and intercostal nerve (T1–T11) take origin from spinal cord and influence the activity of diaphragm and intercostals muscles, respectively.

So if there is a complete transverse section of spinal cord at the level of

- C2 segment person dies of respiratory paralysis.
- C6 person survives because the diaphragmatic respiration continues.

In a normal person, the inspiratory center (IC) appears to generate impulse on its own. During the course of the generation of impulse, it is presumed that the rate of impulse generation goes on increasing till it reaches a certain point and then there will be sudden cessation of impulse generation. Because of this, IC is known to act as a ramp generator. The impulses from the apneustic center have a regulatory influence on the inspiratory center. The apneustic center activity in turn is controlled by the impulses coming from the pneumotaxic center and through the vagus nerve from the stretch receptors of lungs. When the influence by the vagus and pneumotaxic center over the apneustic center is lost, there will be prolonged inspiration and a sudden expiration. This type of breathing is known as apneustic breathing (Fig. 4.26).

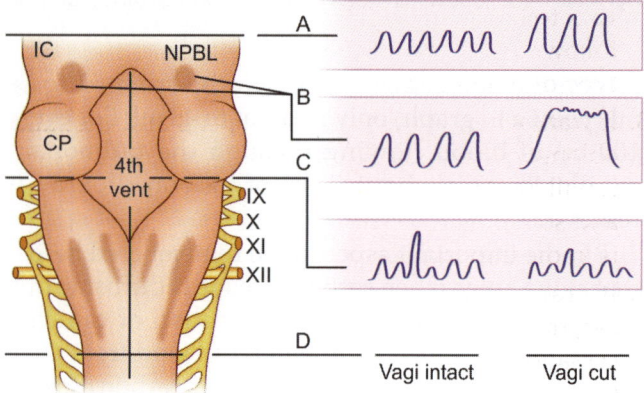

Fig. 4.26: Role of pontine respiratory centers over the medullary centers and also the role of vagus in control of breathing

Sequence of events during normal regulation of respiration by neural mechanism:

- Onset and gradual increase in the number of impulses production in the inspiratory center because of the ramp generator.
- This leads to:
  a. Impulses being sent from IC to spinal cord for stimulation of phrenic and intercostals nerves.
  b. Reciprocal inhibition of expiratory center by IC.
  c. Excitatory impulses from IC sent to pneumotaxic center through multisynaptic pathway.
- When inspiration is going on, there will be gradual inhibition of the apneustic center by the impulses coming from the pneumotaxic center and also from the afferent vagal fibers coming from the distended alveoli.
- Apneustic center influence over the IC ceases completely. Hence the activity of inspiratory center stops and leads to no inhibition influence over the expiratory center (EC). No more impulses from the inspiratory center to motor neurons in the spinal cord.
- The muscles of inspiration start relaxing. This starts the process of expiration which normally lasts for about 3 sec.
- After this, once again the activity in the IC starts, leading to the next respiratory cycle.

Location of the respiratory centers in CNS for rhythmic respiration can be experimentally studied from the following observations:

1. If transection is done above pons, the rhythmic respiration continues as usual.
2. If a mid-pontine section is done along with bilateral vagotomy, there will be a prolonged inspiration followed by a sudden short expiration (apneustic type of breathing).
3. If transection is done between pons and medulla oblongata, though respiration continues on its own, it will be irregular. Sometimes it becomes shallow and sometimes it is deeper. This type of breathing is known as gasping.
4. If transection is done below medulla (at the beginning of the spinal cord), it leads to complete cessation of breathing.

So by the above studies, it can be concluded that the centers are present in brainstem. The pontine centers play role in smooth and rhythmic respiration.

Hering-Brueur reflex: Inflation of alveoli brings about cessation of inspiration and expiration commences. The details are as under:

- Inflation of alveoli
- Leads of stimulation of stretch receptors present in the alveoli.
- Afferent impulses are carried by vagal fibers.
- Inhibit the activity of the respiratory center, cessation of inspiration.
- Leads to relaxation of muscles of inspiration.
- Expiration commences.

This reflex is not very well seen in adults. The reflex probably helps to prevent over distension of the alveoli.

Chemical Influence on Respiration

This is brought about by the chemoreceptors. They are called:

- Peripheral
- Central chemoreceptors.

Peripheral Chemoreceptors (Fig. 4.27)

a. Carotid bodies which are present at the branching of internal carotid artery.
b. Aortic bodies are present in the arch of aorta.

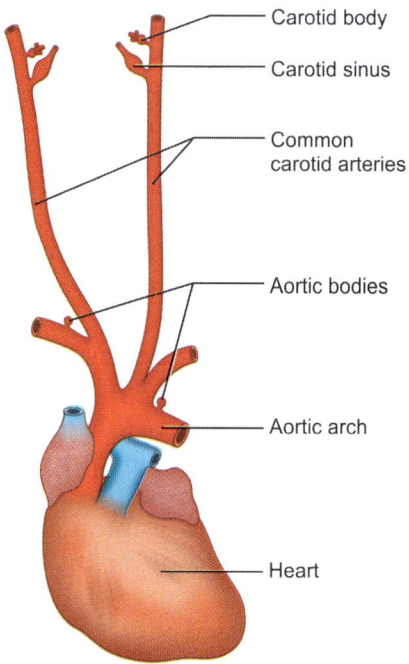

Fig. 4.27: Location of peripheral chemoreceptors

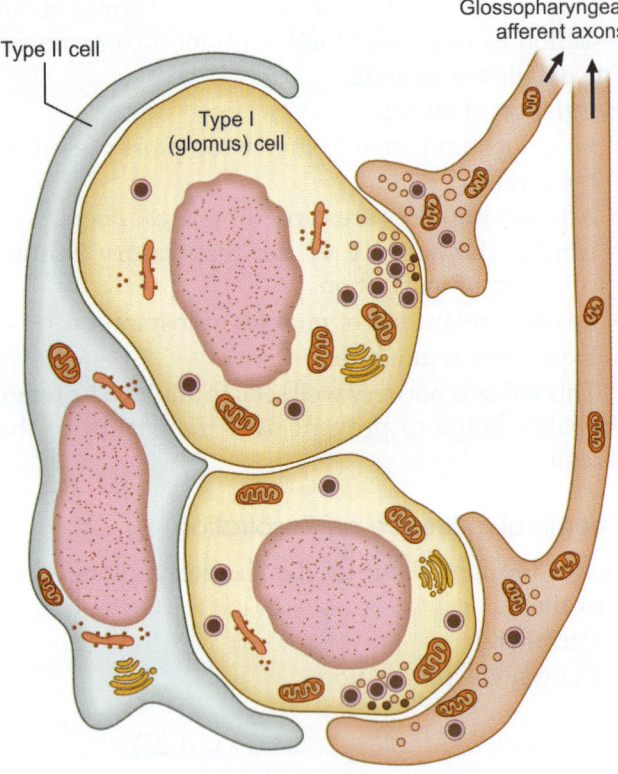

Fig. 4.28: Afferent nerve carrying impulse from carotid body

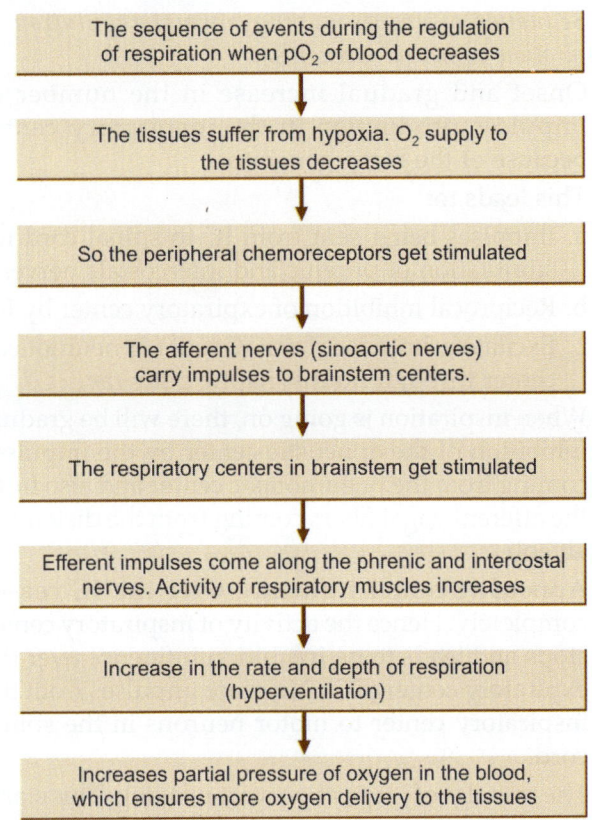

Fig. 4.29: Sequence of events during the regulation of respiration by peripheral chemoreceptors

From the carotid bodies, the afferent impulses will be carried by the sinus nerve (Fig. 4.28) a branch of glossopharyngeal nerve and from the aortic bodies by the aortic nerve branch of vagus nerve.

The peripheral chemoreceptors respond to:
- Decrease in pO_2
- Increase in H^+
- Increase of pCO_2 of blood.

Details of the role of peripheral chemoreceptors in regulation of respiration are shown in Figs 4.29 to 4.33.

Central Chemoreceptors

They are present in the brainstem near the respiratory centers. They are more sensitive to hydrogen ions, but the hydrogen ion of blood cannot stimulate them because the blood brain–barrier is impermeable for the hydrogen ion to diffuse through. Hence, the increase in partial pressure of carbon dioxide forms the stimulus (Fig. 4.34).

Decreased pO_2, increased pCO_2 together (asphyxia) will have an additive effect on chemoreceptors. Hence there will be maximum respiratory response in such

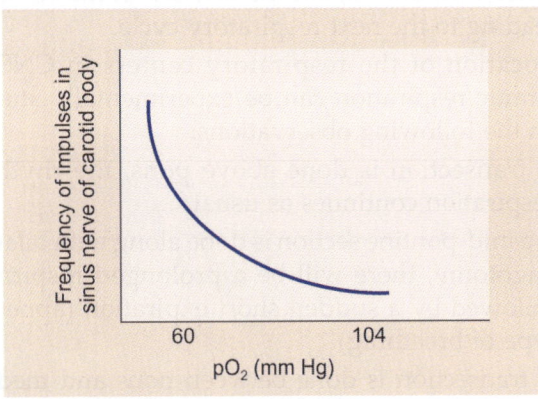

Fig. 4.30: Relationship between pO_2 and frequency of impulses in the sinus nerve from the carotid body

a situation (Fig. 4.35). Asphyxia occurs in conditions, like drowning or strangulation.

Non-chemical influence on respiratory centers pertains to impulses coming from:
- Baroreceptors
- Muscle spindles of respiratory muscles to control depth of respiration.

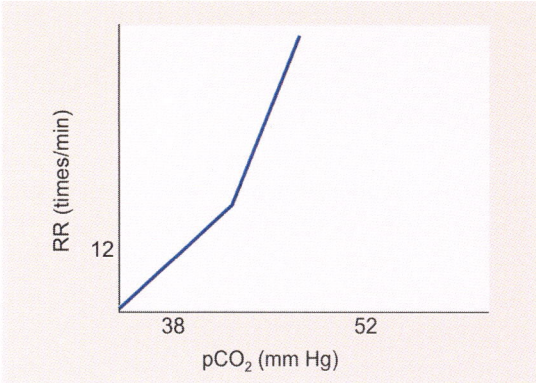

Fig. 4.31: Relationship between pCO₂ and rate of respiration

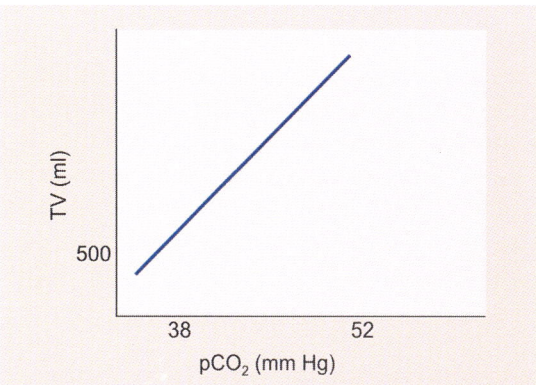

Fig. 4.32: Relationship between pCO₂ and tidal volume

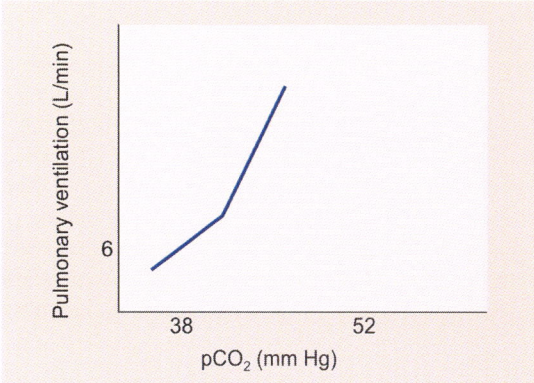

Fig. 4.33: Relationship between pCO₂ and pulmonary ventilation

- Pain receptors
- Intracranial tension
- Irritant receptors stimulation in lungs while coughing.

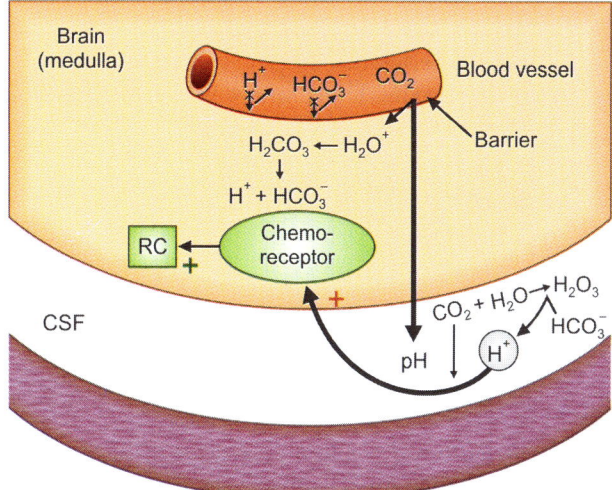

Fig. 4.34: Reactions occurring in the brain and the consequent stimulation of central chemoreceptos

- Higher parts of CNS
- Irritation of nasal mucosa (sneezing)
- Mechanoreceptors in pharynx (deglutition).
- Receptors of muscles and joints.

Depending on the location of the receptors influencing the respiratory centers, there will be appropriate alterations in the respiration.

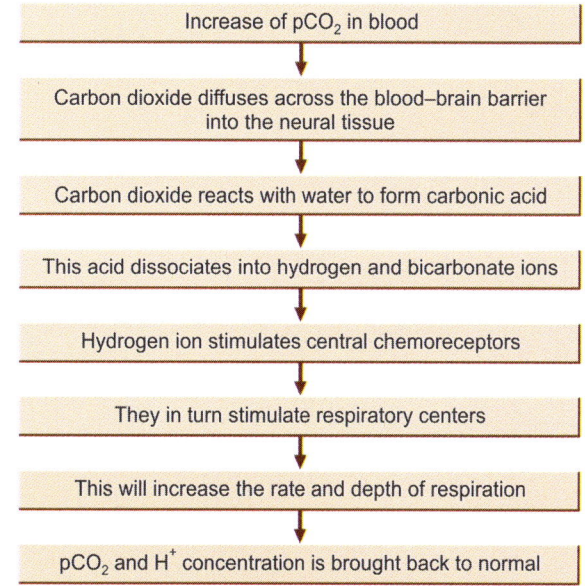

Fig. 4.35: Sequence of events during the regulation of respiration by central chemoreceptors

Hypoxia

When there is deficient oxygen supply to the tissues it is called hypoxia. There are 4 types of hypoxias. They are:

1. Hypoxic hypoxia (hypoxemia)
2. Anemic hypoxia
3. Stagnant hypoxia
4. Histotoxic hypoxia

Some of the characteristic features and causes for different types of hypoxia are given in Table 4.2.

Hypoxic Hypoxia

- Arterial pO_2 and oxygen content will be less than normal because most of the times the problem will be for the diffusion of oxygen at the level of alveolus.
- Hb cannot get oxygenated completely due to faulty diffusion or decreased pO_2 at high altitude, % saturation of Hb is decreased. More amount of reduced Hb (Hb that is not oxygenated) remains in circulation.
- At the level of tissues, reduction of Hb occurs further due to release of oxygen and hence the reduced Hb concentration increases. This leads to cyanosis.

Anemic Hypoxia

- Arterial pO_2 remains normal because diffusion of gas at the alveolus is normal. So the dissolved form of oxygen transported remains normal.
- Arterial oxygen content decreases because of either qualitative (carbon monoxide poisoning) or quantitative (anemia) defect in Hb.

Stagnant Hypoxia

- In this case, both the oxygen diffusion at alveoli and Hb function will be normal. Hence partial pressure, content, % saturation of Hb remain normal in arterial blood.
- Since circulation has slowed down or almost no circulation (cardiac failure) or hypokinetic (obstruction in venous drainage), it results in more oxygen being extracted by the tissues from the capillary blood. It leads more than normal amount of reduced Hb formation, and therefore, cyanosis will be present.

Table 4.2: Types of hypoxia—characteristic features and causes

Type of hypoxia	Arterial blood			Venous blood			Cyanosis	Occurs in conditions
	pO_2 (95 mm Hg)	% satura-tion of Hb (97%)	O_2 content (20 ml%)	pO_2 (40 mm Hg)	% satura-tion of Hb (70%)	O_2 content (15 ml%)		
Hypoxic	↓	↓	↓	↓	↓		Seen	Alveolar hypoventilation (bronchial asthma), pulmonary edema, at high altitude
Anemic	N	N	↓	N	N	↓	No	Anemia, carbon monoxide poisoning
Stagnant	N	N	N	↓	↓	↓	Seen	Cardiac failure, myocardial infarction, venous obstruction for any reason
Histotoxic	N	N	N	↑	↑	↑	No	Cyanide poisoning

Histotoxic Hypoxia

- Alveolar diffusion of oxygen, Hb function and the circulation is normal and hence all the parameters in arterial blood remain normal.
- Since there is poisoning of the enzyme system (cytochrome oxidase), the tissues are unable to take up oxygen from blood. The amount of oxygen used by the tissue gets decreased. So, less amount of reduced Hb is formed. The venous blood oxygen content will be more than normal. Hence A-V oxygen difference will be less than normal (parameters in the venous blood will be increased when compared to any normal situation).

Dyspnea

It means difficulty to breathe. The point at which a conscious necessity to increase the breathing occurs is known as dyspnea point. Dyspnea is seen in bronchial asthma, pneumothorax, respiratory and cardiac disorders. It can also be seen in physiological condition like in severe muscular exercise.

Cyanosis

a. Cyanosis is the bluish discoloration of skin and mucous membrane.
b. It occurs due to an increase in the concentration of reduced hemoglobin in capillary blood.
c. The concentration of reduced hemoglobin when exceeds 5 g%, there will be cyanosis.
d. Cyanosis can be central or peripheral.
e. Usually it is obvious in lips, nail beds, tongue, and finger tips.
f. Cyanosis occurs in hypoxic hypoxia and stagnant hypoxia.
g. It can occur due to diseases of lungs or heart.

Mountain Sickness

When people living at higher barometric pressure areas/low altitude get exposed suddenly to higher altitude, they are exposed to lower barometric pressure environment. Because of this, they will suffer from certain problems. All the symptoms are basically due to acute hypoxia especially on the neurons of central nervous system. The neurons of cerebral cortex are most susceptible for hypoxic effects when compared to either the brainstem or spinal cord. Some of the milder symptoms of mountain sickness are:

- Drowsiness
- Confusion
- Headache
- Nausea
- Impairment of judgment.
- Alteration of behavior.
- Motor incoordination.

Severe symptoms include cerebral and pulmonary edema, loss of consciousness, which may lead to death. To avoid such symptoms, people are advised to climb slowly so that body can get acclimatized to the atmosphere.

Acclimatization

Acclimatization can be defined as the physiological changes that are brought about to adjust for an altered atmosphere when exposed for prolonged duration.

Some of the physiological changes occur when the body is exposed to high altitudes are:

- Increase in rate and depth of respiration due to hypoxic stimulus acting through the peripheral chemoreceptors. However, the increase in rate and depth of respiration brings about washout of carbon dioxide. This reduces pCO_2 (respiratory alkalosis) and the fall in pCO_2 depresses the respiratory center activity. Hence there will be final increase of ventilation.
- There will be increased production of 2–3 DPG which helps for shifting of oxygen dissociation curve to right even though pCO_2 is less than normal.
- There will be increase in the diffusion capacity. Normal diffusion capacity is about 21 ml/min/mm Hg. Increase in diffusion capacity is because of increased surface area available for diffusion due to opening of the normally dormant capillaries and further distension of the already functional alveoli.
- Increase in myoglobin content to store as much of oxygen as possible.
- Increase in cytochrome oxidase enzyme activity to extract as much of oxygen from blood as possible.
- Increase in mitochondria to increase the supply of energy.
- Increase of red blood cell count because of hypoxic stimulus increasing the secretion of erythropoietin.
- Increase of cardiac output.

All the above changes help the person to sustain life easily even at a higher altitude.

Decompression Sickness/Caisson's Disease/Dysbarism

It occurs when people exposed to high barometric pressure suddenly get exposed to low atmospheric pressure. Usually, it is seen in divers who are exposed to high pO_2 below sea level. At high pressures, more gas will have gone into the dissolved state in all the tissues of body including blood. Among the gases, nitrogen which is neither utilized nor excreted also will be dissolved more in the tissues. It escapes from blood and enters organs and tissues. As it is fat-soluble, comparatively more of nitrogen is dissolved in fatty tissue and one of the vital organs in which a lot of nitrogen goes into dissolved state is brain.

When such people ascend up (come back to sea level) all of a sudden, nitrogen is decompressed. The gas starts escaping from the tissues at a faster rate leading to bubbling. When these bubbles enter blood vessels, it may obstruct the blood flow producing embolism. Because of the bubbling of gases either in tissues or in blood, it can lead to certain problems. Some of the features of the condition are:

- Compression in chest (chokes)
- Pain in the joints (bends)
- Pain at the back
- At times there can be damage to brain tissue as well, which may lead to paresis/paralysis.

Treatment

1. Avoid ascending up suddenly.
2. Promote recompression in a chamber and perform slow decompression.

Apnea

Apnea is temporary cessation of breathing. The different types are:
- Deglutition apnea (during deglutition) occurs during 2nd phase of swallowing.
- Voluntary apnea when breath is held voluntarily. Holding of breath cannot continue beyond a particular time. This is because, when breath is held, carbon dioxide accumulates in blood. This increases pCO_2 in circulation. The increased pCO_2 will override the voluntary breath holding effort and the person respires. The point at which the override effect is observed is known as breaking point.
- Hyperventilation apnea is because of washout of carbon dioxide leads to fall in pCO_2. The pCO_2 in

arterial blood can be as little as 15 mm Hg from a normal value of 40 mm Hg.
- Vagal apnea
- Adrenaline apnea

Asphyxia

Asphyxia is a condition in which simultaneously there will be hypoxia (decrease in pO_2) and hypercapnia (increase in pCO_2) occurring in the body. Asphyxia occurs in strangulation, drowning, obstruction to the airway, etc. Asphyxia also occurs when newborn infant fails to breath. Since this condition could be fatal, immediate intervention to restore normal respiration must be initiated.

Periodic Breathing

Periodic breathing is when the breaths are interposed with some amount of apnea. The different types of periodic breathing are (Fig. 4.36):
- Cheyne-Stokes
- Biot's

Effects of hyperventilation: The increase in the rate and depth of respiration will bring about certain alterations in the body. They are:

- Decreased arterial pCO_2 which can fall to as low as 15 mm Hg.
- Increased arterial pO_2, which can be as high as 140 mm Hg.
- The increased voluntary hyperventilation cannot go for any length of time, because the washout of CO_2 from the body decreases the stimulatory influence on the respiratory center.

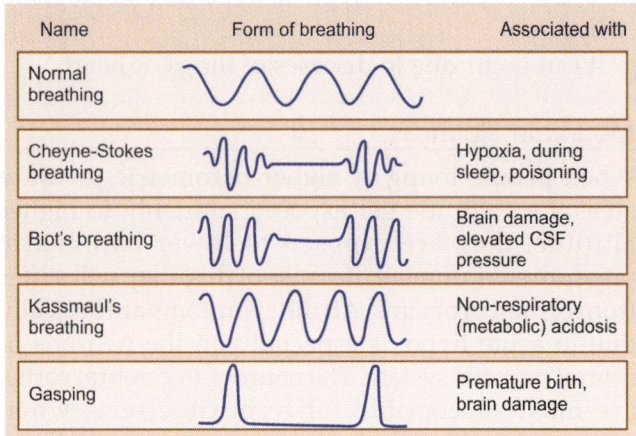

Name	Form of breathing	Associated with
Normal breathing		
Cheyne-Stokes breathing		Hypoxia, during sleep, poisoning
Biot's breathing		Brain damage, elevated CSF pressure
Kassmaul's breathing		Non-respiratory (metabolic) acidosis
Gasping		Premature birth, brain damage

Fig. 4.36: Periodic breathing in different conditions

- When pCO_2 has fallen down to around 15 mm Hg, the respiration arrests for some time. This is known as hyperventilation apnea.
- Because of more of CO_2 elimination from the body, the pH of blood increases. In order to maintain the pH of blood, H^+ from the plasma proteins get liberated. Now the sites occupied by the H^+ are free. To these sites, the ionic calcium binds. This leads to decreased concentration of ionic calcium circulation. Hence can lead to tetany.
- The washout of CO_2 decreases the pCO_2 in blood. The vasodilator effect of carbon dioxide on the cerebral vessels decreases. There will be vasoconstriction in cerebral vessels and leads to decreased blood flow. This can lead to dizziness and loss of consciousness.

Artificial Respiration

When normal breathing has stopped for any reason, it is very essential to induce artificial respiration as early as possible. It is because if oxygen is not supplied to the brain for more than 3 minutes, it causes irreversible damage to brain. Artificial respiration has to be continued till the automatic respiration resumes.

There are different methods of artificial respiration. They can be broadly classified into:
1. Manual methods
2. Instrumental methods.

Some of the important manual methods are:
a. Mouth to mouth breathing.
b. Arm lift back pressure method (Holger Nielsen method)
c. Sylvester's method.
d. Eve's rocking method.

The most important advantage of manual methods is they can be employed anywhere and everywhere without any time delay. But the disadvantage will be they cannot be continued for longer duration. Each one of the manual methods has certain advantages and disadvantages.

Instrumental method: They are mechanical ventilators and basically are of two types, namely:
1. Positive pressure ventilator (air is forced into lungs from the respirator by positive pressure)
2. Negative pressure ventilator (air is made to enter lungs as the negative pressure applied by the respirator will act on the chest wall and bring about the expansion of same)

In both the type of methods, expiration will be brought about by a passive process.

The biggest advantage of the instrumental methods is they can be employed to continue artificial respiration for any length of time. On the other hand, these methods are available only at bigger hospitals and expensive and hence may not be within the reach of common man.

5
CHAPTER

Digestive System

Gastrointestinal Tract

Gastrointestinal tract can be described as a specialized tube communicating with the external environment both at its upper and lower ends. There is regional specialization suited for the local functions. The main functions of GIT are:

1. Secretion: Exocrine—enzymes; endocrine—hormones of GI tract
2. Motility
3. Absorption
4. Storage and excretion of undigested waste materials.

The functions of gastrointestinal tract are controlled by both neural and hormonal mechanisms.

Motility of GIT is mainly the function of the smooth muscle found in most part of the GIT. The movement helps in two ways:

1. Local mixing of the food components
2. Forward propulsion of the food materials

GIT can be described as a barrier between blood and the components of food that has been eaten. Unless the nutrients, vitamins, minerals and other substances pass through the wall of the GIT into the blood, they are not useful to the body. Absorption is, therefore, the process by which the nutrients, minerals, vitamins, water and other substances pass into the blood across the wall of the GIT. The wall has got four layers (Fig. 5.1):

1. *Serous coat:* Contributed by visceral peritoneum throughout except mouth, pharynx, esophagus,

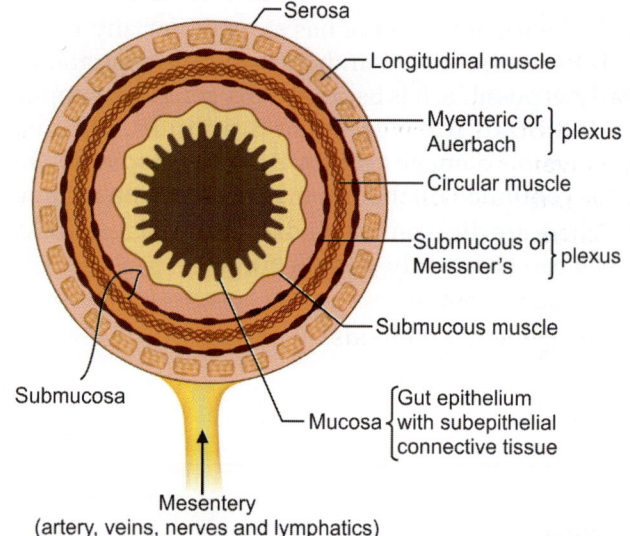

Fig. 5.1: Transverse section of small intestine showing various muscle layers and nerve plexus

rectum and anal canal, where the serous coat is replaced by fibrous tissue.

2. *Muscular coat:* Contributed by smooth muscles arranged generally in two layers; an outer longitudinal and an inner circular muscle. The latter is thickened in the region of sphincters. Between the two layers of muscles, there is the myenteric or Auerbach plexus formed by sympathetic and parasympathetic fibres.

3. *Submucous coat:* Formed of fibrous tissue, lymphatic and blood vessels. Between the muscular and submucous coats is another nerve plexus namely sub-

mucous or Meissner's plexus formed by sympathetic and parasympathetic nerves and also fibers from myenteric plexus.

4. *Mucous coat* has three important components:
   a. Musuclar mucosa formed of smooth muscles
   b. *Lamina propria* which is connective tissue support structure for the epithelium
   c. Epithelium besides lining the GIT is also modified into special glands.

The entire digestive processes namely secretion, motility and absorption are under dual control.

1. *Neural regulatory mechanism:* Mainly through autonomic nervous system controlled by hypothalamus (Figs 5.2 and 5.3), various parts of limbic system and cerebral cortex.

2. *Hormonal regulation:* In this, the GIT hormones as well as the hormones from other specialized endocrine glands outside the GIT, help to regulate the GIT functions.

The various physiological aspects discussed on GI tract are:

a. Mastication (chewing)
b. Salivary secretion
c. Deglutition (Swallowing)
d. Gastric secretion

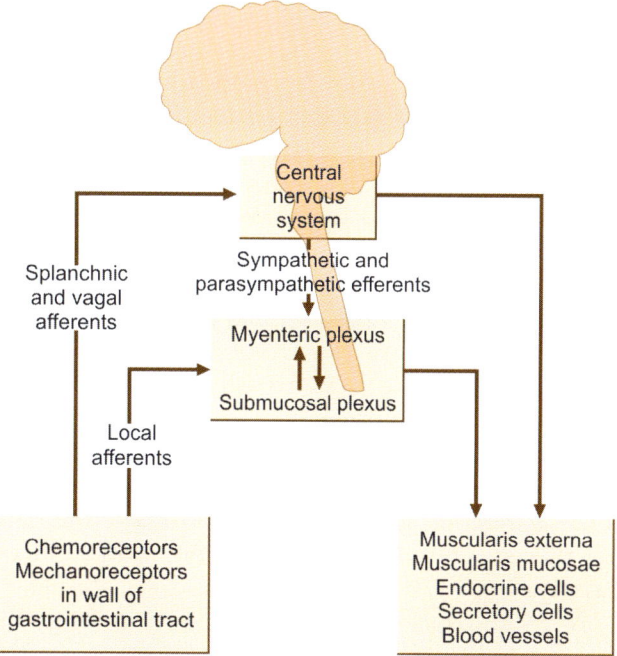

Fig. 5.3: The receptors of GIT, local afferents, splanchnic and vagal afferent, CNS control over the functions of GIT through autonomic nerves

e. Gastric motility
f. Pancreatic secretion
g. Biliary secretion
h. Intestinal motility
i. Functions of colon including movements
j. GI hormones secretion and their actions
k. Digestion and absorption

Salivary Secretion

Saliva is the first digestive juice to come in contact with food. Saliva is secreted by three major salivary glands namely:
• Parotid
• Submandibular (submaxillary)
• Sublingual

Apart from these, there are minor salivary glands in the floor of the mouth, pharynx, tongue and cheeks.

Structure of Salivary Gland

Secretory unit of salivary gland is an acinus. There are two types of acini in the salivary glands namely serous and mucous type.

Parotid gland is mostly made up of serous type, sublingual is predominantly mucous type, sub-

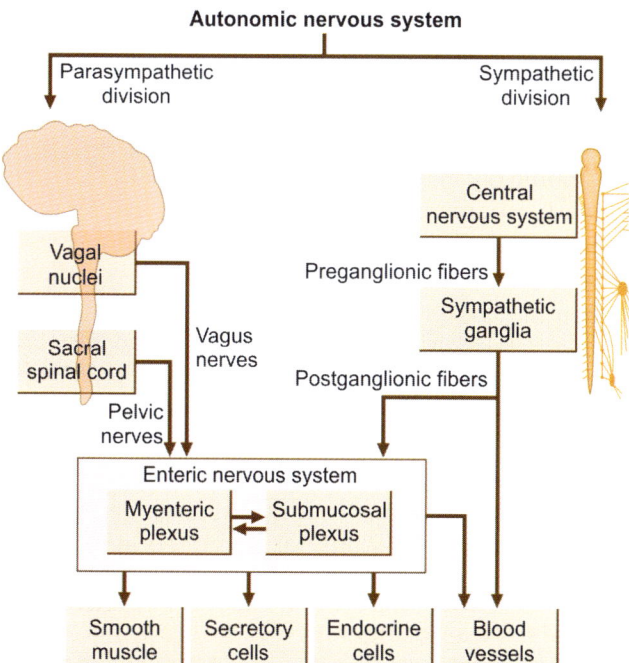

Fig. 5.2: The autonomic nervous system influence on GI tract functions through muscle, secretory and endocrine cells

mandibular is both, but more of serous than mucous type.

Each acinus is lined by glandular epithelium secretion of which enter the lumen which later on continues as intercalated duct (Fig. 5.4). A serous acinus contains cells, the nucleus of which is more towards the base and they have zymogen granules. These granules are precursors of salivary enzyme ptyalin which is also known as salivary amylase.

Mucous acini have cells which contain mucinogen granules which are precursors of mucin. These granules do not take up stain easily and hence appear translucent under normal hematoxylin stain.

In submanidular gland, another type of acini known as seromucous acini are present. In this type, there is mucous acinus, on top of which serous cells are placed. The salivary glands have profuse blood supply.

As for the duct system, each acinus drains into the intercalated duct. The intercalated ducts of various acini drain into striated ducts. These ducts are so-called because their epithelium possesses numerous infolding at the base and hence appear striated. They also have numerous mitochondria; several striated ducts unite to form an excretory duct. Excretory ducts join to form the main collecting duct.

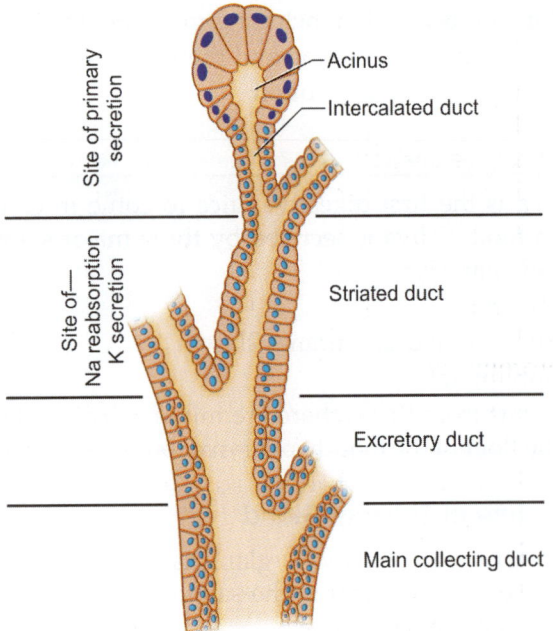

Fig. 5.4: Histology of salivary gland showing the primary and secondary areas of secretion

The duct of each parotid gland, known as Stenson's duct and this opens into the mouth opposite the upper 2nd molar tooth.

The duct of each submandibular gland, known as Wharton's duct, and this opens into the mouth by the side of frenulum lingue.

From the sublingual gland, 5–15 ducts open into the floor of the mouth and these ducts are known as ducts of Rivinus.

Nerve Supply

The acini, myoepithelial cells and the blood vessels of salivary glands are well supplied by sympathetic and parasympathetic nerve fibers.

Parasympathetic: These fibers are important because they are known as the secretomotor fibers to the salivary gland. On stimulation, they bring about (1) secretion from the glands and (2) increase the blood flow to salivary glands.

There are two nuclei in the medulla known as superior and inferior salivary nuclei. From the superior salivary nucleus, the secretomotor fibers for submandibular and sublingual glands take origin. The preganglionic fibers travel in the chorda tympani nerve which is a branch of the facial nerve. The fibers of chorda tympanic nerve synapse in the sub-mandibular ganglion. The postganglionic fibers supply the submandibular and sublingual salivary glands (Fig. 5.5).

From the inferior salivary nucleus, the pre-ganglionic fibers for the parotid gland arise and travel in the tympanic branch of glossopharyngeal nerve. This nerve forms tympanic plexus and continues as the lesser superficial petrosal nerve. The preganglionic fibers then synapse in the otic ganglion. From the otic ganglion, postganglionic fibers travel as the auriculo-temporal nerve and supply the parotid gland. Since parasympathetic nerve is involved in the salivary secretion, the secretion can be blocked by atropine.

It is interesting to note that the chorda tympani (branch of VII) and IX cranial nerves carry taste sensations from the tongue. The deep association between taste and salivation is very well known.

Sympathetic: Preganglionic nerve fibers take origin from the lateral horn cells of T1, T2 segments of spinal cord. They relay in the superior cervical ganglion from where the postganglionic fibers take origin and reach

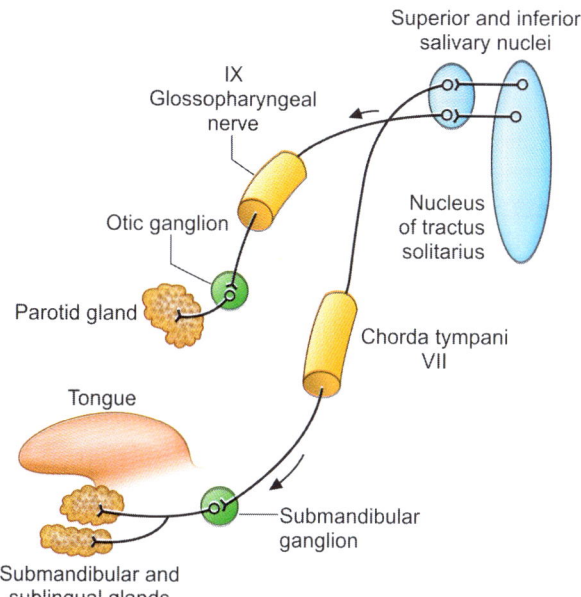

Fig. 5.5: The efferent parasympathetic innervations from salivary nuclei to salivary glands

the glands along the blood vessels supplying the gland.

Composition of Saliva

On an average, the rate of secretion of saliva is about 1 ml/minute.
- Total volume/day = 1–1.5 liters
- pH—slightly acidic
- Hypotonic to plasma
- 99.5% water
- 0.5% solids
- Electrolytes: Na^+, K^+, Ca^{++}, Cl^-, HCO_3^-, PO_4

Organic
- Salivary—ptyalin (salivary amylayse)
- Proteins—mucin
- Lysozome
- Kallekrein
- Blood group substance
- Amino acids
- Urea
- Uric acid
- Creatinine
- Cell debris

Mechanism of Secretion of Saliva

There are two theories that try to explain the mechanism of salivary secretion:

a. *Active secretion:* Secretion of saliva is an active process because it involves increased metabolism, utilization of energy substrate and increased oxygen consumption. The secretion from the acini is called the primary secretion. It contains water and electrolytes similar in composition to plasma besides the other salivary proteins. Unlike other glands, the duct system of salivary glands is actively involved in modifying the composition of saliva, e.g. in the striate duct of the epithelium reabsorbs Na^+ in exchange for K^+. This epithelium also actively secretes HCO_3^-. Therefore, the final saliva reaching mouth has more K^+ and HCO_3^- and less of Na^+ and Cl^- compared to the primary secretion.

b. *Ultrafiltration:* According to this theory, saliva is an ultrafiltrate of plasma, very much like glomerular filtrate in the kidney. The pressure for filtration is provided by arterial blood pressure. This theory is not accepted because even when the pressure in the salivary gland is higher than the arterial blood pressure, the salivary secretion continues.

The saliva that is collected from the mouth is contributed by all the salivary glands and the fraction from the different glands will be 70% from submandibular, 25% from parotid and 5% from sublingual.

Regulation of Secretion of Saliva

Salivary secretion regulation is brought about by both neural and the hormone (hormonal) mechanisms. Salivary secretion is a spontaneous process subject to modification by other factors. Effect of stimulation of nerves supplying salivary glands

a. *Parasympathetic secretomotor fibers:* As the name secretomotor implies, parasympathetic stimulation increases the volume of salivary secretion profoundly.

The secretion is rich is ptyalin. This is because of two reasons:
  i. The parasympathetic nerve fibers stimulate the acinar cells directly.
  ii. They cause vasodilatation in the salivary gland increasing the blood flow.
    a. The mechanism of vasodilatation by the parasympathetic nerves in salivary gland is brought about by acetylcholine.

b. Parasympathetic stimulation also liberates VIP (vasoactive intestinal polypeptide). This can also cause vasodilatation.

c. Parasympathetic stimulation also secretes kallikrien, an enzyme found in the acini, kallikrien acts on two globulins of plasma and forms bradykinin which is a very powerful local vasodilator. Increase in the blood flow is not abolished by atropine suggesting that acetylcholine is not responsible for vasodilatation.

b. *Sympathetic stimulation:* Sympathetic stimulation causes vasoconstriction and reduction in blood supply to the salivary glands.

As far as the direct action on acini is concerned, the sympathetic stimulation has no effect on parotid gland in man. In the case of submandibular gland, in man there is increase in secretion but the amount is small and the secretion is thick and viscous due to high mucin content. Sympathetic stimulation causes contraction of myoepithelial cells.

Reflex Regulation

Salivary secretion is brought about by reflex action.

a. *Unconditioned reflex:* This reflex is present at birth. This is due to the stimulation of receptors in the mouth by chemical substances which are present in food and even mechanical stimulation brought about by food in mouth. Presence of food in the mouth brings about immediate secretion.

Exclusive mechanical stimulation of oral cavity by any means also stimulates salivary secretion. For example, maneuver of oral cavity by dentists, movement of tongue thereby coming in contact with cheeks.

The most important stimulus is the presence of food in the mouth. The details of the influence of unconditioned stimulus on salivary secretion is detailed in Fig. 5.6.

b. *Conditioned reflex:* This reflex is acquired during the life. Here, the stimulation process originates not from the mouth but from the organs of special senses, especially sight and smell, to a certain extent even hearing. In the case of human beings, the previous experiences associated with the supply of food like the sight, smell can give rise to secretion of saliva. In animals, the conditioned reflex for secretion of saliva can be experimentally produced for sight, sound or smell of food.

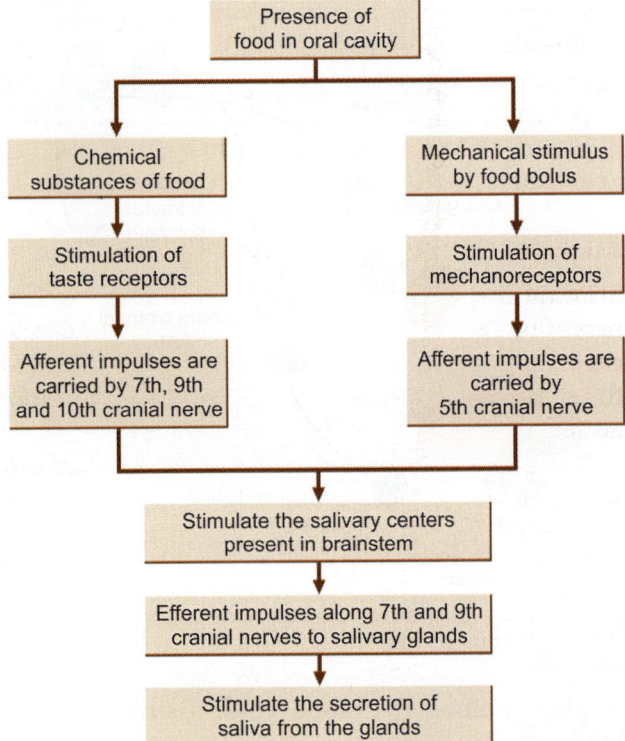

Fig. 5.6: Flow chart detailing the unconditioned salivary secretion

Pavlov demonstrated conditioned salivary secretion in dogs. Every time a dog was served with food, after ringing of bell. After few days, just the ringing of the bell alone without food being served causes secretion of saliva. During the training period, the dog learns to associate ringing (sound) of bell with supply of food.

Paralytic Salivary Secretion

When the chorda tympani nerve supplying the submandibualr and sublingual glands is cut, although these fibers are the secretomotor fibres, still the two glands secrete saliva initially less in volume but it starts increasing to a maximum by about the 7th or 8th day after the nerve is cut. This rate of secretion remains constant for about 3 weeks and by about 6 weeks the secretion almost stops. The reasons for the paralytic salivary secretion are:

1. *Chorda tympani*, the parasympathetic nerve cutting, means cutting the preganglionic fibers. The postganglionic fibers remain active and secrete acetylcholine for some time.

2. *Increased excitability of sympathetic fibers:* On cutting the parasympathetic nerve, the excitability of

sympathetic fibers increases and they get stimulated more easily.

3. *Denervation hypersensitivity:* Cutting of the parasympathetic chorda tympani nerve makes the gland more sensitive to circulating chemical substances, like acetylcholine.

Augmented Salivary Secretion

Stimulation of sympathetic and parasympathetic nerve fiber supplying the salivary glands simultaneously causes an increase in secretion which is far more than the summated effects of individual nerve stimulation added.

Taste is not essential for salivation. Substances which are insipid also stimulate the secretion of saliva. But the rate of secretion of saliva is affected by taste. Substances having sour taste bring about a greater volume of secretion. Composition of saliva whether it is rich in enzymes, mucin or water can be varied according to the food that is presented.

Functions of Saliva

Salivary glands are not essential for life. The functions of saliva are:

a. *Lubrication of food:* Assisted by chewing, saliva gets mixed with food in the mouth; the mucin which is a sticky substance helps to form bolus. Saliva prepares the food for swallowing forming a slippery coat over the bolus.

b. *Solvent action:* Taste is a chemical sense. Any substance, the taste of which has to be perceived, has to be in dissolved state to stimulate the taste receptors present in taste buds thoroughout the oral cavity. Saliva acts as the solvent and thereby helps for perception of taste.

c. *Cleansing action:* The continuous flow of saliva keeps the mouth clean, free from food particles; shed epithelial cells and foreign bodies. Moreover, the lysozyme present in saliva helps to kill certain bacteria. The evidence of this action is obvious during fever. In most of the fevers, the salivary secretion is diminished.

d. *Digestive function:* Salivary amylase or ptyalin is a carbohydrate splitting enzyme. It acts at a pH of 6.8. It can act only on cooked starch. When the starch is boiled, the cellulose covering of starch granules break and amylase can penetrate cellulose. *Cooked starch is digested by ptyalin in the following manner:*

$$\text{Cooked starch}$$
$$\downarrow$$
$$\text{Erythrodextrin + Maltose}$$
$$\downarrow$$
$$\text{Achrodextrin + Maltose}$$
$$\downarrow$$
$$\text{Isomaltose + Maltose}$$

Small amount of glucose may also be formed. The duration for which food remains in the mouth is not sufficient for all these steps to be completed. Once the food reaches the stomach, the pH of stomach is highly acidic and hence not conducive for ptyalin action. Yet the action of ptyalin continues in the deeper part of food bolus even in the stomach.

e. *Excretory function:* Several substances can be excreted in saliva, e.g. heavy metals like mercury, lead, iodides, alkaloids like morphine, antibiotics like penicillin, streptomycin, microorganisms like viruses causing mumps, measles, polio, etc. But most of the times, the saliva formed is being swallowed. Thus it may not serve much of excretory function.

f. *Helps in speech:* The moistening action of saliva in the mouth helps in articulation of speech. Those who speak for a long time sip a little water in between to facilitate articulation of speech.

g. *Role in regulating water content in body:* Since saliva contains 99.5% water and daily secretion of saliva is 1 liter or more, decrease in body water content decreases salivary secretion and results in thirst sensation.

h. *Buffering function:* Saliva contains bicarbonate, phosphate, proteins, etc. They act as buffers to keep the salivary pH within the normal limits. Decreased pH predisposes to caries whereas increase in pH will be responsible for tartar material and destroys the alveogingival margin.

Disorders of Salivary Secretion

a. *Hyposalivation* is decrease in the volume of salivary secretion. It can be caused by anxiety, excitement or irradiation.

b. *Hypersalivation or sialorrhea:* This can occur in pregnancy and parotitis (e.g. mumps), tumors in oral cavity.

c. *Xerostomia (dry mouth):* This is a rare condition in which the salivary glands are deficient or absent right from birth. So there may be scanty secretion of saliva.

d. *Chorda tympani syndrome:* Sometimes the chorda tympani nerve may be cut accidentally. When the fibers regenerate, they miss their normal target and instead innervate the sweat gland of skin in the submandibular region. In such a case, whenever there is stimulation for salivation, say while eating, there is also significant sweating of skin in sub mandibular region. It must be noted that now the sweat glands are also supplied by some parasympathetic nerve fibers that were supplied to salivary glands earlier.

Mastication or Chewing

Mastication or chewing is the first mechanical process to which the food is subjected in the GIT.

The objectives of this mechanical process are 3-folds:

a. The action of teeth and mandible breaks down larger food particles into smaller one.

b. Enables saliva to mix with the food so as to provide lubrication and form a bolus which is a preparatory step for swallowing.

c. To enable the contents of saliva, especially ptyalin to mix uniformly with the food.

There are different muscles involved in the movement of mandible. The muscles of mastication are:

- Masseter
- Temporalis
- Pterygoid—medial pterygoid and lateral pterygoid

Temporalis and masseter help in the closure of the jaw. Pterygoids help in side to side movement of the mandible. Opening of the mouth is mainly aided by:

- Digastric
- Myelohyoid
- Gravity

Mastication is also helped by another muscle known as buccinator.

Masseter, temporalis and the pterygoids receive nerve supply from mandibular division of trigeminal nerve.

Mastication is a voluntary process. However, stimulation of certain areas in the medulla and cerebral cortex can elicit chewing movements.

Deglutition or Swallowing

Deglutition is complex and coordinated physiological process by which food placed in the mouth moves down into the stomach by passing through pharynx and esophagus.

Stages of Deglutition

There are three important stages:

1. *Oral or buccal stage:* In which food passes from mouth to pharynx.
2. *Pharyngeal stage:* In which food passes from pharynx to esophagus.
3. *Esophageal stage:* In which, food passes through esophagus to stomach.

Of these three stages, the 1st stage is voluntary initially but later on becomes involuntary. 2nd and 3rd stages are exclusively involuntary and, therefore, occur by a reflex action (Fig. 5.7).

- Swallowing can be considered as a reflex
- *Receptors* are situated around the oropharynx.
- *Afferents:* Through V, IX and X cranial nerves.
- *Center:* The swallowing center (deglutition center) is located close to the respiratory centers in the floor of the 4th ventricle of medulla oblongata.

Anatomists believe that nucleus ambiguus and nucleus of tractus solitarius act as the swallowing centers.

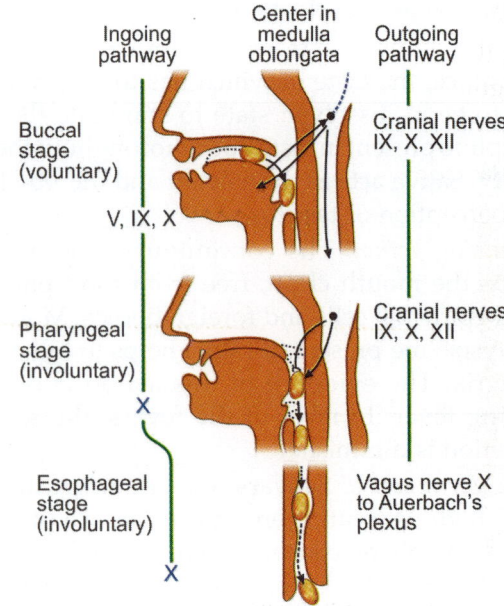

Fig. 5.7: Afferent and efferent nerves involved in different phases of deglutition

Efferent: 9th , 10th and 12th cranial nerve for first and second stages, 10th nerve for the 3rd stage.

Effectors: Muscles of the tongue, palate, pharynx, esophagus (upper one-third esophagus has skeletal muscle while lower two-thirds has smooth muscle).

1. Buccal or Oral Stage

By the action of tongue, and muscles contracting against the palate, the food is converted into bolus which is lubricated by saliva. The bolus is then pushed by the tongue to the posterodorsal aspect of the tongue. This is called the preparatory position. In this process, the tongue moves upwards and backwards pressing against the hard palate.

From the preparatory position, the rest of the first stage of swallowing is by a reflex action, wherein the following muscles of the tongue are involved.

- Myelohyoid
- Styloglossus
- Hypoglossus

The above muscles contract, and push the food into the pharynx. The first stage thus gets completed. The oral phase of deglutition is affected in the following diseases affecting tongue, lips, palate, etc.

- Inflammatory
- Neoplastic
- Congenital anomalies
- Paralytic

2. Pharyngeal Stage (Very Important) (Fig. 5.8)

During this stage, food has to pass from pharynx into esophagus avoiding the respiratory tract in the process.

The objectives of this stage are: (a) protective, (b) propulsive

Food in the pharynx can take any of the four directions, namely:

a. Back into the mouth
b. Up into the nose
c. Forwards and downwards into the larynx and respiratory tract
d. Down into the esophagus

Except for movement down into the esophagus, normally entry of bolus into all the three other regions will be prevented.

1. Movement back into the mouth is blocked by the tongue compressing against the hard palate and blocking the passage.
2. The soft palate moves upwards and backwards closing the posterior nasal aperture. The muscles in the soft palate which contract are:
   - Tensor veli palatini
   - Levator veli palatini
3. Due to inhibition of respiration and approximation of the vocal cords which close the larynx and also the epiglottis forming a hood over the larynx, food is prevented from entering into larynx. During the second stage of deglutition, respiration is reflexly inhibited and speech is interrupted.
4. Since all the other three routes are blocked, food can easily go into the 4th outlet namely esophagus. During deglutition, the cricopharyngeal muscle (upper esophageal sphincter) relaxes and facilitates the entry of bolus from pharynx into the esophagus.

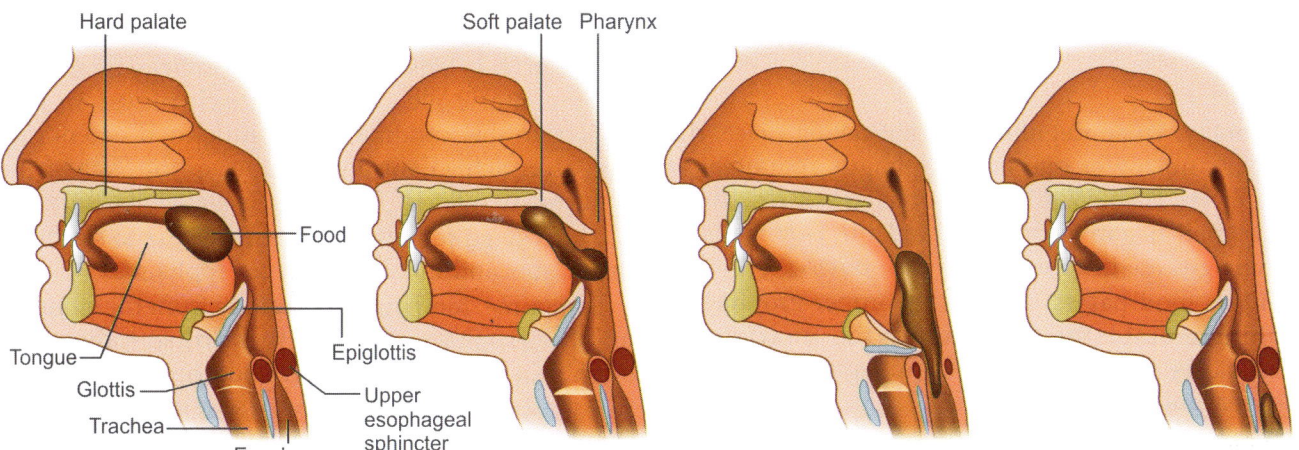

Fig. 5.8: Passage of bolus from pharynx to esophagus during the pharyngeal phase of deglutition

Propulsive aspect: Once the food is in the pharyngeal area the muscles of the pharynx act on it. The important pharyngeal muscles brought into action are: Superior, middle, inferior—constrictors of the pharynx.

Superior and middle constrictors go into powerful contraction known as pharyngeal peristalsis. Inferior constrictor is also known as cricopharyngeus. This is located at the pharyngoesophageal junction forming the upper esophageal sphincter or cricopharyngeal sphincter.

Once the pharyngeal peristalsis starts, cricopharyngeal sphincter relaxes as a part of the swallowing reflex and lets the food pass into the esophagus.

The upper esophageal sphincter has a length of about 4 cm and when there is no deglutition, it is in a state of powerful contraction. Second stage of swallowing is further helped by upward and forward movements of larynx, the epiglottis helping to divert the food to the sides of larynx.

Disturbances of second stage: Conditions affecting larynx, pharynx, soft palate are:
- Inflammatory
- Neoplastic
- Congenital anomalies
- Paralytic

The two stages are well made out especially when solids are swallowed. Very often while swallowing liquids, 1st and 2nd stages are merged into one called the buccopharyngeal stage, i.e. the pharyngeal stage hardly takes a second.

The temporary cessation of breathing which occurs during swallowing is called deglutition apnea.

3. Esophageal Stage

Normally, when deglutition is not taking place, the upper and lower ends of esophagus remain in a contracted state. Within the esophagus, at rest, there is a small negative pressure and the two walls of esophagus are in contact with each other.

Once food passes through the upper esophageal sphincter into the esophagus, the pharyngeal peristalsis continues in the esophagus as primary esophageal peristalsis.

Peristalsis is a coordinated phenomenon in which a wave of contraction will be preceded by a wave of receptive relaxation and travels down a hollow organ (or viscera) and as a rule, this wave travels from oral towards the aboral direction.

If a primary wave is unable to propel the bolus into the stomach, then secondary peristaltic wave starts in the esophagus and completes the act of swallowing. This is brought about by distension of wall of esophagus due to the presence of food.

Tertiary esophageal contractions are irregular contractions usually found in the lower part of esophagus. The cause and nature of these contractions are not well understood. These are not normally seen in human beings. Factors influencing third stage of deglutition are:
- Consistency of food
- Vagal stimulation
- Gravity

Helped by these peristaltic contractions and in the erect posture facilitated by gravity also to a certain extent, the food reaches the esophagogastric junction. This junction is guarded by a physiologic sphincter known as cardiac sphincter. Cardiac sphincter extends above and below the diaphragm by about 1–2 cm. Normally, this area remains contracted but during the third stage of swallowing the sphincter relaxes to allow the food to enter stomach. The relaxation thus produced is known as receptive relaxation.

The cardiac sphincter is relaxed by vagal stimulation, action of acetylcholine, secretin and VIP (vasoactive intestinal polypeptide). It is powerfully contracted by action of gastrin.

Difficulty in swallowing in any stage is known as dysphagia.

Achalasia cardia: In this condition, the food is held up in the lower region of esophagus which is in a state of spasm. It is believed to be due to degeneration of the myenteric plexus or Auerbach plexus in that region. In this condition, very little food enters into the stomach. Esophagus above the spasm is abnormally dilated. Treatment is usually by surgery.

Third stage can also be disturbed due to stricture, neoplasms and inflammation of esophagus.

Sometime, food may regurgitate from the stomach into the esophagus because the cardiac sphincter is often in a relaxed state. This is detrimental because the acid contents of stomach can damage the esophageal wall which is normally not exposed to acid. This condition is called reflux esophagitis. This causes typical burning pain behind the sternum. The pain of reflux esophagitis is called heart burn as the pain is felt behind the sternum. In hiatus hernia also, there can be heart burn.

Stricture of esophagus due to consumption of strong alkali or acid is associated with dysphagia. Dysphagia also occurs in esophageal carcinoma.

Belching: It is the involuntary expulsion of swallowed air. Air is normally swallowed during food intake.

Some hysterical people swallow too much of air "Aerophagia". Once air collects in the upper part of the stomach, the intragastric pressure may increase so much that the cardiac sphincter relaxes resulting in the expulsion of air through esophagus and mouth.

Gastric Secretion

Functions of Stomach

1. *Temporary storage organ:* It acts as a temporary storage organ. Because of this, the frequency of eating is reduced.
2. *Secretory function* (Fig. 5.9): It secretes HCl and pepsin apart from other things including mucus. The G cells of pyloric region secrete gastrin hormone which is one of the GI tract hormones.
3. *Digestive function* is because of pepsin enzyme. It is a proteolytic enzyme.
4. *Protective function* is because of high acidic medium due to presence of HCl, many of the micro-organisms die. Thereby it protects the GI tract from getting invaded by the microorganisms.

5. *Hemopoietic function* is because of the intrinsic factor which is secreted by gastric glands. Intrinsic factor is essential for absorption of vitamin B_{12} in the ileum region.
6. *Absorptive function* is also one of the functions of stomach. Some amount of water and alcohol is absorbed in the stomach region.

Structure of Gastric Mucosa

The gastric mucosa is normally covered by a thick layer of mucous. Once this layer is removed, one can make out a number of pores known as gastric pits. Each pit is the out let for 3–7 gastric glands (Fig. 5.10). The gastric glands are tubular glands which extend from the pit up to the muscularis mucosa. Each gland has got isthmus, neck, body and base. The characters of the gastric glands vary from the cardiac to the body and fundus and in the pyloric regions. They have five different types of cells.

1. *Mucous neck cells:* Secrete soluble mucin whereas the mucous cells lining the surface of the stomach which are derived from mucous neck cells secrete insoluble or visible mucin. This visible mucin is the one that coats the inner surface of stomach. The mucous cells also secrete bicarbonates. The mucous secretion is alkaline.
2. *Chief/peptic/zymogen cells:* These secrete the enzymes of gastric juice, most important of which is pepsiongen. So these cells have Golgi apparatus, mitochondria and endodplasmic reticulum, all of which are responsible for protein synthesis.

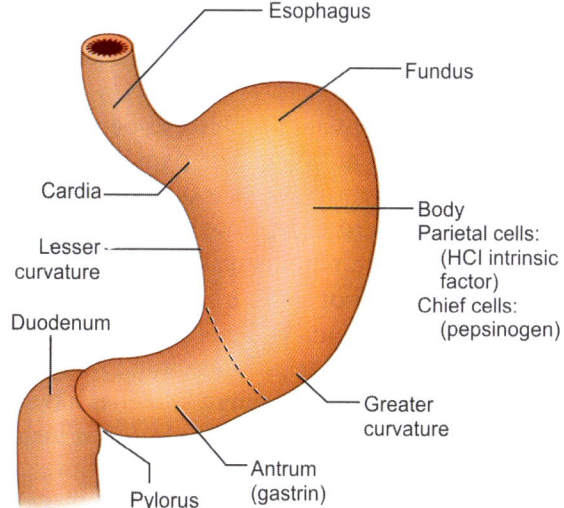

Fig. 5.9: Main parts of stomach and the some important cell types involved in gastric secretions

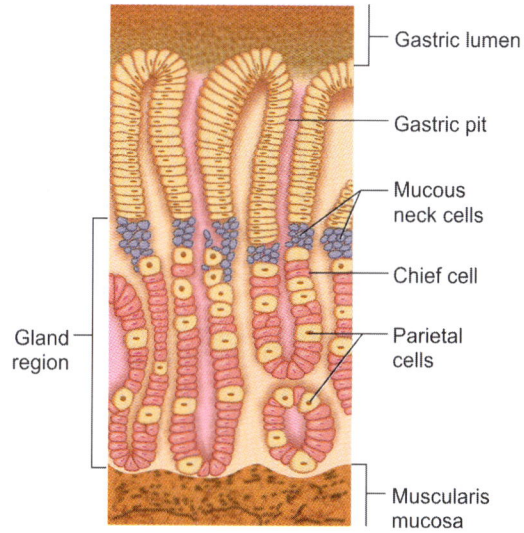

Fig. 5.10: The various cell types in gastric glands

3. *Parietal or oxyntic cells:* Located in the side walls of the gland. These cells secrete HCl and intrinsic factor of Castle. These parietal cells have got well-developed intracellular canaliculi, tubulovesicular system and a large number of mitochondria. Their secretion gets into the lumen of the gland by flowing in between the chief cells. The presence of canaliculi and other structures are meant for secretion of HCl.

4. *The G cells* present in the pyloric antral region secrete gastrin, one of the important hormones of GI tract with few important actions.

5. *Undifferentiated cells:* These are believed to be undifferentiated and are believed to be the precursors of the parents of parietal cells, chief cells and enteroendocrine cells.

Gastric glands of cardiac region are shorter and are predominantly mucous cells.

In the pyloric region, again the mucous cells predominate. There are very few chief and parietal cells in the above regions.

Innervation of Stomach

Parasympathetic: It is through the right and left vagi. The preganglionic fibers arise from the dorsal motor nucleus of vagus in medulla. The ganglia are found in myenteric and submucosal plexus. Postganglionic fibers are very short and supply mucous membranes, gastric glands and muscles.

- Left vagus supplies anterior aspect of stomach
- Right vagus supplies posterior aspect of stomach
- The efferent fibers are secertomotor to the stomach. Vagus also contains afferent fibers which carry afferent impulses from the stomach to the medulla.

Stimulation of efferent vagi supplying the stomach increases the volume of gastric secretion which is rich in HCl, pepsinogen and also increases the contraction of the gastric muscles. This enhances the peristaltic contractions in stomach and hence emptying of the contents of stomach.

Sympathetic nerve supply are from lateral horn cells of T5–T10 segments of spinal cord. These are preganglionic fibers. Few of them synapse in the ganglia of the sympathetic chain while most of them synapse with cells of celiac ganglion. The post-ganglionic fibers accompany the arterial supply to the stomach.

Effects of sympathetic stimulation on gastric secretion are not definite. Indirectly, it diminishes gastric secretion by reducing blood flow by bringing about vasoconstriction. It is also known that sympathetic stimulation causes an increased alkaline mucoid secretion from the glands. Like vagus sympathetic nerves also carry efferent and afferent fibers to and from the stomach.

Composition of Gastric Juice

- Gastric juice is the secretion of gastric glands.
- Total amount secreted: 1, 200–1.500 ml per day.
- Night secretion (during sleep) alone is 400 ml/day.
- Acidity of gastric juice: 40–60 mEq/liter
- pH: 0.9–1.5
- Water content—99.45%
- Total solids—0.55%
- Specific gravity—1.002–1.004
- *Solids:* Inorganic: 0.15% (NaCl, KCl, CaCl, calcium phosphate, magnesium phosphate, bicarbonate, etc.)
- *Organic:* 0.4%
  - Mucin, blood group, substances, intrinsic factor of castle
  - *Enzymes:* Pepsinogen, gastric lipase, rennin (absent in adult human beings, may be present in infants)
- Characteristic component of gastric juice is HCl.

Enzymes of Gastric Juice

Pepsinogens: Three different pepsinogens have been discovered. Pepsinogen I, II and III. Molecular weight is about 46,000.

- Pepsinogen is activated by HCl to pepsin; pepsin itself can cause activation of pepsinogen (auto-catalysis). Activation involves only the removal of a short peptide from pepsinogen.
- Molecular weight of pepsin: 35,000
- Pepsin acts at pH of 1.5–3.5
- Being a proteolytic enzyme, it converts larger proteins into smaller polypeptides by attaching peptide bonds involving phenylalanine or tyrosine.
- A small amount of pepsin is excreted in urine as uropepsin.
- *Rennin:* If present has got an action on milk by clotting it. This is nothing but conversion of soluble caseinogen into insoluble calcium caseinate. Since

rennin is mostly absent in human beings, pepsin performs the same action.

- *Gelatinase:* It is a very useful enzyme for the digestion of gelatin. The gastric enzymes are not essential for life. Most important gastric enzyme is pepsin and what pepsin can do; the pancreatic trypsin does equally well.
- *Gastric mucins:* There are two types of mucin. Soluble mucin from the mucous neck cells and the insoluble mucin from the surface epithelium of stomach.

Functions of Mucin

a. Mucin along with the bicarbonate protects the gastric walls from the action of gastric HCl and pepsin.

b. The mucin lining the mucous membrane of the stomach forms a mechanical barrier preventing HCl and pepsin to come in contact with gastric mucosa. A breakdown of this barrier can easily result in formation of peptic ulcers.

Peptic ulcers can be defined as ulcers in the gastric wall caused by acid peptic digestion. (Ulcers in general mean a discontinuity in skin or mucous membrane.)

Nowadays, it is be believed that more than the mucin barrier, the very structure of gastric mucous membrane with its tight intercellular junctions forms a more effective barrier to the action of HCl and pepsin. Gastric mucin secretion is stimulated by any type of chemical or mechanical irritation of the stomach. The drug aspirin, alcohol, etc., can break the mucin barrier and increase the susceptibility (vulnerability) to peptic ulcer.

Functions of HCl

a. Activation of pepsinogen to pepsin.
b. Provides an acid medium for the action of pepsin.
c. Being a strong acid, it can kill many bacteria that have entered stomach along with the food.
d. HCl in the duodenum can stimulate and increase the secretion of bile from liver and the exocrine secretion from pancreas.

Mechanism of secretion of HCl (Fig. 5.11): HCl is secreted by the parietal cells. Pure parietal cell secretion has (H^+) –150 mEq/liter whereas (H^+) of plasma is 0.00004 mEq/liter. It means that the parietal cells have to secrete H^+ ions actively. The concentra-

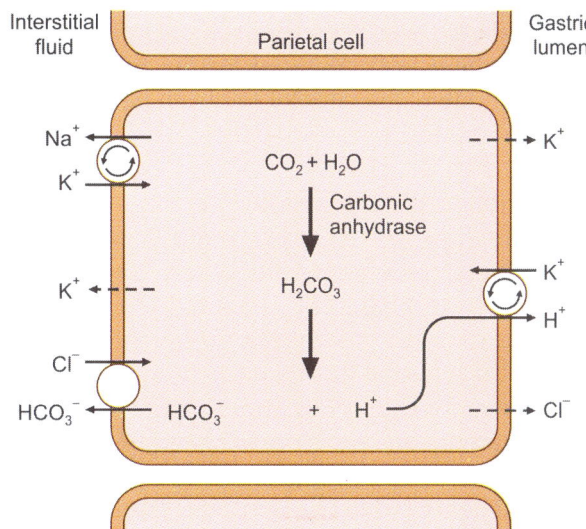

Fig. 5.11: Reactions involved in the process of secretion of HCl by parietal cells

tion of H^+ ions secreted is directly proportional to the number of parietal cells.

There are two views regarding the source of H^+ ions for HCl secretion:

1. *Davenport's view:* According to this, a high energy compound is oxidized to yield H^+ ion and an electron. The electron is processed in the mitochondria by the cytochrome system and is accepted by an O_2. In the process, OH^- is formed and energy is liberated. The H^+ ion formed initially uses the energy liberated to form HCl. Cl^- for this reaction comes from plasma.

2. *Modern view:* States that H^+ ions in the parietal cells are obtained by active ionization of water yielding H^+ and OH^- ions OH^- should not be allowed to accumulate inside the cell. It is neutralized in the following manner: CO_2 produced inside the cell and also contributed from plasma combines with water in presence of carbonic anhydrase (CA) to yield H_2CO_3. H_2CO_3 dissociates to yield H^+ ion and HCO_3^- ion. This H^+ ion neutralizes the OH^- ion. H^+ and OH react to form water.

If carbonic anhydrase action is blocked, the entire HCl secretion is inhibited. One of the drugs used to block the action of carbonic anhydrase is acetazolamide (diamox).

The H^+ ion formed because of ionization of water is pumped into the intracellular canaliculus in exchange for K^+. This H^+–K^+ pump activity requires the energy supply. ATP is readily available from metabolism of carbohydrates inside the parietal cells to supply the energy required for the activity of the pump. Cl⁻ enters the parietal cell from plasma in two ways:

   i. In exchange of HCO_3^-
   ii. By independent diffusion.

Thus it is proved that H⁺ and Cl⁻ are actively secreted into the canaliculus where the coupling occurs to form HCl. The canaliculus is in direct continuation with gastric gland which enters the stomach through the gastric pit.

Immediately following a meal, pepsin and HCl secretion are increased. More H⁺ ions being utilized, more HCO_3^-, ions secreted outside. HCO_3^- will enter blood and hence pH of blood becomes more alkaline. This phenomenon is called post-prandial alkaline tide. Following a meal, kidney excretes more of alkaline urine for short period to maintain the pH of blood.

HCl secretion by parietal cells is stimulated by vagus, gastrin, and histamine (Fig. 5.12). Parietal cells have receptors for the above chemicals. The receptor activity can be selectively inhibited to decrease acid secretion in patients who are secreting excess HCl leading to peptic ulcer formation. HCl secretion is inhibited by:

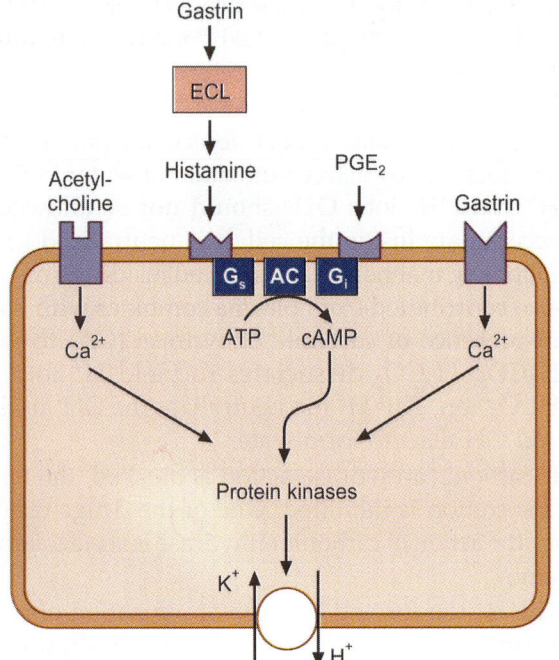

Fig. 5.12: Receptor sites for binding of various chemical substances for modulation of the activity of parietal cells

  a. Acid in the pyloric antrum
  b. Acid in the duodenum
  c. Fat in the duodenum
  d. Hyperosmotic particles in the duodenum
  e. Emotional problems, like depression, disappointment

Methods to Study Gastric Secretion

There are several methods available in experimental animals and in man to collect gastric juice, enabling us to study the various aspects of gastric secretion and their regulation.

a. In Experimental Animals (usually in dogs)

1. *Pavlov's pouch:* This pouch is made out of the stomach in the dog in such a way that the pouch opens through the skin to the exterior and is still connected to the main body of the stomach by a bridge. The pouch helps in the collection of pure gastric juice uncontaminated by food. Being a part of the main stomach, Pavlov's pouch retains both parasympathetic and sympathetic nerve supply. Pavlov's pouch is very useful in the study of various phases of gastric secretion and their regulation.

2. *Heidenhain's pouch:* This pouch is constructed in a way similar to Pavlov's pouch. The only difference is that Heidenhan's pouch does not have vagal supply. It has got sympathetic nerve supply and blood supply. It is also very useful in study of gastric secretion. Especially to study the effect of absence of vagal influence on gastric secretion. Secretion will be influenced by only the hormones.

3. *Bickel's pouch:* It is nothing but Heidenhain's pouch without sympathetic supply. Totally denervated pouch.

4. *Pavlov's sham feeding:* In this experiment, esophagus of the dog is exposed in the neck. A complete cut is made transversely and the two cut ends of esophagus are made to open one below the other through the skin of the neck. Therefore, any food placed inside the mouth once swallowed, does not enter the stomach. It comes out through the upper cut end of esophagus. The animal gets all the pleasure of eating (sensation but the food does not reach the stomach. That is why this procedure is called SHAM or mock feeding). To make the animal survive, it is fed through the lower cut end of esophagus. This is very useful to study the cephalic

phase of gastric secretion. The lower end is also useful to collect gastric juice from stomach with the help of a tube.

b. In Man

a. *Through Ryle's (nasogastric) tube:* A thin flexible rubber tube is passed through the nose or mouth and gastric juice can be collected from stomach by aspiration.

b. *Gastric fistula:* Fistula is a communication between one hollow organ and another or a communication between a hollow organ and the exterior.

c. *Gastroscopy:* Gastroscope is an instrument through which the interior of the stomach can be easily visualized. This is particularly done to determine ulcers, cancerous growths, etc.

Phases of Gastric Secretion and their Regulation

There are four phases of gastric secretion:

1. Cephalic phase
2. Gastric phase
3. Intestinal phase
4. Interdigestive phase

Cephalic Phase of Gastric Secretion

Presence of food in the mouth stimulates gastric secretion through the taste pathways. This is an inherent reflex. Sight, smell and thought of food also stimulate gastric secretions through conditioned reflexes acquired during childhood. For all these stimuli to evoke gastric secretion, efferent vagus nerve should be intact. Since all the above stimuli act through higher centers in CNS, this is known as cephalic phase (Fig. 5.13).

Within 3–5 minutes of stimulation, the gastric secretion starts. In about 30 minutes, it reaches the peak, the volume of secretion being 30–150 ml in 20 min.

This phase can be very well demonstrated in sham fed dogs.

In sham fed animals, if both the efferent vagi supplying the stomach are cut, the cephalic phase of gastric secretion is abolished. The gastric juice produced by sight, smell and thought of food, i.e. food not being in stomach or mouth at all, is called appetite or psychic juice. Good music, pleasant surroundings, neatly dressed servers can influence the volume of juice secreted during this phase.

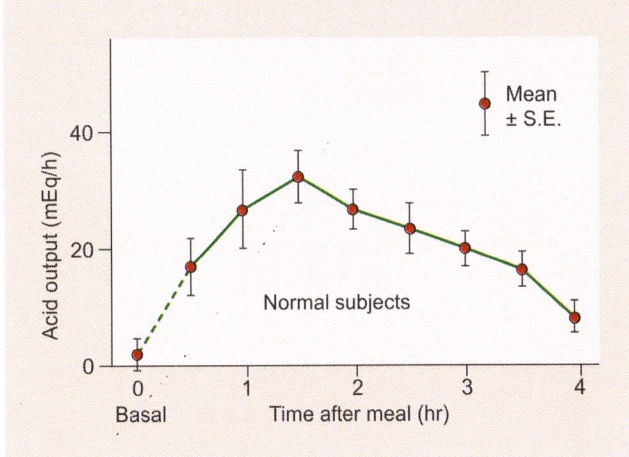

Fig. 5.13: Time required for maximal acid output after ingestion of food

Appetite is anticipation of pleasure of eating. This significance of cephalic phase is that the stomach prepares itself to receive the food.

Emotional factor also acts through cerebral cortex. Feelings of anger and aggression increase gastric secretion. Chronic fear, depression, grief or sorrow all diminish gastric secretion. Most of the stimuli of cephalic phase act through different areas of cerebral cortex one of which is the limbic lobe including the hypothalamus. From here, the stimuli reach the dorsal motor nucleus of vagus from where the preganglionic fibers take origin and reach stomach. The post-ganglionic fibers from the plexus stimulate the chief and parietal cells in different ways: (a) through acetylcholine which directly acts in gastric glands, (b) stimulates G cells of pyloric antrum through Bombesin. G cells in turn produce gastrin which acts on gastric glands (Fig. 5.14).

Parietal and chief cells have got separate receptors for acetylcholine, gastrin and histamine.

Gastric Phase

It is also called chemical or hormonal phase. Presence of food in the stomach stimulates gastric secretion. Secretion starts within 15 minutes of arrival of food in the stomach. The volume of secretion is 225 to 350 ml in 5 hrs. Specific stimuli responsible for this phase are:

a. Mechanical distension of stomach by the food

b. Proteins and derivatives in the food

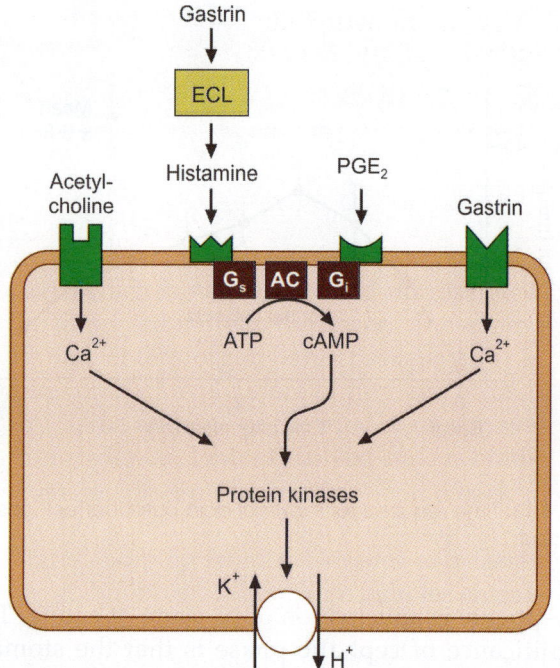

Fig. 5.14: Chemical substances acting on the parietal cells and intracellular reactions involved during the process of secretion of hydogen ion which later on reacts with chloride ion to form hydrochloric acid

These stimuli act locally within the stomach. Their receptors are in the gastric mucosa and the efferent are local vagal fibers which stimulate the ganglion cells in submucosal plexus from where the post-ganglionic fibers stimulate the gastric glands.

Although vagus and gastrin can act independently on the gastric glands (parietal and chief cells), they potentiate the action of each other or have synergistic action.

Gastrin: It is a very important GI hormone. It is a polypeptide.

Site of production: G cells or APUD cells (Amine precursor uptake and decarboxylation cells) located in the pyloric antrum. Similar cells are found in duodenum also.

The hormone secreted by these cells in response to specific stimuli, enters the systemic circulation and reaches gastric glands.

Types of gastrin: There are different types of gastrin. The most important ones are:
- G-17 LITTLE gastrin.
- G-14 MINI gastrin
- G-34 BIG gastrin

Gastrin is in use for studying gastric secretion. Pentagastrin has got last 4 amino acids of G-17 and one more amino acid. Pentagastrin has all the actions of G-17. All the gastrins are inactivated in liver and kidney

Regulation of gastrin secretion: Stimuli that release gastrin:
a. Mechanical distension of stomach
b. Partially digested food proteins
c. Vagal stimulation releasing Bombesin
d. Blood-borne factor, like epinephrine
e. Ca^{++} ions.
f. Alcohol

Factors that inhibit gastrin release are:
a. HCl in pyloric antrum or in duodenum (anytime when the pH of gastric contents falls below 2).
b. Hormones from duodenum, e.g.:
   - GIP (gastric inhibitory polypeptide)
   - VIP
   - Secretin
   - Enterogastrone
   - Glucagon

Actions of gastrin: Physiological actions:
   i. Stimulates secretion of gastric juice rich in HCl and pepsin
   ii. Stimulates gastric motility
   iii. Promotes the growth of gastric mucosa.
   iv. Increasing the tone of esophageal sphincter.

Intestinal Phase of Gastric Secretion

Presence of food in the small intestine stimulates gastric secretion.

Specific stimuli: Partially digested proteins and polypeptides stimuli are supposed to act through release of gastrin in duodenum. Duodenal gastrin can also be released by alcohol. Duodenum in response to presence of HCl, partly digested fat, hyperosmolar solutions in its lumen, inhibits gastrin release from pyloric antrum and thereby diminishes gastric secretion. This inhibitory action is believed to be brought about through certain hormones examples of which are:
- Enterogastrone (hypothetical hormone)
- GIP
- VIP

- Secretin
- Glucagon from duodenum

Intestinal phase takes about 2 hrs to start and volume of secretion is 200–300 ml.

Interdigestive Phase

Small quantity of gastric juice is continuously produced and is known as interdigestive phase secretion. The mechanism of this phase is not well understood. Emotional conditions and conditioned reflexes may be responsible for this phase.

Rate of secretion is 30–60 ml/hr.

Other gastric stimulants: Secretogogues

Secretogogue is any substance which increases the gastric secretion.

Histamine is a very powerful stimulant of gastric secretion, especially HCl. It is as powerful as gastrin and vagal nerve stimulation. It binds to specific receptors on the parietal cells known as H_2 receptors. Cyclic AMP is also involved in the action.

Combination of histamine with H_2 receptors can be blocked by drugs, e.g. cimetidine which is very useful in treatment of peptic ulcers.

Although histamine is produced in large quantity by stomach wall from mast cells, its physiological role is not very clear.

Factors Stimulating Gastric Secretion

1. Condiments (flavoring agents)
2. Vegetable extracts like soup
3. Alcohol (ethyl alcohol) very powerful stimulant of gastric secretion. Probably acts by liberation of histamine and gastrin in stomach.
4. Caffeine (coffee extract) very good stimulant of gastric secretion
5. *Parasympathetic agents:* Such as acetylcholine, etc are stimulants.
6. *Cigarette smoking:* Nicotine of tobacco in small doses stimulates autonomic ganglia. Vagal stimulation increases gastric juice secretion rich in acid and enzymes.

Depressants of Gastric Secretion

1. Drugs that act against acetylcholine, e.g. atropine
2. *Anti-H_2 drugs,* e.g. cimetidine
3. Antacids, e.g. $Mg(OH)_2$

i. Aluminium hydroxide
ii. Sodium bicarbonate ($NaHCO_3$)
iii. Calcium carbonate
   All these neutralize HCl.

Other Hormones that Influence Gastric Secretion

1. *ACTH and glucocorticoids:* They stimulate gastric secretion. The hormone secretion is increased during stress. It is well documented that people undergoing chronic stress develop peptic ulcer.
2. *Insulin:* By causing hypoglycemia. Stimulates hypothalamus which in turn stimulates vagus leading to gastric secretion. For this to be effective, blood sugar level should fall to 50 mg% of the normal. This principle is made use of in a gastric function test (insulin test or Hollander's test).
3. *Somatostatin:* It is a hormone secreted by the neurons in the hypothalamus. Though its primary action is to inhibit GH release from anterior pituitary, it also inhibits gastric secretion by inhibiting gastrin release.

Tests for Gastric Secretory Function in Man

Total and free acidity: Gastric juice is collected using Ryle's tube. HCl in this juice is in two forms: free H^+ ions called free acidity (20–60 mEq/liter) and a part of the acid is in combination with proteins.

This can be determined by titration of gastric juice against N/10 NaOH. Titrate to pH 3.5 using Topfer's indicator. It gives free acidity. On continuing titration to pH 7.4 using phenolphthalein will give total acidity.

Absence of acid in gastric juice is achlorhydria: Decrease in acid content below normal is hypochlorhydria and increase above normal is called hyperchlorhydria.

Achlorhydria can be true or false. In true achlorhydria, HCl is absent from gastric juice even after injection of histamine or pentagastrin. This occurs in pernicious anemia and gastric cancer.

Hypochlorhydria can be produced in gastritis.

Total and free acidity is usually estimated either from gastric juice collected overnight or basal secretion (early in the morning).

Over the years, it has become a practice to study the effect of specific stimulants on gastric secretion. Initially, a carbohydrate meal in the form of porridge or toast and coffee is given. Gastric juice is collected before and after the meal and analyzed for HCl, pepsin activity, etc. Such a test is known as fractional test meal (FTM). This will also facilitate the person performing the test to understand the gastric motility and emptying time.

This was replaced by *augmented histamine test*. In this, instead of giving a meal, histamine is injected 0.04 mg/kg body weight to stimulate gastric secretion. To make histamine act only on the H_2 receptors of stomach, the other unwanted side effects of histamine are blocked by antihistamine drugs.

Because of the side effects, this test is also given up. Now pentagastrin is used. Pentagastrin is injected 5 µg/kg body weight. Gastric juice is collected before injection and every 15 min after the injection. In a normal response, the HCl secretion reaches a peak of 25–40 mEq/hr within 15 min; the peak is maintained for another 15 min and acidity comes back to normal value 30 min later.

The peak acid output after pentagastrin may be raised in duodenal ulcer. The peak may be lowered in gastritis or other diseases where gastric mucosa is damaged.

Hollander's test (insulin test): Insulin test is effective only in the presence of vagus. This test is very useful to confirm the success of vagotomy, a common operation done for peptic ulcer.

Peptic ulcer: Refers to the chronic type of ulcer caused due to acid peptic digestion of gastric or intestinal mucosa. The classical sites of peptic ulcer are:

a. On the lesser curvature just proximal to pyloric region. This is known as gastric ulcer.
b. When the very beginning part of duodenum is involved, it is known as duodenal ulcer.

The factors that may be involved in the production of ulcers are:

1. Breakdown of gastroduodenal mucous barrier.
2. Excess of secretion of HCl.
3. In gastrinoma which is tumor of D cells, there is very high level of gastrin leading to increased HCl and pepsin secretion leading to peptic ulcer. This clinical condition is known as Zollinger-Ellison syndrome and there is hyperplasia of D cells of pancreas in this condition.

Other factors which may predispose the development of peptic ulcer are:

a. Chronic stress

b. *Helicobacter pylori* infection
c. Dietary factors, like spicy food
d. Alcohol
e. Smoking
f. Steroid administration
g. Administration of aspirin group of drugs.

Treatment of peptic ulcer:

1. Antacids
2. Cimetidine, ranitidine, famotidine, etc. which are H_2 blockers
3. Omeprazole which is a proton pump blocker
4. Proglumide drug which inhibits the action of gastrin on G receptors
5. Bland diet
6. Meditation
7. Vagotomy
8. One of the surgical procedures is gastro-jejunostomy (by passing duodenum).

Motor Functions of Stomach

The movement of stomach serves important objectives namely:

1. It enables the stomach to act as a temporary reservoir of food.
2. The movements of stomach converts solid food into a fluid paste called chyme and delivers this in small quantities to duodenum for proper digestion in small intestine.

Anatomical basis of gastric motility: The movement of stomach depends on the arrangement of smooth muscle in the wall. The arrangement is as follows:

a. Outer longitudinal muscle layer.
b. Inner circular muscle layer.
c. Oblique muscle which is inner to the circular muscle layer and restricted to upper part of stomach.
d. The muscularis mucosa present in the submucosa.

All the muscles are supplied by vagus and sympathetic fibers.

Types of Movements

1. *Receptive relaxation:* As the food fills the stomach, the smooth muscle undergoes relaxation increasing the capacity of the stomach to accommodate the incoming food. This is called receptive relaxation. This is in accordance with LaPlace's law which states that in a cylindrical structure

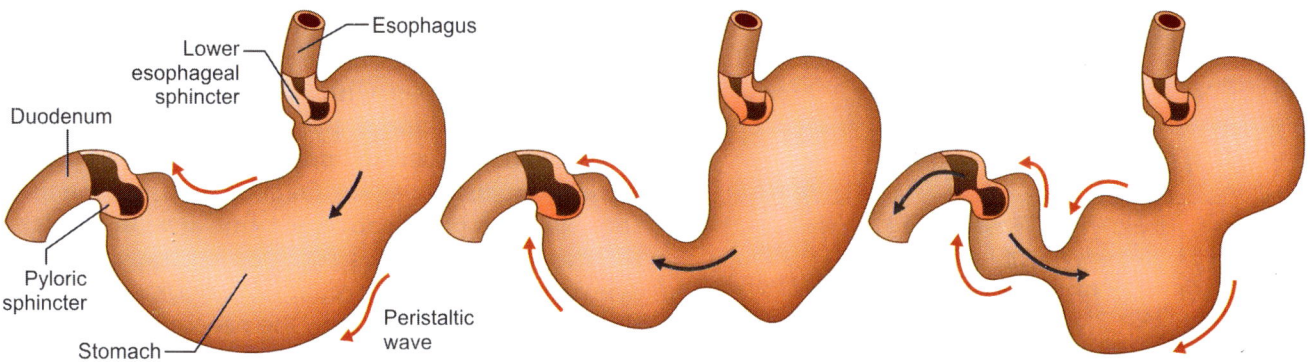

Duodenum

Lower esophageal sphincter

Esophagus

Pyloric sphincter

Stomach

Peristaltic wave

Fig 5.15: Passage of peristaltic contractions from the body of stomach toward the pyloric region

$P = T/r$

P = Pressure

T = Tension

r = Radius

An increase in the tension should, therefore, cause increase in the pressure. During receptive relaxation, the relaxation of the stomach increases its radius and hence increase in the tension due to stretching of the muscle will not lead to increase in pressure. This facilitates consumption of large quantity of food. The receptive relaxation of gastric smooth muscle is influenced by impulses coming along the vagus nerve.

2. *Mixing and propulsive movements:* The conversion of solid food into the fluid chyme and transit of food through the stomach into duodenum is due to gastric peristalsis (a wave of contraction preceded by wave of relaxation). For peristalsis to originate in the stomach, there is slow wave of depolarization starting from the greater curvature. This is known as gastric slow wave or basal electrical rhythm. It is suggested that upper part of greater curvature acts like a pacemaker for gastric peristalsis. The rate of peristalsis is about 3/min. The contractions are slower in the body of stomach but become stronger and faster in the pyloric antrum (Fig. 5.15). The pyloric orifice leading to duodenum is quite narrow.

The peristaltic contractions of pyloric antrum act like a powerful pump pushing the chyme into pyloric canal. Since the canal is narrow, only a small part of chyme is made to pass through. And the rest of chyme is pushed back (squirting movement) into the cavity of stomach. This retropulsion helps breaking larger particles into smaller one and also mixing of food with gastric juice. Vagal stimulation increases peristalsis while sympathetic stimulation depresses peristalsis. Therefore, after vagotomy, peristalsis become weaker or abolished.

Gastric emptying time and control: The normal gastric emptying time for mixed diet is about 2–4 hours. The gastric emptying time depends on the force of peristalsis which is again under the control of factors operating in stomach and duodenum (Fig. 5.16).

Gastric factors:
  i. *Role of nerves:* Vagal stimulation increases peristalsis and shortens gastric emptying time. Sympathetic stimulation has opposite effect.
 ii. Diet rich in carbohydrate is emptied faster than diet rich in proteins or fats.
iii. Fluids emptied faster than solids.
 iv. Quantity of food and gastric emptying time has inverse relationship.
  v. *Emotional factors:* Excitement hastens gastric emptying while grief and sorrow delays it.

Duodenal factors (Fig. 5.16): Mechanical distension of duodenum, presence of emulsified fats and fatty acids, products of protein digestion, sugars, hyperosmolar substances, HCl, etc., in duodenum delays gastric motility through a reflex known as enterogastric reflex. The reflex is an example for vagovagal reflex. Even if vagal connection between stomach and duodenum is cut, fats in duodenum can still delay gastric emptying. It is brought about by hormonal factor and the hormones involved secretin and CCK-PZ (cholecystokinin pancreozymin), GIP, etc. Duodenum has got specific receptors for HCl, fats, osmolar substances, etc.

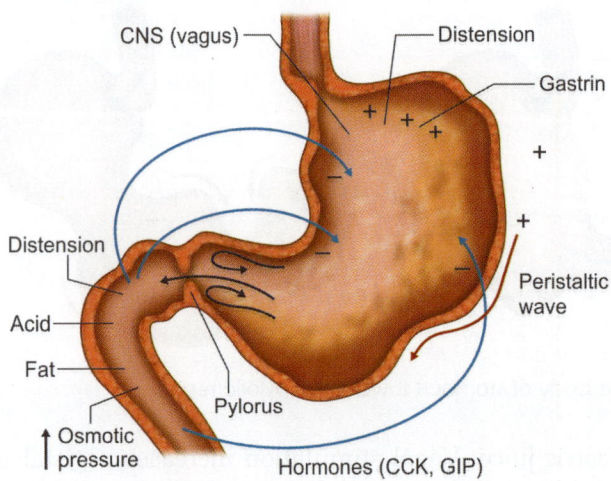

Fig. 5.16: Factors influencing gastric emptying time

Significance of duodenal inhibition of gastric motility:
1. Small amount of chyme is presented to small intestine for better digestion and absorption.
2. Acidity of the chyme needs to be neutralized by alkaline pancreatic juice and bile. Some time is needed for these juices neutralize hydrogen ions.

Contractions of empty stomach: Empty stomach is capable of contractions called hunger contractions or hunger pangs. Hunger pangs appear, if fasting is there for more than 12 hours. Hunger pangs disappear once food is taken in. Impulses from hypothalamus and the vagus are responsible for initiating these contractions.

Pancreas

Structure of Pancreas

Pancreas is a dual organ. It has endocrine portion and exocrine portion.

The exocrine part resembles the salivary glands in histology; being formed of acini arranged into lobules. Cells of the acini contain numerous mitochondria, a nucleus and granular cytoplasm. The zymogen granules are located more towards the apex and contain enzyme precursors of pancreatic juice. Each acinus drains into a duct. The cells lining the intra-acinar portion of the duct are called centroacinar cells. The acinar cells secrete various enzymes of the pancreatic juice while the centroacinar and duct cells contribute to the secretion of electrolytes, most important of which is HCO_3^-. All the minute ducts

from the various lobules unit to form main pancreatic duct of Wirsung. This duct opens into the second part of duodenum along with bile duct. In most of the normal people, there is also an accessory pancreatic duct of Santorini which opens into the second part of duodenum just above the main duct. In this manner, the exocrine pancreatic secretion drains into the duodenum. Pancreas is supplied by the vagus and sympathetic fibers from celiac ganglion, just like heart, the ganglia for vagus are in the pancreas itself.

Composition of Pancreatic Juice

Pancreatic juice is a colorless, odorless, highly alkaline fluid of low viscosity, pH = 8– 8.4. Alkalinity is because of HCO_3^-. The important components of pancreatic juice are (Figs 5.17 to 5.19):
- H_2O
- *Cations:* Na^+, K^+, Mg^{++}, Ca^{++}
- *Anions:* HCO_3^-, Cl^-, SO_4^-, HOP_4^-

Enzymes
1. Trypsinogen
2. Chymotrypsinogen
3. Procarboxypeptidase A   } Proteolytic enzymes
4. Procarboxypeptidase B
5. Proelastase
6. Lipase
7. Cholesterol esterase   } Lipolytic enzymes
8. Prophospholipase

Others:
1. Amylase
2. Deoxyribonuclease
3. Ribonuclease

Miscellaneous:
- Immunoglobulins
- Albumins
- Kallikrein
- Trypsin inhibitor
- Co-lipase

Functions of the Individual Components

Bicarbonates make the pancreatic juice alkaline and alkaline medium is essential for the pancreatic enzymes to perform their digestive functions.
1. The chyme received from the stomach is acidic and acidity is harmful to duodenal mucosa and also does not permit pancreatic and intestinal enzymes

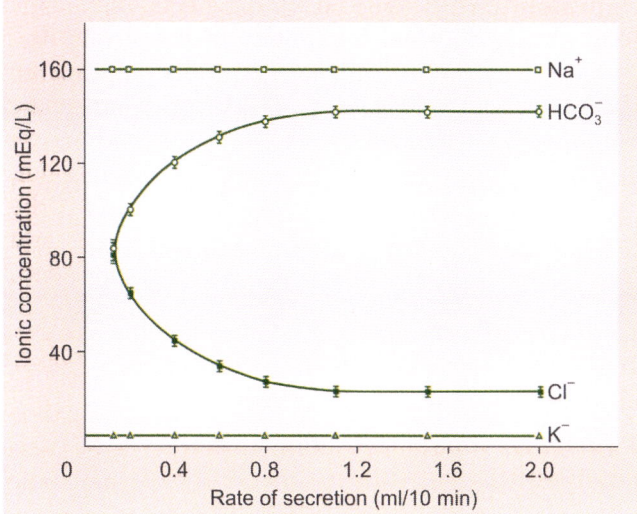

Fig. 5.17: Level of various ions in pancreatic juice depending on the rate of secretion. When the rate of secretion is high, level of bicarbonate is more compared to chloride ions

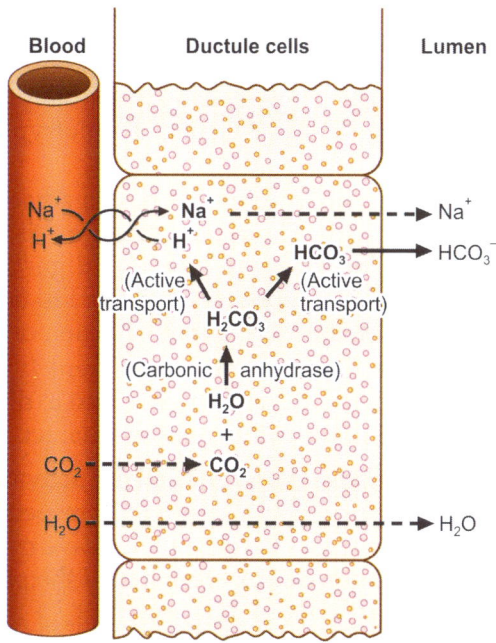

Fig. 5.19: Process of secretion of bicarbonate and water

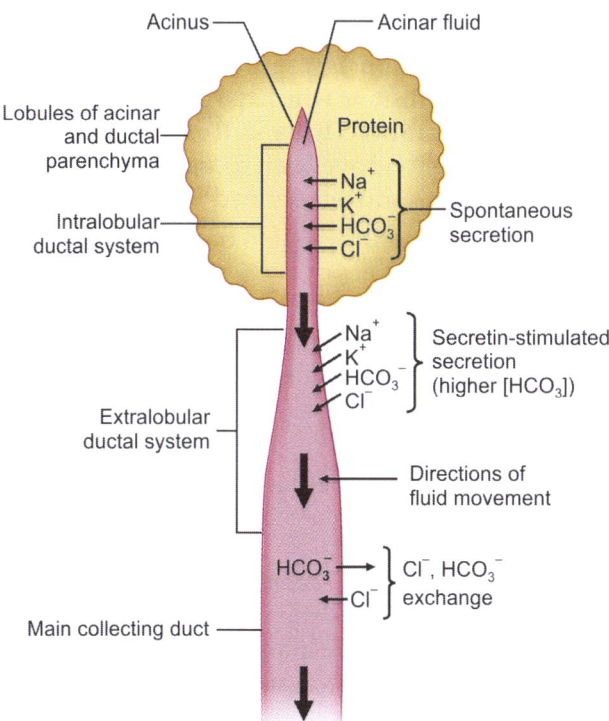

Fig. 5.18: Modification of the composition that is brought about during the process of secretion of pancreatic juice from the acini into the collecting duct of the gland

to act. HCO_3^- neutralizes the acidity rendering the pH of intestinal contents between 7 and 8 which is essential for digestive processes to occur in the small intestine.

2. HCO_3^- inactivates pepsin because pepsin being a proteolytic enzyme will digest all pancreatic enzymes.

Normal HCO_3^- content of pancreatic juice: 80–120 mEq/liter

Enzymes: Proteolytic Enzymes

Trypsinogen: Trypsinogen is the inactive form of trypsin.

$$\text{Trypsinogen} \xrightarrow{\text{Enteropeptidase}} \text{Trypsin}$$

It is activated by another enzyme known as enteropeptidase (also called enterokinase) secreted by intestinal mucosa.

It activates trypsinogen to trypsin. Once trypsin is formed, trypsin by itself activates trypsinogen. This type of a reaction is known as an autocatalytic reaction.

Trypsin is a powerful endopeptidase because it acts inside the protein molecule and breaks the peptide bonds adjacent to arginine or lysine; thereby breaking larger protein molecules into smaller polypeptides. It requires a pH of 7–8 for its action. Other actions include a weak coagulting action on milk.

All the enzymes of pancreatic juice are secreted into duodenum in the inactive form, if not enzymes themselves will digest the entire pancreas.

Besides this, trypsin has got a specific inhibitor in the pancreas itself.

Chymotrypsinogen: This is also an endopeptidase. Chymotrypsinogen is activated to chymotrypsin by trypsin.

Chymotrypsin breaks peptide bonds adjacent to aromatic amino acids. The pH required for this action is about 7–8. This enzyme helps to digest large proteins into smaller peptides. Compared to trypsin, it has got more powerful coagulating action on milk.

Some believe that there are 6 different types of chymotrypsinogen and one of these is used to dissolve the lens capsule in the eye to remove cataract.

Procarboxypeptidase A and B: Both are activated by trypsin into carboxypeptidase A and B, respectively. They are exopeptidases because they cleave or break peptide bonds at the carboxy terminal of the protein.

Carboxypeptidase A, breaks peptide bonds of carboxy terminal attached to branched aliphatic amino acids. Whereas B attacks and breaks peptide bonds of carboxy terminal attached to basic amino acids. These exopeptidases help to form or break individual amino acids from peptides produced by the action of trypsin and chymotrypsin.

Proelastase: Activated to elastase by trypsin. An elastase acts on the protein elastin attacking peptide bonds adjacent to aliphatic amino acids.

Lipolytic Enzymes

Pancreatic lipase: It is the most important fat splitting enzyme in the GIT. It acts on emulsified fats, emulsification having been brought about by bile salts in the presence of lecithin and monoglycerides. Bile salts activate pancreatic lipase.

Although from the reaction, it is seen that triglycerides can be broken down by lipase into glycerol and fatty acids, actually since the final two steps are slow, the usual products of lipase action are 2 monoglyceride and fatty acids.

Lipase also requires alkaline pH of 7–8 for the action. Colipase helps to expose the triglyceride molecule which has formed a complex with bile salts. This exposure is necessary for lipase to hydrolyze the triglyceride. If pancreatic lipase is absent either due to complete destruction of pancreas because of disease or removal of entire pancreas surgically, the digestion and absorption of fats and fat-soluble vitamins is significantly disturbed and more fat is excreted in fecal matter. Normal fat content of feces is up to 5 g/day. If lipase is completely absent, fat content increases to 40–50 g/day. Presence of abnormal amounts of fatty stool is called steatorrhea.

Prophospholipase: This is activated by trypsin to phospholipase. Phospholipase converts lecithin into lysolecithin by splitting of fatty acid and later can be absorbed.

Cholesterol esterase: This enzyme hydrolyses cholesterol ester to yield free cholesterol which is absorbed along with fatty acids.

Pancreatic amylase: Actions similar to salivary amylase.

Deoxyribonuclease: This converts DNA into the respective nucleotide.

Ribonuclease: This hydrolyses RNA to the respective nucleotide.

Regulation of Pancreatic Secretion

Pancreatic secretion is regulated by neural and hormonal mechanism of which hormonal mechanisms is more important. Three different phases for pancreatic secretion have been recognized in animals and these are not so well defined in man. The three phases are:

1. Cephalic Phase

Taste of food stimulates pancreatic secretion. In addition to this, sight or smell also can also stimulate.

2. Gastric Phase

Presence of food in the stomach by way of mechanical distension and chemical composition stimulates pancreatic secretion.

Distension of stomach causing pancreatic secretion of enzymes is called gastropancreatic reflex.

Cephalic and gastric phases are controlled by vagus. Stimulation of vagus promotes pancreatic secretion which is rich in enzymes, yet pancreatic secretion can go on in the absence of vagus. The action of vagus is through acetylcholine.

3. Intestinal Phase

Presence of food, HCl, etc., in the small intestine promotes pancreatic secretion through mechanical

distension as well as chemical composition. This very important phase is brought about two hormones, viz:
a. Secretin and
b. Cholecystokinin-pancreozymin (CCK-PZ)

Secretin: This is the first hormone ever to be discovered (and synthesized) in the year 1902 by Bayliss and Starling.

This is a polypeptide hormone having 26 amino acids. This GI hormone is secreted by specialized cells in the mucosa of duodenum and jejunum.

Stimuli for release: The most important stimulus is the presence of HCl in the duodenum (Fig. 5.20). Whenever pH of chyme in the duodenum falls to less than 4.5, secretin is released into the portal vein and then returns to GIT through the circulatory system.

Actions (functions): Secretin increases the volume of pancreatic juice which is rich in HCO_3^- and water. Therefore, its main site of action is centroacinar and duct cells of pancreas.

- It potentiates action of CCK-PZ on pancreas.
- Increases secretion of bile from hepatocytes.
- Inhibits gastric motility and delays gastric emptying by contraction of pyloric sphincter.
- Inhibits gastrin release and gastric secretion.
- Inhibits gastric motility and delays gastric emptying by contraction of pyloric sphincter.
- Releases insulin from beta cells of islets of Langerhans.

Cholecystokinin-pancreozymin (CCK-PZ) initially discovered as the separate hormones: pancreozymin and cholecystokinin, former acting on pancreas and the latter on gallbladder. Subsequently, they were found to be one and the same. This polypeptide GI hormone has got 33 amino acids and is produced from mucosa of duodenum and jejunum.

Stimuli for release of CCK-PZ (Fig. 5.21): Presence of food in duodenum and jejunum stimulates secretion of this hormone. Although products of protein, fat and carbohydrate digestion all can release CCK-PZ, amino acids form the most powerful stimulus and the next potent stimulus is fatty acids. HCl is a weak stimulus for CCK-PZ

Actions (functions): CCK-PZ acts on pancreatic acini to produce pancreatic juice rich in enzyme content.

While secretin acts through cAMP, CCK-PZ acts not only through cAMP but also increases intracellular Ca^{++} concentration in the acini which is necessary for release of pancreatic enzyme.

CCK-PZ promotes contraction of gallbladder. This results in expulsion of bile from the gallbladder into duodenum. An agent that causes contraction of gall-bladder is called cholegogues. CCK-PZ is a very powerful cholegogue.

1. Potentiates action of secretin on pancreas
2. Promotes secretion of bile.
3. Inhibits gastric motility and, therefore, delays gastric emptying.
4. Promotes release of insulin in from the B cells of islets of Langerhans.
5. Promotes pancreatic cell growth.

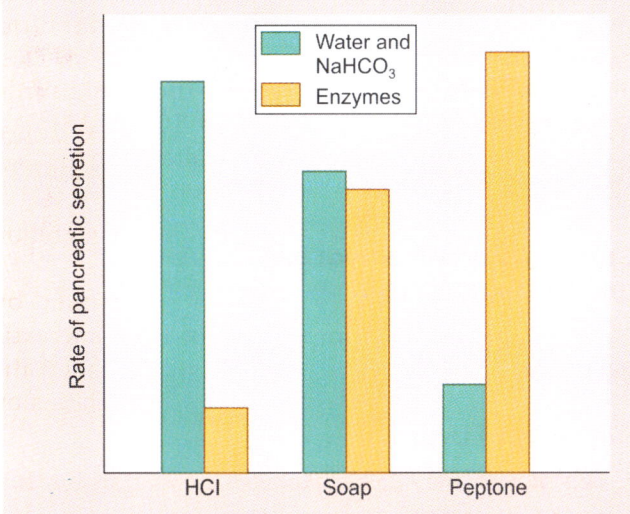

Fig. 5.20: Variation in the composition of pancreatic juice depending on the type of stimulus acting

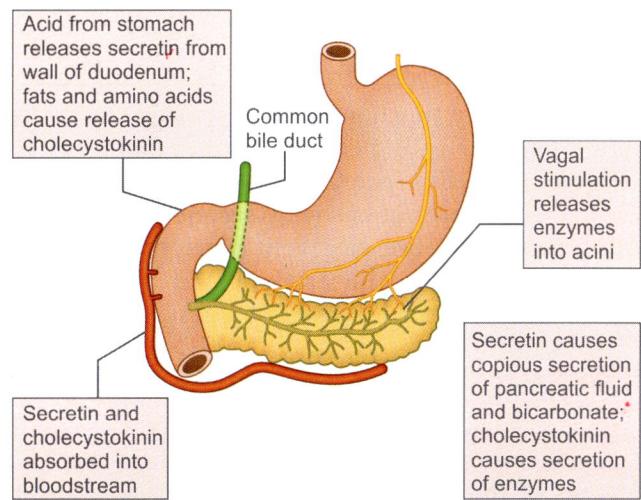

Fig. 5.21: Factors influencing the secretions of pancreatic juice

Pancreatic Function Test
(Only for exocrine pancreas)

It is now possible to collect pure pancreatic juice right from the pancreatic duct by passing a thin catheter through the mouth into the duodenum with the help of an instrument called duodenoscope.

Pancreatic juice is collected and analyzed for HCO_3^- content and trypsin activity. After collecting the morning initial sample, with the individual in fasting condition, an injection of secretin and CCK-PZ is given. A few minutes after the injection, pancreatic juice is again collected at intervals of 10 minutes and HCO_3^- content and trypsin activity are estimated every time. If pancreas is normal, secretin should cause an increase in HCO_3^- content and PZ should increase in tryspin activity. If pancreas is not functioning normally, both will be reduced.

Effect of Total Pancreatectomy

This is sometimes done for the carcinoma of the pancreas. Removal of pancreas leads to following abnormalities:

1. Diabetes mellitus
2. Abnormalities in digestion and absorption of lipids and proteins, but carbohydrates digestion is not affected significantly because salivary amylase and enzymes present in intestinal secretion keep carbohydrate absorption and digestion normal. Diminished digestion and absorption of lipids causes steatorrhea while impaired digestion and absorption of proteins is reflected by increased nitrogen content of stool which is normally up to 1 g/day.

Liver and Bile Secretion

Liver has many functions. One of them is to secrete bile. The liver cells per day secrete about 600 to 1000 ml of bile. Bile secretion is a continuous process. Certain substances are actively secreted and certain other substances are passively transported. Water molecules follow the transported substances mechanism.

Histology of Liver

Figure 5.22 shows basic histology of liver.

Stages of Bile Secretion

Bile secretion occurs in two stages:

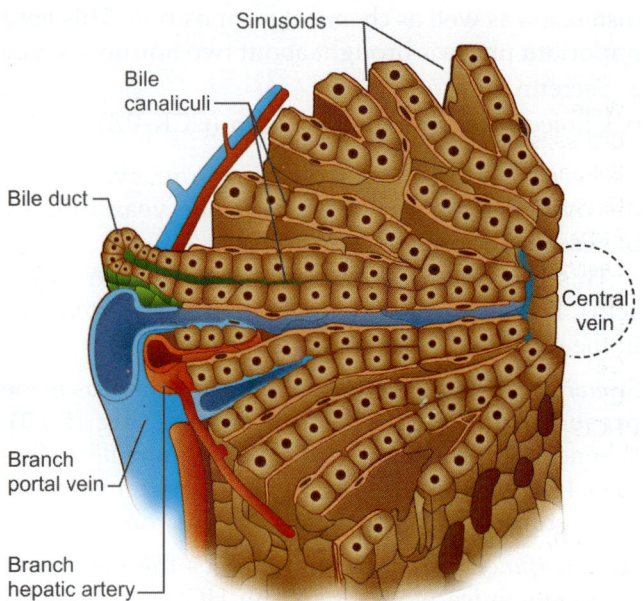

Fig. 5.22: Basic histology of liver

Primary secretion: Occurs at the level of the hepatocytes. This initial secretion is rich in bile acids, cholesterol, bile pigments and other organic materials. From the cells, these substances are secreted into the bile canaliculi. This bile then enters the bile ducts. Here, sodium and bicarbonates are added by active secretion under the influence of the hormone secretin. The bile that has entered the hepatic duct normally flows along the cystic duct and gets stored in the gall-bladder for sometime. During this time, the composition of the bile gets changed again. Sodium, bicarbonates, chlorides and water get absorbed. This brings about concentration of the remaining substances to the extent of about 10 to 14 times (secondary secretion—composition alteration in gall-bladder).

Composition of the Liver Bile and Gallbladder Bile

Table 5.1 shows the composition of liver bile and gallbladder bile.

Functions of Liver

1. *Secretion of bile:* The hepatocytes are responsible for secretion of bile.
2. *Synthetic function:* All the plasma proteins except gamma globulin fraction are synthesized in liver.

Table 5.1: Composition of bile		
	Liver bile	*Gallbladder bile*
Water	97.5 g/dl	92 g/dl
Bile salts	1.1 g/dl	6 g/dl
Bilirubin	0.04 g/dl	0.3 g/dl
Cholesterol	0.1 g/dl	0.3 to 0.9 g/dl
Fatty acids	0.12 g/dl	0.3 to 1.2 g/dl
Lecithin	0.04 g/dl	0.3 g/dl
Na^+	145.04 mEq/L	130 mEq/L
K^+	5 mEq/h	12 mEq/L
Ca^{++}	5 mEq/L	23 mEq/L
Cl^-	100 mEq/L	25 mEq/L
HCO_3^-	28 mEq/L	10 mEq/L

3. *Storage function:* Many of the vitamins, glycogen, iron, etc. are stored in liver.
4. *Excretory function:* Cholesterol, bile pigments, and alkaline phosphatase are excreted along with bile.
5. *Hemopoietic function:* In fetal life liver, liver is one of the sites of erythropoiesis.
6. *Detoxification function:* Several drugs, toxins, are detoxified in liver. Detoxification may involve oxidation, reduction, hydrolysis, etc.
7. *Inactivation of hormones:* Most of the hormones especially steroidal group of hormones is inactivated in liver.

Composition of Bile

- Bile is golden yellow aqueous solution.
- Volume secreted per day is about 600–1000 ml.
- pH is around 8.

Composition
- Water 97%
- Solids 3%

Organic constituents: Bile salts, bile pigments, cholesterol, alkaline phosphatase, etc.

Inorganic constituents: Sodium, hydrogen ion, calcium, bicarbonate, etc.

Bile Salts

They are derived from bile acids. The two important bile acids are cholic acid and chenodeoxy cholic acid which are produced in the liver from cholesterol. These acids are conjugated with glycine or taurine and then form salt with sodium or potassium. Hence bile salts are nothing but sodium or potassium glycocholate or taurocholate.

Bile salts enter jejunum along with bile. In the intestine, bile salts are subjected to bacterial actions. This brings about the formation of lithocholic acid and deoxycholic acid. About 95% of bile salts that have reached the intestine are returned to liver (Figs 5.24 and 5.25) by enterohepatic circulation (portal circulation). The absorption of bile salts into entero-hepatic circulation occurs in the terminal part of ileum and at the beginning of large intestine. Enterohepatic circulation is repeated about 4–8 times per day. The total pool of bile salts in the body is about 1.6 g.

Regulation of secretion of bile (Fig. 5.23): Neural influence is through the vagus nerve. This influence is not much on secretion of bile.

Hormonal influence: Hormones secreted from duodenum stimulate secretion of bile. Any agent which stimulates the secretion of bile is known as choleretic. Apart from bile salts some of the other choleretic agents are:
a. Secretin
b. Acetylcholine

Functions of the Gallbladder

1. It stores bile. It can store about 30–60 ml of bile.
2. *Absorption:* While it is being stored sodium, chloride, bicarbonates and water are reabsorbed.

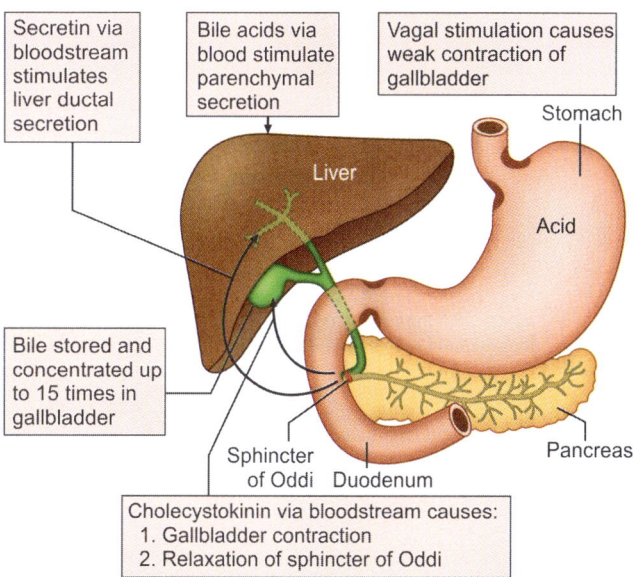

Fig. 5.23: Factors affecting bile secretion and gallbladder contractility

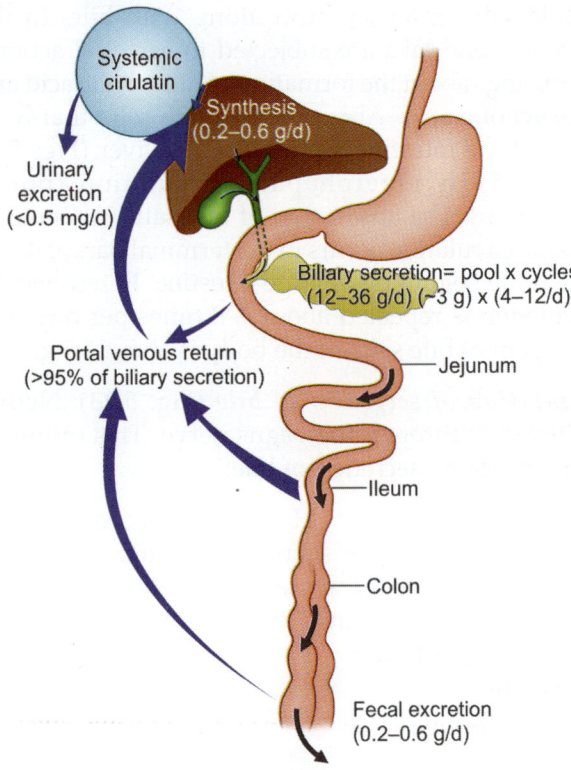

Fig. 5.24: Recycling of bile salts along portal circulation that have got absorbed from the ileum region

3. By absorption of water, it tries to maintain a low pressure in the biliary tree so that the bile secretion remains a continuous process.
4. By absorption of water, it maintains a high concentration ratio between bile salts and cholesterol. This prevents the precipitation of cholesterol and, therefore, the formation of gallstones (Fig. 5.26).
5. *Expulsion of bile:* Contraction of the gallbladder will bring about expulsion of the bile into the intestine.

Any substance that brings about the contraction of the gallbladder and releases or increases the bile flow into the intestine is known as a cholagogue substance. Bile salts, CCK-PZ are very powerful cholagogues.

Fate of bile salts: Bile acids are synthesized in the liver from cholesterol by hepatocytes. Bile acids are cholic acid and chenodeoxycholic acid. They combine with glycine or taurine to form glychocholic or taurocholic acid. This in turn combines with sodium or potassium to form sodium and potassium salts of glychocholic or taurocholic acid. Contraction of the gallbladder leads to entry of bile salts into the duodenum.

Functions of the Bile/Bile Salts

1. Bile salts are very powerful surface tension lowering agents. This helps in the emulsification

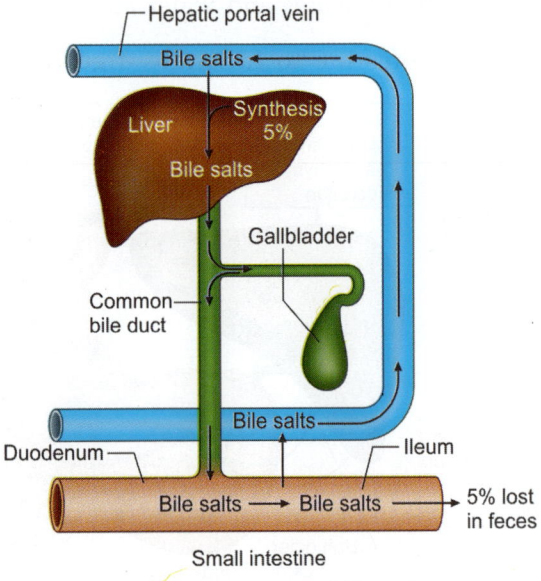

Fig. 5.25: Recycling of bile salts

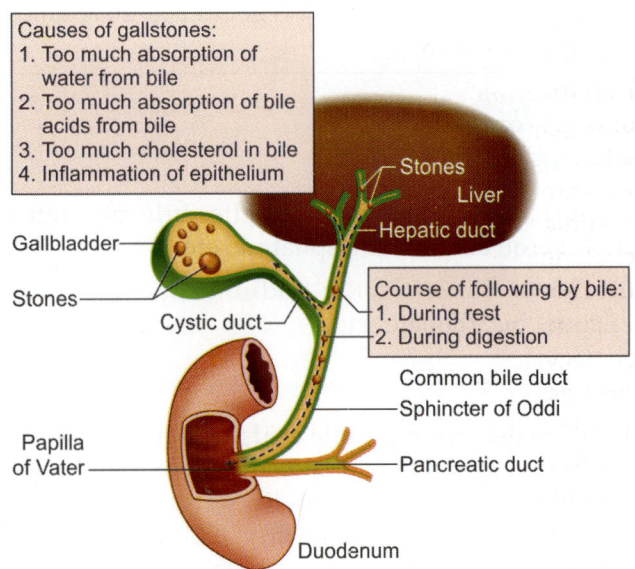

Fig. 5.26: Factors affecting gallstones formation and the course of bile secreted by liver until it reaches duodenum

Due to water absorption, the bile in the gallbladder gets concentrated by about ten to fourteen times.

of fats. The larger fat molecules are broken down to smaller ones so that larger surface area is made available for the pancreatic lipase to act.

2. Bile salts with phospholipids, cholesterol, free fatty acids and monoglycerides form micelles and help in the absorption of fats.

3. They also help in the absorption of fat-soluble vitamins A, D, E, and K.

4. They are very powerful choleretic agents. Choleretic agents are those substances, which increase the secretion of bile from the liver cells.

5. They activate pancreatic lipase.

6. They also act as mild laxative agents.

In the small intestine, about 90 to 95% of the bile salts are absorbed into the portal circulation. The site of absorption is the ileum, and the process involved is an active process. Rest of it enters the large intestine, gets converted into secondary bile salts—deoxycholic acid and lithocholic acid. A part of it is lost in the stools. About 200 to 600 mg of the bile salt is lost in the stools per day. This quantity synthesized by the liver daily and added to the bile salt pool so that the total quantity of bile salt constant is kept constant.

Cholecystography: It is a radiological procedure to visualize gallbladder. In oral cholecystography, radiopaque dye (tetroiodophenolphathalene) is given orally. This dye gets secreted by liver cells. So the dye reaches gallbladder along with bile. In the gallbladder, dye is concentrated due to absorption of some amount of water from bile. About 2–3 hours after giving the dye, if X-rays are taken, the details of its passage from liver through gallbladder and biliary duct can be made out. To facilitate the contraction of gallbladder, usually a fatty food (cheese) is given. When the radiopaque substance is injected intravenously and the radiographic study of gallbladder is done, it is known as cholangiography. Gallbladder can be visualized by ultrasonography.

Removal of the gallbladder is known as cholecystectomy, and this has no harmful effect on the person. The effects of cholecystectomy are:

1. Bile ducts undergo enlargement to accommodate bile in the absence of concentration function of gall-bladder.

2. If sphincter of Oddi does not have adequate tone, bile may dribble into intestine.

3. If the tone is high in sphincter of Oddi, accumulation of bile in the biliary tract leads to back pressure development and may affect the functions of hepatocytes.

Movements of Small Intestine

Motility of small intestine: The movements of small intestine are brought about by the smooth muscle present in its wall.

a. Wall of small intestine has an outer longitudinal and an inner circular layer.

b. The movements are subjected to neural control through the plexus of nerves, namely myenteric and Meissner's plexuses, through the influence of extrinsic autonomic nerves. Movements are subjected to hormonal control and to local control as well.

Aims of Small Intestinal Motility

1. *Agitation of food or chyme:* This helps in three ways:
   a. Mixing the food with the enzymes of pancreatic and intestinal juice thus facilitating enzyme action.
   b. Breaks the food into very small particles which again helps in digestion and absorption.
   c. Renewal of the layers in contact with the villi which helps in absorption.

2. *Propulsion:* The chyme is moved over the large area of small intestine to facilitate digestion and absorption and the residues are propelled downwards to the ileocecal junction to reach the large intestine, mostly for excretion.

In man, the time taken for the food to travel in the small intestine as well as in stomach can be easily estimated radiologically with the help of barium meal. It takes about 2–12 hours for the food to travel from pylorus to ileocecal junction.

Types of Intestinal Movements

Rhythmic Segmentation Contractions (Figs 5.27 and 5.28)

Ability of the muscle to contract, stretch when the walls are distended and generation of impulse almost at regualr intervals (rhythmicity) are the fundamental properties of visceral smooth muscle all over GIT. Rhythmic segmentation contractions are ring like contractions a few cm long as small segments in small intestine.

Site of first contraction

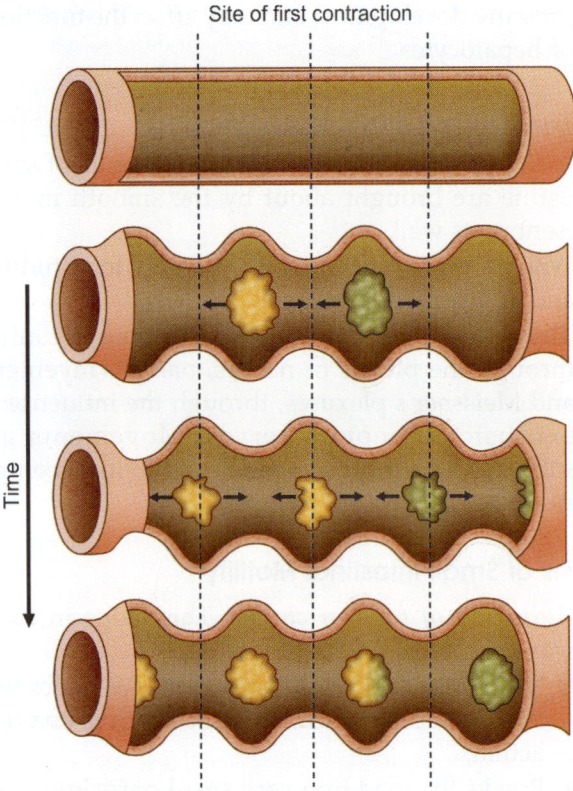

Fig. 5.27: Rhythmic contractions in small intestine

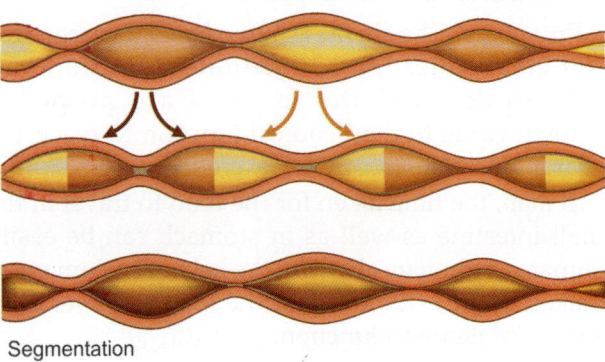

Segmentation

Fig. 5.28: Segmentation contractions

These contractions are caused by distension of walls due to chyme. The contractions are so organized that in a given segment, contractions and relaxations alternate and at the next instant, contracted segment relaxes and relaxed segment goes into contraction. This type of movement chops the food and helps in mixing food with intestinal secretions. These contractions depend on the presence of myenteric

plexus. They can occur even when the extrinsic vagus and sympathetic are cut. These contractions occur at a faster rate in the duodenum (12/min) and slow down towards the ileum (8/min). Parasympathetic stimulation increases these contractions and sympathetic stimulation inhibits them.

Peristalsis

It is defined as a wave of contraction preceded by a wave of relaxation which travels down a hollow organ. In the intestine, the contractions proceed towards aboral region.

Peristaltic wave always travels in the aboral direction is called law of the intestine which is dependent on myenteric reflex (Fig. 5.29).

Stimulus: Usually distension of intestine caused by food. Sometimes chemical irritation also can act as stimulus.

- *Receptor:* Stretch receptors in the mucous membrane of small intestine.
- *Afferent:* Short vagal fibers in the intestinal wall itself
- *Center:* Ganglion cells of myenteric plexus
- *Efferent:* Short parasympathetic fibers in the intestinal wall itself.
- *Effector:* Circular muscle of the wall.

Response: Contraction of circular muscle resulting in peristalsis.

In the genesis of peristalsis, the wave of contraction occurs a few centimeters prior to the part of intestine where food (chyme) is present and the receptive relaxation occurs beyond the area of chyme. This sort of movement helps to propel the food, so peristalsis

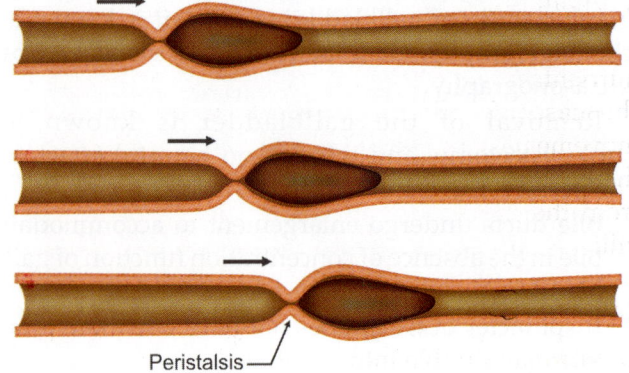

Peristalsis

Fig. 5.29: Process of peristaltic contractions passage towards the ileum from the duodenum

is more of propulsive movement. It can also occur in absence of extrinsic nerve supply. Sympathetic stimulation inhibits it and parasympathetic stimulation promotes it. Peristaltic movements are more frequent in the upper small intestine (12/min) and less so in the lower intestine (8/min). This leads to a postulation that there is a pacemaker in the duodenum (similar to the one in the heart), which directs the peristalsis down towards the ileocecal junction. Theoretically, distention by food can result in a peristaltic wave traveling in both directions but the one towards the mouth dies out.

Thus it is believed that it is due to pacemaker function located in the duodenum.

Peristalsis in the reverse direction is called *antiperistalsis*.

There is an interesting experiment where a small loop of small intestine is cut and anastomosed in the reverse direction. The food does not cross the segment the area of anastomoses and stop. This experiment proves the directional integrity of myenteric plexus is essential for peristalsis and the propulsion of food.

Pendular Movements

Here, long segments of about 20 cm move forwards and backwards, up and down helping mainly agitation of food. These and peristalsis are superimposed on rhythmic segmentation contractions. These can also occur in absence of extrinsic nerve.

Movements of Villi

These are due to contractions of muscularis mucosa which extend into each villus. There are two types of movements:

a. Lashing movement
b. Rhythmic shortening and elongation of the villus.

These movements help in the absorption of nutrients into the blood vessels as well as lacteals. In the case of villi, parasympathetics inhibit the movement, sympathetics promote it. It is believed that there is hormone villikinin (yet to be isolated) secreted from the duodenum and promotes contractions of villi.

Regulation of Intestinal Motility

1. *Neural:* Except in the case of villi, vagal stimulation promotes intestinal movements whereas sympathetic stimulation inhibits them. Yet intestinal

movements can go on without the influence of extrinsic nerves. Certain emotional factors influence intestinal motility, e.g. grief inhibits the movements and causes constipation. Similarly fear causes stimulation of movements and causes diarrhea.

These emotional factors act through cerebral cortex and autonomic nervous system.

Gastroileal reflex: Intake of food into the stomach stimulates intestinal movement and empties the contents from ileum and other parts of large intestine. This may be acting through vagal connections between stomach and small intestine.

Peristaltic rush: Here, extreme distension or irritation of small intestine by food leads to exaggerated peristalsis in which, in one sweep of a movement the food from duodenum reaches the ileocecal junction.

2. *Hormonal:* Acetylcholine, 5-HT cause contractions of small intestine. These are local hormones.

Among general hormones, thyroid hormone stimulates intestinal motility. So in hyperthyroidism, there is diarrhea. In hypothyroidism, there is constipation.

3. *Local regulation:* In the absence of extrinsic nerves the presence of food alone by way of distension or chemical stimulation can cause intestinal movements. This is more important mechanism of regulation.

When the person is fasting, the GIT is completely empty, the small intestine exhibits peristalsis-like movements called migrating myenteric complexes. This shows that smooth muscle of small intestine is always active.

Ileocecal Junction

The junction between ileum and cecum is guarded by a sphincter known as ileocecal sphincter which is normally in contracted state. Moreover, the ileal opening into the cecum is having a valve-like mechanism (similar to uterus—cervix and vagina) which normally permits entry of chyme into the cecum and not in the reverse direction.

Functions of Ileocecal Sphincter

1. It regulates the entry of chyme into the cecum so that enough time is spent by the chyme in small intestine to complete digestion and absorption.

2. It prevents the reflux of bacteria-laden contents of the large intestine into the sterile small intestine.

Regulation of Ileocecal Sphincter

1. Parasympathetic stimulation relaxes it while sympathetic stimulation contracts the sphincter.
2. Gastroileal reflex helps to relax the ileocecal sphincter enabling the chyme to pass into the colon.
3. ACh and gastrin relax the ileocecal sphincter while secretin contracts it.

Large Intestine

Functional Anatomy

The mucosa has no villi. It has short glands containing numerous goblet cells. The smooth muscle is made up of two layers: the inner circular similar to what is present in rest of the gastrointestinal tract, whereas the outer longitudinal is arranged in three bands called tenia coli. Since these bands are shorter than the entire length of the colon, the colon is compressed to form puckering or haustrations.

Functions of Large Intestine

1. *Secretion:* The glands secrete a watery fluid containing H_2O and HCO_3^- to which mucin is added from globlet cells. Mucin is meant for lubrication of chyme.
2. *Absorption:* About 1–2 liters of chyme enter the colon. This volume is reduced to less than 200 ml by the time is reaches rectum mainly by active reabsorption of Na^+, water and Cl^- following passively. The ability of colonic mucosa is made use of in administration of drugs especially in children by way of suppositories and also enemas usually for constipation.
3. *Synthesis:* Colon has got a variety of bacteria. These bacteria are in a way beneficial because they can synthesize vitamins of B complex group, vitamin K. This fact is taken into consideration when broad-spectrum antibiotics are administered. B-complex vitamins are always given with broad-spectrum antibiotics because the latter also kills the beneficial bacterial flora of intestine.
4. *Movements:* The presence of smooth muscle in the colon is responsible for colonic motility. There are two major types of movements:

   a. *Mixing movement:* Rhythmic segmentation contractions occur as a result of circular muscle activity while tenia coli cause haustral contractions. These contractions roll the colonic wall back and forth against the contents helping in the absorption of Na^+ and water and reducing the bulk of chyme. These are also called kneading movements.
   b. *Mass peristalsis (movements):* Peristalsis does not occur in large intestine the way it occurs in small intestine. Instead, mass peristalsis is found. It occurs a few times in a day usually in the hour after breakfast lasting for duration of 10 minutes. It can start in any part of the colon, it occurs usually in the transverse or descending colon.

   When it occurs, it propels the colonic contents right up to the rectum. Once the rectum is filled up the desire for defecation is felt. The mass peristalsis is initiated by following factors:

   i. *Gastrocolic reflex:* Food in the stomach through neural pathways (may be vagus) stimulates mass peristalsis in the colon.
   ii. *Duodenocolic reflex:* Distension of duodenum with food can stimulate mass peristalsis.
   iii. Irritation of colon due to infection
   iv. Over distension of colon, e.g. enema
   v. Parasympathetic stimulation

5. *Storage and expulsion of feces*

   Composition of feces:
   - Weight/day = 75–170 g/day
   - pH: 7–7.5
   - Color is due to stercobilinogen
   - Odor is due to indol and skatol and also by bacterial action in the intestine

   Actual composition: 75% water and 25% solids

Other important constituents are:

1. *Fiber:* Cellulose, hemicellulose, lignin, pectin, enzymes to digest any of these components of vegetarian diet. They add up to the bulk of the food. Being undigested, they add up to the bulk of feces. This is important because feces should be bulky enough to stimulate smooth muscle of large intestine which result in defecation.
2. Bacteria
3. Fats and fatty acids
4. Desquamated mucous cells

5. Unabsorbed digestive juices containing small quantities of enzymes
6. Mucin
7. Inorganic substances particularly Ca^{++} and phosphates.

Defecation

Defecation is a reflex which results in the expulsion of feces and is normally under voluntary control in adult. In infants, it is purely a reflex action. The desire for defecation is felt when the finally formed feces enter the rectum. Continuous escape or dribbling of feces is prevented by presence of two sphincters.

a. *Internal anal sphincter:* Formed of smooth muscle supplied by parasympathetic and sympathetic stimulation, the former relaxes it while the latter contracts the sphincter. Thus it is involuntary.
b. *External anal sphincter* is formed by the skeletal muscle fibers and supplied by pudendal nerve which is somatic and is, therefore, activity is under voluntary control.

Defecation reflex has following:

- *Stimulus:* Distension of rectal wall by the feces.
- *Receptors:* Stretch receptors in the mucosa of rectum. These receptors can distinguish between fluid and gas.
- *Afferents:* Pelvic splanchnic (parasympathetic) nerves.
- *Center:* S2, S3 and S4 segments of spinal cord controlled by impulses from the higher centers.
- *Efferent:* Parasympathetic pelvic splanchnic nerves.
- *Effectors:* Smooth muscle of rectum and internal anal sphincter.
- *Response:* Contraction of the rectum and relaxation of internal anal sphincter.

When the desire of defecation is felt, the individual can voluntarily postpone the same by the act the contractions of the external anal sphincter, if the time and place are not socially acceptable. This voluntary control is lacking in infants. They develop the habit and control by training. External anal sphincter can withstand pressure up to 55 mm Hg.

Once the act of defecation is postponed, it remains inhibited for some time. When the time and place are socially acceptable, the act of defecation can be carried out by straining efforts. This consists of a deep inspiration followed by forced expiration against closed glottis—Valsalva maneuver.

During straining, the downward movement of diaphragm and contraction of abdominal muscle and voluntary relaxation of external anal sphincter help in the act of defecation. Levator ani also contracts pulling the anal canal up over the fecal matter so that the fecal matter can pass through.

Gas in the Intestine

Gas in the intestine is in the form of O_2, N_2, CO_2, H_2, H_2S, and CH_4.

O_2, N_2, CO_2 are respiratory gases of the swallowed air.

Others are formed by bacterial action on foodstuff. Some of these are absorbed while others are expelled through canal as flatulence. When there is large bowel obstruction, the patient does not pass feces as well as flatulence.

Effect of Colectomy

Sometimes most of the large intestine has to be removed especially in cancer. In that case, the ileum is made to open to the exterior through anterior abdominal wall. The individual can still survive provided his diet and water electrolyte balance are properly maintained (ileostomy)

Constipation

Diminished frequency of defecating is called constipation. The frequency of defecation varies from individual to individual. It is usually due to faulty habit, sometimes due to diseases of the colon. Chronic constipation leads to loss of appetite, abdominal distention. Constipation is the most important symptom of intestinal obstruction (pain, vomiting, and constipation).

Hirschsprung's Disease or Megacolon

In this congenital disease, a short segment of distal colon becomes spastic due to absence of ganglion cells in submucous and myenteric plexus. Colon above the segment is dilated.

Important symptom will be constipation.

Treatment: Surgery which includes resection of spastic segment and continuity between normal proximal and distal colon is reestablished by anastomosis.

Diarrhea

Diarrhea is increased frequency of defecation, usually due to infection. It leads to loss of water and electrolytes resulting in dehydration and electrolyte imbalance. This will become a serious problem if diarrhea is severe. Loss of K^+ in particular is detrimental to the cardiac function.

Vomiting or Emesis

Vomiting is the expulsion of gastric contents to the exterior through the esophagus and mouth. Sequence of events during vomiting is as follows:

1. Nausea
2. Increased salivation
3. Sweating
4. Tachycardia
5. Rapid, deep, irregular breathing
6. *Retching:* Uncoordinated contractions of inspiratory muscle that is diaphragm moves down during expiration.
7. Glottis is closed.
8. Soft palate contracts and blocks the nasopharynx to prevent the vomitus from entering the nose.
9. Powerful contractions of pyloric antrum with simultaneous relaxation of body of stomach, cardiac contents travel upwards through the relaxed stomach and esophagus into the mouth. The downward movement of the diaphragm and powerful contractions of abdominal muscles also have a compressing effect on the stomach to aid in the vomiting processes.

Vomiting is a reflex and the vomiting center is situated in the reticular formation of medulla.

Impulses for vomiting can arise not only from stomach but also from small intestine, kidney, uterus, heart (in myocardial infarction) and vestibular apparatus (inner ear—responsible for motion sickness).

Some of the drugs, like morphine, digitalis, can also cause vomiting by stimulating the vomiting center through a group of neurons in the medulla called chemoreceptor trigger zone.

Agents which cause vomiting are called emetics and the agents that suppress the same are called antiemetics.

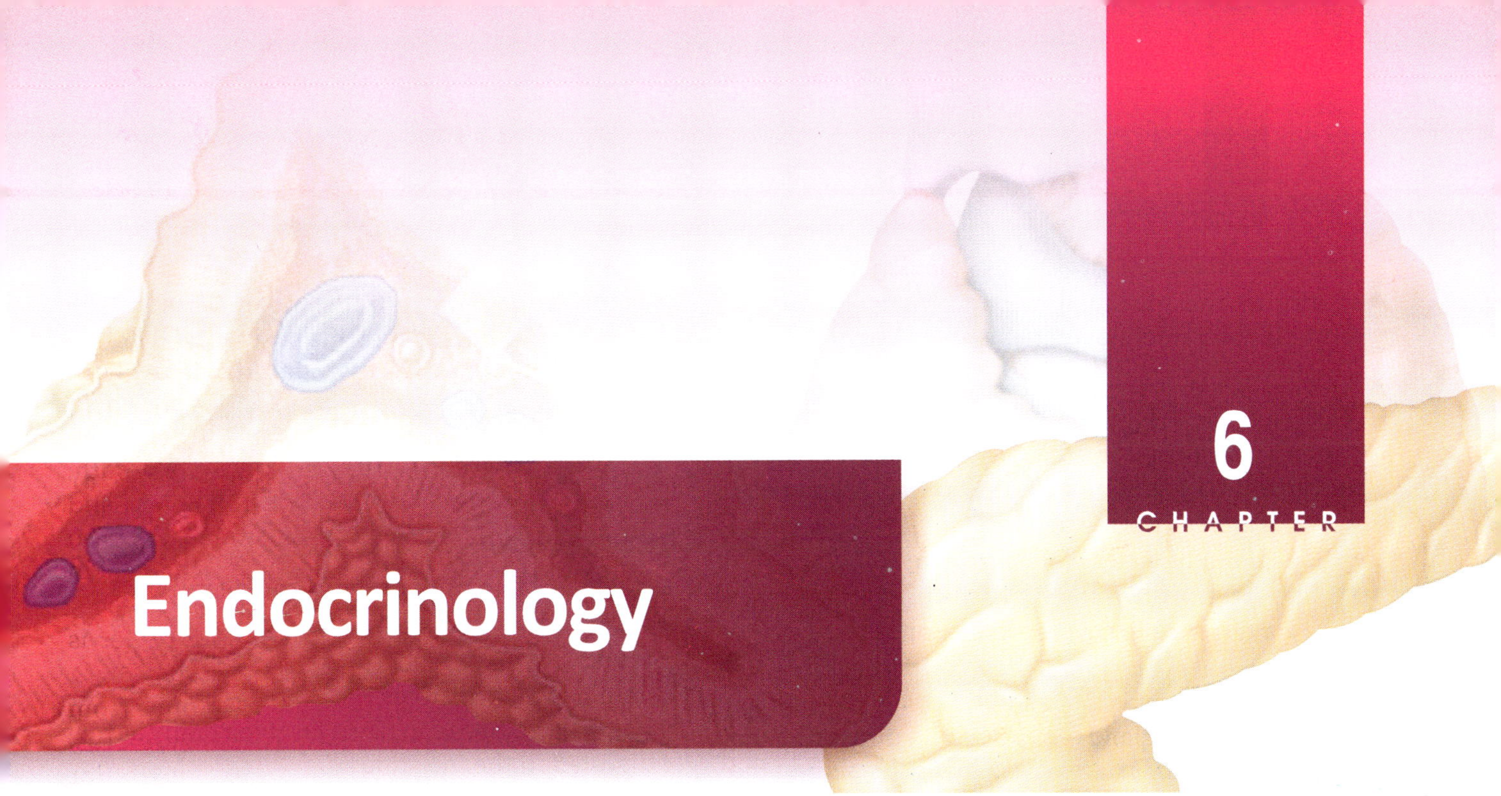

Endocrinology

Introduction

The study of hormones secreted by specialized glands that are ductless is known as endocrinology. Hormones are special chemical messengers constantly present in circulation. The organ/tissue on which the hormone acts is known as target organ. The hormones carry chemical messages to almost all the parts of the body (Fig. 6.1) and hence are important along with nervous system for regulation of functions of the body.

Apart from the hormones, certain other chemical signals are also secreted by cells. These are termed as:

a. Autocrine
b. Paracrines
c. GI tract hormones

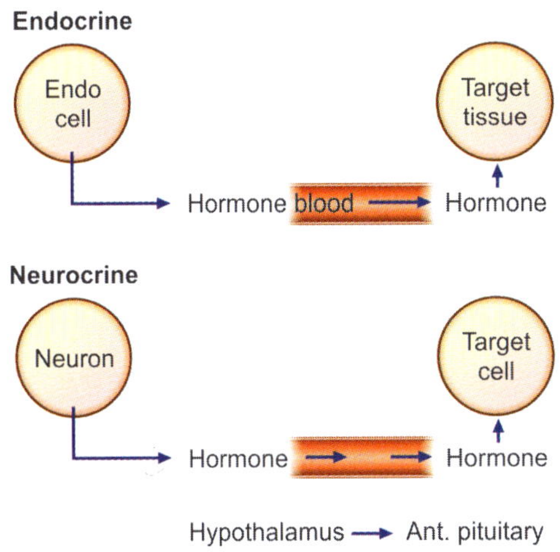

Autocrines are chemical signals produced by the cell and influences the activity of the cell itself (Fig. 6.2). Autocrine effects are more important for growth and sustenance of cancer cells. In a hostile environment, normal cells cannot grow but the cancer cells grow and proliferate.

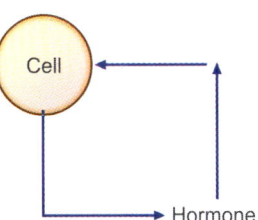

Fig. 6.2: Autocrine concept

Paracrines are chemical signals produced by a cell and diffuse in the surrounding area and act on the cells in the vicinity without entering circulation (Fig. 6.3). Somatostatin which regulates the secretion

Endocrine

Neurocrine

Hypothalamus → Ant. pituitary

Fig. 6.1: Endocrine and neurocine concepts

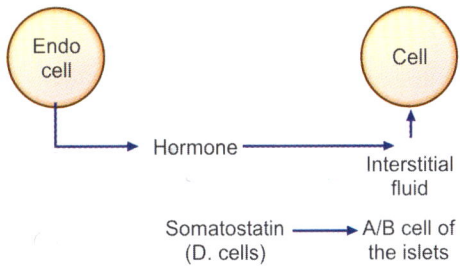

Fig. 6.3: Paracrine concept

of insulin and glucagon in pancreas is a classical example for paracrine.

GI tract hormones are not included under classical endocrinology. The hormones of GI tract act on the structures in the GI tract and alter the secretion and movements. The hormonal functions in the body are:

- Regulation of the metabolism
- Regulation of water and electrolyte content
- Help for growth
- Also necessary for the reproduction
- In certain situations, they help the body to withstand the stressful stimuli.

The endocrine glands are present in different parts of body. Few of them are paired like adrenals and the others are unpaired like pituitary (Fig. 6.4).

  i. Hypothalamus
 ii. Anterior and posterior pituitary
iii. Islets of Langerhans
 iv. Adrenal cortex and adrenal medulla
  v. Thyroid
 vi. Parathyroid
vii. Testes/ovaries

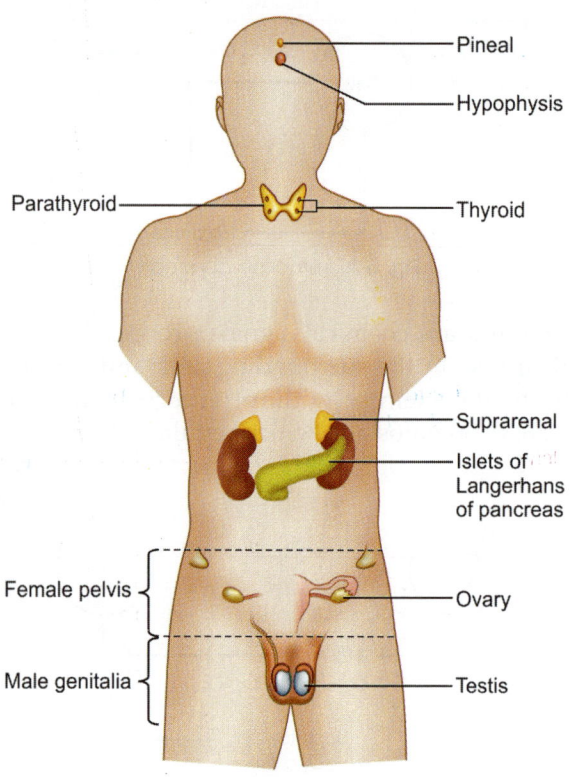

Fig. 6.4: Location of endocrine glands in the body

Essential endocrine glands mean without the secretions from these glands the basic survival of the person is not possible. The essential endocrine glands in the body are:

- Parathyroid
- Adrenals

Chemical Nature

The biochemical nature of the hormone can be:

- Peptide/protein
- Steroid
- Amino acid derivatives

Peptide hormones can never be given orally as they get digested in the intestine.

1. Amino acid derivatives—thyroxin, catecholamine
2. Protein—insulin

   Peptides—glucagon, parathyroid hormone, pituitary hormones

3. Steroids—hormones of adrenal cortex, sex steroids

Transport

Hormones are circulated in bloodstream in two forms:

- Free form
- Protein bound form (with plasma proteins).

The amount of free form in circulation is very less but still is important as it exerts all the biological actions of the hormone. The protein bound form acts as a reservoir and gets released into free form as and when required. Apart from this, the protein bound form cannot get filtered in the kidneys and hence hormones loss from the body is minimized.

Degradation of Hormones

Most of the hormones get metabolized in the target organs. Hormones belonging to steroid group are metabolized in the liver.

1. By the target tissue
2. By the liver/kidney—conjugated either by glucuronyltransferase system or by SO_4.

Tropic Hormone

The hormones, which are essential for the regulation of growth and secretion of some other endocrine glands, are known as tropic hormones.

All the tropic hormones are secreted by the anterior pituitary gland. They are:

- TSH (thyroid-stimulating hormone)

- ACTH (adrenocorticotropic hormone)
- FSH (follicular-stimulating hormone)
- LH (ICSH) (luteinizing hormone or interstitial cell stimulating hormone)
- To a certain extent even growth hormone also can be considered as a tropic hormone.

The tropic hormone secretion from anterior pituitary gland is under the influence of neuro-hormones secreted by the hypothalamus.

Mechanism of Action

Second messengers: Peptides and catecholamine:
- Formation of cyclic-AMP
- Calcium
- Inositol triphosphate
- Diacyl glycerol

Hormones in general act as first messenger.

Proteins and peptide hormones can bind to the cell membrane receptors. Hence when they act on the receptors, in the intracellular fluid part there will be alteration in the concentration of substances, like cAMP, Ca^{++} or inositol triphosphate. These substances act as second messengers and exert all actions of the hormone in the intracellular fluid region.

Steroid hormones can enter the cell through the cell membrane and bind to the receptors present in the cytoplasm or the nucleus. This increases the formation of mRNA by a process known as transcription and helps for synthesizing new proteins. Thyroxin hormone binds to the receptors present on the nucleus.

Receptors

Receptors for the hormonal actions can be present at three different places in the target organ/cells (Fig. 6.5).
1. Cell membrane bound receptors are for all peptide hormones and catecholamine.
2. Cytosolic receptors for steroid hormone group.
3. Nuclear receptors for thyroxin hormone.

Regulation of receptor number in the target organ depends on the concentration of the hormone in circulation.

Down regulation is brought about when almost all the receptors are occupied by the hormone. There will be almost nil receptors available for binding with fresh molecules of the hormone. This normally occurs in hypersecretory state of the hormone.

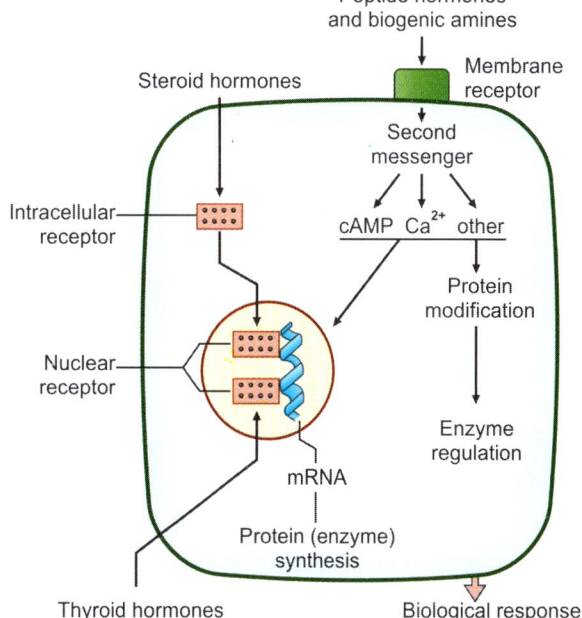

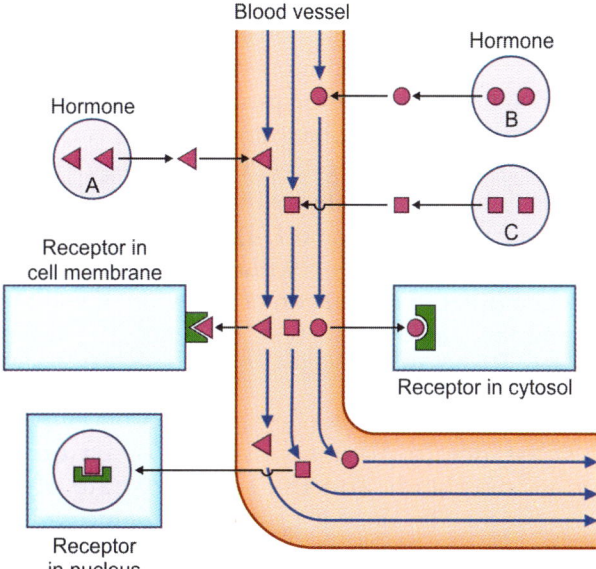

Fig. 6.5: Location of receptors for various class of hormones

Up regulation occurs when less amount of hormone available for binding with the receptors. In other words, in this situation most of the receptors are free to bind with hormones. This normally occurs in hyposecretory state of the hormone. Whatever little hormone is available, the receptors want to bind with it.

Estimation of hormones: Can be done by:
- Radioimmunoassay

- Spectrophotometer methods
- Bioassay.

How to establish the function or actions of hormones in the body?

1. Remove the suspected gland and look for signs and symptoms.
2. Prepare an extract and inject.
3. Inject extract in larger amounts.
4. Correlate with signs and symptoms in clinical conditions
5. Synthesis.

Regulation of Secretion of Hormones

It can be brought about by different ways.

Feedback control wherein, the concentration of the hormone in circulation regulates its own secretion by acting through the hypothalamus or anterior pituitary or both. The feedback control may be negative or positive. In negative feedback, increase in the free form of hormone in circulation brings about decreased secretion of the same hormone by acting through the hypothalamus or anterior pituitary gland or both, whereas in positive feedback it will be vice versa. One of the examples for negative feedback regulation of hormone secretion is thyroxin (refer Regulation of Secretion; page no. 173 and 174). One of the examples for positive feedback regulation is secretion of estrogen (refer to Regulation of Secretion of Estrogen around the Day of Ovulation; page no. 201) around the day of ovulation.

Concentration of substances in plasma: Concentration of substance in plasma can directly act on the endocrine glands and the secretory rate of the hormone may be altered, e.g. the blood glucose level regulates insulin secretion. (More is blood glucose; more will be secretion of insulin.)

Neural influences: The activity of the nervous system can also regulate the secretion of some hormones, e.g. catecholamine and prolactin secretion is regulated by neural activity. The neuroendocrine reflex can also be included here (for details refer to Oxytocin Secretion Regulation; page no. 160).

Stressor influences: They can also alter the secretion of hormones. Any sort of stress either alters the internal environment or threaten to alter the homeostasis. Common examples of stress include:

a. Surgery, accidents, burns, etc.
b. Mental stresses, like death of near and dear ones, certain apprehensions, etc. If the stressful situation is not combated, it may become fatal. In such a situation, hormonal secretion does altered, e.g. increased secretion of cortisol in any stress situations.

Diurnal variation: During 24 hours of the day, the rate of hormone secretion varies depending on the time, e.g. secretion of ADH is more during the night than during daytime. Even cortisol secretion has diurnal variation and is more during daytime when compared to night-time (Fig. 6.6).

Half-life of hormone is the time required for the hormone level to fall to 50% of its original level. The half-life varies with the hormones. Catecholamine has very less half-life of about 20 seconds whereas thyroxine has half-life of about 7 days. The half-life of a hormone will also depend on whether the hormone is present in free form only or both in free form and protein bound form. In case the hormone is present only in free form, the duration of half-life is very less (e.g. catecholamine).

Endocrine Dysfunction

Hyperfunction

a. *Neoplastic:* Benign/malignant, e.g. pituitary adenomas, cancer of any gland
b. *Ectopic:* SIADH, ACTH
c. *Autoimmune:* Graves' disease
d. *Iatrogenic:* Cushing's disease, hypoglycemia

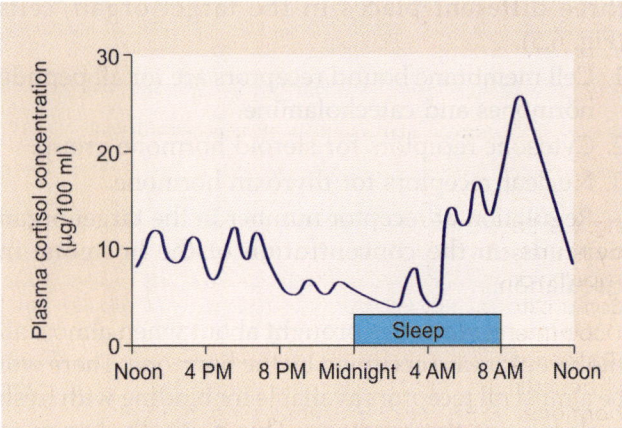

Fig. 6.6: Diurnal variation of cortisol secretion

Hypofunction

a. *Autoimmune:* Hashimoto's thyroiditis, type I diabetes, Addison's disease
b. *Iatrogenic:* Radiation-induced, surgical, drug-induced
c. *Infectious:* Addison's disease
d. *Enzyme deficiency:* Especially which belong to steroid hormone group
e. *Hemorrhage/infarction:* Sheehan's syndrome

Anterior Pituitary Gland

- It is also known as adenohypophysis.
- Secretes a number of hormones which are generally termed as tropic hormones.
- The secretion of hormones from anterior pituitary is regulated by the factors secreted by the hypothalamus (Fig. 6.7). The hypothalamic factors are of two types, namely:
  a. Releasing factors or releasing hormones.
  b. Releasing inhibiting factors or release-inhibiting hormones.
- The anterior pituitary is connected to the hypothalamus by hypothalamohypophyseal portal system. The factors secreted by the hypothalamus reach the anterior pituitary gland through this vascular connection (Fig. 6.8).
- The cells of the anterior pituitary are grouped into two types namely the chromophobes and chromophils. The chromophils are further divided into acidophils and basophils. Chromophils are the cells which secrete the factors of the hypothalamus which in turn influence the activity of the anterior pituitary gland.
- The chromophil cells of the anterior pituitary are named based on the hormone they secrete. Examples are:
  a. Somatotropes which secrete growth hormone.
  b. Lactotropes which secrete prolactin.
  c. Thyrotropes which secrete thyroid-stimulating hormone.
  d. Gonadotropes which secrete follicular-stimulating and luteinizing hormones.
  e. Corticotropes which secrete adrenocorticotropic hormone, beta lipotropins and beta endorphins.

Growth Hormone

Growth hormone (GH) also known as somatotropic hormone and is a peptide hormone secreted by acidophils of the anterior pituitary gland. GH is stored in large, dense granules present in acidophil cells. It is a single chain polypeptide with molecular weight of 22,000 having 191 amino acids and two disulphide

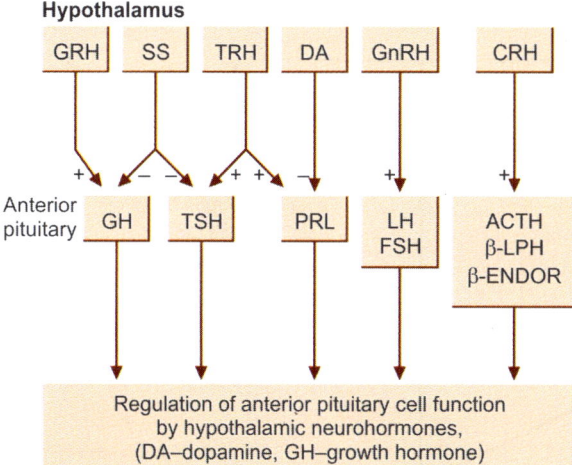

Fig. 6.7: Regulation of secretion of anterior pituitary hormones by the releasing and release-inhibiting hormones secreted by hypothalamus. GRH—Growth hormone releasing hormone, SS—Somatostatin, TRH—Thyrotropin-releasing hormone, DA—Dopamine, GnRH—Gonadotropic-releasing hormone, CRH—Corticotropin-releasing hormone, GH—Growth hormone, TSH—Thyroid-stimulating hormone, PRL—Prolactin, LH—Luteinizing hormone, FSH—Follicular-stimulating hormone, ACTH—Adrenocorticotropic hormone, βLPH—βLipotropin, βENDOR—βEndorphin

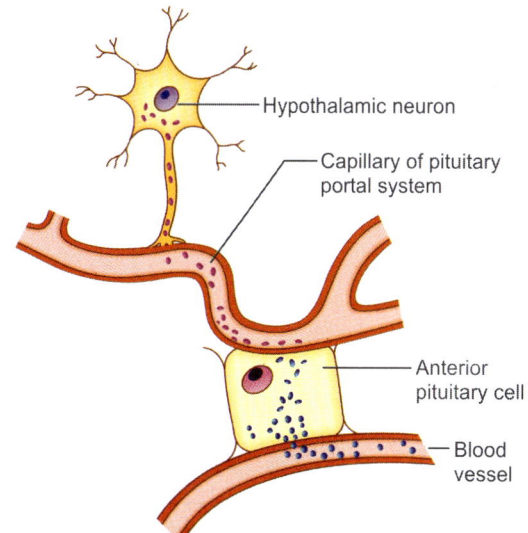

Fig. 6.8: Connection between hypothalamus and anterior pituitary gland (vascular connection—hypothalamohypophyseal portal system)

bridges. As the name indicates, its action is on the growth of the body. It stimulates somatic growth and development and helps to maintain lean body mass and bone mass in adults.

Mechanism of Action

- Receptors for growth hormone are present on the plasma membrane of cells.
- Belong to cytokine family of receptors.
- Presence of excess of GH down regulates the synthesis of its receptors.
- Many hours must elapse after administration of GH before anabolic and growth-promoting actions of the hormones to become evident.
- Most of the actions of GH require the production of GH induced somatomedin C or insulin-like growth factor (IGF).
- The plasma half-life of IGF is much longer than that of GH.

Actions of the hormone can be broadly classified into two types:

a. Indirect growth promoting action
b. Direct anti-insulin action.

1. **Indirect growth promoting action** (Figs 6.9 and 6.10) is due to the action of growth hormone on liver. When the hormone acts on liver, liver secretes

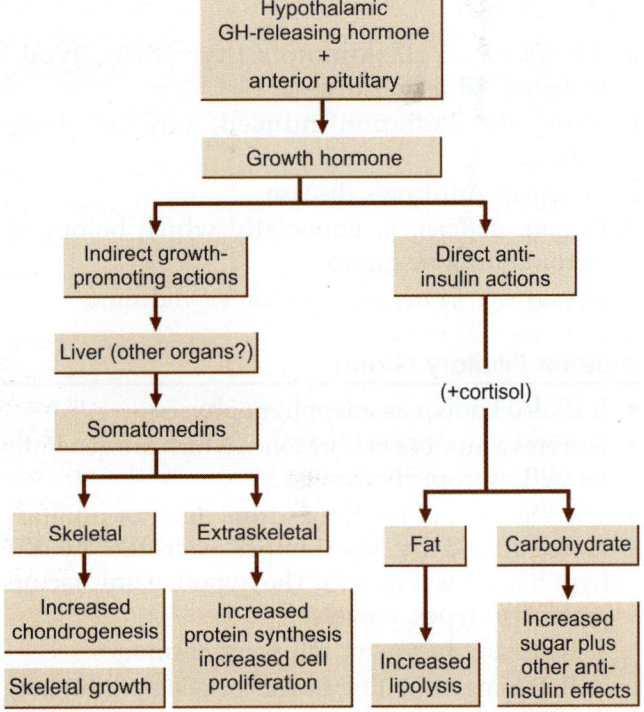

Fig. 6.9: Composite diagram showing actions of GH

somatomedin C or insulin-like growth factor (IGF-I). This substance acts on skeletal and extraskeletal compartments.

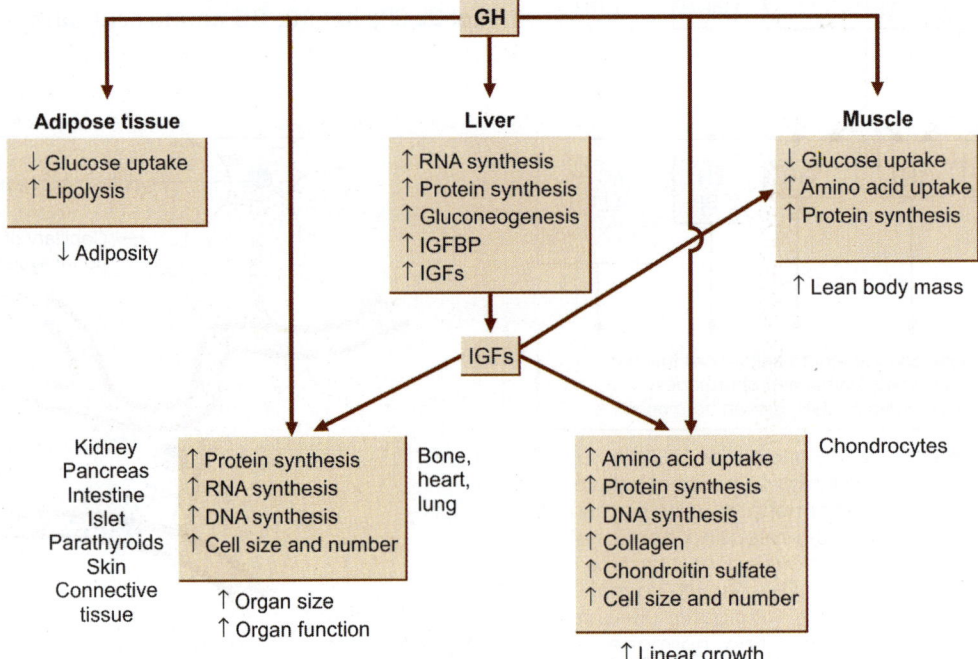

Fig. 6.10: Highlighting various intracellular actions of GH in the body

- *Skeletal compartment:* When somatomedin acts on epiphyseal plate present between the long bones, the epiphyseal plate gets widened. This gives space for the chondrogenesis of the long bones. The long bones grow linearly. Hence, the height of the person increases. The long bones can grow only up to the age of about 18–20 years beyond which the epiphyseal plates get fused with long bones and there can be no more linear growth of body.

- *Extraskeletal compartment:* This in general refers to the growth of organ and tissues. The growth is brought about by hyperplasia (stimulating mitotic cell division and hence increase in cell number) and hypertrophy (increase cell size). The various tissues in the body grow. There will be increased protein synthesis because of which it brings about positive nitrogen balance. The proteins synthesized are incorporated for the growth of the organs.

The various parts of the body do not grow in equal proportion at the same time. The growth of the different parts of the body based on chronological age has been shown in Fig. 6.11.

2. *Direct anti-insulin action:* This can be brought about in the target organs in presence of cortisol (permissive action of cortisol is required.

Details of permissive action can be got from actions of cortisol; page no 162).

- *On carbohydrate metabolism:* It is a hyperglycemic agent. Increases the blood glucose level by:
  a. Decreasing the peripheral utilization of glucose.
  b. Increased gluconeogensis in liver.
  Metahypophyseal diabetes: Uncontrolled secretion of GH for a long time brings about increase in blood glucose level. This leads to increase stimulation of beta cells of islets of Langerhans to secrete insulin. After sometime, due to constant stimulation, the beta cells get exhausted and lead to development of diabetes mellitus.

- *Fat metabolism:* Acts on the adipose tissue. Neutral fats and triglycerides are broken down to release the free fatty acids. They are utilized for energy supply to the tissues.

This can lead to increased production of keto acids. Growth hormone also promotes the retention of sodium, potassium, calcium and phosphate since these substances are required for the growth of the body.

Regulation of Secretion

It is mainly by the negative feedback control by the free form of the hormone level in circulation.

Growth hormone releasing hormone (GRH) secreted from the hypothalamus acts on anterior pituitary gland and stimulates the secretion of growth hormone, which in turn increases insulin-like growth factor (IGF) I or somatomedin C secretion from liver. When IGF I level in circulation increases, it acts on hypothalamus to stimulate the secretion of somatostatin (SS). SS on reaching anterior pituitary decreases the secretion of growth hormone (Fig. 6.12).

IGF I also acts directly on anterior pituitary and exerts inhibitory influence on the secretion of growth hormone.

GH secreted by the anterior pituitary gland is able to reach the hypothalamus through circulation and on reaching hypothalamus it stimulates the secretion of somatostatin. Somatostatin on reaching anterior pituitary inhibits further secretion of growth hormone.

Some of the other factors that increase the secretion of growth hormone are:

- Increase in amino acids in circulation
- Hypoglycemia

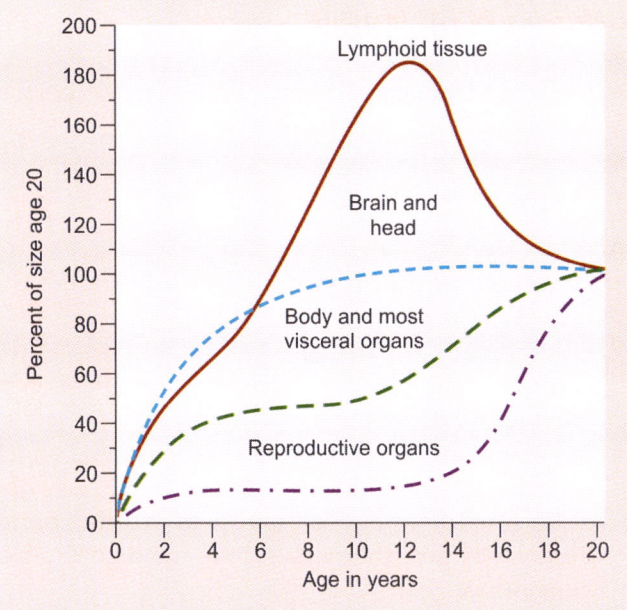

Fig. 6.11: Extent of growth of various tissues at different ages

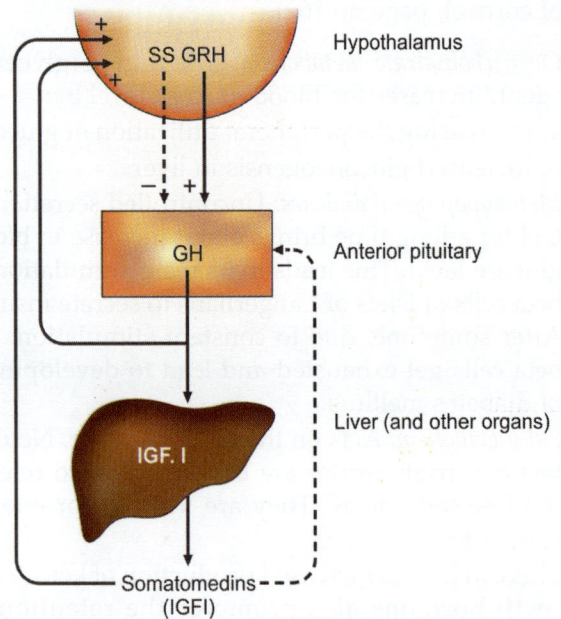

Fig. 6.12: Regulation of secretion of GH by feedback mechanism

- Free fatty acid decrease
- Exercise
- At puberty
- Stage IV sleep.

The factors which inhibit the GH secretion are:
- Dreaming or rapid eye movement (REM) sleep.
- Glucose increase.
- Cortisol.
- Obesity.

Applied aspects

Deficiency of GH in children
- Hypothalamic dysfunction
- Pituitary destruction
- Defective GHRH receptor
- Biologically incompetent GH or GH receptor
- Failure to produce IGF
- GH receptor deficiency
- GH receptor unresponsiveness: Laron dwarfism

Dwarfism
- It s because of hyposecretion of GH from childhood.
- Person will have short stature. There will be a generalized stunted growth of the body.
- The person will have normal reproductive development.

- There will not be any mental abnormality and will have normal intelligent quotient (IQ).
- Facial changes correspond with chronological age.
  Achondroplasia is the most common form of dwarfism. The characteristic feature will be short limbs and normal trunk.

Laron dwarf
- It will be due to insensitivity of the tissues to GH.
- The receptors are non-responsive to GH.
- There can be normal or elevated level of GH in circulation.

Progeria: Deficiency of growth hormone in adult. The person appears older at an younger age. Dwarfism could also be due to:
- Cretinism—thyroxine deficiency
- Gonadal dysgenesis
- Kaspar Hauser syndrome—psychosocial dwarfism
- Achondroplasia—child born to aged father

Frolich dwarf: Destructive disease of part of anterior pituitary. At times may include post-pituitary and hypothalamus.
- Stunted growth.
- Obesity
- Decreased sexual development
- Somnolence
- Mentally subnormal

Deficiency of GH in adult
- Decreased muscle
- Decreased muscle strength and exercise performance
- Decreased lean body mass
- Decreased bone density

Acromegaly (Fig. 6.13)
- Hypersecretion of growth hormone after the puberty.
- Enlargement of hand and feet (acral parts of the body only can grow because of the ossification of the long bones).
- There will also be enlargement of mandible which results in prognatism. There will also be enlargement and protrusion of frontal bone. Because of this, the person may have gorilla-like appearance.
- Certain osteoarthritic changes are also observed leading to kyphosis.

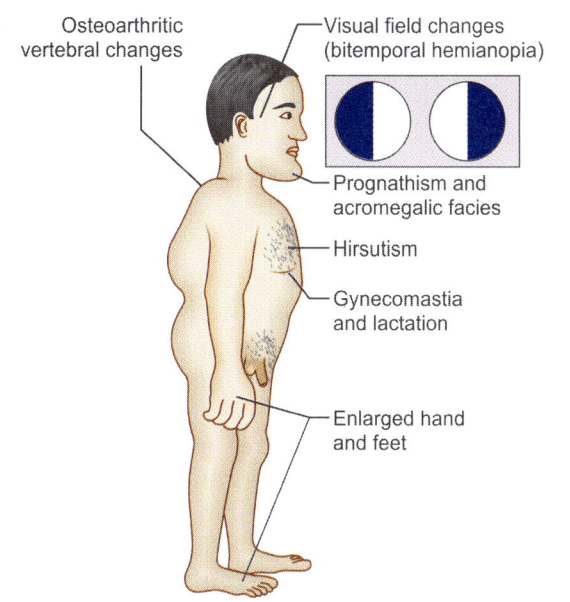

Osteoarthritic vertebral changes

Visual field changes (bitemporal hemianopia)

Prognathism and acromegalic facies

Hirsutism

Gynecomastia and lactation

Enlarged hand and feet

Fig. 6.13: Some of the important features of acromegaly

- There can be enlargement of viscera especially that of heart and may lead to cardiomegaly.
- There can be hirsutism (increased hair growth on anterior part of trunk) and gynecomastia (enlargement of breasts even in males) and lactation (secretion of milk).
- The person may suffer from bitemporal hemianopia (a type of visual field defect) due to the compressing on the medial part of optic chiasma by enlarged pituitary gland.

Gigantism
- Hypersecretion of hormone from childhood.
- Size of the person is pathologically big, but the person will be weak. Hence, the person is known as weak giant. There will not be proportionate growth of the contractile proteins in the muscles. Hence muscles are weak.
- The person is prone to develop early diabetes. This is because since growth hormone has hyperglycemic action, the sustained increase in blood glucose level may lead to exhaustion of beta cells of islets of Langerhans. So the person develops diabetes.
- The longevity of these people is restricted and die early.

Sheehan's syndrome
- Observed in female. Due to postpartum hemorrhage, there can be ischemic necrosis of pituitary gland.

- The pituitary gland secretion in general gets decreased.
- Symptoms include lethargy, sexually inactive, unable to withstand stress. Growth is inhibited and thyroid function is depressed.
- There can be atrophy of gonads. The menstrual cycle stops.
- When there is general deficiency of all the hormones of anterior pituitary gland, this condition is known as panhypopituitarism.

Hyperprolactinemia: It could be due to administration of dopamine antagonist/prolactin secreting adenomas. Features:
a. Amenorrhea
b. Galactorrhea
c. Decreased libido
d. Impotence
e. Hypogonadism
f. Testosterone level low

Posterior Pituitary Hormones

Posterior pituitor, gland is also known as neurohypophysis. The hormones of posterior pituitary gland are synthesized in the neurons of the hypothalamus. The two different groups of neurons in the hypothalamus, which synthesize these hormones are, supraoptic and paraventricular nuclei (they are also known as magno cellular neurons in general).

The hormones are transported from the hypothalamus to the posterior pituitary gland through the axoplasmic flow (Fig. 6.14). Supraoptic and para- ventricular nuclei of the hypothalamus are connected to the posterior pituitary gland through hypothalamo- hypophyseal tract. When impulses come through this tract to the posterior pituitary gland, the stored hormones in the gland are released into the circulation (Fig. 6.15).

Supraoptic nucleus predominantly secretes antidiuretic hormone (ADH/vasopressin) and para ventricular nucleus predominantly secretes oxytocin hormone. Both are peptide hormones.

Actions of Antidiuretic Hormone

As the name indicates, the hormone decreases the volume of water lost in the urine and thereby helps to maintain body water content by conservation of water. The sites of action are kidney and smooth muscle of blood vessels.

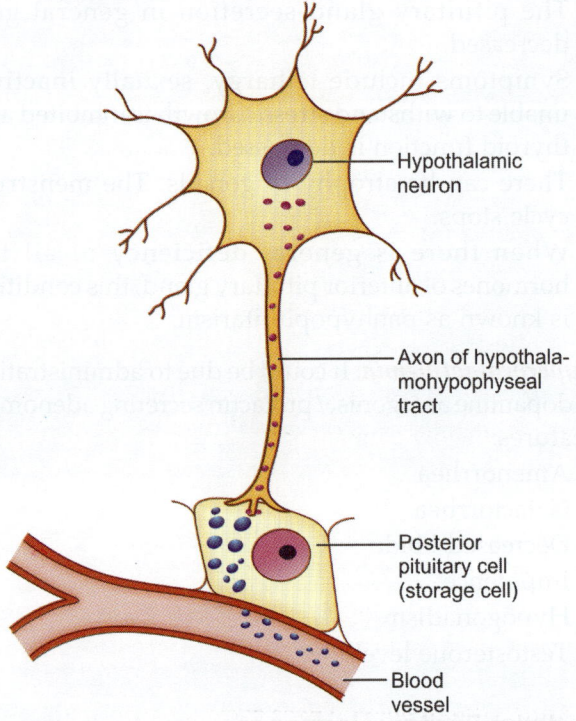

Fig. 6.14: Connection between hypothalamus and posterior pituitary gland (neural connection—hypothalamohypophyseal tract)

1. *Water reabsorption* (Fig. 6.16)
   - It acts on the epithelial cells lining the collecting duct and also distal convoluted tubule through V_2 receptors.
   - This brings about the insertion of water channels (aquaporins) in the epithelial cells.
   - Through these channels, water gets reabsorbed.
   - Water reabsorbed in these parts of the nephrons is under the influence of this hormone.

2. *Urea movement:* It facilitates the rate of urea recycled from the collecting duct. Because of reabsorption of water from DCT and CD, the concentration of urea increases in fluid present in tubular lumen. Due to the concentration gradient between the tubular lumen and interstitium in renal medulla, urea diffuses into the interstitium from the lumen. From the interstitial region of renal medulla along the concentration gradient, urea diffuses back into the fluid present in the ascending limb of loop of Henle.

3. *Rate of blood flow through vasa recta:* It reduces the rate of blood flow through the vasa recta and increases the time available for the operation of countercurrent system. Decreased rate of blood

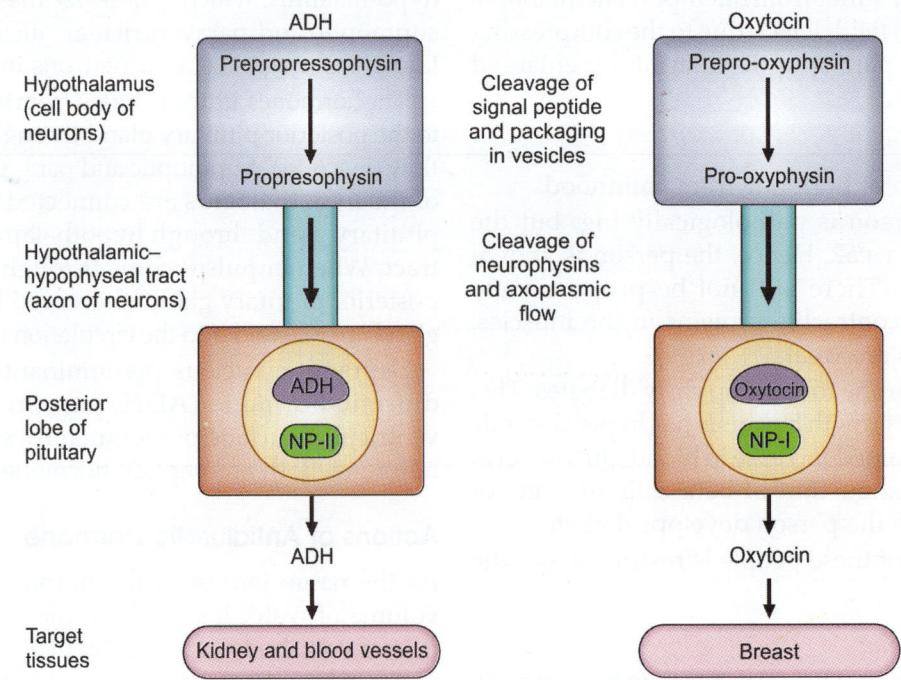

Fig. 6.15: Process involved in the secretion of active form of posterior pituitary hormones

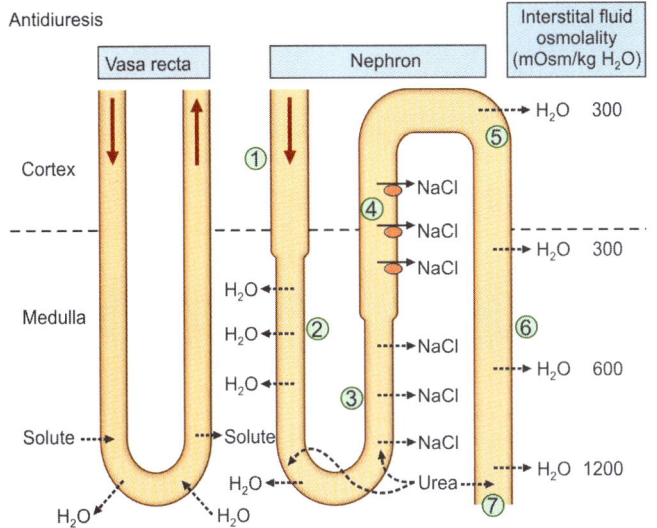

Fig. 6.16: Actions of ADH on kidney during water conservation

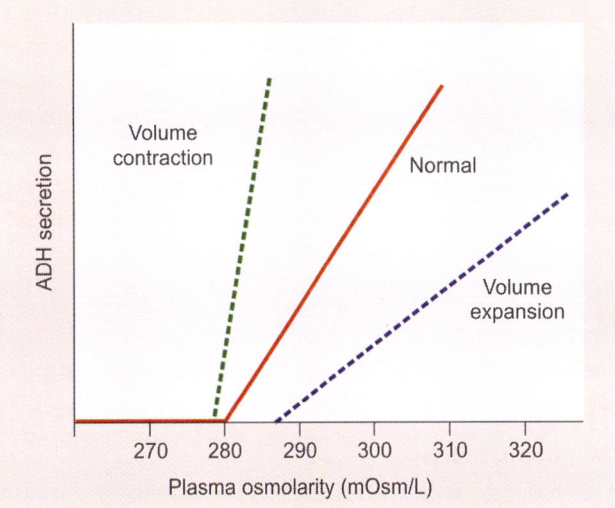

Fig. 6.17: Difference in the amount of ADH secreted for a given osmolarity depending on the volume variations

flow through vasa recta is essential concentration of urine.

All the three aforesaid actions help in concentration of urine.

4. *Vascular smooth muscle:* In addition to the above actions, ADH in large doses acts on the smooth muscle of blood vessels through the V_1 receptors and brings about vasoconstriction. Because of this, there will be increase in peripheral resistance and hence increase in diastolic blood pressure.

Regulation of Secretion

Regulation of secretion is brought about by two important mechanisms. There is involvement of osmoreceptors and volume receptors in regulation of secretion (Fig. 6.17).

1. *Osmoreceptors:* They are present in the hypo-thalamus near the supraoptic nucleus. When the plasma osmolality increases (normal is 300 mOsm/L water), by exosmosis water moves out of osmoreceptors into the interstitium. This leads to shrinkage of the osmoreceptors and consequent stimulation of the receptors. This in turn stimulates the supraoptic nucleus. From the supraoptic nucleus, more impulses are sent to posterior pituitary through the hypothalamohypophyseal tract. Because of this, more antidiuretic hormone will be released into the circulation. This helps for increased retention of water through the kidneys and normalizes the osmolality of the plasma.

2. *Volume receptors:* Volume receptors are present in the walls of the great veins and in the walls of the right side of heart. These receptors are also known as low pressure receptors. Increase in blood volume stretches the walls of great veins and the right side of heart and stimulates these receptors. Afferent impulses from the receptors reach the hypothalamus and inhibit the activity of supraoptic nucleus. This decreases the frequency of impulses along the hypothalamohypophyseal tract to posterior pituitary gland. So less amount of antidiuretic hormone is released from the posterior pituitary gland into circulation. This decreases the volume of water reabsorbed from the renal tubules. Increased urine output will restore the blood volume.

Some of the other factors that can alter secretion of the hormone are:
- Alcohol
- Pain
- Surgery
- Trauma.

Applied Aspect

Diabetes insipidus: It occurs due to deficiency of anti-diuretic hormone secretion. Some of the features are:
- *Polyuria:* Increased volume of urine excretion due to loss of concentrating ability in kidney.

- *Polydypsia:* Increased thirst center activity due to decrease in body water content. Person drinks more water.
- Glucose will be absent in urine and blood glucose level will be normal.
- Specific gravity of the urine will be less due to excretion of more dilute urine most of the times.

Actions of Oxytocin

On the breasts: It acts on the myoepithelial cells of the breasts. This causes the ejection of milk from the alveolar ducts of the breasts.

On myometrium

- It acts on the myometrium of the uterus and causes severe contraction of the myometrium. This leads to the parturition or delivery of the fetus due to increase in the intrauterine pressure.
- In the non-pregnant woman, oxytocin is believed to bring about minute myometrial contractions which facilitate movement of sperm along the uterus to reach fallopian tubes.
- In males, it is believed to bring about contraction of smooth muscles in vas deferens and facilitate sperm movement in the genital system.

Regulation of Secretion

Regulation of secretion is brought about by neuro-endocrine reflex. In this reflex, part of the reflex pathway is neural and part is hormonal. Milk ejection and parturition reflexes are classical examples of neuroendocrine reflex.

Suckling of the breasts brings about the stimulation of the touch receptors present on the nipple and areola. Afferent impulses are carried to the hypothalamus through the ascending tracts in spinal cord and stimulate the paraventricular nucleus. The nucleus stimulation leads to more impulses along the hypothalamohypophyseal tract to posterior pituitary gland. This brings about the release of the hormone from the posterior pituitary gland into the circulation. The hormone on reaching breasts brings about milk ejection by acting on the myoepithelial cells.

When head of the fetus presses on the cervix, the stretch receptors present in the walls of cervix are stimulated and the afferent impulses from these receptors reach the hypothalamus along the ascending tracts in spinal cord. This brings about the stimulation

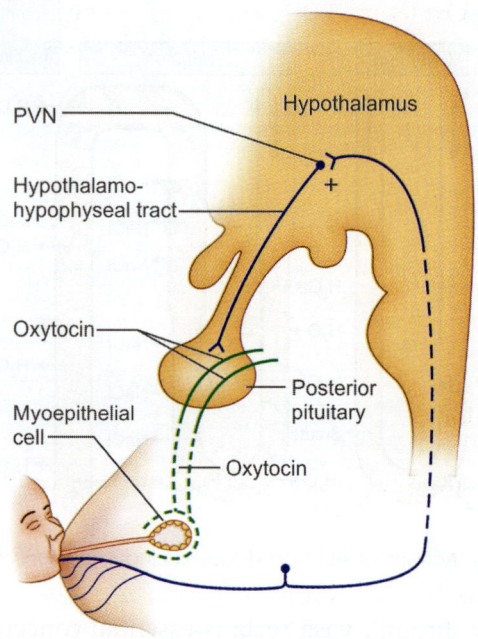

Neuroendocrine reflex

Fig. 6.18: Pathway involved in milk ejection reflex

of the paraventricular nucleus in the hypothalamus. More impulses conveyed along the hypothalamo-hypophyseal tract to the posterior pituitary gland. This leads to the release of the hormone into circulation. The hormone acts on the myometrium present in the walls of uterus to bring about contractions of the uterus resulting in parturition (delivery of fetus).

Milk ejection reflex (Fig. 6.18):

Suckling of breasts
↓
Stimulates touch receptors present around nipple and areola
↓
Afferent impulses reach hypothalamus along ascending tracts in spinal cord
↓
Stimulation of paraventricular nucleus
↓
More impulses along hypothalamohypophyseal tract to posterior pituitary gland
↓
Release of oxytocin into circulation
↓

Oxytocin brings about contraction of myoepithelial cells in the breasts
↓
Ejection of milk

Parturition reflex

Head of fetus pressing on cervix
↓
Stimulates stretch receptors present in walls of vagina
↓
Afferent impulses reach hypothalamus-along the ascending tracts in spinal cord
↓
Stimulation of paraventricular nucleus
↓
More impulses along hypothalamo-hypophyseal tract to posterior pituitary gland
↓
Release of oxytocin into circulation
↓
Oxytocin brings about contraction of myometrium in the uterus
↓
Delivery of the baby

ENDOCRINE FUNCTION OF ADRENAL CORTEX

The adrenals are made up of two parts. Outer zone known as adrenal cortex and the inner core region is adrenal medulla. The hormones secreted by adrenal cortex are collectively known as corticosteroids whereas the medullary hormones are known as catecholamine. Apart from this difference, even during the embryonic life, they get developed from entirely different regions and the medullary region is nothing but the modified ganglion of the sympathetic nervous system.

Adrenal Cortex

It is divisible into three different layers, from outwards within will be:
- Zona glomerulosa
- Zona fasciculata
- Zona reticularis.

All three layers secrete the hormones.
Zona glomerulosa secretes mineralocorticoids of which the most important is aldosterone.

Zona fasciculata and *reticularis* together secrete glucocorticoids of which the most important are cortisol and corticosterone. The layers also secrete sex steroids, of which adrenal androgen is most important. Both the glucocorticoids and mineralocorticoids can exert the action of the other group as well especially when the concentration of the hormone is very high.

Principal hormones of renal cortex have been enumerated in Table 6.1, and the relative efficacy of glucocorticoid and mineralocorticoid and certain other substance actions have been compared in Table 6.2.

Biosynthesis of Hormones (Figs 6.19 and 6.20)

Genetic defects in cortisol biosynthesis have important consequences. A defect in 21 or 11-hydroxylase

Table 6.1: Principal adrenocortical hormones in adult humans[a]

Name	Synonyms	Average plasma concentration (free and bound)[a] (µg/dL)	Average amount secreted (mg/24 h)
Cortisol	Compound F, hydrocortisone	13.9	10
Corticosterone	Compound B	0.4	3
Aldosterone		0.006	0.15
Deoxycorticosterone	DOC	0.006	0.20
Dehydroepiandrosterone sulfate	DHEAS	175.0	20

[a] All plasma concentration values except DHEAS are fasting morning values after overnight recumbency

Table 6.2: Relative efficacy of actions of adrenocortical hormones

Steroid	Glucocorticoid activity	Mineralocorticoid activity
Cortisol	1.0	1.0
Corticosterone	0.3	15
Aldosterone	0.3	3000
Deoxycorticosterone	0.2	100
Cortisone	0.7	0.8
Prednisolone	4	0.8
9α-Fluorocortisol	10	125
Dexamethasone	25	~0

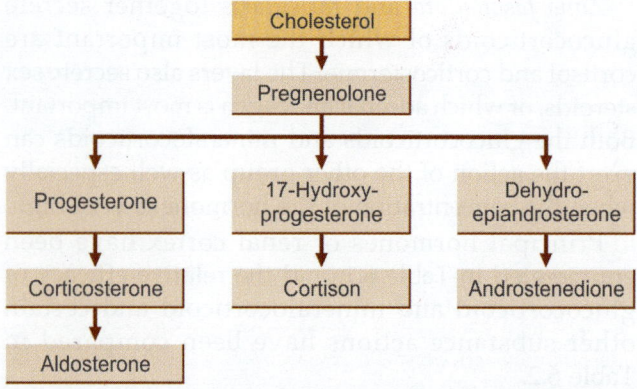

Fig. 6.19: Major steps involved in biosynthesis of adrenocortical hormones

enzyme gene leads to overproduction of androgenic steroids from the precursors. Hence there will be production of excess of androgens and this causes masculinization of female fetuses' in utero and early secondary sexual changes in male infants and young boys.

Cortisol is transported in circulation. A major part of it is in the protein bound form along with globulin (cortisol binding globulin—CBG). The level of this protein increases in pregnancy because of which in the initial stages, the free form of hormonal level in circulation decrease. This in turn stimulates more of secretion of the hormone by increased secretion of ACTH from the anterior pituitary gland. Levels of CBG decrease in cirrhosis of liver and in nephrosis.

Actions

Permissive Action

Cortisol should be present in the target organs for the action of certain other hormones, e.g. the catecholamine can exert the vasoconstrictor effect on vascular smooth muscle only in the presence of cortisol. The vasoconstrictor effect is necessary to maintain peripheral resistance and hence blood pressure. Permissive action of cortisol is also required for certain actions of growth hormone and glucagon.

Metabolic Actions (Fig. 6.21)

a. **Carbohydrate metabolism:** It is a hyperglycemic agent and increases blood glucose level.
- By decreasing peripheral utilization of glucose in almost all parts of body except heart and brain.

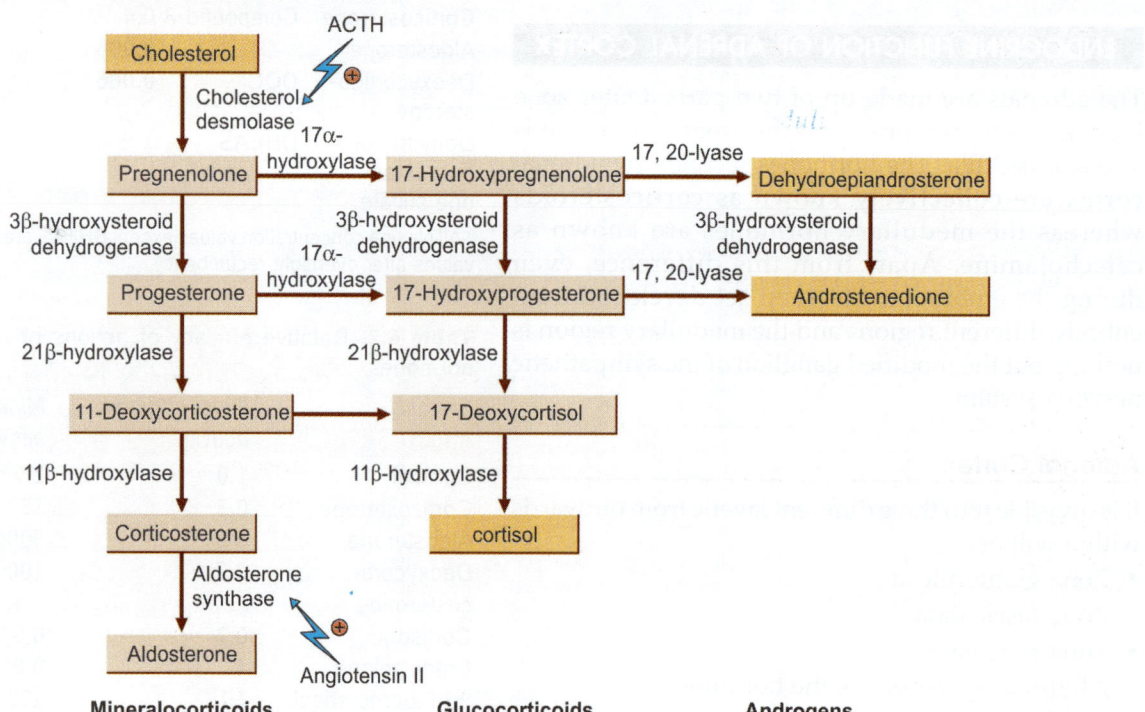

Fig. 6.20: Steps involved in biosynthesis of adrenocortical hormones and the enzymes affecting the respective hormonal synthesis

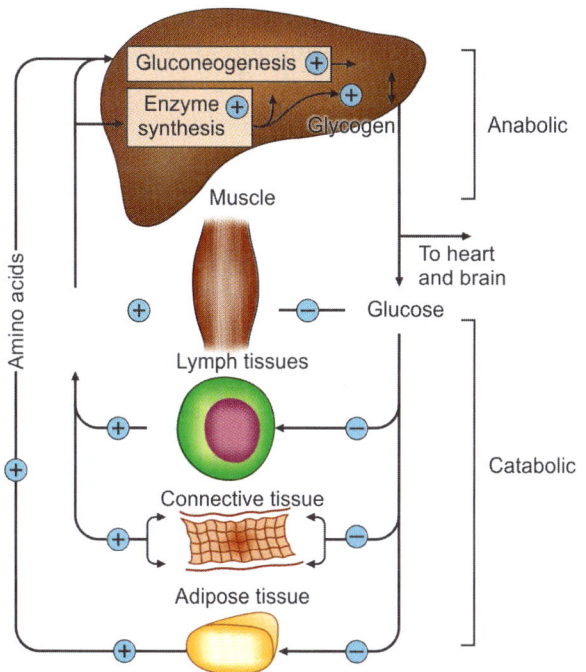

Fig. 6.21: Some of the important metabolic actions of cortisol

- By increasing the gluconeogenesis and glyco-genesis in liver.
- Excessive use of cortisol as therapeutic agent may lead to exhaustion of beta cells of pancreas and cause metasteroid diabetes.

b. *Protein metabolism:* In large doses, it enhances the protein breakdown especially in the lymphoid tissue, muscles, and bones.
  - Leading to decreased immunity
  - Muscular weakness
  - Weight loss
  - Susceptibility of the bones for fracture.
  - The amino acids released due to protein break-down are used for gluconeogenesis in the liver.

c. *Fat metabolism:* The hormone generally increases the lipolysis in adipose tissue. So brings about the breakdown of neutral fats and triglycerides. This will result in increase in free fatty acids and glycerol in circulation.
  - The free fatty acids are used both for energy supply to the tissues and gluconeogenesis in the liver.
  - There will be redistribution of fats in the body.
  - Fats are removed from the peripheral parts and deposited in the more central parts of body

resulting in moon face, buffalo hump and pendulous abdomen.

d. *Mineral metabolism:* Excess of cortisol can also exert some amount of action like aldosterone. Hence it increases the sodium reabsorption in the distal convoluted tubule and in exchange for this, potassium excretion in the urine increases. Reabsorption of sodium increases water retention, so blood volume and blood pressure are increased.

e. *Water metabolism:* Person with low levels of cortisol has defective water regulation in the body. This could be because of the increase in the plasma antidiuretic hormone level (ADH degradation rate is slowed) and decreased glomerular filtration rate. Both of these contribute for delayed water excretion. The retention of water by the body can lead to water intoxication.

On Organs

1. *CNS:* It increases the activity of the neurons in central nervous system and hence the patient may have euphoria. It will also increase the irritation of neurons because of which, administration of this as drug to any patient susceptible to / suffering from epilepsy should be borne in mind. Administration of this drug may worsen the condition.

2. *GIT:* In large dose, increase the gastric acid secretion and damages the mucus barrier. So the people are more prone to develop peptic ulcer.

3. *Skeletal muscle:* Excess of cortisol leads to muscular weakness promoting protein catabolism and insufficiency also causes muscular weakness.

4. *Blood:* Cortisol insufficiency leads eosinophilia, lymphocytosis, etc. whereas excess of cortisol brings about eosinopenia, lymphocytopenia. Eosinophil count is decreased because of sequestration of the cells in liver. Increased protein breakdown in the lymphoid tissue may lead to decreased antibodies in circulation and the person is more susceptible for infections.

5. *Bone:* Excess of cortisol impedes development of cartilage and causes thinning of epiphyseal plates. There will also be defective synthesis protein matrix and deposition of calcium salts. Because of these things, osteoporosis occurs in Cushing's syndrome.

Pharmacological actions occur only when the levels are far in excess.

Anti-inflammatory Action

In some people, acute inflammation can cause more damage to the tissues. Inflammation is due to increased:

a. Blood flow due to increased metabolic rate of the bacteria at the site of infections
b. Permeability of the capillaries
c. Emigration of leukocytes to the site of infection from the blood vessels
d. Lysozyme release from the cells leading to proteolysis.

Cortisol counters the aforesaid effects by decreasing

a. Metabolic rate of bacteria
b. Capillary permeability
c. Emigration of leukocytes and stabilizing the lysozymes.

Cortisol should never be administered alone in bacterial infection as anti-inflammatory agent. It should always be combined with antibiotics to take care of the bacteria otherwise it can lead to spread of the bacteria, without the overt reaction of the body due to infection. This can lead to severe problems.

Antiallergic Activity

Especially in organ or tissue transplantation sometimes the recipient's body resists or rejects the new organ/tissue. Cortisol can be used to decrease the immunosuppression reactions. This helps to prevent rejection of the transplanted tissues. Suppresses immune responses by:

• Decreasing the eosinophil, and lymphocyte count.
• Decreasing the eosinophil count by sequestration of the cells in liver and spleen.
• Decreasing the lymphocyte percentage by catabolism of proteins in lymphoid tissue. Hence it will decrease the concentration of circulating antibodies in course of time.

Regulation of Secretion

By the negative feedback mechanism and there is involvement of hypothalamo–pituitary–adrenal axis. Increase free form of hormone in circulation acts on hypothalamus and anterior pituitary gland. From the hypothalamus, secretion of corticotrophin releasing factor (CRF) decreases, so it leads to decreased secretion of ACTH. Cortisol also acts directly on the anterior pituitary gland and inhibits secretion of

ACTH. Decreased ACTH leads to less of cortisol secretion from the adrenal gland. Apart from this, stress and circadian rhythm directly act on hypothalamus to alter the secretions (Figs 6.22 and 6.23).

Cortisol as a drug when used one has to be careful at the time of discontinuation of the drug. Unlike many drugs, which can be stopped all of a sudden, this cannot be done with cortisol. When exogenous cortisol is administered, the increased level of free

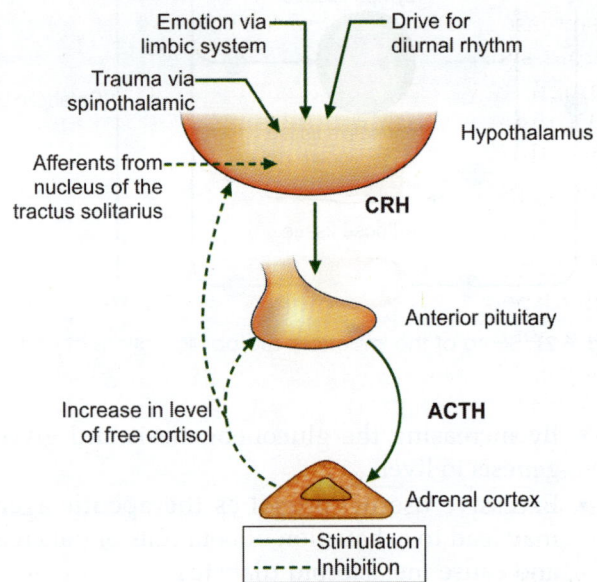

Fig. 6.22: Regulation of secretion of cortisol by negative feedback mechanism and factors influencing

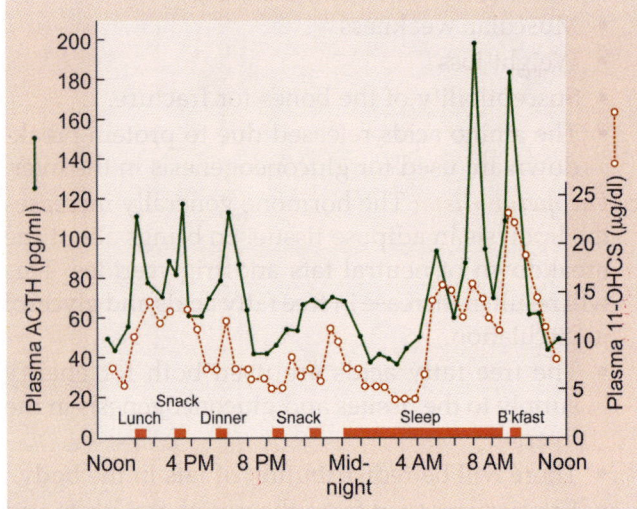

Fig. 6.23: Diurnal variation in the secretion of ACTH and 11-OHCS

form of cortisol in circulation constantly inhibits the hypothalamus. This brings about the depression of the hypothalamopituitary–adrenal axis function. If cortisol is withdrawn suddenly, the axis cannot get revived immediately and patient may develop a crisis. If cortisol is withdrawn slowly and steadily (tapering dose), more time is provided for the regaining of the activity of the hypothalamopituitary–adrenal axis and the restoration of the endogenous secretion of cortisol can start once again (Fig. 6.24).

Aminoglutethimide is a potent inhibitor of desmolase reaction and thereby decreases all adrenal steroid synthesis. This drug has been used to treat women with breast cancer. Ketoconazole an antifungal agent also inhibit several steps in biosynthesis of the hormones and thus effective in treating patients having excess of cortisol secretion.

Adrenal Androgens

Dehydroepiandrostenedione (DHEA) and androstenedione are weak androgens. In the peripheral tissues, they get converted to potent androgen, testosterone. In female, the action of adrenal androgens will be:

- Sustaining of normal pubic and axillary hair.
- In menopausal stage, estradiol of adrenal origin is important source of estrogen activity.

In normal male, the amount of testosterone secreted by the testis far exceeds the adrenal androgens and not much role to play by the adrenal androgens. If the adrenal androgen secretion becomes abnormally high especially in children, it can lead to precocious puberty.

Aldosterone

As stated already, the most important mineralocorticoid is aldosterone, which is secreted by the zona glomerulosa.

Actions

On the Kidney

It acts on the distal convoluted tubule and increases the sodium reabsorption. In exchange for this, there will be increased secretion of either potassium or hydrogen ion. Sodium reabsorption will be coupled with chloride and water reabsorption as well. This will increase the extracellular fluid volume and hence blood volume.

On the epithelial cells of the kidney when aldosterone acts, it facilitates the Na^+–K^+ pumps activity at the basolateral surface and increases sodium movement from the cells into the interstititum and finally into the blood vessels.

Regulation of Secretion (Fig. 6.25)

a. Concentration of K^+ and Na^+ in circulation can act directly on the gland to alter the secretion. Of the two, the most potent is increase in the concentration of potassium. The normal plasma K^+ level is low (5 mEq/L water) when compared to Na^+ (150 mEq/L water). So, small alteration in K^+ level will have a profound effect on the rate of secretion.

b. *Angiotensin II:* This is formed due to activity of renin–angiotensin system can directly act on the adrenals and enhance the secretion of the hormone.

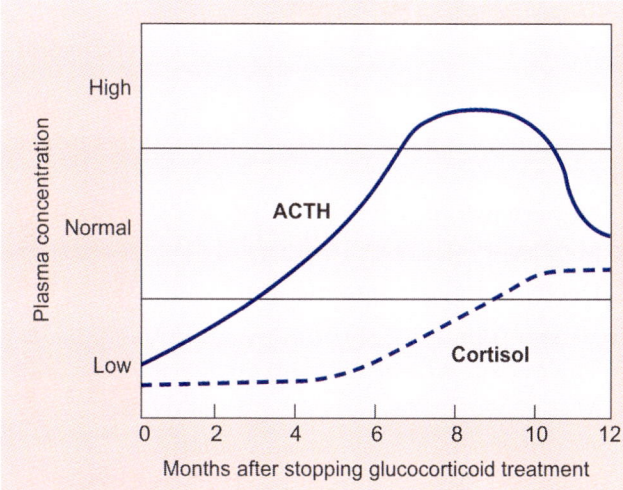

Fig. 6.24: Duration required for resumption of normal endogenous secretion of ACTH and cortisol

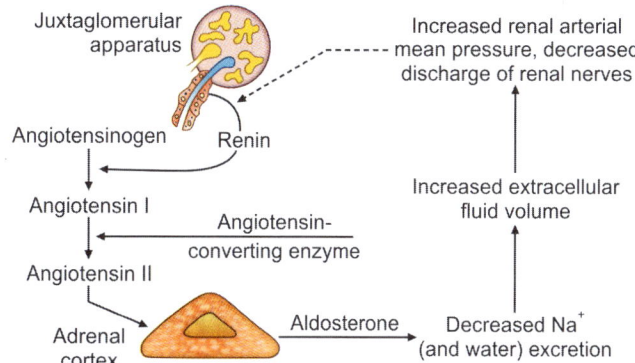

Fig. 6.25: Role of renin–angiotensin in the regulation of secretion of aldosterone

c. Some of the other factors which can increase the secretion of aldosterone are anxiety, physical trauma and hemorrhage.

Cushing's syndrome (Fig. 6.26) is due to hypersecretion of cortisol. Hypersecretion could be because of problem in adrenal cortex (primary), anterior pituitary (secondary) or in hypothalamus (tertiary).

Addison's disease is hyposecretion of all hormones of adrenal cortex.

Adrenogenital syndrome is due to hypersecretion of dehydroepiandrosterone. The features of a female suffering from adrenogenital syndrome have been shown in Fig. 6.27.

Virilism is due to deficiency of 21β hydroxylase enzyme which leads to lot of secretion of sex hormones from adrenal cortex. In boys, it leads to precocious sexual development and in female leads to pseudohermophroditism. In adult female, it leads to the development of adrenogenital syndrome.

Conn's syndrome: Conn's syndrome is due to primary hyperaldosteronism. Secondary hyperaldosteronism can be due to liver disease, stenosis of renal artery, etc. Whether it primary or secondary cause, there will be abnormal increase in the secretion of aldosterone.

Cushing's syndrome (Increased cortisol secretion)
• Redistribution of fat—moon face, bufello hump, pendulous abdomen • Thin extremities—protein catabolism • Poor wound healing • Muscular weakness • Personality changes • Hyperglycemic • Hypertension

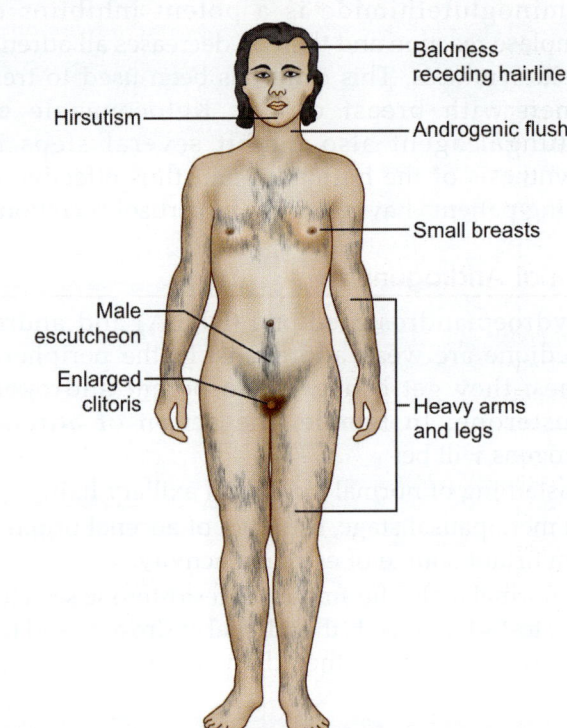

Fig. 6.27: Features of adrenogenital syndrome in a female

Features of Conn's syndrome/hyperaldosteronism are:

1. Hypertension.
2. Increased total body sodium.
3. Decreased plasma potassium.
4. Urine acidic
5. The person will suffer from alkalosis.
6. Muscle weakness, fatigue and paralysis.
7. At times person may develop tetany.
8. Polyuria
9. No edema because of sodium escape phenomenon.

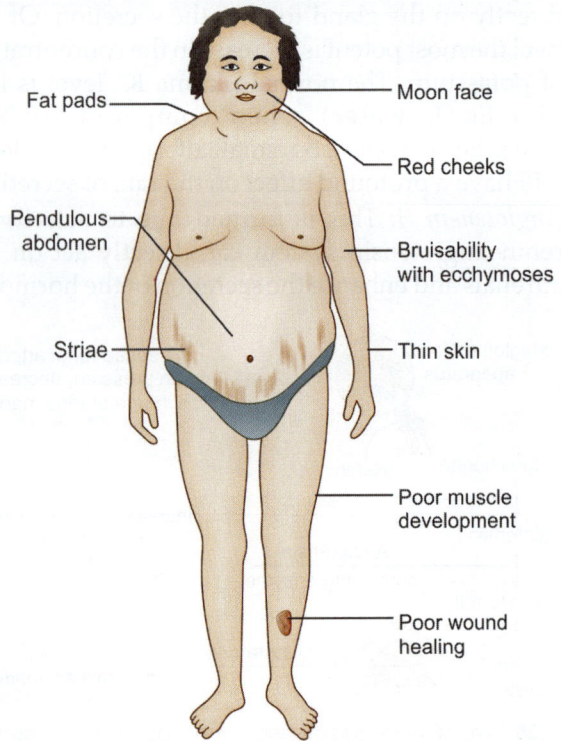

Fig. 6.26: Some of the important features of Cushing's syndrome

Disorders of adrenocortical functions

1. Hypofunction—Addison's disease signs and symptoms due to decreased aldosterone and decreased cortisol
2. Excersive pigmentation (due to increased ACTH)
3. Anorexia, nausea, diarrhea and vomiting
4. Mental confusion
5. Decreased ability to withstand stress
6. Dehydration, hypotension, loss of weight

Adrenogenital syndrome (Fig. 6.27)

- Excessive secretion of DHEA
- Women develop male sec. sex characters (adrenal virilism)
- Deepening of voice
- Amenorrhea
- Enlarged clitoris
- Hair growth—masculine distribution
- Increased muscle mass

Congenital adrenal hyperplasia (virilism) due to enzyme dificiency (congenital) mostly due to lack of 21β hydroxylase. Hyperplasia is due to increased secretion of ACTH. Signs and symptoms—due to increased secretion of DHEA

a. In boys—Precocious sexual development testes remains infantile (infant hercule)
b. Women—Genetically female external genitalia looks like a male child. Pseudohermophroditism
c. Adult women—Adrenogenital syndrome

Disorder of Adrenal Cortical Functions— Addison's Disease

a. Hypofunction of adrenal cortex (primary adrenal insufficiency)
- Decreased secretion of cortisol and aldosterone
- Hyperpigmentation of skin and buccal mucosa
- Anorexia, nausea, diarrhea and vomiting
- Confusion
- Unable to withstand stress
- Dehydration, hypotension and loss of weight
- Hyperkalemia, salt wasting, metabolic acidosis

b. Secondary and tertiary adrenal insufficiency
- No hyperkalemia
- No metabolic acidosis
- No volume contraction
- No hyperpigmentation
- Congenital adrenal hyperplasia

Enzyme deficiency and consequent hormonal abnormality and symptoms (Table 6.3).

21 beta hydroxylase—most common form of congenital adrenal insufficiency:
a. Decreased cortisol and aldosterone
b. Increased ACTH
c. Hyperplasia of zona fasciculata and reticularis
d. Increased adrenal androgens
e. Virilization in women
f. Hypotension
g. Hyperkalemia
h. Hyponatremia

17 alpha hydroxylase deficiency:
a. Decreased glucocorticoid and androgens
b. Increased ACTH
c. Increased aldosterone
d. Hypoglycemia
e. Metabolic alkalosis, hypokalemia, hypertension
f. Lack of axillary and pubic hair

Endocrine Function of Adrenal Medulla

It secretes the hormones of emergency. The secretion is stimulated in conditions, like fight, flight or fright. For the synthesis of the hormone, the amino acid

Table 6.3: Problems associated with enzyme deficiency in the biosynthetic pathway

Enzyme	Steroid abnormality	Symptoms
21 β hydroxylase	Deficiency of cortisol and aldosterone, increased androgens	Salt loss, masculinization
11 β hydroxylase	Decreased cortisol and aldosterone, increased DOC and androgen	Hypertension, masculinization
3 β hydroxysteroid dehydrogenase	Decreased cortisol and aldosterone, increased androgen (DHEA)	Salt loss, masculinization
17 α hydroxylase	Decreased cortisol and androgen, increased DOC, aldostrone, and corticosterone	Sexual infantalism, hypertension, hypokalemic alkalosis

required is phenylalanine. Catecholamine group includes the hormones adrenaline, noradrenaline and dopamine. In human beings, about 80% of the hormone secreted from this region is adrenaline.

Biosynthesis of Hormones (Fig. 6.28)

The precursor of tyrosine is phenylalanine amino acid (essential amino acid). Phenylalanine on hydroxylation by the enzyme phenylalanine hydroxylase is converted to tyrosine.

Degradation of Hormones (Fig. 6.29)

Metanephrine, normetanephrine and VMA are excreted from the body along with urine.

Most of the hormone will be degraded in the target organs and the end products of the metabolites are excreted along with the urine in the form of vanillyl-mandelic acid and as conjugates.

The receptors through which the hormone acts are termed as adrenergic receptors. The types of receptors

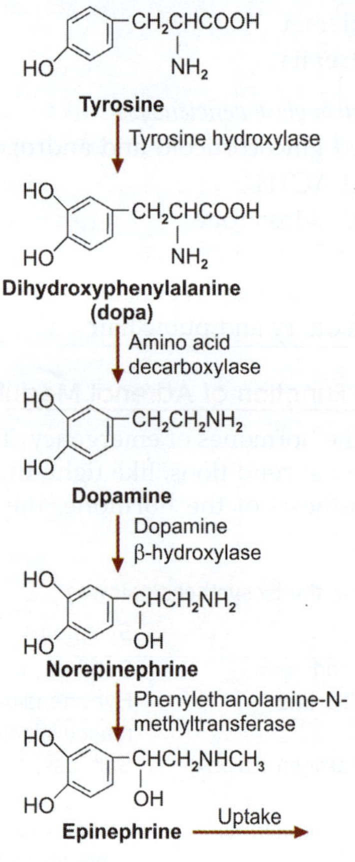

Fig. 6.28: Steps involved in the biosynthesis of adrenal medullary hormones

are alpha and beta. They are further divided into alpha 1 and alpha 2 and beta 1 and beta 2. The action of the hormone on the target organ depends on the type of receptor through which the action is mediated.

Actions

On Vascular Smooth Muscle

In the presence of cortisol, catecholamine is able to act on the smooth muscle of blood vessels especially in the arteriolar regions. Due to this, some amount of vasoconstriction is maintained all the time and hence peripheral resistance. Peripheral resistance is the factor that is responsible for the diastolic blood pressure. Noradrenaline is a powerful vasoconstrictor.

On Heart and Blood Vessels

It is able to increase both the heart rate and force of contraction. This action is mediated through the beta receptors present in cardiac muscle. It exerts both chronotropic and inotropic actions. Hence it increases cardiac output and systolic blood pressure in general.

On the Blood Vessels (Fig. 6.30 and Table 6.4)

Noradrenaline: Alpha receptors are present on the smooth muscle of arterioles and when it exerts its influence there will be vasoconstriction. Noradrenaline predominantly acts through this group of receptors and hence there is an increase of total peripheral resistance in the body. This is going to increase the diastolic blood pressure and hence there will be a secondary increase of systolic pressure as well. Increase in diastolic BP increases mean arterial pressure. The increase will stimulate the baroreceptors and hence there will be a reflex bradycardia and fall of cardiac output after sometime.

Adrenaline: It acts through both alpha and beta receptors present on the smooth muscle of blood vessels.

When it acts through the alpha receptors, it brings about vasoconstriction and through beta receptors it brings about vasodilatation. Since the beta receptors present in the blood vessels of skeletal compartment, there will be an enormous amount of vasodilatation when compared to vasoconstriction. The net effect will be vasodilatation in the body. Due to this, there will be a fall of peripheral resistance and hence the diastolic BP decreases. So the mean arterial pressure would

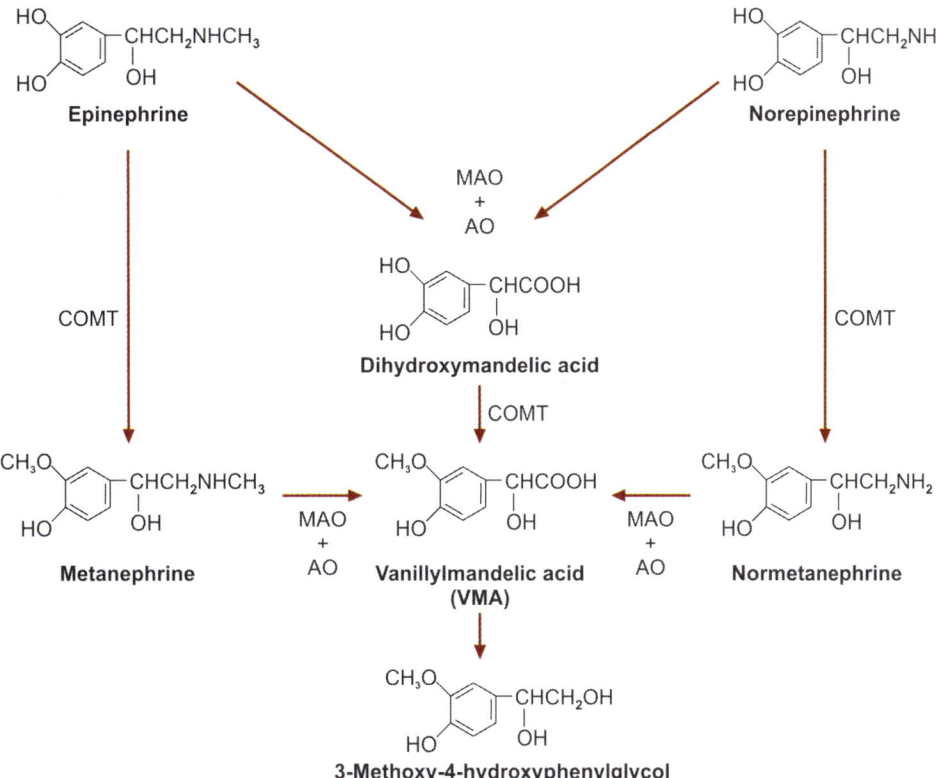

Fig. 6.29: Steps involved in the catabolism of adrenal medullary hormones. MAO–monoamino oxidase, AO–aldehyde oxidase, COMT–catechol-O-methyltransferase

remain almost normal, because of which there would not be any change in the activity of the baroreceptors.

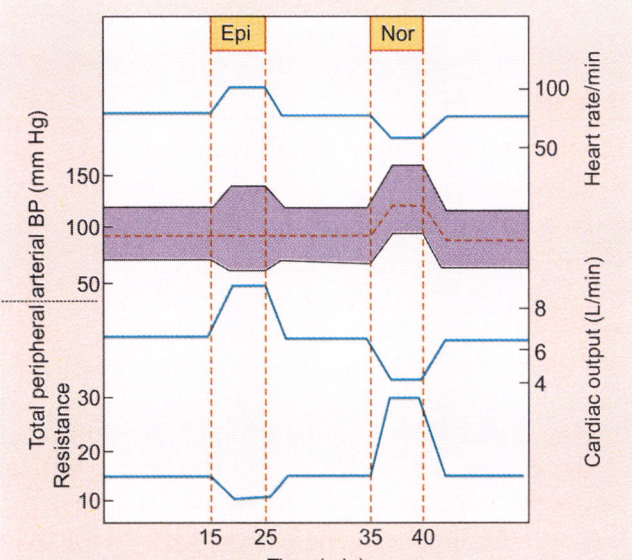

Fig. 6.30: Comparative actions of adrenaline and noradrenaline on cardiovascular parameters

Since Adrenalin also exerts its influence on heart through the beta receptors, there will be an increase of cardiac output and hence even the systolic BP is increased.

On Brain

Increases the activity of the neurons of central nervous system and person becomes more alert. But if the amount acting on the brain is very much, it brings about the inhibition of spinal reflexes.

On Bronchial Smooth Muscle

Brings about the bronchodilation and relieves a person suffering from bronchial asthma.

On Skeletal Muscle

It increases the blood flow and help to sustain the increase in the muscular activity.

On Iris

It acts on the dilator pupillae muscle and hence there will be dilation of pupil.

Norepinephrine	Parameter	Epinephrine
	Table 6.4: Relative efficiency of epinephrine and norepinephrine	
Decreased (due to reflex bradycardia)	Cardiac output	Increased
Increased	Peripheral resistance	Decreased
++++	Mean arterial pressure elevation	+
++++	Free fatty acid release	+++
++++	Stimulation of CNS	++++
+++	Increased heat production	++++
+	Increased blood sugar (β)	++++
+	Dilation of bronchioles	++++

Metabolic Effects

It acts as hyperglycemic agent and increases blood glucose level by stimulating the glycogenolysis in liver and muscle and gluconeogenesis in liver.

It also increases the lipolysis and increases the free fatty acid release and also the metabolic rate of the tissue. Since it enhances the rate of metabolism, it is termed as a calorigenic agent. This increases the metabolic rate in the body and hence there will be increased heat production. Because of this, they have an important role to play when person needs immediate heat production when exposed to colder situations. There will also be more amount of blood flow to the cutaneous region to facilitate increase in heat loss.

GIT

It stimulates the activity of the sphincters and relaxes the smooth muscle due to which there will be decreased motility of the GIT.

Regulation of Secretion

Adrenal medulla has efferent nerve supply from the sympathetic nervous system only.

The activity of the autonomic nervous system (parasympathetic and sympathetic) is under the influence of the activity of the neurons present in hypothalamus.

When the neurons present in the hypothalamus which control the activity of the sympathetic nerves get stimulated, impulses from hypothalamus reach the neurons present in the lateral horn cells of spinal cord. From the neurons of the lateral horn cells, the efferent sympathetic fibers taken origin and hence these neurons when get stimulated, will lead to increase in the sympathetic activity.

This increases the secretion of adrenal medulla.

Adrenal medullary secretion specially gets increased when a person is in fight/flight/fright situation, because of enormous increase in sympathetic activity.

Pheochromocytoma

- It is because of tumor in adrenal medulla.
- There will be an abnormally high amount of secretion of hormones from this region.

  Some of the features of this condition are:
  - Sustained severe hypertension.
  - Palpitation.
  - Headache.
  - Sweating.
  - Hyperpnea.
  - Nausea and vomiting.
  - Anxiety and muscular weakness.

Thyroid Gland

The hormones secreted by this gland are:

- Thyroxine (T_4)
- Triiodothyronine (T_3)
- Thyrocalcitonin (calcitonin)

Among the three hormones, the follicular cells of the gland secrete the first two hormones (T_3 and T_4) and the last one (thyrocalcitonin) is secreted by the parafollicular cells. T_4 is also known as tetraiodo-thyronine and gets converted to T_3 at the time of action in the target organ. Calcitonin hormone will be discussed along with calcium metabolism.

Biosynthesis of hormone is regulated by the activity of TSH secreted from the anterior pituitary gland. Since it is a tropic hormone, TSH regulates the growth and functioning of thyroid gland.

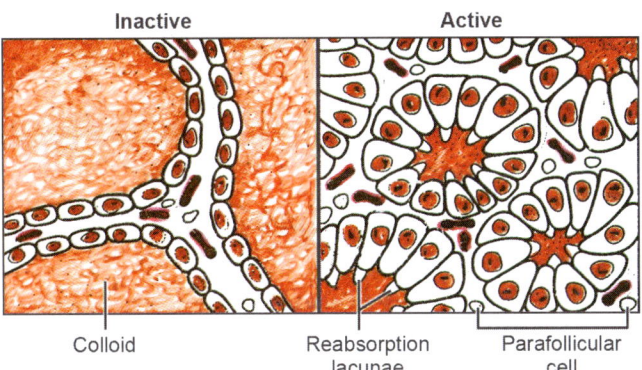

Inactive   Active

Colloid   Reabsorption   Parafollicular
                 lacunae   cell

Fig. 6.31: Amount of colloid in the inactive and active state of the gland

The following diagram indicates the action of TSH on thyroid gland (Fig. 6.32).

The steps in the biosynthesis of the hormone are (Fig. 6.33):

- *Iodide trapping* that is the uptake of iodide by the follicular cells from the plasma against the electrochemical gradient. The hormone TSH secreted by the anterior pituitary gland affects this step. Substances, like thiocyanate, pertechnetate and perchlorate that are examples of antithyroid drugs can inhibit iodide trapping.

- *Oxidation of iodine:* Occurs inside the follicular cells by the action of the enzyme peroxidase. Drugs like thiouracil and carbimazole can inhibit this step and act as antithyroid drugs.

- *Organification:* Iodine gets incorporated to tyrosine amino acid present in the colloid and leads to the formation of MIT (Monoiodotyrosine). On further iodination of MIT, there is formation of DIT (Diiodotyrosine).

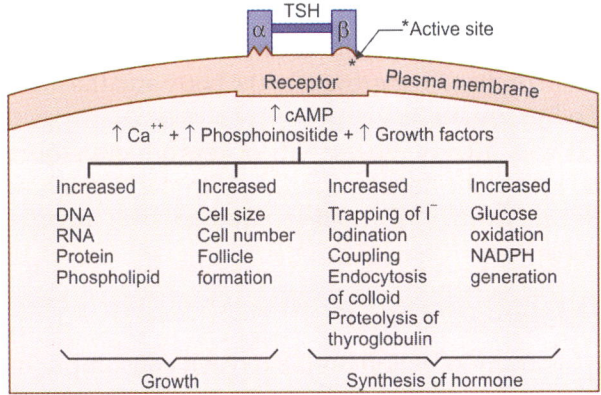

Fig. 6.32: Actions of TSH on the thyroid gland

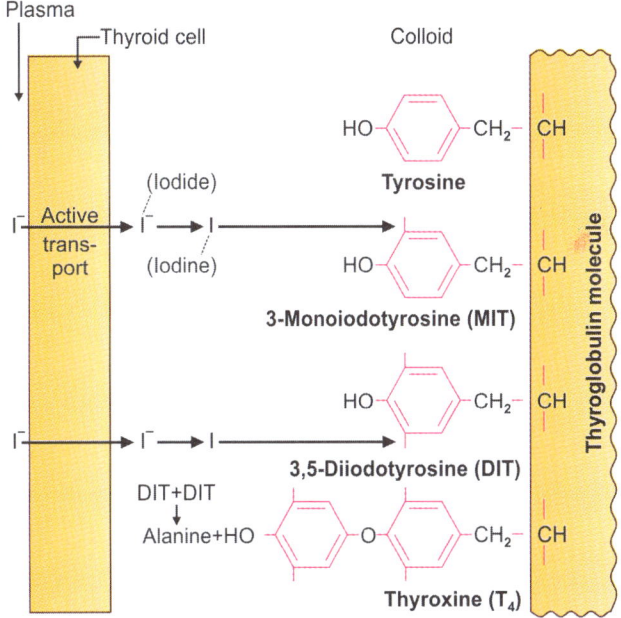

Fig. 6.33: Steps in the biosynthesis of thyroxine

- *Coupling:* Coupling of 2 DIT will lead to the formation of T_4 and 1 MIT with 1 DIT will results in T_3.

After the synthesis, the hormone with thyroglobulin is stored in the colloid.

There are many substances which have the ability to decrease the amount of thyroxin secreted by the gland. These drugs will be of choice when there is a necessity to decrease the amount of thyroxine secretion in certain pathological situations. Table 6.5 shows the list of antithyroid drugs.

Steps involved in hormonopoiesis of thyroxine
1. Iodide trapping (active process)
2. Conversion of iodide to molecular iodine. Peroxidase is the enzyme involved.
3. Organification of tyrosine to form MIT and DIT—*iodinase*.
4. Oxidative coupling of MIT + DIT—to form T_3. DIT + DIT—to form T_4
5. Proteolytic separation of T_3 and T_4 from thyroglobulin—*deiodinase*

Table 6.5: List of antithyroid drugs
1. Perchlorates and thiocyanates negatively charged. Compete with iodides
2. Thiouracil group of drugs inhibit peroxidase enzyme activity
3. Iodides in high (mg) dosage

Table 6.6: Transport of thyroxine in plasma

Proteins available	Quantity of proteins (mg/dl)	Affinity	Transported bound %	
			T_4	T_3
TBG	2	+++++	67	46
TBPA	15	++	20	1
Albumin	3500	+	13	53

At the time of release of the hormones into circulation, the acinar cells will engulf the thyroglobulin along with the hormones by endocytosis.

In the cells, the hormone will be separated by proteolysis and released into the circulation and thyroglobulin will be retained for further use.

Most of the hormone in circulation is in protein bound form along with thyroid binding globulin (TBG), albumin (TBA), thyroid binding pre-albumin (TBPA) (Table 6.6).

Actions of the Hormone

1. Calorigenic Action

It increases the oxygen consumption in almost all the tissues of the body except adult brain, gonads, lymphoid tissue. Increased metabolic rate increases the heat production in the body. The unit to measure heat energy is calorie (Fig. 6.34).

In normal adult male, the basal metabolic rate (BMR) is about 40 Kcal/sq m BSA/Hr ±15%.

In hyperthyroidism, it can be as much as + 60 to 100%.

In hypothyroidism, it can fall by –40 to –60%.

Hence estimation of BMR forms one of the thyroid function tests.

2. Nervous System

For the growth of the nervous system in the first three years of even during the postnatal period, the action of the thyroxine on brain is essential. The growth of the brain occurs only during this phase after birth. The growth of the brain includes:
- Formation of the synapses.
- Growth of axon and dendrites and arborization of these processes.
- Increase in the number of glial cells.
- Myelination of nerve fibers.

In cretin (when thyroxine is deficient from childhood):
1. The brain remains smaller than normal.

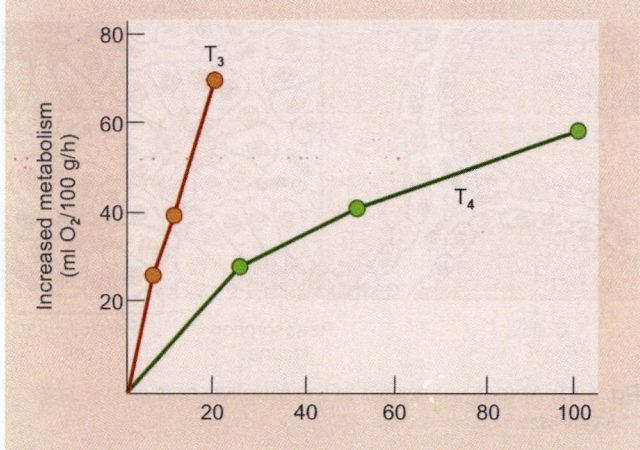

Fig. 6.34: Graph comparing the metabolic rate action of triiodothyronine and thryoxine

2. Number and size of the nerve cells reduced.
3. Arborization of the dendrites is less profuse.
4. Net effect in the child will be marked decrease in IQ.
5. Myelination will be defective.
6. CSF protein content is increased.

Because of these reasons, the action of hormone on the brain is very crucial in the first two to three years of postnatal life. If there is deficiency of the hormone during this period, it can lead to mental retardation. This is associated with delayed milestones during the growth of the infant.

3. On Growth and Development

It affects the growth and development of other parts of body as well.

The general growth is influenced by the growth hormone of the anterior pituitary gland but thyroxine potentiates the action of the growth hormone and hence the summated effect of these hormones is very much for the linear growth of the body and the growth of other organs.

It also affects the growth of reproductive organs and lack of the hormone may lead to sterility, infantile sex organs in adults and in adult females menstrual problems.

4. Metabolic Actions

Apart from its action on the oxygen consumption by the tissues, it also influences the metabolism of carbohydrate, fats and proteins.

a. *Carbohydrate metabolism:* It acts as a hyperglycemic agent. It increases the blood glucose level by increasing gluconeogenesis and glycogenolysis in the liver. It also enhances the peripheral utilization of glucose.

b. *Protein metabolism:* It has both anabolic and catabolic effects. Excess of hormonal level in circulation, catabolism predominates and leads to loss of body weight and muscular weakness. In hypothyroidism, the anabolism suffers and again leads to muscular weakness.

c. *Fat metabolism:* It increases lipolysis. Cholesterol synthesis and degradation are both affected by this hormone. The degradation is more dependent on thyroxine than synthesis and hence in hypothyroidism the serum cholesterol level is increased.

d. *On mucopolysaccharides:* The excretion of substances, like hyaluronic acid and chondroitin sulphate, is affected by the action of this hormone. Hence, in hypothyroidism, they get deposited in the subcutaneous region giving rise to myxedema.

5. On Systems

The hormone affects functioning of the different systems of the body. Some of the systems on which the actions are more pronounced are:

a. *CVS:* It increases both the heart rate and force of contraction. It increases the number of beta receptors and affinity of the beta receptors for catecholamine. Hence, the resting heart rate will be more in hyperthyroid subjects. The increase in cardiac output leads to increase of systolic blood pressure (systolic hypertension). It also increases the blood flow to the skin in order to facilitate the heat loss from the body. It is essential as the hormone increases basal metabolic rate and hence increased heat production. As a result of this cutaneous vasodilatation, the peripheral resistance decreases which will result in fall in diastolic BP.

b. *GIT:* Hormone is required for normal secretory aspects and movements of gastrointestinal tract. In hyperthyroidism, the patients suffer from diarrhea and in hypothyroidism the patient may develop constipation.

c. *Nervous system:* In adult, it affects the velocity of impulse conduction in the nerve fibers. In hyposecretion state, it results in increased reflex time and vice versa in hyperthyroidism.

Regulation of Secretion of Hormone

It is brought about by the negative feedback mechanism. There is involvement of hypothalamo-pituitary-thyroid axis (Fig. 6.35).

Increase in free form of hormone in circulation acts on hypothalamus and anterior pituitary gland. Acting on hypothalamus, it decreases the secretion of thyrotropin-releasing hormone (TRF/TRH) and this acts on anterior pituitary decreases secretion of TSH.

Net effect will be decreased TSH from anterior pituitary gland. This decreases the secretion of thyroid hormones from the gland.

Many of the other chemical influences acting on TRH-TSH-Thyroxine (hypothalamo-pituitary-thyroid axis) secretions have been shown in Table 6.7.

Alteration in the temperature can directly act on the hypothalamus to alter the secretion of the hormone.

Thyroid Function Tests

1. Determination of BMR.
2. Blood cholesterol level.
3. Estimation of protein bound iron (PBI)
4. ^{131}I uptake studies (Figs 6.36, 6.37)
5. Estimation of free T_3, T_4 and TSH in plasma.

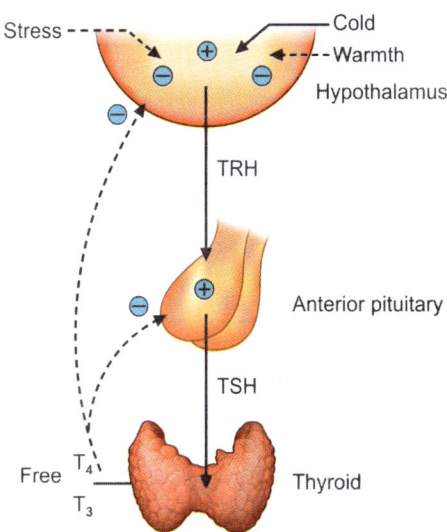

Fig. 6.35: Regulation of secretion of thyroxine (by nagative feedback mechanism)

Table 6.7: Thyroid hormone feedback

Hypothalamus	Stimulatory	Inhibitory
Decreased TRH	Alpha adrenergic agonists	Alpha adrenergic blockers
		Tumors
Anterior pituitary	*TRH*	*Somatostatin*
Decreased TSH	Estrogen	Dopamine
		Glucocorticoids
		Chronic illness
Thyroid gland	*TSH*	*TSH receptor blocking antibody*
Decreased T$_3$ and T$_4$	TSH receptor stimulating antibody	Iodine, lithium

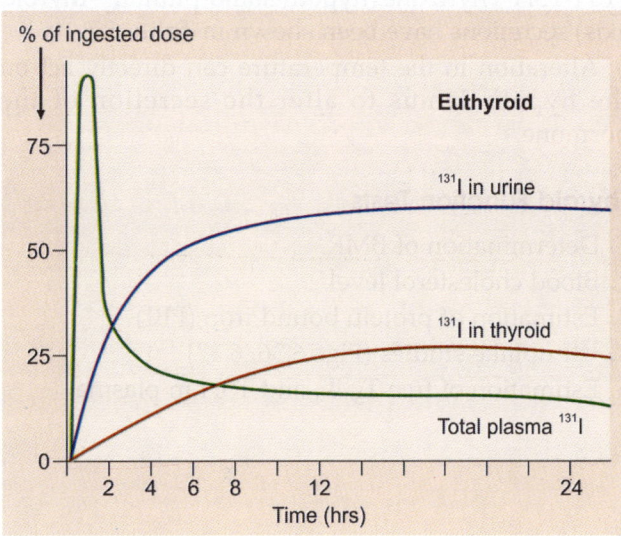

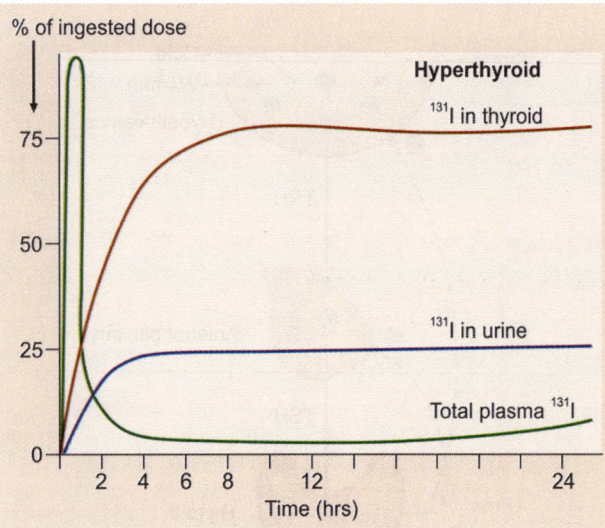

Fig. 6.36: Graphs comparing the radioactive iodine levels in thyroid, urine and plasma in 24 hours period in euthyroid and hyperthyroid state

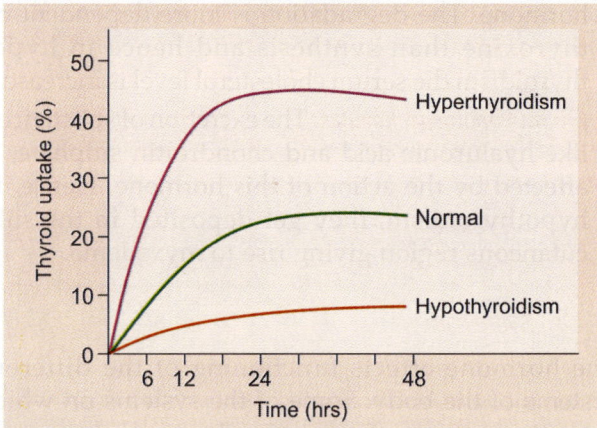

Fig. 6.37: Graph comparing radioactive iodine uptake by thyroid gland in normal, hyperthyroidism and hypothyroidism

Applied Aspects

Cretinism (Fig. 6.38 and Table 6.8)
- Hyposecretion of thyroxine from infancy.
- Skeletal growth will be stunted and hence short stature.
- Mental retardation due to poor growth of nervous system.
- Milestones in the development of child get postponed.
- Thick protruding tongue and pot belly.
- Even after attaining the adolescence, there will not be development of sex organs and hence the sex organs remain infantile.
- Facial changes will not correspond with chronological age.

Congenital hypothyroidism could be due to:
- Maternal iodine deficiency.
- Fetal thyroid dysgenesis.

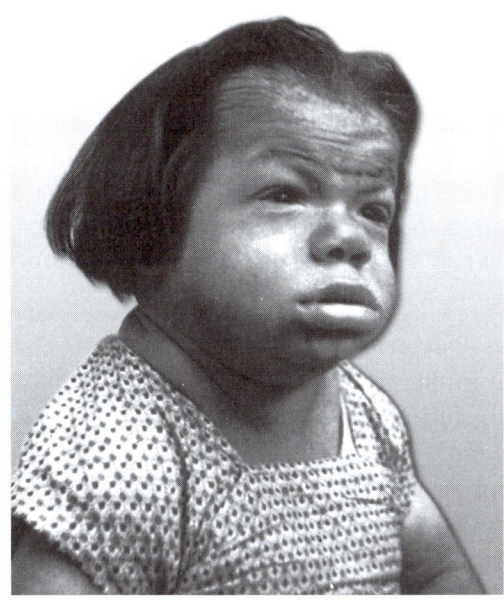

Fig. 6.38: Picture of cretin

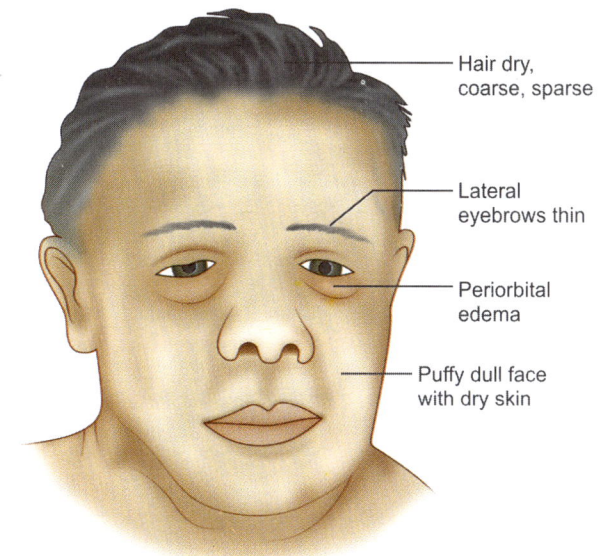

Fig. 6.39: Some of the features in patient suffering from myxedema

Table 6.8: Features of cretinism
• Are dwarfs
• Mentlly retarded—low IQ
• Pot belly, enlarged tongue
• Delayed milestone
• Peculiar cry

• Inborn errors in thyroid hormone synthesis.
• Maternal antithyroid antibodies crossing.
• Fetal hypopituitary hypothyroidism.

Myxedema (Fig. 6.39 and Table 6.9)
• Hyposecretion of thyroxine in adults.
• Person's basal metabolic rate is grossly reduced. It can be as little as –40 to –60%.
• Person cannot withstand cold stress.
• Cold dry skin with sparse hair.
• There will be accumulation of chondroitin sulfate and hyaluronic acid in the subcutaneous region. These substances are osmotically active and hence this results in retention of water also in the subcutaneous region. This results in non-pitting edema (puffiness of face, legs, etc.).
• Person will have bradycardia and blood pressure also will be less than normal.
• The activity of CNS becomes dull, thereby it may lead to loss of memory and dulling of intelligence and reaction time is prolonged.

Table 6.9: Features of myxedema	
Myxedema	*Hypothyrodism in adults*
Problems may be with	Thyroid gland
	Pituitary gland
	Hypothalamus
Signs	Low BMR
Hair	Coarse and sparse
Skin	Dry and yellow
Cold	Poorly tolerated
Voice	Hoarse
Mentation	Slow, sluggish

• There will be increase in the serum cholesterol level.
• The reproductive ability of the person suffers and the females may suffer from menorrhagia.

Myxedema could be due to:
• Hashimoto's thyroiditis.
• Hypothalamic or pituitary destruction.
• Nodular goiters.
• Surgical removal.

Graves' disease (Fig. 6.40 and Table 6.10)
• Hyperthyroidism in adult stage.
• Person may show exophthalmos.
• Tachycardia and palpitation.
• The person may suffer from systolic hypertension.

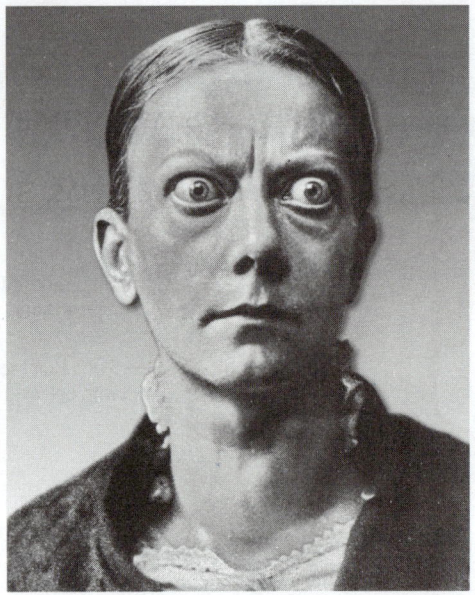

Fig. 6.40: Typical face in a patient suffering from hyperthyroidism

Table 6.10: Features of hyperthyroidism
• Nervousness
• Weight loss inspite of hyperphagia
• Heat intolerance
• Increased pulse pressure and heart rate
• Tremors—fine
• BMR— ↑ +60 to + 100%
• Exophthalmos may be present

• Negative nitrogen balance with loss of wasting of muscle tissue.
• CNS symptoms include tremors, hyperreflexia, and psychosis.
• The basal metabolic rate may be increased to as much as plus 60 to 100%.
• The person cannot withstand heat stress.
• Skin will be warm and wet.
• Serum cholesterol level will be less than normal.
• The person may suffer from loss of libido and infertility.

The disease may be because of autoimmunity. The body starts producing antibodies which are known as thyroid-stimulating immunoglobulins (TSI) or long-acting thyroid stimulators (LATS). These antibodies bind to the receptors where TSH normally binds. They imitate the action of TSH on the gland and hence bring about increased secretion of thyroxine. Since the thyroxine level in circulation is increased, this exerts more negative feedback regulation on anterior pituitary. So TSH secretion from anterior pituitary gland is decreased. This results in decreased concentration of TSH in circulation.

Goiter means enlargement of thyoriod gland. Goiter can be due to hypo- or hyperthyroidism. Endemic goiter (hypothyroidism) usually occurs due to deficiency of iodine (Fig. 6.41). Exophthalmic goiter occurs due to hyperthyroidism.

Features of hyperthyroidism in adult
• Heat intolerance.
• Tachycardia and palpitations.
• Hyperactivity and irritability.
• Tremors.
• Warm wet skin.
• Diarrhea.
• Oligomenorrhea.
• Lid retraction and lid lag.
• Weight loss.

Features of hypothyroidism in adult
• Cold intolerance.
• Bradycardia.
• Poor memory and increased reaction time.
• Cold dry skin.
• Constipation.
• Menorrhagia.
• Diffuse alopecia.
• Weight gain.

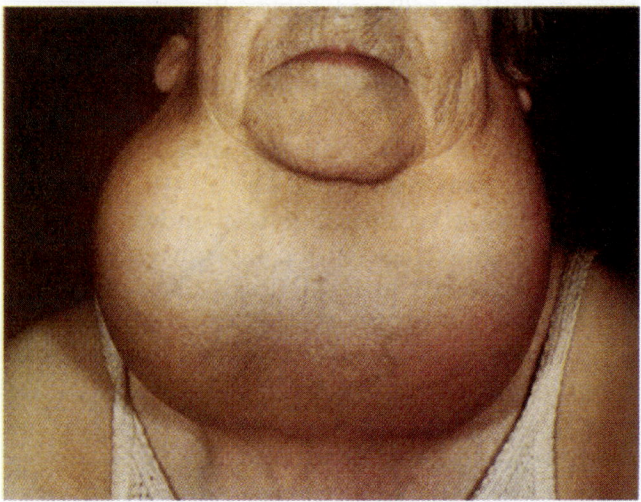

Fig. 6.41: Massive enlargement of thyroid gland in endemic goiter

- Hoarse voice.
- Carpal tunnel syndrome.

Thyroid storm: Serious thyrotoxicosis. Features are:
a. Fever.
b. Tachycardia.
c. Psychosis.
d. Confusion.
e. GI tract symptoms.

Endocrine Pancreas

Pancreas is a unique gland having both the exocrine and endocrine functions. The exocrine function is contributed by the acini present in pancreas and has been dealt in great detail in GI physiology. In this chapter, only the endocrine function of pancreas has been dealt.

Endocrine function of pancreas is performed by the islets of Langerhans, which is spread out throughout the pancreas and more concentrated in the tail. There are approximately 1 to 2 million islets. The islets are made up of different types of cells can be made out by Mallory stain and they are (Fig. 6.42):

1. Alpha cells or A cells which secrete glucagon
2. Beta cells or B cells which secrete insulin
3. Delta cells or D cells which secrete somatostatin
4. F cells which secrete pancreatic polypeptide

When pancreatectomy was done on dogs by Von Mering and Minkowski and later on by Banting and Best, the following features were observed in the animals:

1. Hyperglycemia followed by glycosuria.

Cells can be separated

1. By electonmicroscopic studies
2. By using mallory stain

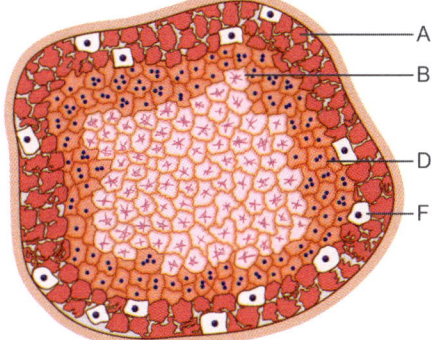

Fig. 6.42: Different types of cells in islets

Cells in Islet

B—Cells—60–70%
  Located in the center
A—Cells—20% (surrounding B cells)
D—Cells ⎱
F—Cells ⎰ Rest
B—Cells—granules are of different sizes (polymerises with zinc)
A—Cells—granules are of equal size

2. Polyuria, polydypsia and polyphagia.
3. Loss of body weight, early fatigue, weakness and poor growth.
4. Delayed wound healing and repeated infections and negative nitrogen balance.
5. Increased lipolysis and decreased lipogenesis
6. Formation of ketone bodies—acetoacetic acid, beta-hydroxybutyric acid and acetone.

Insulin

- Beta cells secrete insulin.
- It is the only hypoglycemic hormone secreted in the body.
- It is a polypeptide hormone made up of two chains namely A and B.
- A chain is smaller than B chain; the two chains are linked to each other by disulphide bridges.
- Intravenous injection of insulin decreases the plasma glucose level to as low as 30 mg%.
- It is not only an anabolic hormone; it is an anti-catabolic hormone as well.

Actions of Insulin (Figs 6.43, 6.44)

1. On carbohydrate metabolism
2. Fat metabolism
3. Protein metabolism
4. On plasma potassium.

Action on Carbohydrate Metabolism

- It is a hypoglycemic agent.
- Decreases the blood glucose level.
- The normal fasting blood glucose level is in the range of 60–90 mg%.

The actions of insulin on carbohydrate metabolism are:

a. Increasing the peripheral utilization of glucose: In most of the tissues of the body, for transfer of

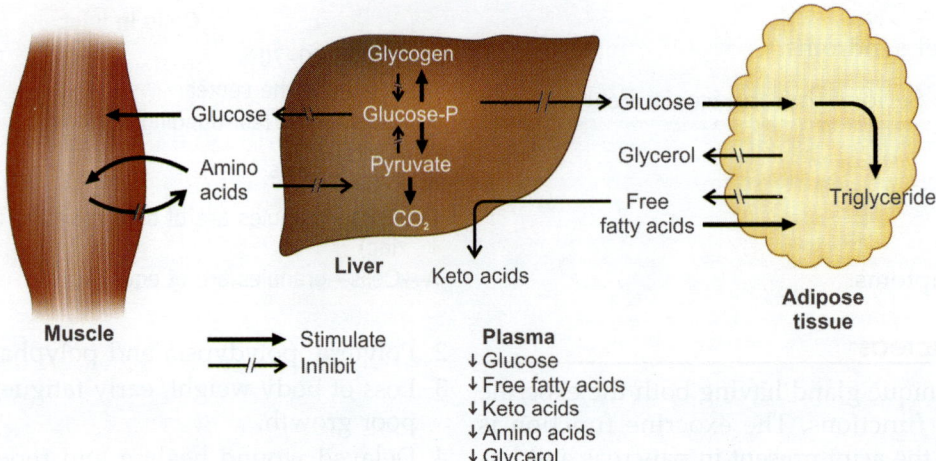

Fig. 6.43: Actions of insulin in liver, muscle and adpose tissue

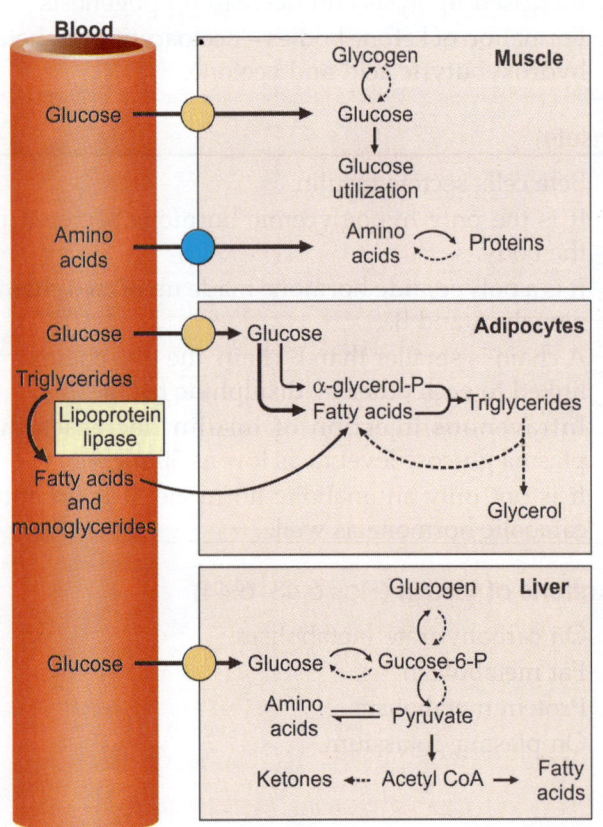

Fig. 6.44: Metabolic actions of insulin on liver, muscle and adipose tissue

glucose from ECF to ICF and glycolysis to be brought about inside the cell, insulin is essential. Some of the tissues which do not require insulin for peripheral utilization of glucose are whole of brain except satiety center, RBCs, renal tubules and mucosa of gastrointestinal tract. During the movement of glucose from ECF to ICF, potassium will also be transferred from ECF to ICF. Because of this, plasma potassium level falls. It is for this reason, when insulin is administered in large doses as done in the treatment of diabetic ketoacidotic coma, along with insulin, potassium should be administered to prevent hypokalemia and its deleterious effects. Insulin can be also administered, if one has to treat cases of severe hyperkalemia but since insulin is a very powerful hypoglycemic agent, in the treatment of hyperkalemia, along with insulin glucose also must be given to prevent patient developing hypoglycemia and its consequences.

b. Utilization of glucose to supply energy spares the proteins from getting catabolized. This is known as protein sparing effect.

c. It also increases the glucose uptake by the liver and enhances the conversion of glucose to glycogen. This is brought about by enhancing the activity of glycogen synthase. This glycogen gets stored in liver.

d. It also decreases glycogenolysis in liver and muscle tissue. So the breakdown of glycogen to glucose will be less.

e. It decreases gluconeogenesis that is formation of glucose from non-carbohydrate sources, like amino acids and fatty acids.

On Protein Metabolism

It facilitates the transfer of amino acids from ECF to ICF. The amino acids that have entered the ICF will be utilized for protein synthesis. At the same time, it will also decrease the breakdown of proteins. Incorporation of amino acids into proteins leads to retention of nitrogen in the body and brings about positive nitrogen balance. The proteins synthesized will be used for growth of tissues and organs. This facilitates the growth, repairing of wounds, adequate resistance against infections (because of immuno-globulins) and gain of weight. In case, the child suffers from juvenile diabetes, growth of the child decreases because of loss of aforesaid actions of insulin on protein metabolism.

On Fat Metabolism

It is a lipogenetic agent. It acts on the adipose tissue and increases the activity of lipoprotein lipase and decreases the hormone sensitive lipase activity. This leads to increased lipogenesis and decreased lipolysis. The fatty acids are transferred from ECF to ICF in adipose tissue. These fatty acids are converted to neutral fats and triglycerides and stored in adipose tissue. Deposition of fats will increase the weight of the person. Absence of insulin brings about increase in the free fatty acid levels in circulation. When glucose cannot be utilized to supply energy, the fatty acids are metabolized to supply energy. This brings about increased formation of ketone bodies. Such situation is called as ketoacidosis.

On Plasma Potassium

Since insulin is involved in transfer of potassium from ECF to ICF, it decreases plasma potassium level.

Regulation of Secretion of Insulin

1. One of the important factors which regulate insulin secretion is plasma glucose level (Fig. 6.45). More is the plasma glucose level more will be the amount of insulin secreted. The amount of insulin secreted for the same amount of glucose, depends whether glucose is administered orally or intravenously. Administration of glucose through oral route brings about enhanced insulin secretion than intravenous administration. This is because of the influence of some of the GI tract hormones and vagus nerve influence on the beta cells in islets.

2. Some of the other factors which enhance insulin secretion are amino acids, keto acids, exercise, GI tract hormones, ACh, etc. (Table 6.11).

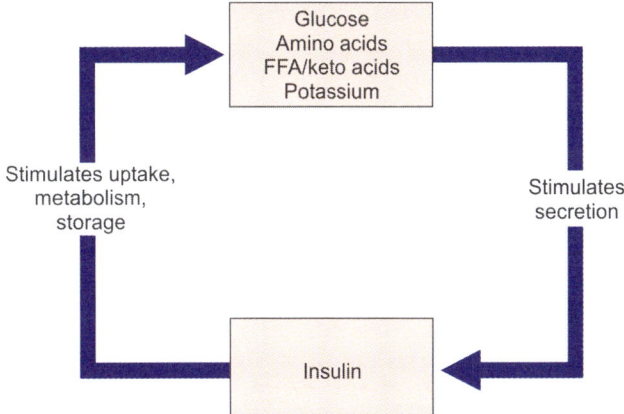

Fig. 6.45: Role of glucose, amino acids and free fatty acids in secretion of insulin

Table 6.11: Factors affecting insulin secretion

Stimulators	Inhibitors
Glucose	Somatostatin
Amino acids	α-adrenergic stimulating agents
GI hormones (gastrin, secretin, (CCK-PZ, glucagon)	K-depletion
	Alloxan
Keto acids	
Acetylcholine	
Glucagon	
β-adrenergic stimulating agents	

3. Some of the factors which decrease insulin secretion are somatostatin, potassium depletion, alpha adrenergic stimulation, etc.

Insulin Lack

- Administration of toxic substances, like alloxan, streptozotocin, destroys the beta cells of islets of Langerhans and thus lead to insulin lack.
- Lack of insulin results in increased blood glucose (hyperglycemia) level.
- When blood glucose level exceeds 180 mg% (renal threshold), it leads to glycosuria. That is glucose appears in urine. Hence the condition is known as diabetes mellitus.
- When glucose is excreted, since glucose is an osmotically active substance, it drags water also with it. This will give rise to polyuria.
- In the hypothalamus, there are two centers namely hunger center which is located in the lateral hypothalamic nucleus and ventromedial nucleus

which acts as satiety center. Normally, the hunger center activity is under constant inhibitory influence from the satiety center. The utilization of glucose by satiety center is dependent on insulin. When insulin is absent, the activity of satiety center is depressed. Because of this, the inhibition on the hunger center by satiety center is decreased (disinhibition). Now, the hunger center activity becomes unopposed and gives rise to increased hunger and hence polyphagia.

Pathophysiology of Diabetes Mellitus

Diabetes mellitus can be of two types namely type I or insulin-dependent diabetes mellitus (IDDM) and type II or non-insulin-dependent diabetes mellitus (NIDDM).

Type I
- Younger age of onset.
- Severe or absolute insulin deficiency.
- Less genetic predisposition.
- Loss of beta cells.
- More prone to ketoacidosis.

Type II
- Late onset, >40 years.
- Relative insulin deficiency.
- Reduced sensitivity of tissue to insulin.
- Genetic predisposition is more.
- Normal beta cell mass.
- Non-ketotic hyperosmolar coma.

Whatever may be type of diabetes, there will be fault in glucose metabolism. Decreased peripheral utilization and increased hepatic glycogenolysis brings about an increase of blood glucose level.

- Increased blood glucose (above renal threshold of 180 mg%) level leads to glycosuria.
- Glycosuria leads to polyuria (increased urine excretion) since glucose is an osmotically active substance. This type of polyuria differs from polyuria of diabetes insipidus because in diabetes insipidus, the diuresis is termed as water diuresis and the specific gravity of urine will be low.
- Increased loss of water along with urine leads to dehydration and resulting in stimulation of thirst center and hence there will be polydypsia (increased drinking).
- Unopposed activity of hunger center results in polyphagia (increased eating).

Glycosuria
- Polyuria, polydypsia, polyphagia
- Weightloss inspite of polyphagia
- 3 polys are very characteristic features of DM.

- Since the blood glucose level is more and body protein content is less, the person is more susceptible to infection and poor wound healing.
- Increased protein catabolism leads to weight loss and poor growth. The amino acids which are the end products of protein catabolism will be used for gluconeogenesis.
- In the absence of glucose getting metabolized to supply energy, fats catabolism increases and this gives rise to lipolysis. The beta oxidation of fatty acids brings about increased formation of ketone bodies and lead to ketoacidosis. Ketone bodies can be excreted along with expired air and hence the breath of these patients will have characteristic apple odor.

The cardinal symptoms of diabetes mellitus are shown in Fig. 6.46.

Tests for Diabetes Mellitus

1. Test for glucose in urine.
2. Test the fasting blood glucose level.
3. Perform oral glucose tolerance test (GTT).

Coma is one of the serious problems of glucose metabolism. The person may get into coma both because of hyperglycemia or hypoglycemia. One of the examples of hypoglycemic coma is improper management of diabetic patients especially when the antidiabetic drug is taken but diet is compromised or drug taken may be more than the required dose. Among the two types of coma, hypoglycemic coma is more dangerous.

The signs and symptoms of hypoglycemic coma are:

1. Dizziness and nervousness due to increased autonomic discharge.
2. Palpitation.
3. Sweating.
4. Weakness.
5. Ataxia that is incoordination of movements.
6. Confusion.
7. Nervousness and apprehension.
8. Tremors.

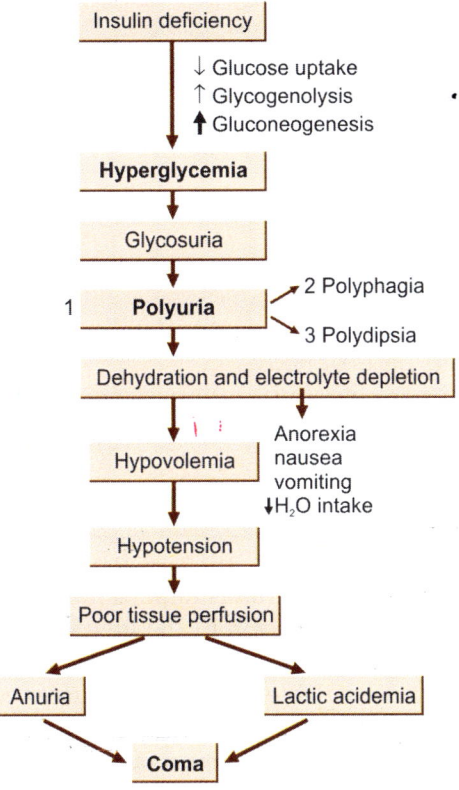

Fig. 6.46: Effects of insulin deficiency

9. Slurred speech.
10. Convulsions.

How to differentiate whether coma is because of hypo- or hyperglycemia?

When comatose patient is brought into the emergency room, time should not be wasted. Treatment to the patient has to be started as fast as possible. One of the first and foremost things to be done is, when it is not certain that coma is due to hypo- or hyperglycemia,

infuse glucose intravenously to the patient. If coma is because of hypoglycemia, the patient recovers without any further procedure. If coma is due to hyperglycemia, the patient will not recover and infusion of glucose would not harm the patient anymore. Now the treatment has to be initiated to manage the hyperglycemic coma.

The differences between hyperglycemic and hypoglycemic coma has been detailed in Table 6.12.

Some of the conditions in which glycosuria occurs are:
1. Diabetes mellitus due to problem in glucose metabolism.
2. Renal glycosuria due to problem in function of renal tubules.
3. Alimentary glycosuria occurs in hyperthyroidism. In hyperthyroidism, the rate of absorption of glucose from GI tract is enhanced and this may lead to glycosuria.
4. Picquare glycosuria in which constant stimulation of brainstem area leads to glycosuria.

Glucagon

- It is a peptide hormone.
- Secreted by alpha or A cells of islets of Langerhans.
- Unlike insulin which is a hypoglycemic agent, glucagon is a hyperglycemic agent.

Actions

1. Carbohydrate metabolism
2. Fat metabolism

On Carbohydrate Metabolism

- It is a hyperglycemic agent and hence increases blood glucose level.

Table 6.12: Coma in diabetes mellitus		
	Hyperglycemic	*Hypoglycemic*
Unconciousness	+++	+++
Dangerous	Less	More dangerous (medical emergency)
CNS	Depressed	Stimulated
Blood glucose	Increased (high)	Low
Glucose in urine	+++	Absent
Ketone bodies in urine	+++	– –
Treatment	Insulin, correct acidosis, correct fluid, balance K^+ administration	Glucose intravenous infusion
Cause	Poor management of diabetes mellitus	Over dosage of insulin

- Brings about glycogenolysis in liver only. Glucose produced by glycogenolyis is added on to circulation.
- Increases gluconeogensis in liver.

On Fat Metabolism

- It is a lipolytic agent.
- Acts on adipose tissue and increases the activity of hormone sensitive lipase.
- This brings about increase lipolysis. Free fatty acids are added on to circulation due to breakdown of neutral fats and triglycerides.
- Utilization of fatty acids to supply energy may lead to ketone body formation.

Regulation of Secretion

The concentration of blood glucose affects the secretion of hormone. Decrease in the blood glucose level will increase the secretion of glucagon and vice versa when level of glucose is increased in circulation. Apart from this, some of the other factors which can affect the secretion of glucagon are: Stimulators:

- Ingestion of proteins.
- Sympathetic stimulation

One of the important factors which decrease the secretion of glucagon is somatostatin.

Features of Excess of Glucagon

- Glucose level increased and keto acids in circulation.
- Gluconeogenesis markedly increased.
- Generalized reduction in AA level and decreased excretion of nitrogen.
- Loss of weight.

Glucose Homeostasis

Glucose homeostasis is brought about by:
a. Actions of hormones on metabolism and glucostatic role of
b. Hypothalamus
c. Liver

Actions of Hormones on Metabolism

Many of the hormones have role to play and there are five hyperglycemic hormones and only one hypoglycemic hormone. The hormones having hyperglycemic action are:

1. Growth hormone
2. Thyroxine
3. Glucagon
4. Adrenaline and noradrenaline
5. Cortisol.

The only hormone having hypoglycemic action is insulin.

Glucose homeostasis is brought about by the action of aforementioned hormones on various parts of body, like liver, muscle, and peripheral utilization of glucose in various parts of body.

As far peripheral utilization is concerned, it is not confined to any tissue or organ. This is because most of the times the cells in tissues require constant supply of energy to take care of the metabolic activity which is provided by the metabolism of glucose. It is not just the movement of glucose from ECF to ICF (facilitated diffusion) that is important; it should also bring about the activation of the glycolytic pathway to metabolize glucose to supply energy. In case glucose is not available, alternative sources of energy will be looked into.

Gluconeogenesis is brought about only in liver. And hence any of the hormones which either enhance/inhibit gluconeogenesis should act on the liver and alter the activity of the various enzymes involved in this process. For gluconeogenesis to be brought about, there is requirement of fatty acids and amino acids. These acids are made available for gluconeogenesis by increased lipolysis or proteolysis in various parts of body.

Glycogenolysis can take place either in liver or muscle or both. The stored glycogen in these structures will be broken down to release glucose into circulation. This is aided by enhancing the activity of the enzymes involved in the breakdown of glycogen.

Glycogenesis also occurs in liver. Glucose is removed from circulation, converted to glucose and stored in liver and muscle.

Hormones having influence on peripheral utilization are:
1. Insulin
2. Thyroxine
3. Cortisol
4. Growth hormone

Hormones having influence on glycogenolysis are:
1. Insulin
2. Glucagon.
3. Adrenaline and noradrenaline.

Hormones having role on glycogenesis are:
1. Insulin
2. Cortisol

Hormones having influence on gluconeogenesis are:
1. Insulin
2. Thyroxine
3. Cortisol
4. Growth hormone
5. Glucagon.

The role of hypothalamus is equally important in glucose homeostasis. The functioning of both the hypothalamic nuclei and the actions of insulin in tandem is very much essential for normoglycemic situation to prevail. In the hypothalamus, there are two important nuclei that try to maintain glucose homeostasis. They are:
1. Ventromedial nucleus
2. Lateral hypothalamic nucleus.

Ventromedial nucleus is also known as satiety center and lateral hypothalamic nucleus is termed as hunger center. The whole of the brain does not require insulin for peripheral utilization of glucose except the ventromedial nuclear area. And another special aspect of these nuclear regions of hypothalamus is, the lateral hypothalamic nucleus is believed to be constantly active on its own.

Under normal conditions, when insulin is able to exert its usual action, glucose from ECF enters ICF of neurons of ventromedial nucleus and gets metabolized. This results in ventromedial nucleus to become active. The ventromedial nucleus now inhibits the activity of lateral hypothalamic nucleus and hence the person stops eating.

In diabetes mellitus, since the peripheral utilization of glucose is affected, the ventromedial nucleus is unable to utilize glucose. So the inhibitory influence of this nucleus on the lateral hypothalamic nucleus is lost (there will be disinhibition). Now the activity of the lateral hypothalamic nucleus goes unopposed, because of which the person develops polyphagia. Hence one of the cardinal symptoms of diabetes mellitus is polyphagia.

Parathyroid Gland and Calcium and Phosphate Metabolism

Ionic calcium plays an important role in our body. Hence its concentration has to be very well regulated.

Total calcium present in the body in a young human adult is about 1100 g. Of this about 99% is present in bone. The plasma calcium level is about 9–11 mg%. Approximately 50% of this is in ionic form and the rest is present in bound form bound either to plasma proteins or as citrates (Fig. 6.47).

Functions of Ionic Calcium (Table 6.13)

1. *Maintenance of RMP:* Because of this, the excitability of neuron and muscle is maintained. A decrease in calcium ion level increases the excitability and vice versa when calcium ion level decreases.
2. *N-M transmission:* It plays an important role in conduction of impulse across neuromuscular junction. The amount of ACh released is directly dependent on the number of calcium ion influx at the presynaptic terminal.
3. *Maintenance of excitability and contractility of cardiac muscle:* The plateau phase of action potential of cardiac muscle and for contraction of cardiac muscle calcium ion is necessary.
4. *Blood coagulation:* In many of the steps of blood coagulation, calcium ion is required. Removal of calcium ion, blood fails to clot.

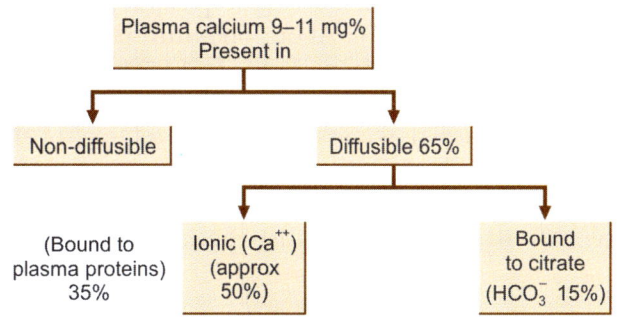

Fig. 6.47: Plasma calcium in various forms

Table 6.13: Functions of ionic calcium

1. Maintenance of resting membrane potential and hence excitability of nerve and muscle tissue
2. Release of ACh at NMJ
3. Excitation–contraction coupling
4. Rhythmicity and contractility of cardiac muscle
5. Blood coagulation
6. Formation of bone and teeth
7. Release of certain hormones
8. Activation of certain enzymes (ATPase, lipase)
9. Formation of intercellular matrix (ground substance)

5. Development of bone and teeth
6. It is required for activation of certain enzymes.
7. It is required for release of certain hormones.

Calcium is actively transported from GI tract. The most important factor influencing calcium absorption is 1,25-dihydroxycholecalciferol. The other factors which can also influence calcium absorption are growth hormone, and acidic pH in duodenum. Calcium absorption is decreased in old age. Large amount of calcium is filtered in the kidneys and about 99% of filtered calcium is reabsorbed. About 60% of reabsorption occurs in PCT and the rest from DCT.

Calcium present in the bone are two types namely rapidly exchangeable compartment and in a much stable compartment. The calcium that is present in plasma and bone are in equilibrium. When the plasma calcium level increases suddenly, calcium is removed from plasma to get deposited in the bone along with phosphate. When the plasma calcium level falls, calcium is removed from bone matrix by a process of demineralization and this calcium enters plasma (Figs 6.48 and 6.49).

Phosphate

Total body phosphate is about 500–800 g, of this 85–90% is present in bones. The total plasma phosphate level is about 12 mg%. About one-third of this is in inorganic form mostly as PO_4^-, HPO_4^- and H_2PO_4. About 3 mg of phosphate enters the bone everyday and an almost equal amount of this is removed from the bone.

Phosphate is filtered into the renal tubules and 85 to 90% of this gets reabsorbed. Most of this

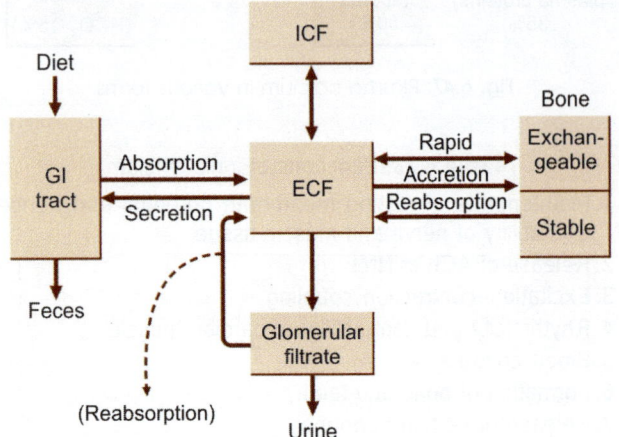

Fig. 6.48: Fate of ingested calcium in ECF and bone and the excretion of calcium from the body

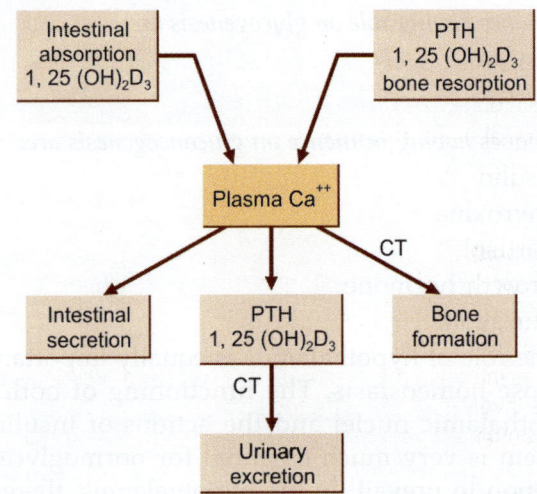

Fig. 6.49: Effect of various hormones on calcium metabolism in the body. PTH—parathormone, CT—calcitonin

reabsorption occurs at PCT and is by an active process. When parathormone acts on the renal tubules, the amount of phosphate reabsorbed is decreased. In the GI tract, phosphate absorption occurs both actively and passively in duodenum. Factors that increase calcium absorption also increase phosphate absorption.

Features of Phosphate Depletion

- Skeletal muscle weakness.
- Cardiac and respiratory muscle dysfunction.
- Loss of red blood cell membrane integrity.
- Abnormal formation of bone.

Bone is a special form of connective tissue. On collagen framework, calcium and phosphate is deposited in the form of hydroxyl appatite crystals. Deposition and resorption of calcium and phosphate ions goes on continuously in the bone matrix. In young people, deposition of salts occurs to a greater extent than resorption and in elderly people it is reversed.

The cells responsible for bone formation are osteoblasts. The osteoclasts are responsible for bone resorption. Osteoclastic activity is associated with increase in the alkaline phosphatase.

The third type of cell found in bone matrix is osteocyte. The cells are responsible for transferring large amount of calcium from the interior to the exterior (ECF) is known as osteocytic osteolysis.

Parathyroid Glands

Parathyroid glands are four in number. Two are in the superior and two are in the inferior poles of

Phosphate

Total body phosphates:
- Skeleton—530 gm
- Skeletal muscle—59 mg
  Lot of it is present in the nervous tissue.

Functions of PO_4

1. *Component of nucleic acid:* Takes part in protein synthesis, cellular reproduction and genetic phenomenon.
2. Major role in carbohydrate metabolism as hexose PO_4 creatine PO_4
3. In the intermediary metabolism of carbohydrates; proteins, fats involved in energy transfer
4. As buffers

thyroid gland in the posterior aspect. Parathyroid glands are essential for basic survival. Removal of the gland can lead to the death of the person. This is because, removal of the gland decreases plasma calcium level and there will be increase in the excitability and contractility of nerve and muscle tissue. The increased excitability will lead to tetany, laryngeal muscle spasm, asphyxia and death.

Histology of Parathyroid Gland

Two different types of cells are seen:
1. Chief cells
2. Oxyphil cells.

The chief cells are responsible for secretion of parathormone (PTH).

PTH is a polypeptide hormone with a molecular weight of about 9500 and contains about 84 amino acids.

Actions

It is a hypercalcemic and hypophosphatemic agent. Hence increases the plasma calcium level and decreases plasma phosphate level. The important sites of actions of PTH are:
1. Bone
2. Kidney
3. GI tract in an indirect way.

PTH and Bone (Figs 6.50, 6.51 and Table 6.14)

It acts on the bone matrix mobilizing calcium and phosphate by resorption of the osseous tissue. To start with, it is supposed to increase the activity of osteocytes. This is followed by increase in the number

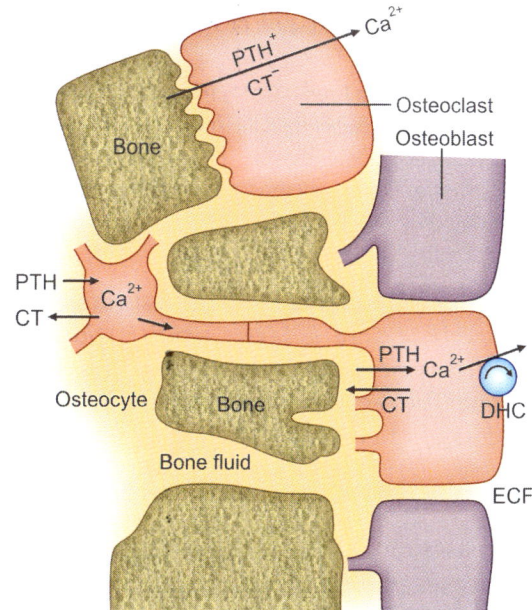

Fig. 6.50: Effect of hormones on calcium metabolism in bones

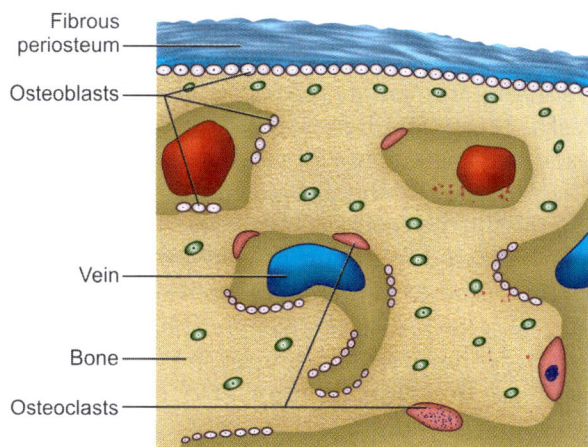

Fig. 6.51: Osteoblastic and osteoclastic activity in bone

of osteoclasts. This increases the osteoclast cells activity. During this process, the hydrogen ion concentration of the bone fluid is increased. This brings about solubility of the calcium and phosphate and they are removed from protein matrix. This brings about osteoporosis. Continued action of PTH on bone will lead to pathological fractures.

Initially, PTH acts on osteocytes and increases the transfer of calcium ions from bone fluid into ECF. A slow but a more sustained way it acts on the osteoclasts which are responsible for resorption of calcium and phosphate from the more mature bone.

Table 6.14: Actions of PTH on bone
Directly acts
Bone resorption: Mobilizes—Ca^{++}, PO_4^-
By ↑ osteoclastic activity
↑ the number of osteoclasts
Mechanism of action by increasing the production of cyclic AMP (thorough ↑ adenylate cyclase activity)

Activity plus the number of osteoclasts are increased by PTH (citric acid + lactic acid) production is increased, this increases the H^+ (proton) concentration in the bone. The resultant increase in the H^+, facilitates the process of calcium and phosphate removal.

PTH and Kidney (Table 6.15)

1. It increases the calcium reabsorption from DCT.
2. It decreases phosphate reabsorption from PCT.
3. It stimulates the activity of 1 alpha hydroxylase activity, which in turn brings about increased formation of 1,25-dihydroxycholecalciferol (active form of vitamin D).

Increased reabsorption of calcium from DCT and the action is immediate. cAMP is involved in this process. More of filtered fraction of calcium is reabsorbed. The amount of calcium excreted in the urine decreases. As the plasma calcium is increased much, the filtered load also increases. This may give rise to increased excretion of calcium in the urine which may lead to formation of renal stones.

Decreases the reabsorption of phosphate from PCT. Therefore, there will be increased excretion of phosphate in urine. It may also decrease the reabsorption of sodium and bicarbonate.

Increases production of 1,25-dihydroxycholecalciferol (1,25-DHCC).

PTH and GI Tract (Table 6.16)

The action on GI tract is an indirect one. The increased formation of 1,25-DHCC in turn facilitates more of absorption of calcium from duodenum.

Table 6.15: Action of PTH on kidney
1. Increases reabsorption of Ca^{++} from DCT
2. Decreases the reabsorption of PO_4^- from PCT
Mechanism of action through increased fromation of cyclic AMP
3. Increases the formation of 1,25 $(OH)_2CC$

Table 6.16: Indirect action of PTH on GIT
• Action is indirect through 1,25 (OH_2) DHCC
• Increases the absorption of Ca^{++}

Regulation PTH and Calcitonin Secretion (Fig. 6.52)

Decrease in plasma calcium level increases PTH secretion and when plasma calcium level increases, there will be increased secretion of calcitonin.

Apart from the plasma calcium level, some of the other factors which can affect the secretion of PTH are:

1. Decreased plasma magnesium level.
2. Increased plasma phosphate level
3. 1, 25-DHCC inhibits the PTH secretion.

Hyperparathyroidism

In primary hyperparathyroidism, increased secretion of PTH is associated with hypercalcemia and hypophosphatemia. This results in decreased excitability of neuromuscular tissue. Associated with this will be pathological fractures, osteoporosis, removal of calcium from gingival margin, formation of renal stones, and deposition of calcium in the soft tissues and along the blood vessels.

Secondary hyperparathyroidism is due to chronic renal diseases associated with excessive calcium loss. Decreased calcium level in plasma stimulates excessive secretion of PTH.

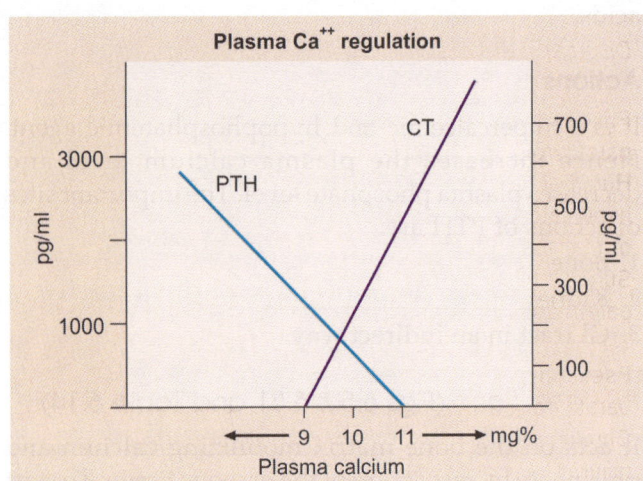

Fig. 6.52: Regulation of secretion of parathormone and calcitonin by plasma calcium levels

Hyperparathyroidism

- Osteitis fibrosa cystica
- Hypercalciuria
- Renal stones
- Hypercalcemia
- Hypophosphatemia
- Demineralization of bones

Details of primary and secondary hyper- and hypoparathyroidism including pseudohypoparathyroidism features and symptoms have been enumerated in Table 60.17.

Hypoparathyroidism

Hypoparathyroidism is due to inadvertent removal of parathyroid glands during thyroidectomy. In rats, removal of the parathyroid glands will result in death of the rats in about 8 hrs. In the case of human beings, there will be hypocalcemic tetany.

Tetany is of two types, namely:

1. Overt tetany and
2. Latent tetany.

In latent tetany, the clinical manifestations of tetany are not obvious, but may be brought out by hyperventilating the lungs. Hyperventilation leads to carbon dioxide washout and this leads to alkalosis (washing out of hydrogen ions from the body). This results into decreased ionic calcium level in plasma.

In latent tetany, mild tapping on the facial nerve at the angle of jaw, leads to contraction of ipsilateral

Hypoparathyroidism (tetany)

Characterized by increased neuromuscular excitability.

- Latent—signs and symptoms are not present.
- Overt—Signs and symptoms—seen Chvostek's sign, Trousseau's sign.
- Tendency towards tetany

$$\frac{[HCO_3^-][PO_4]}{[Ca^{++}][Mg][H^+]}$$

facial muscles. This sign is known as Chvostek's sign. Carpopedal spasm can be produced by applying a BP cuff around the upper arm and increasing the pressure in the cuff. Increasing the pressure in the cuff obstructs the blood flow to the forearm. This sign is known as Trousseau's sign.

In overt tetany, there will be marked increase of neuromuscular excitability with twitching, tonic and clonic contractions of muscle fibers. Contraction of laryngeal muscles will give rise to asphyxia and death.

Features of hypocalcemic tetany are:

1. Numbness—tingling of the extremities (paresthesia).
2. Stiffness of hand and feet.
3. Cramps in the extremities.
4. Convulsions in children.
5. Chvostek's sign
6. Trousseau's sign (carpopedal spasm).
7. Laryngeal spasm.

Disorder	PTH	1, 25-DHCC	Bone resorption	Urine (Ca^{++} and PO$_4$)	Serum Ca^{++}	Serum PO$_4$
Primary hyper-parathyroidism	Increased	Increased	Increased	Both increased	Increased	Decreased
Humoral hypercalcemia of malignancy	Decreased	Increased	Increased	Only phosphate increased	Increased	Decreased
Surgical hypo-parathyroidism	Decreased	Decreased	Decreased	Only phosphate decreased	Decreased	Increased
Pseudohypo-parathyroidism	Increased	Decreased	Decreased	Only phosphate decreased	Decreased	Increased
Chronic renal failure	Increased (secondary)	Decreased	Increased	Only phosphate decreased	Decreased due to decrease in 1, 25-DHCC	Increased

Table 6.17: Pathophysiology of PTH—features and symptoms

Treatment: When the patient arrives with overt tetany, intravenous calcium should be administered. On a long-term basis, a diet rich in calcium and vitamin D must be given.

Hypoparathyroidism
- Hyperexcitability of neurons—hyperreflexia
- Seizures
- Muscle cramps
- Tingling sensation
- Twitching

Vitamin D Deficiency
It could be due to:
- Inadequate sunlight.
- Inadequate dietary sources of vitamin D.
- Elderly institutionalized individuals (lead to osteomalacia).
- Preterm infants who are in air polluted cities and are breastfed.
  Results in rickets characterized by bone deformation.

Excess of vitamin D could be due to over absorption from GI tract. In this condition:
- Increased bone resorption.
- Hypercalcemia.
- Hypercalciuria.
- Renal stones.
- Deposition of calcium in soft tissues.

Osteoporosis could be due to:
- Calcium deficiency.
- Loss of mechanical stress.
- Space flight.
- Increased levels of PTH and 1, 25-DHCC.

Factors leading to osteoporosis are:
- Aging
- Menopause
- Other risk factors

The above problem leads to low bone density and effect is fractures.

Causes of osteomalacia and rickets: Inadequate availability of vitamin D:
- Dietary deficiency or lack of exposure to sunlight.
- Fat-soluble vitamin malabsorption.

Defects in metabolic activation of vitamin D:
- Liver disease.
- Anticonvulsants.
- Renal failure.
- Hypoparathyroidism.

Impaired action of 1, 25-DHCC occurs:
- When patient is on anticonvulsants therapy for prolonged duration.
- Receptor defects for vitamin D.

Calcitonin

In human beings, calcitonin is produced from the parafollicular cells (C cells) of the thyroid gland. Calcitonin is made up of 32 amino acids with a molecular weight of 3500. It is a peptide hormone secreted by the parafollicular cells of thyroid gland.

Actions

It is a hypocalcemic agent and hence decreases plasma calcium level. When thyroid gland is perfused with blood containing high calcium, secretion of calcitonin is increased. This lowers plasma calcium and phosphate levels. Calcium lowering effect of calcitonin is brought about by its action on the bones. It prevents calcium resorption from bone. It inhibits the activity of osteoclasts and increases the excretion of calcium in urine.

Regulation of Secretion

It is directly dependent on plasma calcium level (refer graph given for regulation of secretion of para-thormone on page 186).

Factors which influence calcitonin secretion are given in the following box.

Factors influencing calcitonin secretion
1. Plasma Ca^{++}
2. GI hormones Gastrin CCK   } + on calcitonin (gut factor) Glucagon Secretin

Functions of calcitonin (physiologic role)
1. Hormone production is more in young—may play a role in skeletal development
2. May protect post-prandial hypercalcemia
3. Protect maternal bone during pregnancy and lactation Tendency towards bone loss during pregnancy—due to increased 1, 25 $(OH)_2 D_3$

Hypo- or hypersecretion of calcitonin is not associated with any clinical abnormality. Medullary carcinoma of thyroid gland is associated with increased production of calcitonin, but no signs and symptoms are seen in this hyperstate of secretion of calcitonin. It has been shown that comparatively more hormone is secreted in young individuals. It may be help for deposition of calcium on bone and facilitates bone growth. Diet rich in calcium when given, the gastrin which is released in gastric phase of gastric juice secretion may stimulate the calcitonin release as well. The increased release of calcitonin diverts calcium to bone tissue thus preventing excessive rise in plasma calcium level. It may also protect the mother from excessive drainage of calcium during pregnancy and lactation. The excessive drain of calcium during pregnancy may be due to increased level of 1, 25-DHCC.

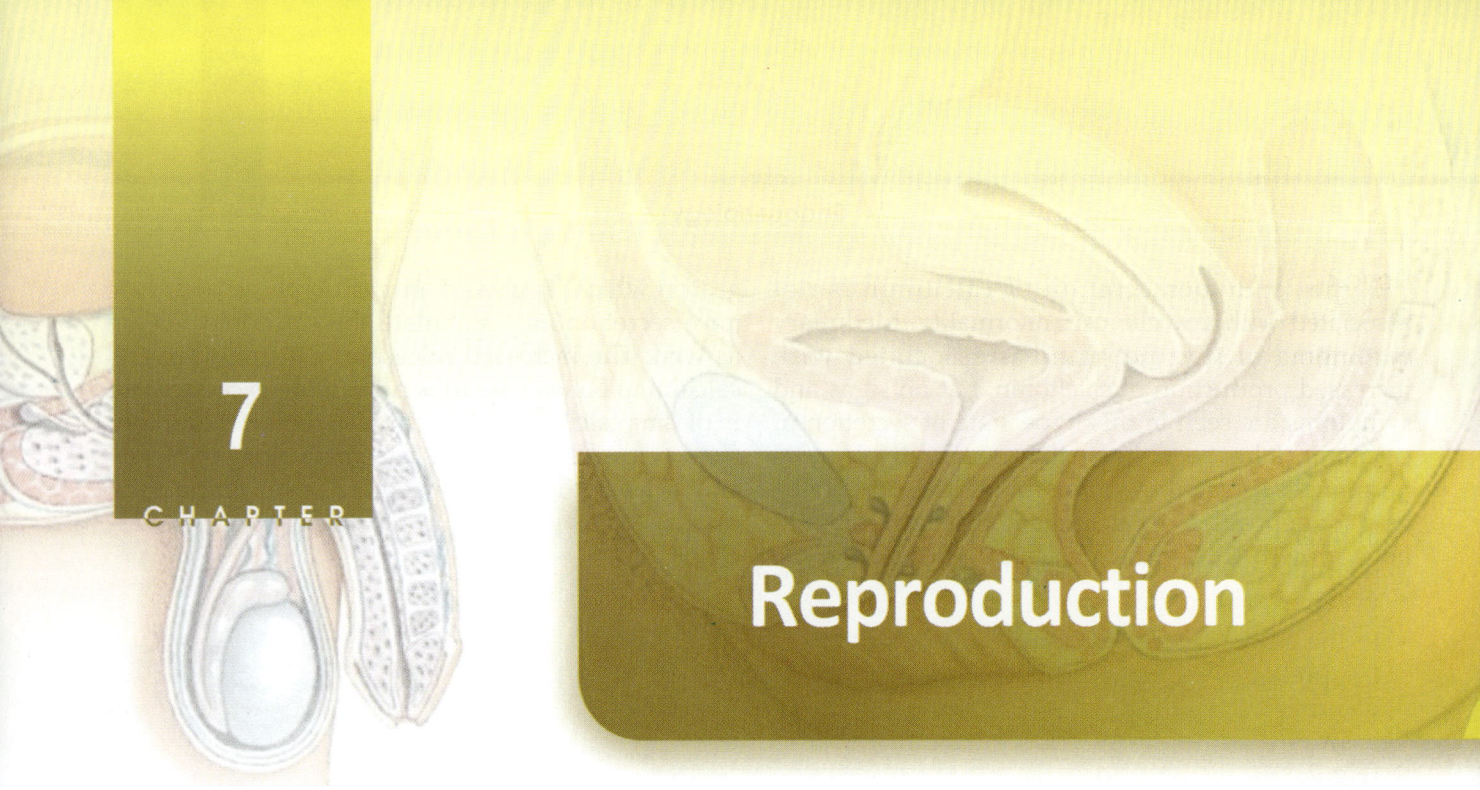

Reproduction

REPRODUCTIVE PHYSIOLOGY

Reproduction is a process of increasing the number of species or propagation of progenies. In the case of human beings, the process of reproduction is sexual. The differentiation of the individual to develop into either male or female with all the reproductive organs designed to carry on their function does occur in the embryonic stage itself. The gametes which are the forerunners of the species will carry the genetic material from one generation to another having all the characteristics of the species in general and that of its own in particular.

Some of the common terminologies in reproductive system are:

1. *Gamete* is the reproductive cell with haploid number of chromosomes (half the number of chromosome the organism will have). The male gamete is known as sperm and female gamete is known as ovum.

2. *Gonad* is the primary organ of sex which has dual function to carryout, namely secretion of sex hormone/s and production of gametes. The different types of cells present in gonad take part in each of this function.

3. *Fertilization* is the fusion of sperm and ovum which results in the development of embryo and finally the fetus.

4. *Accessory organs* of sex will aid in the transfer of gametes from male to female during the course of sexual reproduction. In female, they also help in fertilization to occur and house the developing fetus during pregnancy.

5. *Secondary sexual characteristics* are the apparent features that help to distinguish male from female. They develop at the onset of puberty and persist throughout the rest of the life.

6. *Puberty* is the onset of reproductive ability which normally occurs around the age of 10 to 13 years in males and 8 to 13 years in females.

7. *Menarche* is the first menstrual bleeding that occurs in a female at the onset of puberty.

8. *Menopause* the last menstrual bleeding in a female and beyond which she loses the reproductive ability permanently. Menopause occurs around the age of 45 years.

9. *Amenorrhea* is the absence of menstrual bleeding after the onset of puberty. The common physiological condition where amenorrhea occurs is during pregnancy.

Sex Differentiation and Development

Assigning any person as male or female depends on various criteria;

1. Chromosomal sex wherein male will have one each of XY chromosomes and a female will have two X chromosomes unless there is any aberration.

2. Gonadal sex wherein depending on the gonads present will be either testis or ovary.

Development of Gonads and Reproductive Organs

- Primitive gonad arises from the genital ridge.
- The gonad develops a cortex and medulla. Until sixth week of development, the structures are identical in both sexes.
- Till the 7th week, the genital ducts will be indifferent (Fig. 7.1), that is they can develop either into male or female type depending on the sex of the embryo (Fig. 7.2) .
- In the case of male, around 7th week because of the presence of SRY on the Y chromosome (sex determining region on Y chromosome), medulla grows further into testis and the cortex regresses (Fig. 7.3). In female due to the absence of SRY gene (as female has XX chromosomes), the cortex develops into ovary and medulla regresses (Fig. 7.4).
- When the embryo has functional testis, sertoli cells of testis secrete Mullerian inhibiting substance, which leads to regression of the Mullerian duct and aids in the further development of Wolffian duct into male external and internal genitalia.
- When the embryo lacks functional testis, in the absence of the Mullerian inhibiting factor, the Mullerian duct develops into internal and external genitalia of female type.

- The embryonic testis has the ability to secrete hormones unlike embryonic ovary which cannot secrete any hormone.
- The hormones (testosterone and dihydro-testosterone) secreted by the testis will be responsible for growth of accessory organs of sex and also the differentiation of brain into male type.

Puberty

Immediately after birth, the gonads remain quiescent for some time. The onset of reproductive ability in life is called puberty. It is the time when the gonads develop both endocrine and gametogenic functions. The onset of puberty usually occurs between 10 and 13 years and it occurs slightly earlier in girls than in boys.

Changes Seen at the Onset of Puberty

- Sex hormones are secreted from testis and ovary and due to this; there is increased growth and development of both primary and accessory organs of sex.
- There will be appearance of secondary sexual characters.
- There will be commencement of production sperms or ovum (gametogenic function commences).
- In female, the menstrual cycle starts.

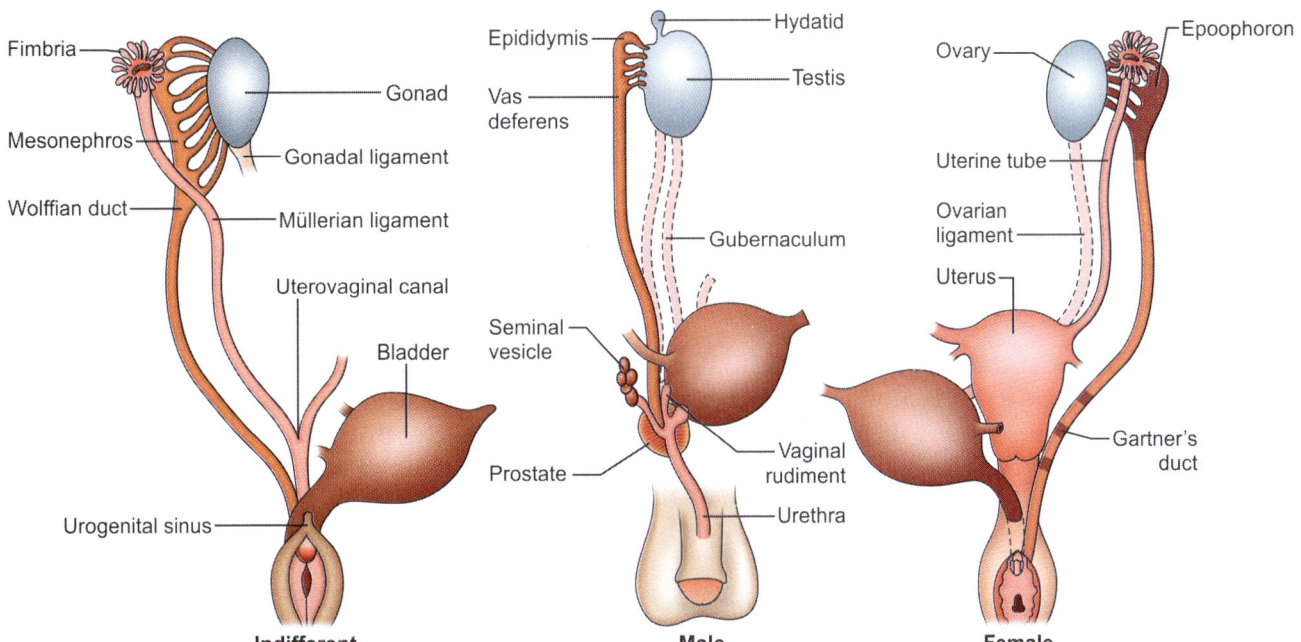

Fig. 7.1: Development of male and female genital organs from indifferent genital ducts

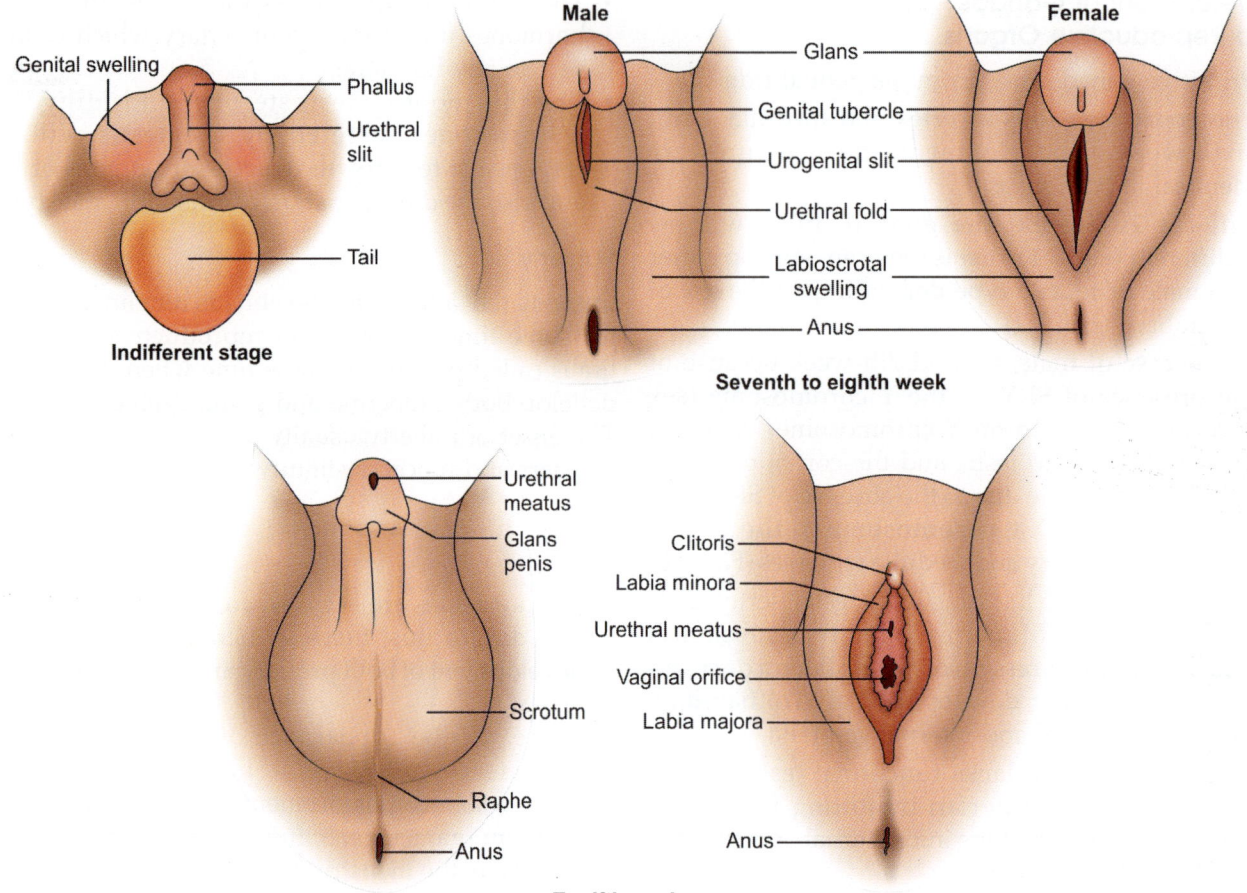

Fig. 7.2: External genitalia in male and female by about seventh and twelfth week of gestation

Changes seen in Boys and Girls at the onset of Puberty (Table 7.1 and Figs 7.5 and 7.6)

Menarche is the onset of first menstrual bleeding at the onset of puberty. This occurs normally around the age of 8 to 13 years. Initial few menstrual cycles occur irregularly and are anovulatory (no ovum).

Menopause is the last menstrual bleeding that is occurs at the termination of reproductive phase of female. It usually occurs around 45 to 55 years.

Primary amenorrhea: It means that the girl has not menstruated even once after attaining the age of puberty.

a. 16 yrs old, never menstruated or 14 yrs old with no secondary sexual features

b. No uterus

c. Congenital problem, if breast development is normal, it can be due to insensitivity to receptors.

Male Reproductive System (Fig. 7.7)

- Primary organ of sex is testis. Testis has two functions namely spermatogenesis (gametogenesis) and secretion of hormones namely testosterone and inhibin.
- The accessory organs of sex are: vas deferens, seminal vesicle, prostate gland, and penis. The accessory organs of sex help for storing sperms, seminal fluid secretions and also passage of sperms along the genital tract.

Functions of Testis (Fig. 7.8)

- Gametogenic function is by seminiferous tubules.
- Endocrine function is by interstitial cells of Leydig.

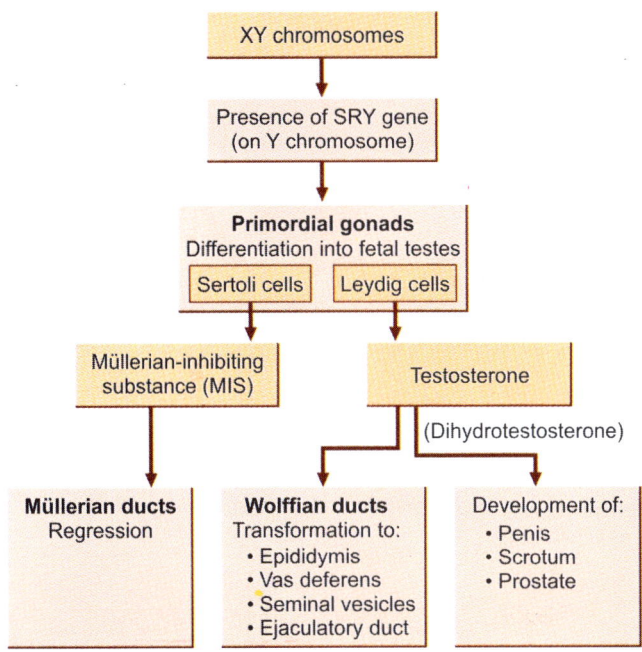

Fig. 7.3: Development of male sex organs based on the presence of SRY gene

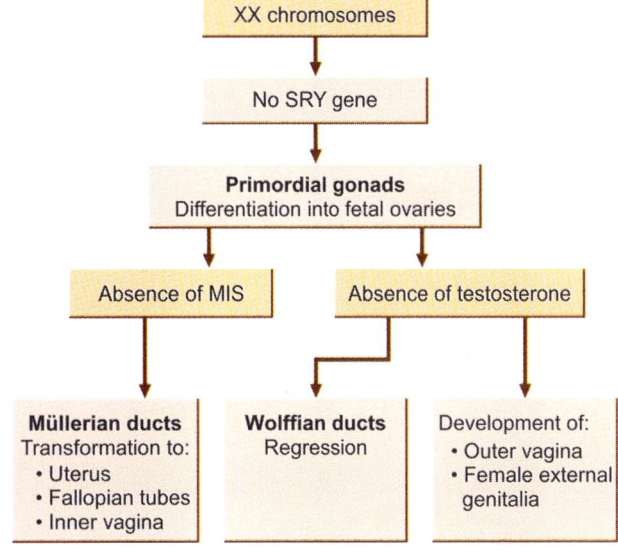

Fig. 7.4: Development of female sex organs based on the absence of SRY gene

Histology of Testis (Fig. 7.8)

Figure 7.8 shows histology of testis.

Spermatogenesis

It is the process of production of mature sperms from the cells of seminiferous tubules (Fig. 7.9). Normally from the starting of the development to complete maturation of sperm, it takes about 74 days. Steps in spermatogenesis are shown in Fig. 7.9.

From one spermatogonium, about 512 sperms are produced.

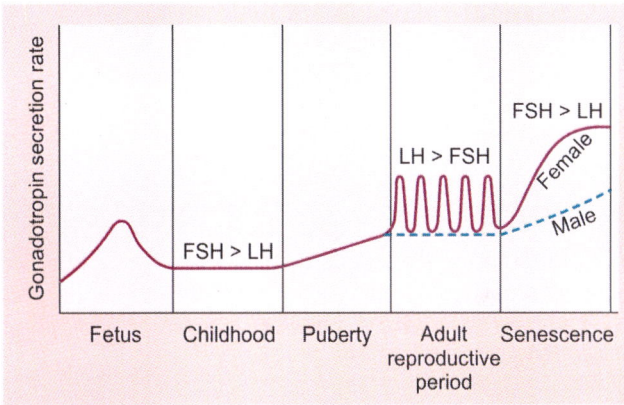

Fig. 7.5: Gonadotropic hormonal levels at different phases of life

Table 7.1: Secondary sex characteristics in male and female		
Character	Boy	Girl
Hair appearance	Beard, mustache, axilla, pubic region	Axilla and pubic region only
Skeletal muscle and body development	More muscular with less fat. Broad shoulder and narrow hips.	Less muscular, more fatty. There will be redistribution of fats in buttocks and breasts. Broad hips and narrow shoulder. Female gyrating movement of hips.
Voice	Breaking of voice due to hypertrophy of laryngeal muscles and increase in the length and thickness of vocal cords.	No breaking of voice. It remains shrill and high pitched.
Deposition of melanin	More melanin deposited and greater tanning of skin.	Lesser tanning of skin.
Emotional changes	More aggressive	Less aggressive
Acne development	Seen	Seen
Sex drive (libido)	Yes	Yes

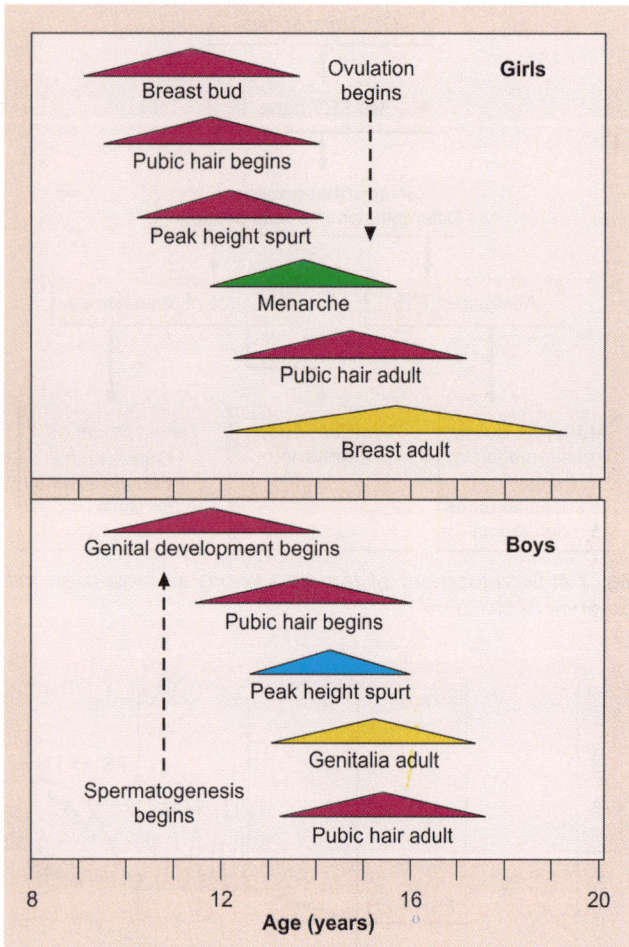

Fig. 7.6: Changes seen the body of boy and girl during the pubertal stage

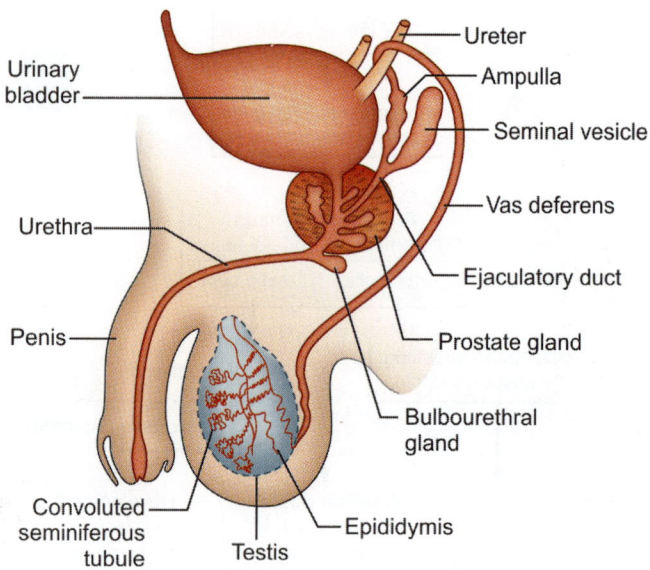

Fig. 7.7: Male sex organs (external and internal)

Exposure to cold, dartos muscles contract, and testis is moved closure to abdomen. In warmth climate, the dartos muscles relax, and testis moves away from abdomen.

Another mechanism is the countercurrent type of blood flow between the testicular artery and pampiniform plexus of veins. Scrotal skin also has a large number of sweat glands.

Vitamins: Vitamin A is important for all the epithelial cells growth including the germinal epithelium. Vitamin E and vitamin D are also essential.

Irradiation: X-ray irradiation brings about the degeneration of the seminiferous tubules. Hence spermatogenesis suffers.

Other factors include alcohol, viral infections, like mumps, gonadal dysgenesis, decrease spermatogenesis.

Cell Types in Testis and their Functions

- Leydig cells
- Sertoli cells

Functions of Sertoli Cells (Fig. 7.10)

1. Synthesize androgen binding proteins.
2. Contribute for blood–testis barrier.
3. Produce inhibin.

Factors affecting Spermatogenesis

Hormones: FSH and LH secreted by the anterior pituitary gland and also testosterone secreted by testis. Germinal epithelium of semineferous tubules is acted upon by the gonadotropic hormone (FSH) from anterior pituitary and final maturation is brought about by testosterone. Hypophysectomy results in atrophy of the semineferous tubules and lack of sperm production. This is restored to normal by administration of testosterone or FSH.

Temperature: The optimum temperature required for spermatogenesis is around 35°C. Since the testes are present in scrotal sac which is outside the abdomen and the activity of the dartos muscle will try to maintain this temperature in scrotal sac for spermatogenesis to occur normally.

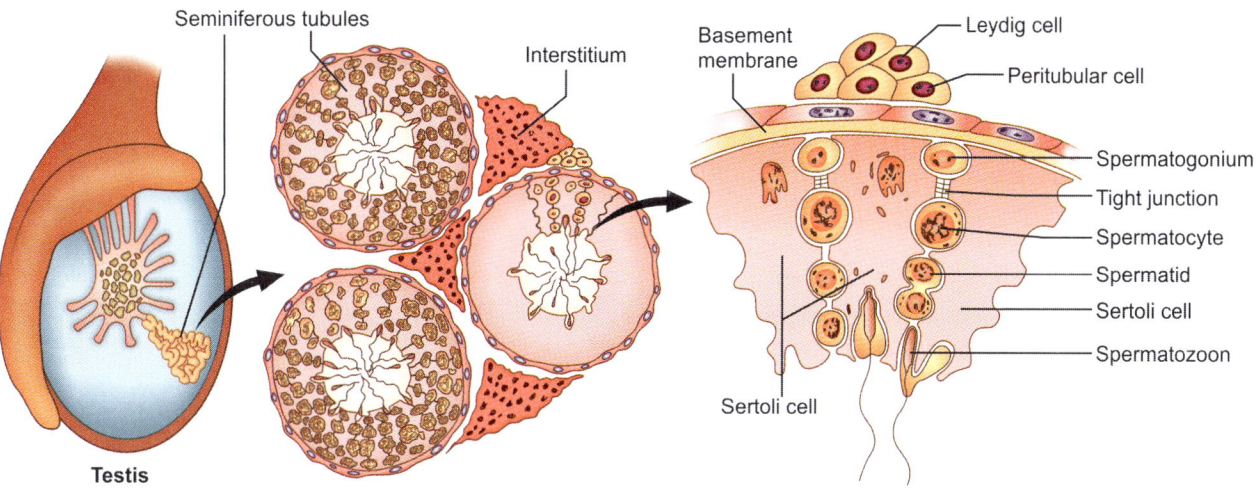

Fig. 7.8: Histology of testis and stages in spematogenesis

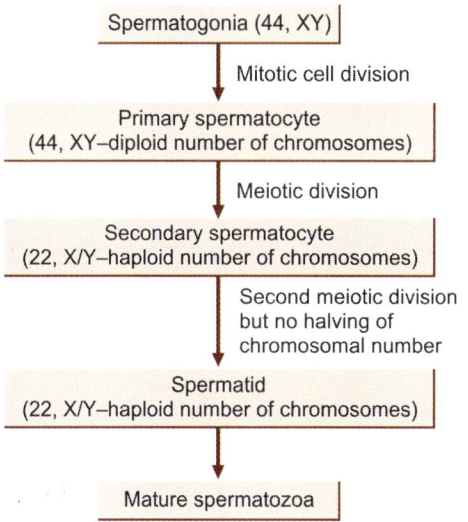

Fig. 7.9: Steps showing stages and changes in spermatogenesis

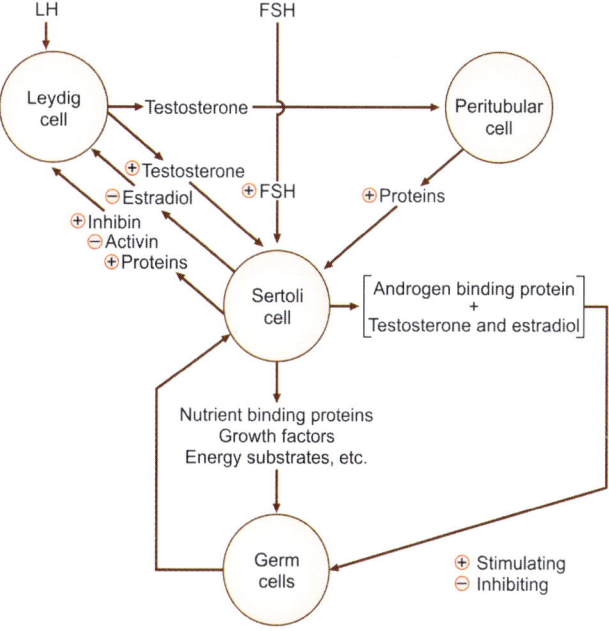

Fig. 7.10: Some of the functions of sertoli cells and the secretion of sertoli cells modifying the secretion from the Leydig cells

4. Synthesize estradiol from testosterone (by aromatase enzyme).
5. Provide nutrition to developing sperms. The sertoli cells are rich in glycogen.
6. Phagocytose malformed sperms.

Actions and Regulation of Secretion of Testosterone

The sex hormone in male is testosterone and is secreted by Leydig cells of testis also known as interstitial cells. In some of the tissues, testosterone is converted to dihydrotestosterone.

Actions

During fetal life:

- Responsible for the descent of testis into the scrotal sac.
- Development of male external and internal genitalia.
- Development of male brain (hypothalamus), which is concerned with secretion of follicular stimulating

hormone and luteinizing hormone. In males, the secretion of the above two hormones will not have any cyclical change, unlike what is observed in females during the reproductive phase.

At the onset of puberty:
- Gametogenesis (spermatogenesis).
- Development of male secondary sexual characteristics and maintenance of some of them.
- Development and maintenance of accessory organs of sex, like prostate gland, semineferous tubules (accessory organs of sex), etc.
- Anabolic and growth promoting effects.
- Initiates spermatogenesis.
- Brings about the development of secondary sexual characteristics as enumerated in Table 7.1.
- Increases the protein anabolism and hence more muscle development and chondrogenesis and collagen synthesis. And also brings about retention of inorganic ions, like sodium, potassium, sulfate, phosphate, etc.
- Promotes early fusion of epiphyseal plates and this brings about cessation of linear growth. Presently it is said that estrogen produced by testis is responsible for this function.
- Indirectly increases production of erythrocytes.
- Exerts negative feedback control over the anterior pituitary gland on the secretion of gonadotropic hormones in general and in particular LH.

During rest of life:
- Maintenance of spermatogenesis.
- Maintenance of accessory organs of sex.
- Maintenance of negative feedback over the anterior pituitary gland over luteinizing hormone secretion.

Regulation of secretion of testosterone (Fig. 7.11):
- Is by negative feedback mechanism.
- Hormones involved are testosterone and inhibin.
- Testosterone exerts negative feedback control over hypothalamus and anterior pituitary.
- Inhibin exerts negative feedback over anterior pituitary only.

Semen

- It is the fluid ejaculated by male almost at the end of sexual act.
- The fluid has secretions from:
  a. Seminal vesicles—60%

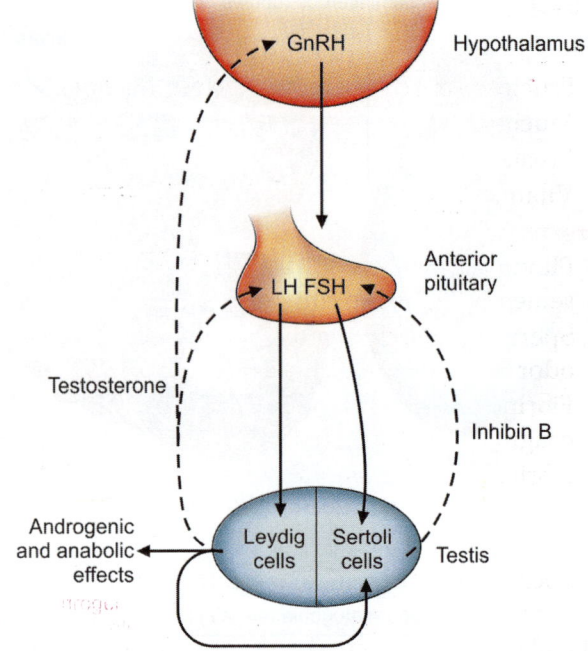

Fig. 7.11: Negative feedback mechanism regulating the secretion of testosterone

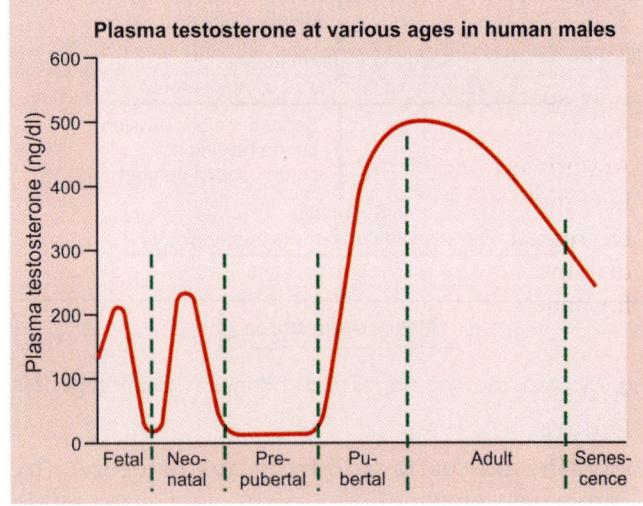

Fig. 7.12: Plasma testosterone levels at different ages (males) and stages

  b. Prostate gland—30%
  c. Spermatozoa—<10%
  d. Bulbourethral glands, vas deferens secretions also contribute.
- pH is around 7.5
- Volume ejaculated 2.5–3.5 ml per ejaculation.
- Each ml of ejaculate contains about 100 million sperms.

Composition of Semen

a. *Seminal vesicle*
- Fructose source of energy needed for nutrition.
- Mucin gives the viscous nature for semen.
- Prostaglandin.
- Vitamin C, etc.

b. *Prostate gland*
- Flavin the yellowish pigment and hence the semen is slightly yellowish.
- Spermine is responsible for the characteristic odor.
- Fibrinogen and thromboplastin responsible for coagulation of semen.
- Fibrinolysin and proteolytic enzymes responsible for semen liquefaction.

c. *Seminiferous tubules*
- Spermatozoa which are the gametes required for reproduction.

The pH of semen is always slightly alkaline in order to neutralize the acidic secretions of vagina. The vaginal secretions are generally acidic and do not facilitate fertilization.

Causes of Infertility in Male

- Low sperm count that is less than 35 million per ml.
- Abnormal shape of sperms (biheaded sperms).
- Less motile sperms.
- Decreased enzymes hyaluronidase and proteases to help for the removal of cell layers from the ovum for penetration of sperm.

Effect of castration before puberty
- Accessory organs of sex do not develop.
- Failure of development of secondary sexual characters.

- Poor muscle development.
- Voice not broken.
- Sparse distribution of hair.
- Impotent, no libido.
- Low BMR and person gains weight.

Effect of castration after puberty (Table 7.2)
- The accessory organs which have developed may undergo atrophy.
- Secondary sex characters will not change. This feature is maintained due to the effect of androgens secreted from adrenal cortex.

Cryptorchidism (Table 7.2): Failure of testis to descend from abdomen into scrotum. Testis continues to remain in the abdominal cavity. Due to high temperature in the abdominal cavity, the seminiferous tubules degenerate and hence there will be no spermatogenesis. However, the interstitial cells of Leydig continue to function normally and hence there will be secretion of testosterone hormone. Because of this, the boys attain puberty and manifest all the changes that are associated with onset of puberty, but they may remain infertile. Chances of malignancy are more in undescended testis.

Effects of bilateral vasectomy, bilateral cryptorchidism and castration after puberty have been compared in Table 7.2.

Female Reproductive System
Introduction and Oogenesis

Production of sperms and release of gonadotropic hormones in male is a continuous process. However, in female, the release of the female gamete and secretion of gonadotropic hormones is cyclical. Gametogenesis occurs in a cyclical fashion. This will prepare the female for the periodic release and fertilization of the ovum and pregnancy.

Table 7.2: Comparing the effects of bilateral vasectomy after puberty with that of bilateral cryptorchidism

	Bilateral vasectomy	Bilateral cryptorchidism	Castration
1. Ejaculation of semen	N	N	↓↓↓
2. Semen volume	N	N	↓↓↓
3. Semen composn. (sperms)	← Sperms absent →		
4. Fertility	← Infertile →		
5. Testosterone prodn	N	N	NIL
6. ACC glands	N	N	Regress
7. 2° sex ch	N	N	N
8. Libido	N	N	N/↓

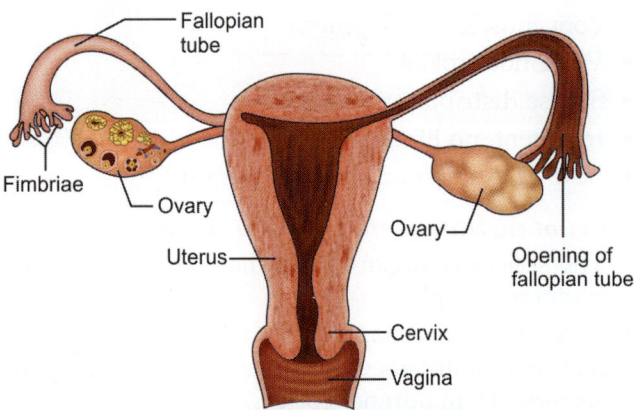

Fig. 7.13: Primary and accessory female sex organs

The parts in the female reproductive system are (Fig. 7.13):

1. Pair of ovaries
2. Fallopian tubes
3. Uterus
4. Vagina

Ovary is the primary sex organ in a female and the functions of the ovary are production of ovum (gametogenesis) and secretion of female sex hormones namely estrogen and progesterone. The cells also produce two hormones namely inhibin and relaxin. The ova are developed from the germinal epithelium. The capsule forms the outer most covering of germinal epithelium. The primordial follicles in the germinal epithelium proliferate to develop into graafian follicle.

In the newborn female infant, there will be about 5×10^6 follicles in both the ovaries. About 5×10^5 will mature and out of which only about 500 may be released in the process of ovulation during the reproductive life of a female.

As stated earlier, the sex hormones in female are estrogen and progesterone. The hormones are secreted in a cyclical fashion throughout the reproductive phase in females. During each cycle, there will be growth and maturation of an ovum from any one of the ovaries. In case there is no fertilization, the onset of next menstrual cycle prepares the female reproductive system to undergo the cyclical changes again.

Changes in Female at the Onset of Puberty

a. The secretion of gonadotropic hormones and sex hormones starts in a cyclical fashion. In female, the gonadotropic hormones are FSH and LH and sex hormones are estrogen and progesterone.
b. Starting of menstrual bleeding which occurs around the age of 8 to 13 years. The first menstrual bleeding is termed as menarche.
c. Development of ovum starts in a cyclical fashion.
d. There will be growth of accessory organs of sex.
e. The secondary sexual characters start developing. The secondary sexual characters in female include:
   1. Sudden spurt in body growth.
   2. Growth of breasts due to deposition of fats, growth of alveoli and ducts.
   3. Pelvic girdle becomes bigger and roomy. Redistribution of fats occurs and more fat gets deposited in the buttocks. This leads to broad hips.
   4. Shoulder will be narrow, and muscle mass is less.
   5. Shrill voice persists.
   6. Psyche: Attraction for the opposite sex
   7. There will be development of hairs in axilla and pubic regions. More hairs in scalp and less in the body.

Menstrual Cycle

The normal average duration of menstrual cycle is about 28 days. However, the duration may not remain the same in each cycle. It can be anywhere between 20 and 45 days. Counting of the days in a cycle begins on the first day the menstrual bleeding starts.

During each cycle, changes will be taking place in the following organs:

a. Ovary
b. Uterus
c. Cervix
d. Vagina

The menstrual discharge contains blood, damaged endometrial cells, damaged endometrial glands and endothelial cells of damaged blood vessels. Ovum will not be present.

In any menstrual cycle, the changes will be taking place simultaneously in:

a. Ovary, termed as ovarian cycle
b. Uterus, termed as uterine or endometrial cycle
c. Changes are also seen in cervix and vagina and is termed as vaginal cycle.

Changes in ovary: Oogenesis is the growth and maturation of an ovum. It occurs in any one of the ovaries during the menstrual cycle. The number of oogonia is fixed at birth.

Stages in oogenesis: Figure 7.14 describes the stages in oogenesis.

Ovarian Cycle

The different stages of ovarian cycle are:
- Follicular phase
- Luteal phase

Follicular Phase (Fig. 7.15)

- Under the influence of the hormone, FSH secreted from the anterior pituitary gland about 5 to 6 primordial follicles start developing.
- Of which only one of follicles grows further and matures. This follicle is known as dominant follicle.
- The remaining follicles start regressing. They are termed as the atretic follicles.
- One of the follicles, which is maturing, develops a cavity and the cavity is known as antrum.

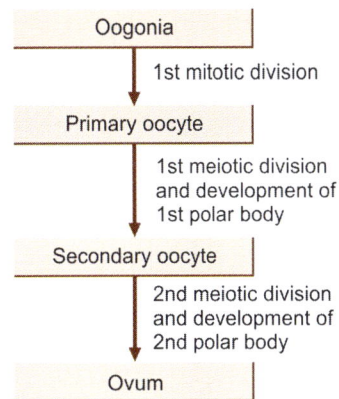

Fig. 7.14: Steps indicating stages and changes during oogenesis

- As the follicle is maturing, the size of the cavity increases and the fluid start accumulating in the cavity.
- All these changes are brought about due to the action of follicular-stimulating hormone of anterior pituitary gland and the estrogen secreted by the theca interna cells of the maturing follicle.

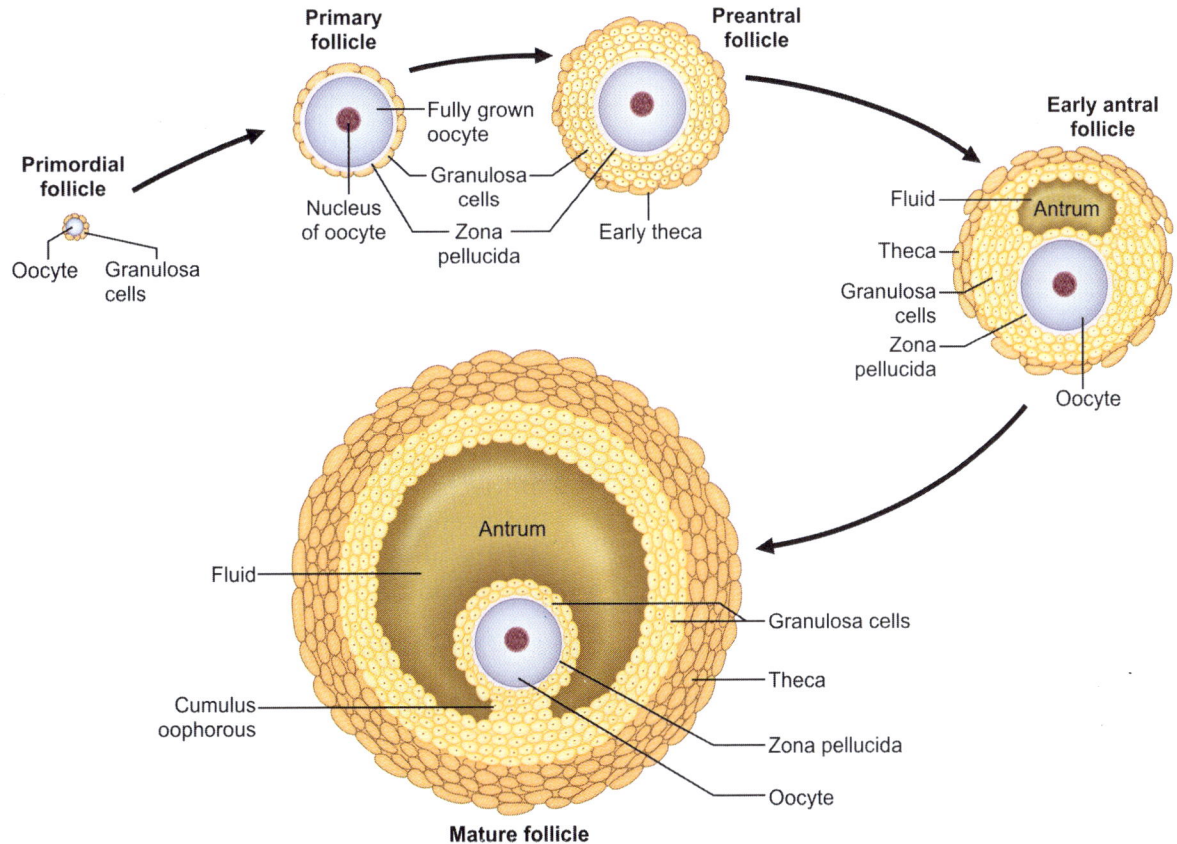

Fig. 7.15: Formation of mature follicle from the primordial follicle

- Around the 14th day in a 28-day menstrual cycle, ovum is liberated from the mature follicle into the abdominal cavity. This process is known as ovulation. The fimbriated ends of the fallopian tube pick up the released ovum from the abdominal cavity.
- The hormone, which is responsible for the ovulation is LH and luteinizing hormone surge is a must. The LH surge is brought about by the positive feedback regulation exerted by estrogen.

Luteal Phase (Fig. 7.16)

- The cavity of the follicle, which has released the ovum, gets filled with small amount of blood. This is known as corpus hemorragicum.
- Around 16th day, the blood spots are replaced by lipid rich luteal cells and hence it is known as corpus luteum.
- The corpus luteum starts secreting estrogen and progesterone until around 24th day.
- In case there is no fertilization, the corpus luteum starts regressing and around 28th day there will be formation of corpus albicans.

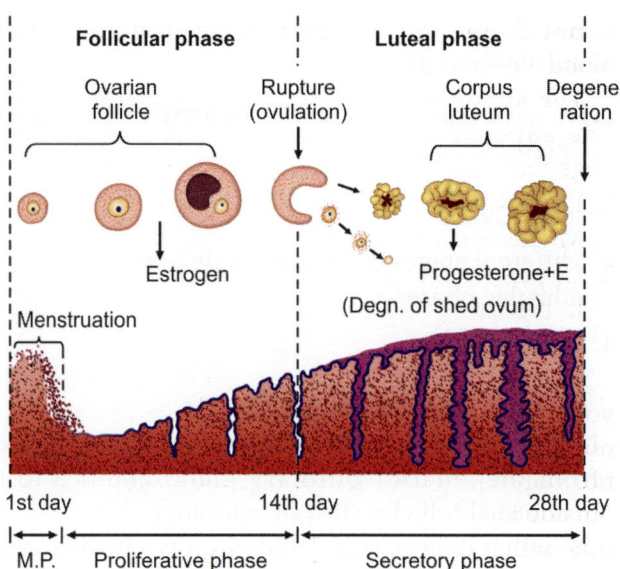

Fig. 7.17: Endometrial and ovarian changes in a menstrual cycle

- The surface epithelium is made up of a single layer of connective tissue cells and tissue fluid.

All the above changes are due to the action of estrogen.

Changes during Secretory (Luteal) Phase

- Uterine endometrium grows further and thickness may be as much as 6 mm.
- Uterine glands increase in size, become tortuous and start secreting. Hence mucus secretion is seen in lumen.
- The endometrium is edematous in appearance due to increase in tissue fluid.
- The spiral arteries increase in length, diameter and endometrium shows increased vascularity.
- Connective tissue cells become larger and store nutrients, like carbohydrate and vitamins, which are essential for the embryo.

All the above changes are due to the action of estrogen and progesterone.

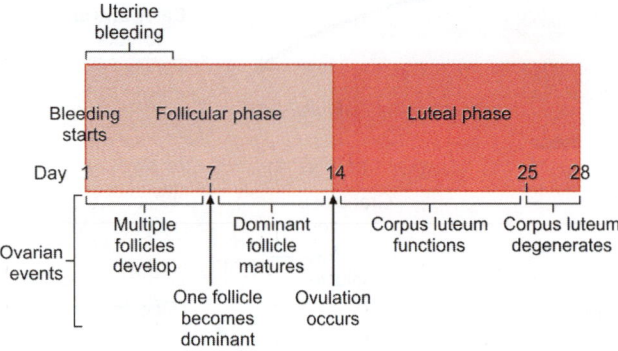

Fig. 7.16: Changes occurring in ovary during the ovarian cycle

Uterine (endometrial) Changes (Fig. 7.17)

During Proliferative (Follicular) Phase

- Lasts from about 4th to 14th day.
- The endometrium thickens and reaches a maximum of 3 mm.
- Uterine glands also grow but do not become tortuous or start secreting.
- Stratum functionale also starts growing resulting in growth of spiral arteries.

Bleeding Phase

This occurs immediately after the secretory phase. The hormonal basis for bleeding is as follows:

If there is no fertilization, there will be sudden drop of estrogen and progesterone levels due to regression of corpus luteum. Progesterone is a vasodilator and now since the vasodilator influence of progesterone is not there, vasoconstrictor spasm occurs in the blood vessels of uterus.

The spasm results in ischemia of endometrium. The superficial one-third layer of endometrium degenerates and the following changes are seen:

1. Epithelial cells and uterine glands break down.
2. Mucus secretion is lost.
3. Upper part of spiral arteries breaksdown resulting in bleeding.
4. Connective tissue cells and tissue fluid are also lost.

All the above appear as menstrual flow. The normal volume of blood lost is about 40 ml. The menstrual blood normally clots inside the uterus and also undergoes fibrinolysis. Hence the menstrual blood does not clot outside the body. If there is heavy bleeding, adequate time will not be available for blood to clot inside the uterus and hence it will clot outside the body.

Changes in Vagina

In the first 14 days, vaginal epithelium shows cornification of epithelial cells and this acts as protection against mechanical injury. During the secretory phase, under the influence of progesterone, thick mucus is secreted and epithelium becomes infiltrated by leukocytes.

Figure 7.18 shows the various hormonal levels including the gonadotropic hormones during one menstrual cycle. Till 10th day in a 28-day cycle, estrogen exerts nepative feedback on FSH and LH secretions. From 11th day until the day of ovulation, estrogen exerts positive feedback and after ovulation estrogen once again exerts negative feedback control over FSH and LH secretions.

Methods to Determine Ovulation

- *Recording of basal body temperature:* Basal body temperature is increased around the day of ovulation by about 0.5°C. So recording of temperature early in the morning before the woman starts the daily work is done to ascertain whether there is any increase in temperature. Usually oral temperature is recorded.
- *Consistency of cervical mucus:* The cervical mucus becomes thinnest around the day of ovulation (less cellular and more watery).
- *Histological appearance of cervical mucus:* A characteristic fern-like pattern is observed around the day of ovulation.

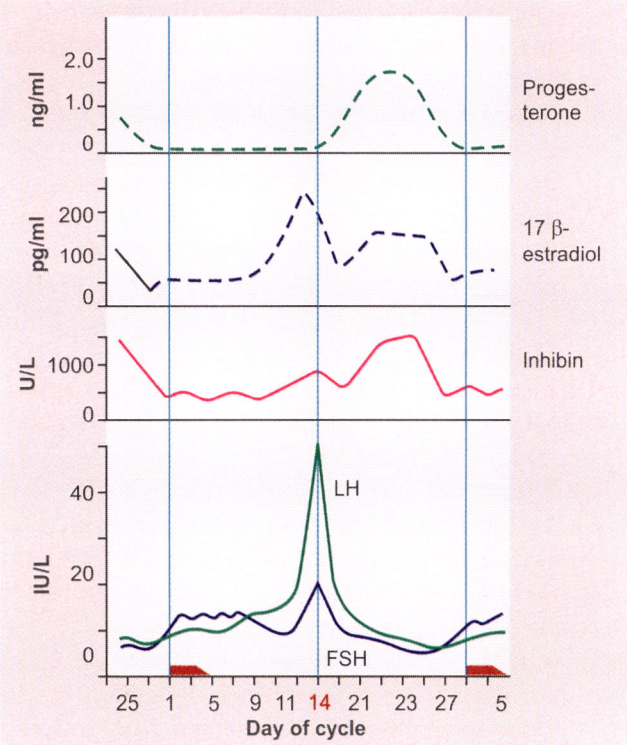

Fig. 7.18: Hormonal changes in a menstrual cycle

Actions of Estrogen

- Sensitizes a single graafian follicle to mature into an ovum. Once sensitized by estrogen, ovulation occurs.
- Growth of accessory organs of reproduction:
  a. Increase in the size of uterus at the onset of puberty and also during the pregnancy.
  b. Changing of vaginal epithelium from single layer to multilayered (cornification) type. This reduces the susceptibility for infection.
  c. Contraction of fallopian tube and number of cilia is markedly increased due to action of estrogen. This facilitates the movement of ovum towards the uterine cavity.
- Increases the size of the mammary gland by increasing the growth and branching of the lacteriferous ducts and also deposition of fats. It is also responsible for pigmentation around areola and nipple.
- It is responsible for development of accessory organs of sex.
- It is responsible for development of all secondary sexual characters at the onset of puberty.

- Responsible for all changes in the uterus and vagina during the follicular phase of menstrual cycle. Changes in the endometrium are:
  a. Increasing the thickness of endometrium.
  b. Increasing the water content.
  c. Increasing the blood flow. It is responsible for growth of vessels in stratum basale.
  d. Responsible for growth of uterine glands.
  e. Increased protein content of endometrial cells.
  f. The cervical mucus secretion becomes thin, watery with more sodium.
- On mineral and water metabolism, estrogen actions are similar to aldosterone actions. It brings about retention of sodium and water in body. This is the cause for premenstrual weight gain.
- On serum cholesterol level, it tends to reduce the cholesterol level and hence susceptibility of the female to heart attack is less when compared to men.
- Its influence on other endocrine glands:
  a. Normal activity of the ovary is dependent on the gonadotropic hormones secreted from anterior pituitary gland. The secretion of gonadotropic hormones is regulated by estrogen level in circulation.
  b. Small amount of estrogen increases prolactin release whereas in large quantity estrogen decreases the prolactin release.
  c. Facilitates release of angiotensins.

Actions of Progesterone

- *On uterus:* It brings about changes in both endometrium and myometrium.
  a. Endometrium grows further and hence the thickness of endometrium is increased.
  b. Uterine glands grow further, become coiled and start secreting. It is because of this, changes occur in the uterus during secretory phase of menstrual cycle. These changes can be brought about only after estrogen has acted on the uterus. This effect is known as priming effect of estrogen.
  c. It decreases the sensitivity of myometrium for the action of oxytocin. This facilitates implantation of zygote in case there is fertilization.
- *On cervix:* The cervical secretions become thick, more cellular and acidic. This decreases the motility of sperms and also the viability of sperms in the female genital tract.

- *On mammary gland:* It stimulates further growth of breasts by increasing the lobules and alveoli.
- *Maintenance of pregnancy:* It is required for:
  a. Embedding the fertilized ovum.
  b. Inhibition of uterine contractions.
- *Thermogenic action:* Because it has slight thermogenic action, around the day of ovulation and during the secretory phase of menstrual cycle, the basal body temperature will be increased by about 0.5°C.
- *On LH release:* The increase in the progesterone levels in circulation exerts a negative feedback influence on pituitary and decreases the secretion of LH.
- *Inhibits the action of prolactin:* The premature secretion of milk is inhibited by progesterone.

Placenta

This is developed at the point of implantation of zygote on the posterior wall of uterus. The placenta has a fetal side and a maternal side. The fetal part has finger-like processes namely chorionic villi which dips into maternal sinusoids. In spite of this, there will be no mixing of maternal and fetal blood.

The placenta is made of the following layers, namely:

a. Endothelial cell lining the fetal capillaries.
b. Chorionic tissue of chorionic villi.
c. Trophoblast cells namely cytotrophoblasts and syncitiotrophoblasts.

Functions of Placenta

- *Respiratory:* Since fetus is not exposed to the outside atmosphere, the fetal lung will be in solid state. The oxygen requirement by the developing fetus and removal of carbon dioxide from the fetal body should be taken care off by the maternal blood. Hence placenta acts as a structure across which these gases can get exchanged. It acts as a fetal lung.
- *Excretory:* Excretion of metabolic waste products, like urea, uric acid and creatinine from fetal to maternal blood, since fetal kidney is non-functional.
- *Nutritive:* Nutrients, like glucose, free fatty acids, get diffused from maternal to fetal blood to meet the demands of the developing fetus. At the same time, the placenta itself acts as fetal liver and synthesizes proteins, since the most of the proteins of mother cannot cross placenta to reach the fetal circulation.

- *Protective:* It prevents transport of certain bacteria and viruses and prevents infection of the developing fetus even though mother may be suffering from the disease.
- *Endocrine* (Figs 7.19, 7.20): It secretes many of the hormones, namely:

  a. hCG

  b. Estrogen

  c. Progesterone

  d. Human chorionic somatomammotropin.

hCG is required to maintain the corpus luteum till placenta per se is able to secrete adequate amount of estrogen and progesterone to maintain the gestation. Normally, it takes about 3 months for the placenta to secrete the required amount of progesterone and estrogen for maintenance of pregnancy.

Physiologic Role of hCG

1. It maintains the corpus luteum. Hence in pregnancy, in the initial two to three months, the corpus luteum continues to function and secretes estrogen and progesterone. When once placenta is fully developed and secretes estrogen and progesterone in adequate quantity, hCG secretion decreases and consequently the corpus luteum starts regressing.
2. It can bring about the growth and development of fetal Leydig cells. This will lead to production of testosterone in fetal life.
3. hCG can be used to facilitate the descent of testis.

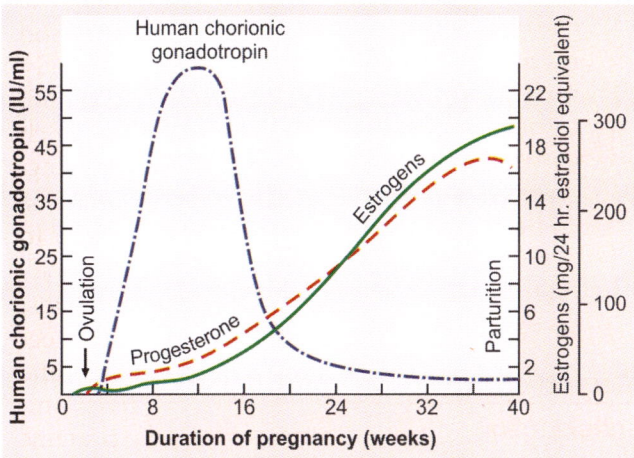

Fig. 7.19: Hormonal levels during pregnancy

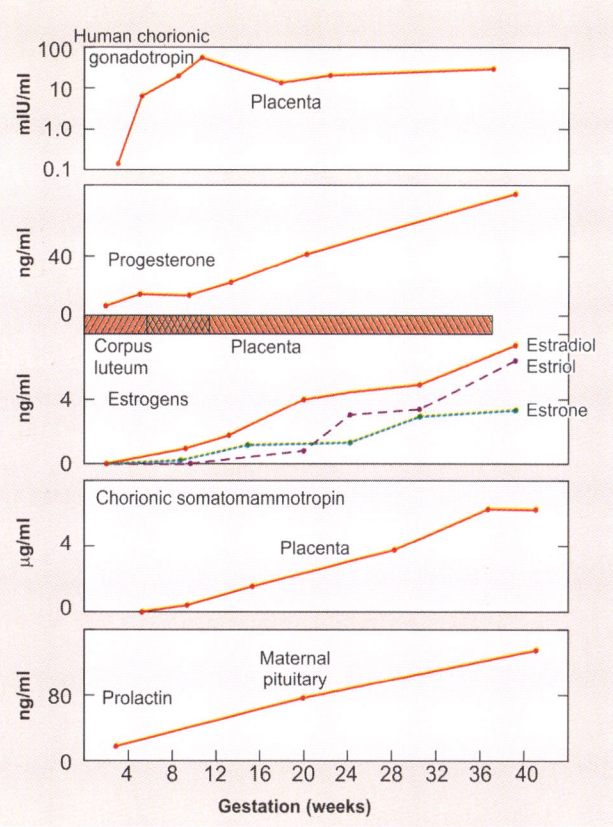

Fig. 7.20: Hormonal levles during gestation

Pregnancy Diagnosis Tests

1. Immunological test/agglutination test:

   a. Accuracy is 99.99%

   b. hCG antibodies are added to a drop of urine of female.

   c. After few seconds, add latex particles coated with hCG.

   d. Wait for few seconds (about 30).

   e. If there is no agglutination of the latex particles, the woman is pregnant. If there is agglutination, then the woman is not pregnant.

The basis for the above test is the presence of hCG in the urine of the female immediately after conception.

Menopause

- Last menstrual bleeding at the termination of reproductive phase in a female. It is opposite of menarche.
- It is also termed as female climacteric.

- It occurs around the age of 45–55 years.
- It is due to unresponsiveness of the ovary to gonadotropic hormones.
- So there will be no secretion of female sex hormones from ovary.
- No more ovulation or menstruation.
- Irritability and the person become more moody.
- Obesity due to decreased caloric expenditure.
- Osteoporosis due to decreasing protein anabolism, causing loss of protein matrix particularly in the vertebral column.
- LH secretion is episodic bursts brings about sensation of warmth spreading from trunk to face. This is known as "hot flushes".
- Decreased secretion of estrogen is responsible for atherosclerosis, osteoporosis and increase in serum cholesterol level.

Maternal Changes during the Pregnancy

1. *Morning sickness* is characterized by nausea and vomiting. It occurs in the first trimester. The exact cause is not known but is presumed to be because of very high concentration of estrogen in circulation.
2. *Placenta*
   - Occurs at the site of implantation of zygote on the posterior wall of uterus.
   - Has maternal and fetal side.
   - At times, the barrier may be broken during pregnancy itself.
3. *Anterior pituitary:* Secretion of FSH and LH becomes almost nil because of increased levels of estrogen and progesterone in circulation. They exert a negative feedback control over the secretion of FSH and LH. However, there will be enormous increase in the secretion of prolactin from anterior pituitary. This is essential for the growth of breasts to take care of milk secretion.
4. *Adrenal cortex:* There will be increased secretion of aldosterone and cortisol.
   Aldosterone is required to conserve sodium since the developing fetus will also require sodium. Hence the loss of sodium has to be restricted. Cortisol secretion also gets increased to cope up with stress the maternal body is experiencing during pregnancy.
5. *Kidneys:* There will be increased secretion of rennin, erythropoietin and 1, 25-dihydroxy-cholecalciferol. In addition to this, there will be more amounts of retention salts and water by the kidney due to the actions of the hormones aldosterone, ADH, etc.
6. *Breasts:* Enlarge and develop mature glandular structure. This is because of the actions of the hormones namely estrogen, progesterone, prolactin and human somatomammotropin.
7. *Blood volume* gets increased. Erythrocyte volume gets increased because of erythropoietin and plasma volume gets increased due to the action of hormones namely aldosterone, and ADH. Since the increase in plasma volume is more than the increase in the erythrocyte volume, the net effect will be a fall of hematocrit value (hemodilution).
8. *Bone turnover* is increased due to increased secretion of parathormone and 1,25-DHCC.
9. *Body weight* on an average few kilograms of weight is gained during pregnancy. The increase in weight is mainly due to retention of water by the body.
10. *Circulation:* There will be increase of cardiac output and systolic blood pressure. However, there will also be fall of total peripheral resistance since there will be dilation of arterioles in uterus, skin, breasts, GI tract, etc. This brings about a slight fall in diastolic BP. Hence the mean arterial pressure remains almost normal.
11. *Respiration:* There would be slight increase in ventilation and this leads to slight fall of partial pressure of carbon dioxide in circulation. The increased ventilation is due to the action of progesterone.
12. *On metabolism:* Metabolic rate in general gets increased. Gluconeogenesis and lipolysis are increased. This may be due to decreased responsiveness of the body for insulin caused by cortisol and human placental lactogen.
13. *Appetite and thirst:* Increased after the first trimester, as the needs of the developing fetus also have to be met with.
14. *Nutritional recommended daily allowance (RDA):* Increased for vitamins, minerals, proteins, etc.

Growth of Population and Contraception

Introduction

- World population has almost trebled in last 60–70 years.

- If the growth of population is not checked, it leads to imbalance between the population and resources available to meet their demands. This would hamper the growth and development of any nation.
- In most of the countries, this is the situation except for certain countries, like Australia, Germany, Sweden, etc.
- The growth of population should be as little as possible and it should not be either on the negative side or too much on the positive side.
- Because of improvement in healthcare, the life expectancy of the individual has increased considerably and nowadays we have more of elderly people in many of the countries around the world.
- At any given time, a balance must be struck between the productive age group and elderly people for healthy growth of any society and country.

Contraceptive Methods

There are many methods that can be employed to check the growth of population. Some of them can be employed:

- Only in males and others only in females. For the methods to be effective, it needs the concurrence and participation of both man and woman.

The contraceptive methods can also be classified into:

1. Temporary
2. Permanent

1. Temporary Methods

The temporary methods of family planning are:

1. Mechanical barriers
2. Introduction of spermicidal jellies
3. Intrauterine contraceptive devises
4. Oral contraceptive pills (hormonal method)
5. Morning after pills

Mechanical Barriers

- In male, it is condoms which cover the penis and does not allow the semen to get deposited into the female genital tract and hence there would not be any chance for fertilization of ovum.
- In female, it is rubber diaphragm or cervical cap which can be inserted into the genital tract and placed on the cervix. It is advisable to use spermicidal jelly along with this for more effective contraception.

Spermicides

- Spermicidal jelly should be applied in the vagina before the intercourse. As the name indicates, it kills the sperms that get ejaculated into the female genital tract.
- Nowadays, there is vaginal cream available in collapsible tubes.
- Foaming tabs when placed in the vagina gives off carbon dioxide which kills sperms.
- Thin plastic film which dissolves when placed in the vagina releasing the spermicidal agents.

Intrauterine Contraceptive Devices (IUCDs)

Commonly used is Copper "T" , Lippe's loop, etc.

Lippe's loop

- It is inserted into the uterine cavity via the vaginal canal.
- Normally, placed in the uterus after two weeks of child birth.
- The loop is coiled and fits well in the uterine cavity.

Copper "T"

- A more recent innovation.
- Thin gauge copper wire is wound around the plastic loop "T".
- It is introduced into the cavity of the uterus.

Mode of action of IUCDs

- Presence of copper or plastic inside the uterus act as foreign body.
- This makes the uterus keep contracting and accelerate the rate of movement of ovum from fallopian tube into the uterine cavity.
- Thereby favorable conditions would not be available for fertilization of the ovum.
- Even if fertilization occurs, implantation of the zygote is prevented because of contractions.

Oral Contraceptive Pills (Hormonal Method)

- Requires taking of tablets having certain amount of specific hormone/s.
- So far the tablets have been made only for the use by female.

- Usually, the tablets have a combination of both estrogen and progesterone hormones in the synthetic form.
- They are taken from day 5 of the cycle to day 25 (21 tablets having hormones).
- The hormonal actions last for about 24 to 36 hours and have a little side effect.
- In the remaining days of the cycle, tablets are taken but they are placebo. The placebos contain iron.

Mechanism of actions

- The exogenous administration of the hormones alters the feedback mechanism over control of gonadotropin hormones secretion from anterior pituitary gland.
- So there will be no LH surge and ovulation may be prevented.
- The rate of movement ovum along the fallopian tubes is increased and conditions may not become conducive for fertilization.
- Even if fertilization occurs, the increase in the movement of uterus may not facilitate the implantation of the zygote.

Permanent Methods

In male: Vasectomy

- More simple procedure.
- The vas deferens on both the sides is cut and ligated.
- Continuity in the vas deferens is lost.
- Sperms will not reach the ejaculatory duct and hence semen will be devoid of sperms completely.
- After vasectomy, the person has to be careful for next 2–3 months sexual life as the sperms stored in the ampulla of Vas before the procedure are viable for about 3 months or so.
- Nowadays, it is possible to bring about recanalization in case of any necessity at a later date.

In female: Tubectomy

- The fallopian tube is cut and ligated or cauterized (laparoscopic sterilization) on both the sides.
- Continuity in the fallopian tube is lost.
- Ovum will not be able to come across the sperms that have entered the female genital tract.
- Nowadays it is possible to bring about recanalization in case of any necessity at a later date.

Other Temporary Methods

Rhythm Method or Safe Period

- The emphasis is on presumable day of ovulation.
- It is based on the viability of ovum, and sperms in the female genital tract.
- Both the sperms and ovum are viable for about 48–72 hours.
- In a 28-day cycle, ovulation may occur on 14th day ±2 days.
- Hence intercourse between 10th and 19th day is not safe in a 28-day cycle.
- But this method is not very reliable as the duration of the cycle and the day of ovulation may vary in each cycle.
- The method is based on the assumption that the duration of the next cycle is of these many days.

Withdrawal Method

- Here penis is withdrawn from the vagina just before ejaculation.
- Hence semen will not be ejaculated into the female genital tract.
- However, during the intercourse, there will be minute amount of semen getting ejaculated and may bring about fertilization.

In most of the temporary methods of family planning, the percentage of success of the method depends. None of the temporary methods of family planning has 100% successful and even in permanent methods as well (Tables 7.3 and 7.4).

Lactation

The hormones which influence the development of breasts are:

a. At puberty, it will be estrogen and progesterone. In addition to these, some of the other hormones which are also required are: thyroxine, growth hormone, cortisol and insulin.
b. During pregnancy, it will be estrogen and progesterone which are secreted in large quantity either from corpus luteum or placenta. Apart from these, the human chorionic somatomammotropin (HCS) secreted by placenta also is responsible for growth of breasts. There is no lactation during pregnancy because, progesterone level is high and it inhibits the release of prolactin.

Table 7.3: Some forms of contraception and mechanism

Method	First year failure rate	Physiological mechanims of effectiveness
Barrier methods Condoms (male and female) Diaphragm/cervical cap (female)	12%	Prevents sperm from entering uterus
Spermicides (female)	20%	Kills sperm in the vagina (after insemination)
Sterilization Vasectomy (male) Tubal ligation (female)	<0.5%	Prevents sperm from becoming part of seminal fluid Prevents sperm from reaching egg
Intrauterine device (IUD) (female)	3%	Prevents implantation of blastocyst
Estrogens and/or progestins Oral contraceptive pill (female) Injectable or implantable progestins (female) Transdermal (skin patch) (female) Vaginal ring (female)	3% <0.5% <1% <1%	Prevents ovulation by suppressing LH surge (negative feedback); thickens cervical mucus (prevents sperm from entering uterus); alters endometrium to prevent implantation of blastocyst

Table 7.4: Contraceptive use and efficacy rates in the United States

Method	Estimated use	Accidental pregnancy in year 1(%)
Pill	32	3
Female sterilization	19	0.4
Condom	17	12
Male sterilization	14	0.15
Diaphram	4–6	2–23
Spermicides	5	20
Rhythm	4	20
Intrauterine device	3	6

c. After delivery, since the concentration of progesterone falls earlier than the estrogen, prolactin secretion starts and lactation commences in about 1–3 days. During this phase, suckling is the most effective stimulus that brings about secretion of prolactin.

"The breasts were more skillful at compounding a feeding mixture than the hemispheres of the most learned professors brain"—Oliver Wendell Holmes

Hormones Influencing Lactation

1. Prolactin: Suckling of breasts not only brings about release of oxytocin (Fig. 7.21), it will also stimulate the secretion of prolactin. For both the hormonal secretions, it is the neuroendocrine mechanism that is involved.

2. Some of the other hormones influencing lactation are thyroxine, and growth hormone. ACTH and glucocorticoids are necessary for maintenance of milk secretion which is known as galactopoiesis.

Emotional conditions, like cry of the baby and condition reflexes, also play an important role in lactogenesis.

Advantages of Breastfeeding

1. Infant gets a well-balanced diet.

2. Stimulation of nipple releases oxytocin. Oxytocin brings about involution of uterus and size of uterus is reduced following parturition.

3. During the time of breastfeeding, ovulation is inhibited. This is because prolactin inhibits the release of luteinizing hormone.

4. The infant gets some amount of passive immunity since milk contains some of the antibodies.

5. Since it is directly coming from mammary gland, contamination is less and chances of child suffering from infantile diarrhea is minimized.

6. It builds psychological bond between mother and child.

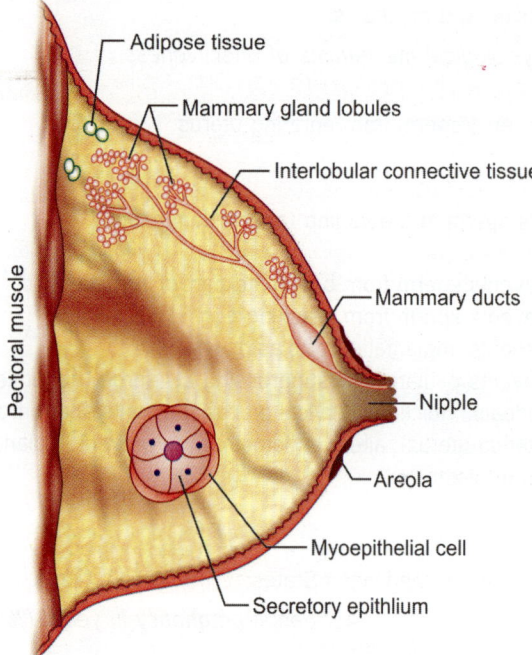

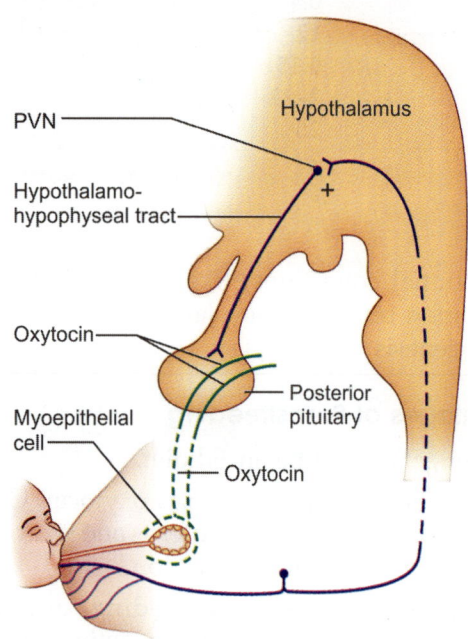

Fig. 7.21: Myoepithelial cells in breast and neuroendocrine reflex during ejection of milk

Gonadal Dysgenesis (Tables 7.5 to 7.7)

Normal sexual development depends on a complex, orderly sequence of events that begin during early embryonic life. The complete development occurs at the onset of puberty. Any deviation can result in infertility, and sexual dysfunction and various degree of intersexuality or hermaphroditism.

A true hermaphrodite possesses both ovarian and testicular tissue, either separate or combined as ovotestes. A pseudohermaphrodite has one type of gonad but a different degree of sexuality of the opposite sex. Disorders of the sexual differentiation can be classified as:

a. Gonadal dysgenesis
b. Female pseudohermaphroditism
c. Male pseudohermaphroditism
d. True hermaphroditism

Gonadal dysgenesis refers to incomplete differentiation of the gonads and is usually associated with sex chromosome abnormalities. These result in the errors in the first or second meiotic division. The most common disorders are:

1. Klinefelter's syndrome—47, XXY.
2. Turner's syndrome—45, XO.

Klinefelter Syndrome

Because of the Y chromosome, Klinefelter's syndrome individual with 47, XXY karyotype and has normal testicular function in utero with AMH (MIF/MIS) and no ambiguity of genitalia at birth. The extra X chromosome may either come from sperm or egg. The extra X chromosome, however, interferes with development of seminiferous tubules and has abnormal Leydig cell function. Testosterone levels will be very low and secondary sexual characteristics will not appear and breast size increases (gynecomastia). They will have high levels of gonadotropins due to loss of negative feedback control. Such males have small testes and azoospermic and often exhibit eunuchoidal features. They can be treated with androgen replacement therapy to increase libido and decrease breast size. However, the normal spermatogenesis will not get restored. Salient features of Klienfelter's syndrome are:

- 47, XXY
- Small testes
- Poorly developed secondary sexual characteristics
- Gynecomastia
- Azoospermic
- Infertile
- Testosterone levels very low
- May be mild reduction in verbal skill
- Frequency 1 in 1000

Table 7.5: Sex chromosome aneuploidies

Syndrome	Main features
Klinefelter (47, XXY)	Small testes, poorly developed secondary sexual characteristics, gynecomastia, infertility. May be mild reduction in verbal skills. Frequency 1 in 1000 male births.
XYY male	Largely asymptomatic. Often tall. May be behavioral problems in later life. Frequency 1 in 1000 male births.
Turner (45, X)	Short stature, webbed neck, primary amenorrhea, lack of secondary sexual characteristics, often coarctation of aorta. Frequency 1 in 5000 female births.
Trisomy x (47, XXX)	Largely asymptomatic, but 20% mildly mentally handicapped. Frequency 1 in 1000 female births.

Table 7.6: Common autosomal aneuploidies

Syndrome	Main features
Down syndrome (trisomy 21)	Flat profile, small nose, upward-slanting eyes, low-set ears. Single palmar (simian) crease in 50%. Floppiness in neonate. IQ usually less than 50. Congenital heart malformations and reduced life expectancy in 40%.
Trisomy 18 (Edwards syndrome)	Characteristic skull with small chin and prominent forehead, low-set ears. Clenched hands with overlapping index and fifth fingers, single palmar crease, rockerbottom feet. Frequent malformations of heart, kidney and other organs.
Trisomy 13 (Patau syndrome)	Cleft lip and palate, polydactyly, small head and close-set tiny eyes, abnormal ears, scalp defects. Frequent congenital heart disease.

Table 7.7: Other examples of abnormal development of reproductive system

Genetic state	Gonad	Mullerian duct	Wolffian duct	External genitalia
XY, loss of X linked gene for androgen receptor	Testis	Regressed	Regressed	Female
XY, deficient testosterone synthesis	Testis	Regressed	Regressed to varying degree	Male or female
XY, deficient 5 alpha reductase	Testis	Regressed	Developed	Male or female
XX, adrenal 11 or 21 hydroxylase deficiency	Ovary	Developed	Regressed	Male or female

Turner's Syndrome

In Turner's syndrome, the individual will have 45 chromosomes with XO karyotype. They will have no gonadal development during fetal life and the person will be phenotypic female at birth. Due to the absence of ovarian follicles, such females have very low levels of estrogen, primary amenorrhea and do not undergo pubertal changes.

Salient Features of Turner's Syndrome

- 45, XO
- Bilateral streak gonads

- Phenotypic female
- Short stature
- Webbed neck
- Primary amenorrhea
- Lack of secondary sexual characteristics
- Frequency 1 in 2500

The XXX karyotype is "super female".

- Trisomy X (47, XXX)
- Largely asymptomatic
- 20% mildly mentally handicapped
- Frequency 1 in 1000

Frequency of incidence is next to XXY (Klinefelter's syndrome).

Non-disjunction of chromosome 21 produces trisomy 21, the chromosome associated with Down's syndrome (mongolism). The incidence increases sharply with advancing maternal age, particularly for mothers over 35 years.

Kallmann's syndrome is a genetic condition where the primary symptom is a failure to start puberty or a failure to fully complete it. It occurs in both males and females and has the additional symptoms of:

- Hypogonadism
- Delayed puberty
- Suffer from anosmia
- Deficiency in FSH and LH secretion
- Cause for deficiency—failure of GnRH neurons to migrate from olfactory bulb to hypothalamus
- May also suffer from color blindness, nerve deafness, renal abnormalities, cryptorchidism, amenorrhea, lack of secondary sex characteristics, and breast development.

Pseudohermaphroditism

Female

1. Congenital virilizing hyperplasia of fetus
2. Maternal androgen excess
3. Virilizing ovarian tumors

Male

1. Androgen resistance
2. Defective testicular development
3. Congenital 17α-hydroxylase deficiency

Precocious Puberty

- More common in girls than in boys
- Hypothalamic tumors
- Precocious pseudopuberty
- No gametogenesis
- Androgen/estrogen secreting tumors
- Congenital virilizing adrenal hyperplasia

Precocious Pseudopuberty

- No gametogenesis
- Androgen/estrogen secreting tumors
- Congenital virilizing adrenal hyperplasia

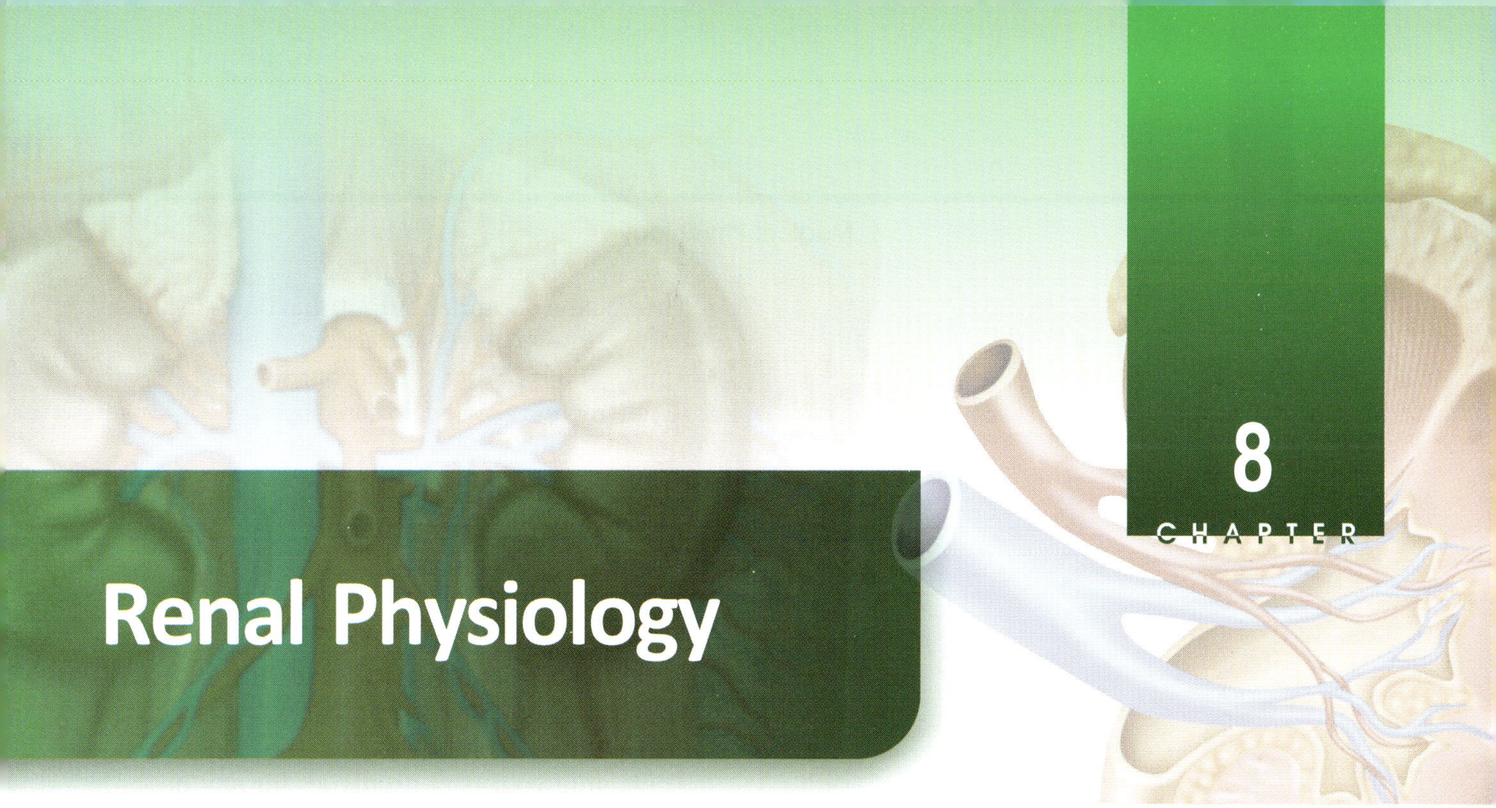

Renal Physiology

Renal physiology deals with the structure and function of kidney and the urinary tract. The structures included in the renal physiology are:

a. Kidneys

b. Ureters

c. Urinary bladder

d. Urethra

The function of the kidney is to maintain homeostasis. Homeostasis includes:

1. Regulation of osmolality and volume of fluids in the body.

2. Regulation of electrolytes concentration.

3. Regulation of acid-base balance.

4. Excretion of metabolic waste products.

5. Secretion of certain hormones like active form of vitamin D, renin and erythropoietin.

Structure of Kidney (Fig. 8.1)

- Each kidney weighs about 150 gm.

- Situated in the abdomen in the posterior part on either side of vertebral column outside the peritoneum (retroperitoneal).

- Kidney is a bean-shaped organ with a hilus directed medially. At the hilus, ureters, renal arteries, renal veins, nerves and lymph vessels either enter or leave the kidney.

- Both the kidneys together receive blood flow of about 1200 ml/min.

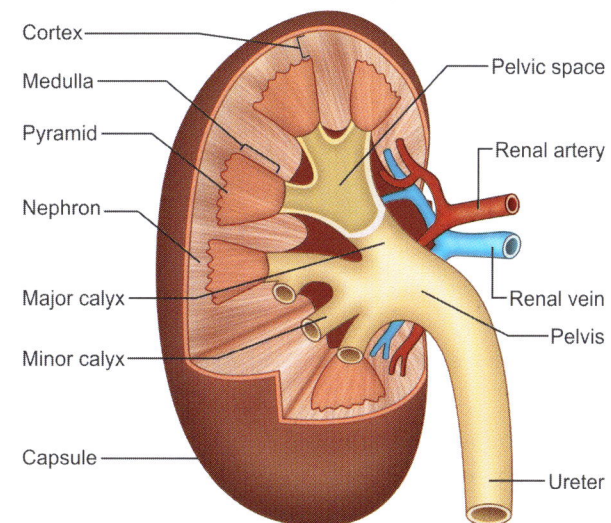

Fig. 8.1: Section of kidney showing important structures

Nephron (Fig. 8.2)

- It is the structural and functional unit of kidney.

- In each kidney, there are about 1 million nephrons.

- The two main parts of nephrons are:
  a. Renal corpuscle, and
  b. Renal tubules.

- The renal corpuscle in turn is made up of
  a. Tuft of capillaries
  b. Bowman's capsule.

Renal tubules are composed of:

a. Proximal convoluted tubule (PCT)

b. Loop of Henle (LH)

211

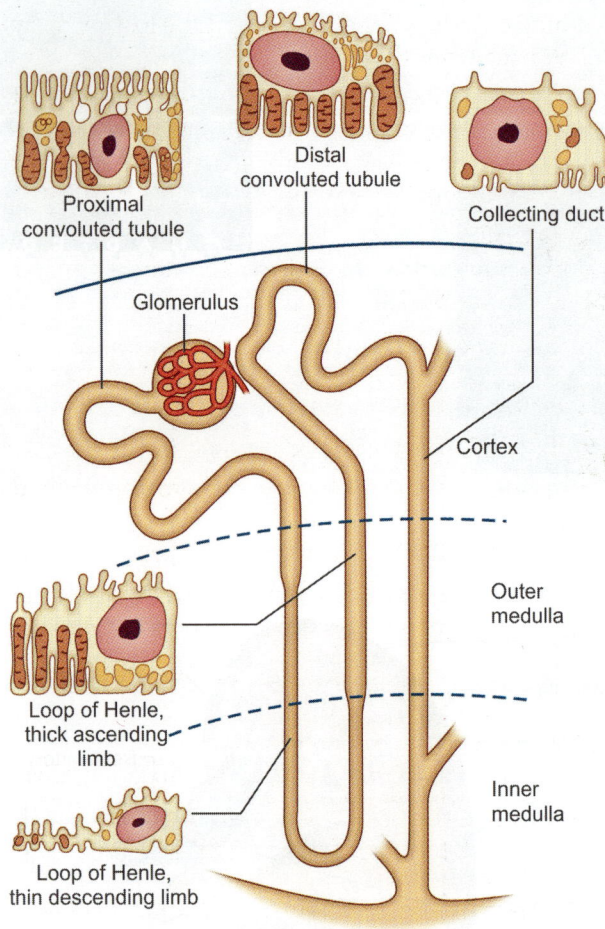

Fig. 8.2: Parts of nephron and epithelial cells lining various parts of renal tubules

c. Distal convoluted tubule (DCT)
d. Collecting duct (CD).

There are two types of nephrons namely cortical and juxtamedullary nephrons (Table 8.1).

Renal Blood Flow

- Kidneys together receive blood flow about 1200 ml/min.

- The fraction of cardiac output, that flows to kidneys only, is known as renal fraction.
- This is about 25% of cardiac output.
  Renal fraction can be calculated using the following formula:

$$\text{Renal fraction} = \frac{\text{Renal blood flow}}{\text{Cardiac output}} \times 100 = ...\%$$

Special Features/Peculiarities of Renal Circulation

1. *Renal fraction* is about 25% and this is essential because kidneys are concerned with homeostasis regulation in the body.

2. There are two sets of capillaries for any nephron. One set namely glomerular capillaries take part in filtration and the other set of capillaries accompanying the renal tubules take part in reabsorption and secretion.

3. *High pressure area in the glomerular capillaries* (Fig. 8.3): Hydrostatic pressure in almost all the capillaries in the body is around 35 mm Hg whereas in the glomerular capillaries it is about 50 mm Hg. This high pressure facilitates better filtration of plasma in the nephrons.

4. *Uneven distribution of blood in kidney* about 90% of blood flows through cortex when compared to medullary region which receives only about 7–9% of renal blood flow. This is essential as most of the nephrons are in cortex and functionally the blood flow is better suited as well.

5. *The efferent arteriolar lumen diameter* is less than the afferent arteriolar lumen diameter and hence this ensures a greater hydrostatic pressure in the tuft of capillaries. This is very essential to achieve filtration.

6. *Has well developed autoregulation* (Figs 8.4 and 8.5): Which is essential in order to prevent excessive

Table 8.1: Differences between two types of nephron	
Cortical nephrons	*Juxtamedullary nephrons*
About 85%	About 15%
Most parts of the nephron is present in cortex	Begins in cortex and most parts of the nephron is in medulla
Length of LH short	Length of LH long
Accompanied by peritubular capillary network	Accompanied by vasa recta
Has not much role in concentration of urine	Has more important role to play in concentration of urine
Exposed to interstitium of 300 mOsm/L water	Exposed to graded interstitium with osmolality from about 300 to 1200 mOsm/L water

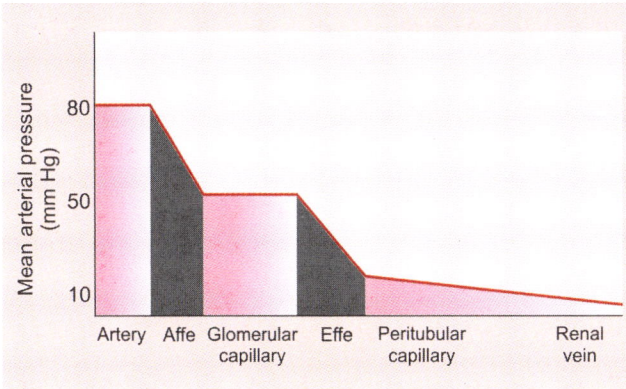

Fig. 8.3: Pressure profile in renal compartment

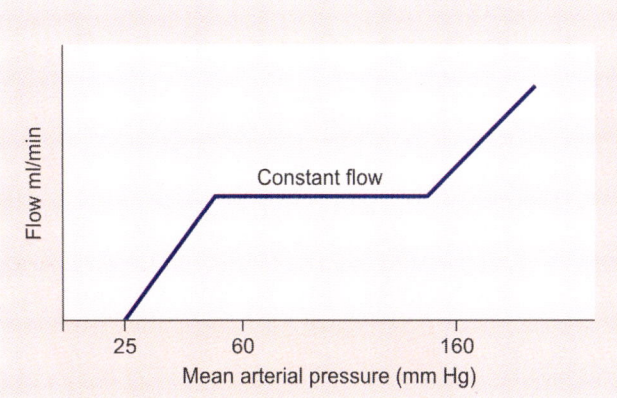

Fig. 8.4: Pressure range around which blood flow remains constant in renal compartment (autoregulation)

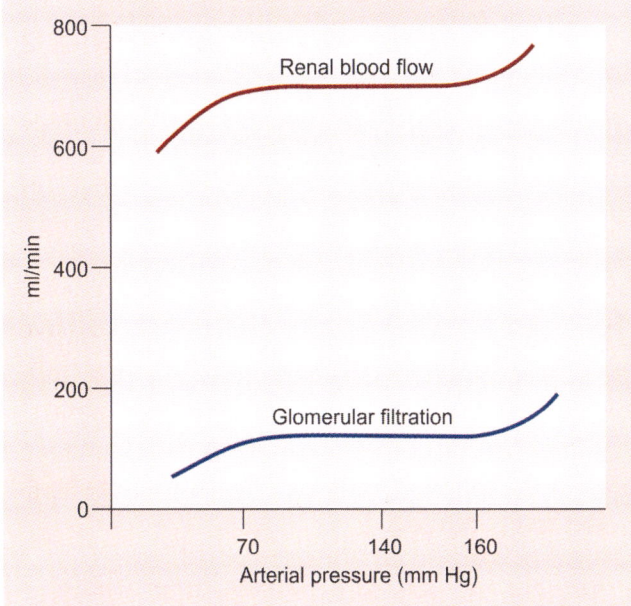

Fig. 8.5: Correlation between renal blood flow and glomerular filtration rate

flushing of kidneys and thereby undue loss of many substances from the body.

7. *The vasa recta accompanying* the loop of Henle of juxtamedullary nephrons contribute for counter-current exchanger mechanism that is a must for concentration of urine.

8. *The specialized myoepithelial cells* of the arterioles contribute for the formation of juxtaglomerular apparatus, which has vital role to play in renin-angiotensin system.

Measurement of Renal Blood Flow

- Can be done based on Fick's principle.
- The substance used is para-aminohippuric acid (PAH).
- Para-aminohippuric acid clearance value has to be calculated first based on the following formula (more details about the clearance concept (value) is given later):

$$\text{Clearance value} = \frac{U \times V}{P}$$

U = concentration of substance in urine (mg/ml)
P = concentration of substance in plasma (mg/ml)
V = volume of urine formed per minute (ml/min)

Assuming that $U = 6.3$ mg/ml, $P = 0.01$ mg/ml and $V = 1$ ml/min

The calculation will be $\dfrac{6.3 \times 1}{0.01} = 630$ ml

Clearance value of PAH is 630 ml/min.

This is known as effective renal plasma flow. In order to calculate the total renal plasma flow, the extraction ratio must be known. To calculate the extraction ratio, the following formula is required:

$$\text{Extraction ratio} = \frac{\text{Quantity of substance extracted}}{\begin{array}{c}\text{Quantity of substance available}\\\text{for extraction}\end{array}}$$

For PAH, it is about 0.9 which means that about 90% of PAH is removed from the circulating plasma and excreted along with urine.

So the total renal plasma flow will be (TRPF)

$$TRPF = \frac{\text{Effective renal plasma flow}}{\text{Extraction ratio}}$$

$$= \frac{630}{0.9} = 700 \text{ ml}$$

From the above we are able to calculate the renal blood flow using the following formula:

$$\text{Renal blood flow} = \frac{TRPF \times 1}{(1 - PCV)}$$

Assuming *PCV* as 40% the calculation will be

$$\frac{700 \times 1}{(1-0.4)} = \text{about 1200 ml/min}$$

Factors influencing blood flow to the kidney are:

- Sympathetic stimulation most important.
- Factors stimulating vasomotor center.
- Bacterial toxins.

Glomerular Filtration Rate

- It is the rate at which filtration occurs in all the 2 million nephrons per minute.
- It is the volume of total plasma getting filtered per minute in both the kidneys.
- The type of filtration is known as ultrafiltration as all substances present in plasma is filtered except for plasma proteins.
- Normally, it is about 125 ml/min (±10%).
- Filtration fraction is the ratio between GFR and RPF (volume of plasma filtered to the volume of plasma flowing through the kidneys per minute) and is about 0.16–0.2.

Filtration Membrane (Fig. 8.6)

1. Innermost layer is the fenestrated endothelial cell lining.
2. Middle layer is basement membrane having negative charges on it.
3. Outer most layer is the epithelial cell lining of Bowman's capsule (finger-like projections called pedicles and hence the name podocytes).

Determination of GFR

- It is based on clearance concept.
- In clinical practice, creatinine clearance value is considered.
- In experimental situation, it can be calculated by determining inulin clearance value.

Clearance concept: It states that the volume of plasma losing (getting cleared off) a particular substance in one minute.

$$\text{Clearance value} = \frac{U \times V}{P}$$

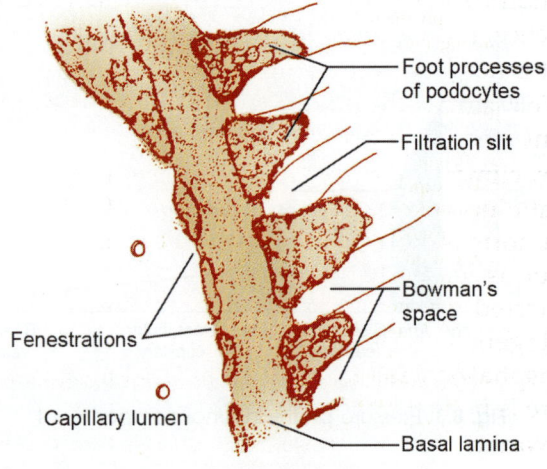

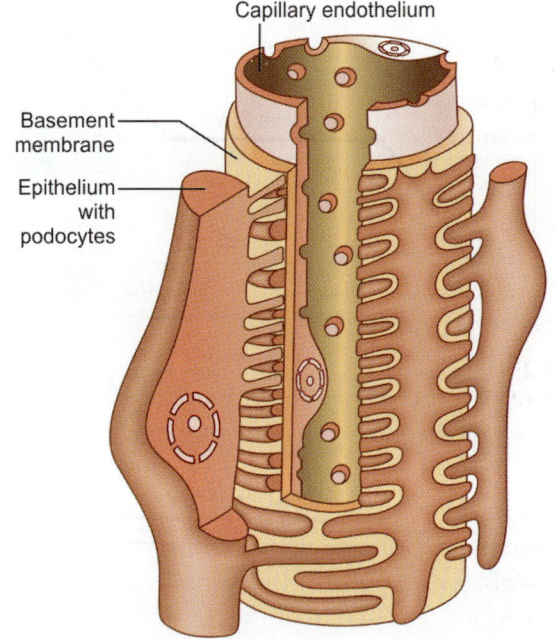

Fig. 8.6: Details of filtration membrane

U = concentration of substance in urine (mg/ml)
P = concentration of substance in plasma (mg/ml)
V = volume of urine formed per minute (ml/min)

Substances used for determination of GFR should possess the following criteria. The substance should:

1. Get freely filtered.
2. Neither reabsorbed nor secreted.
3. Not alter the renal blood flow or GFR.
4. Be non-toxic.
5. Not get metabolized or stored in kidney.

Inulin obeys all the above criteria, but still in clinical practice, it is not used because:

a. It is not produced in the body.

b. To maintain the plasma concentration, it should be injected in a controlled way.

In clinical practice, GFR is determined by using creatinine clearance value and is about 140 ml/min in a normal person. Though the creatinine clearance value is about 10% more than the GFR, still it is preferred for the simple reason that creatinine is an endogenously produced (end product of creatine phosphate metabolism in muscles) substance and there is no necessity to inject in a controlled way.

Normal clearance value of some of the important substances will be as under:

a. Glucose — 0 ml/min
b. Urea — 70 ml/min
c. Inulin — 125 ml/min
d. Creatinine — 140 ml/min
e. Para-aminohippuric acid — 630 ml/min

If the clearance value of any substance is:

- More than that of GFR it means the substance is secreted (partially or completely).
- Equal to that of GFR means the substance is neither reabsorbed nor secreted.
- Less than that of GFR means the substance has got reabsorbed (partially or completely).

Factors responsible/determining GFR:

$GFR = K, S, EFP$

K = permeability constant

S = surface area available for filtration.

EFP = effective or net filtration pressure.

Permeability (Fig. 8.7) of the filtration membrane for any substance to get filtered depends on the:

1. Molecular charge the substance carries.
2. Molecular size of the substance.

Based on the size of the substance, the permeability will be as under:

- <4 nm substance has maximum permeability.
- Between 4 and 8 nm substance has moderate permeability.
- >8 nm substance has least permeability.

Based on the molecular charge, the substance carries the permeability will be:

- Substance carrying +ve charge has maximum permeability.

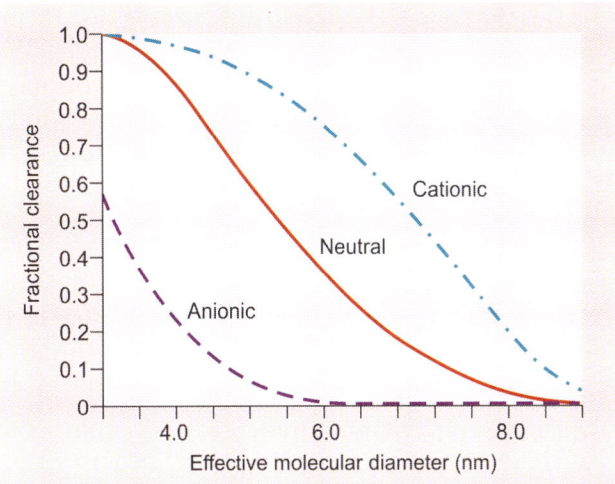

Fig. 8.7: Relative permeability of the substances

- Substance carrying neutral charge has moderate permeability.
- Substance carrying –ve charge has least permeability.

Dextran substance having same molecular size but different charge on it can be used to test the role of molecular charge on the filterability of the substance across the membrane.

Surface area available for filtration is about 0.8 square meters.

Effective Filtration Pressure (EFP) or Net Filtration Pressure

It is the net pressure acting across the filtration membrane and is responsible for filtration.

So, effective filtration pressure is the resultant of the following:

- Hydrostatic pressure in glomerular capillary
- Hydrostatic pressure in Bowman's capsule
- Colloidal osmotic pressure in glomerular capillary
- Colloidal osmotic pressure in Bowman's capsule

The effective filtration pressure can be deduced from the following formula:

$$EFP = (HP_{GC} - HP_{BC}) - (\Pi_{GC} - \Pi_{BC})$$

Wherein

HP_{GC} the hydrostatic pressure in glomerular capillaries, exerted by blood flowing through the capillaries and is the out driving force. This favors filtration.

HP_{BC} is the hydrostatic pressure exerted by the fluid present in the Bowman's capsule and is an opposing force. Hence opposes filtration.

Π_{GC} is the colloidal osmotic pressure exerted by the plasma proteins present in the capillary blood and is also an opposing force like HP_{BC}. Hence opposes filtration.

Π_{BC} is the colloidal osmotic pressure exerted by proteins in the Bowman's capsule and is normally 0 mm Hg as almost all plasma proteins don't get filtered. In case plasma proteins get filtered; the force exerted by the plasma proteins here will favor filtration. Since plasma with all its constituents except plasma proteins get filtered, the process of filtration at nephrons is known as ultrafiltration.

Deducing of effective filtration pressure will be:

$EFP = (HP_{GC} - HP_{BC}) - (\Pi_{GC} - \Pi_{BC})$

$= (50-15) - (25-0)$

$= (35) - (25)$

$= 10$ mm Hg

At the beginning of the filtration membrane, the effective filtration pressure will be around 10 mm Hg. As the filtration proceeds along the filtration membrane, the relative increase in the plasma protein concentration in the tuft of capillaries will also increase the colloidal osmotic pressure and hence the effective filtration pressure goes on decreasing. By the time blood has traversed about 60% length of the filtration membrane, the effective filtration pressure will have become 0 mm Hg (Fig. 8.8). Hence by about 60% of the length of filtration membrane, the equilibration point is achieved and no more filtration is possible beyond this point. The shifting of the equilibration point to right side facilitates more surface area available for filtration in any exigencies.

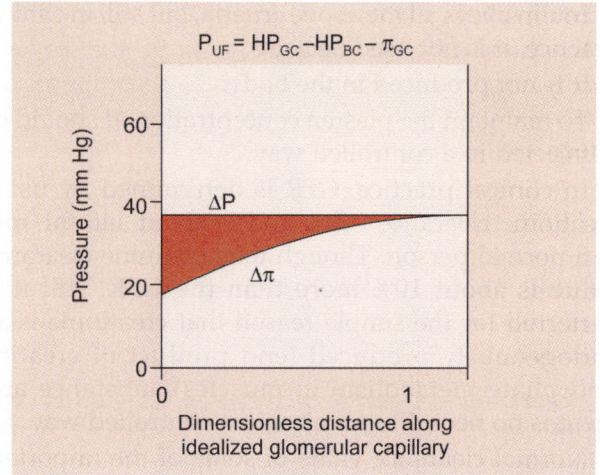

Fig. 8.8: Effective filtration pressure profile along the filtration membrane

Factors affecting Effective Filtration Pressure (Table 8.2)

HP_{GC} whenever increases will increase the GFR. When there is vasoconstriction of the efferent arteriole, it increases HP_{GC} and hence GFR. On the contrary, a decrease of HP_{GC} will decrease the GFR as seen in hemorrhage, dehydration, etc. (hypovolemic state).

HP_{BC} increase will decrease the EFP and hence the GFR. This occurs when there is obstruction to the urinary tract. One of the common conditions in which this occurs is when there is block in ureters due to renal stone (nephrolithiasis).

Π_{GC} decreases in conditions, like nephrotic syndrome, glomerulonephritis, the loss of plasma

Table 8.2: Factors affecting GFR, renal plasma flow and filtration fraction			
Effect	GFR	Renal plasma flow	Filtration fraction (GFR/RPF)
Afferent arteriole constriction	Decreased due to decrease in HP_{GC}	Decreased	No change
Afferent arteriole dilation	Increased due to increase in HP_{GC}	Increased	No change
Efferent arteriole constriction	Increased due to increase in HP_{GC}	Decreased	Increased
Increased plasma protein concentration	Decreased due to increase in	No change	Decreased
Decreased plasma protein concentration	Increased due to decrease in	No change	Increased
Constriction of ureter or urinary obstruction	Decreased due to increase in HP_{BC}	No change	Decreased

proteins in kidney and hence GFR increases. On the other hand in burns due to loss of fluid part of plasma without plasma proteins brings about a relative increase of Π_{GC} and hence glomerular filtration rate decreases.

Strong sympathetic stimulation causes constriction of both the afferent and efferent arterioles. If the afferent arteriolar constriction is more than efferent, it leads to decrease of GFR and vice versa, if efferent arteriolar constriction is more than that of afferent arteriole.

One other important factor, which affects the GFR, is the renal blood flow. But in the renal circulation, there is well-developed autoregulation with respect to renal blood flow. Hence, normally when BP increases from 60 to about 160 mm Hg there will not be any variation in the renal blood flow and hence even the GFR will also be kept constant.

The autoregulation of renal blood flow (Fig. 8.9) across a wide range of pressure can be explained based on the following theory:

1. *Myogenic theory*

BP $\uparrow\to\uparrow$ blood flow $\to$ increases stretching on the walls of blood vessels $\to$ this acts as a mechanical stimulus for the smooth muscle present in the walls of the arterioles $\to$ smooth muscle contracts $\to$ decreases the lumen diameter of blood vessels $\to \uparrow$ resistance and hence decreases the blood flow.

Apart from the above theory, the tissue metabolite theory and tissue fluid pressure theory also try to bring about the autoregulation of blood flow in the renal compartment.

Physiological Control of RBF and GFR

Regulation of renal blood flow can be brought about by:

1. Strong sympathetic stimulation.
2. Hormones like angiotensin II ADH in pharmacological doses and noradrenaline is vasoconstrictor and hence reduces the blood flow. On the other hand prostaglandin, bradykinin, etc. are vasodilators and increase the blood flow.

Autoregulation of GFR can be brought about by tubuloglomerular feedback (Fig. 8.10), according to which when there is:

$\uparrow$ RBF $\to\uparrow$ GFR $\to\uparrow$ filtered load of sodium $\to$ leads to more sodium reaching DCT $\to\uparrow$ activity of JGA $\to\uparrow$ vasoconstriction of afferent arterioles $\to\downarrow$ blood flow through the glomerulus and hence decrease of GFR (Fig. 8.10).

Filtered load: It is the amount of substance getting filtered in all the 2 million nephrons per minute. This can be calculated as follows:

Filtered load = Conc. substance in × GFR (ml/min)
plasma (mg/ml)

Supposing, the plasma glucose level is 100 mg%, the concentration of glucose in 1 ml of plasma will be 1 mg. Assuming that the GFR is 125 ml/min, the filtered load of glucose will be

Filtered load = 1 × 125 = 125 mg/min

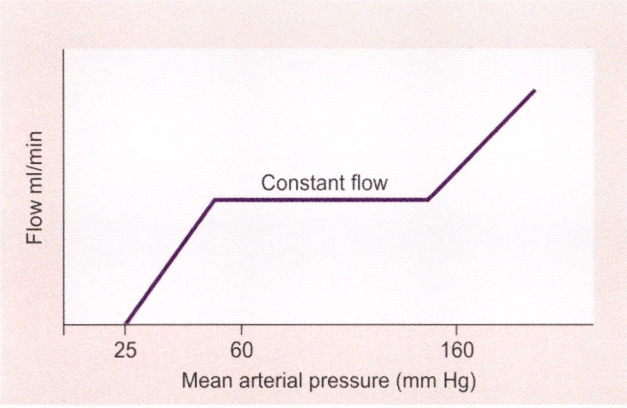

Fig. 8.9: Graph showing autoregulation

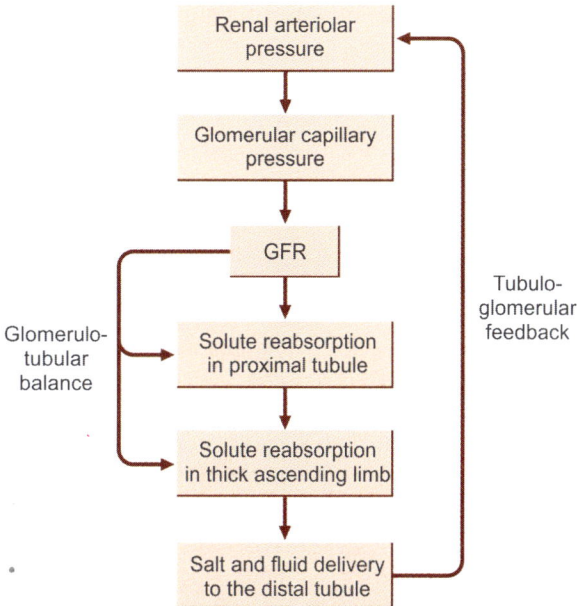

Fig. 8.10: GFR regulation by tubulo-glomerular feedback mechanism

Functions of Renal Tubules

The renal tubules are able to bring about a drastic alteration in the quality and quantity of the filtrate by the following process:

a. Reabsorption.

b. Secretion.

c. Concentration.

d. Acidification.

The ability of the renal tubules is essential for the fine processing of the filtrate which is essential for proper and functioning of the kidneys. Methods available to study tubular functions:

a. *Micropipette technique* wherein small volume of filtrate from the certain parts of the tubules can be taken to assess the composition of the same.

b. *Stop flow technique* in which by certain method, the flow of fluid is stopped and composition of the substance is ascertained before stopping the flow and next after the flow has been reestablished.

c. *Microcryoscopy* in which small slices of kidney tissue are taken starting from the cortical to deep into the medulla is taken and the freezing point of the different slices is checked.

How to calculate the quantity of substance reabsorbed or secreted?

Quantity of substance reabsorbed

    = Filtered load – quantity of sub. excreted

    = ..mg/min

Quantity of sub. secreted

    = Excreted quantity – filtered load

    =.... mg/min

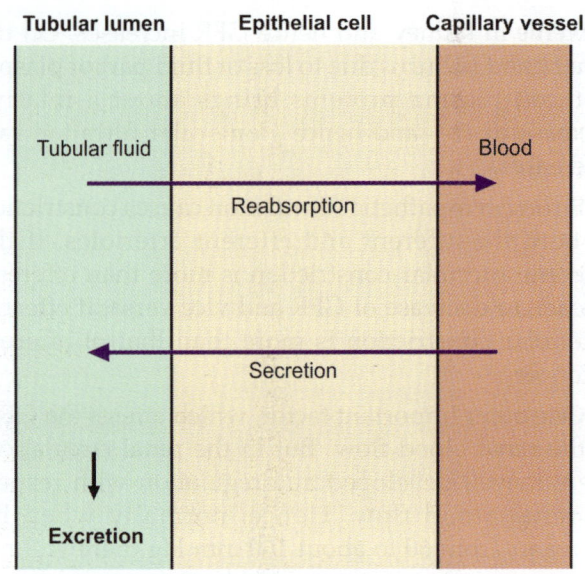

Fig. 8.11: Modulation of filtrate in renal tubules by the process of reabsorption and secretion and final excretion of urine

Concept of Tubular Reabsorption and Secretion (Fig. 8.11 and Table 8.3)

Reabsorption is the process by which substances are brought back into capillary from the tubular lumen.

Secretion is the process by which substances get added on further into the tubular lumen from the accompanying capillary.

Reabsorption of substances in renal tubules can be brought about by any of the following mechanisms:

1. Passive reabsorption is where the reabsorption is along the electrical/concentration gradient or both. Energy is not required here.

Table 8.3: Handling of some of the substances (reabsorption and/or secretion) when the filtrate proceeds through renal tabules

| Substance | Filtered | Per 24 hours | | | |
		Reabsorbed	Secreted	Excreted	Percentage reabsorbed
Na$^+$ (mEq)	26,000	25,850		150	99.4
K$^+$ (mEq)	600	560[2]	50[2]	90	93.3
Cl$^-$ (mEq)	18,000	17,850		150	99.2
HCO$_3^-$ (mEq)	4,900	4,900		0	100
Urea (mmol)	870	460[3]		410	53
Creatinine (mmol)	12	1[4]	1[4]	12	
Uric acid (mmol)	50	49	4	5	98
Glucose (mmol)	800	800		0	100
Total solute (mosm)	54,000	53,400	100	700	98.9
Water (ml)	180,000	179,000		1000	99.4

2. Active reabsorption is where the reabsorption occurs against the electrical/concentration gradient or both. This type of reabsorption requires the expenditure of energy.

3. Simple diffusion wherein there is movement of substances across the cell through the special pores/channels.

4. Carrier-mediated/facilitated diffusion wherein the substance binds to special protein molecules on the cell membrane during their movement into the cell. Carrier mediated may be:

   a. Antiport/countertransport—which brings about the transport of two different substances by the same carrier in opposing directions.

   b. Symport/co-transport—which helps in transport of two different substances by the same carrier in the same direction.

Primary active transport means the energy spent is directly related to the substance that is getting reabsorbed, e.g. sodium reabsorption.

Secondary active transport means the energy spent for the reabsorption of some substance help in reabsorption of certain other substance, e.g. glucose reabsorption (secondary active transport) is due to the primary active reabsorption of sodium.

While reabsorption, substances can pass (Fig. 8.12):
1. Across the cell (transcellular) or
2. At the junction of the adjacent cells (paracellular).

Renal threshold is the concentration of substance in plasma beyond which the substance starts getting excreted in urine.

Tubular maximum (transport maximum) is the maximum ability of renal tubules either to reabsorb or secrete any substance in one minute.

Substances Reabsorbed in PCT

1. Sodium

- About two-thirds of filtered sodium is reabsorbed here. Irrespective of the amount of sodium filtered, the % reabsorption of filtered sodium is constant in PCT. This is termed as glomerulotubular balance.
- An active process brings about sodium reabsorption.
- Some amount of sodium reabsorption is by symport (with glucose) and some amount by antiport (in exchange for H^+) mechanism (Fig. 8.13).

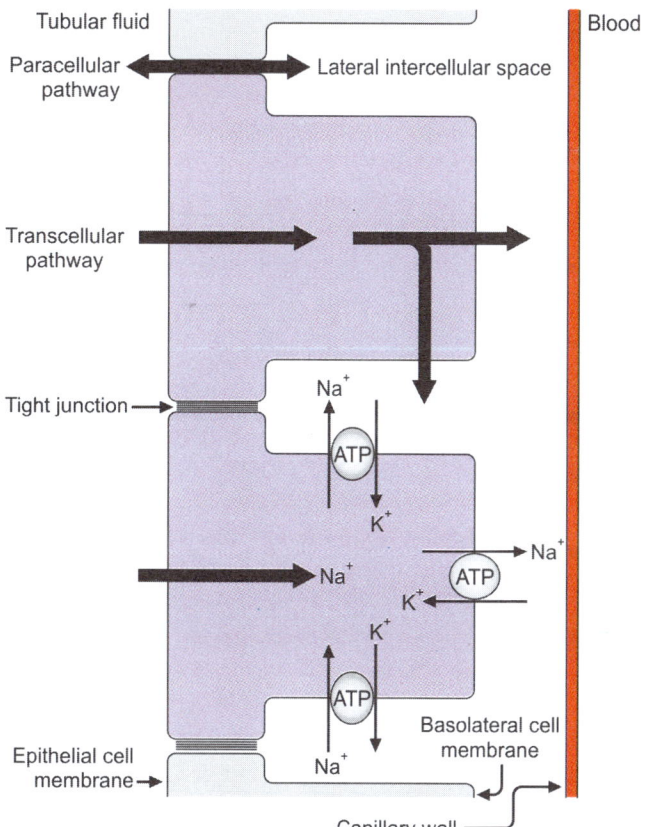

Fig. 8.12: Reabsorption of substances through the transcellular and paracellular pathways across the luminal surface of the epithelial cells in renal tubules

- During reabsorption, sodium moves from the tubular lumen into the epithelial cells along electrochemical gradient.
- From the epithelial cell into the interstitium, an active process involving sodium–potassium ATPase pumps it. For three sodium ions pumped out, two potassium ions are brought in. The sodium–potassium pump activity can be inhibited by ouabain.
- Some amount of sodium ions extruded into the interstitium and chloride moves passively with the sodium. The chloride in the cells will be replenished by the diffusion of chloride from the tubular lumen into the epithelial cells. This pump is known as electrogenic sodium pump. This pump activity can be inhibited by substance, like ethacrynic acid.
- The activity of this pump tries to maintain low sodium inside the cell and also tries to maintain the electrical gradient necessary for the sodium to move from the lumen into the epithelial cell.

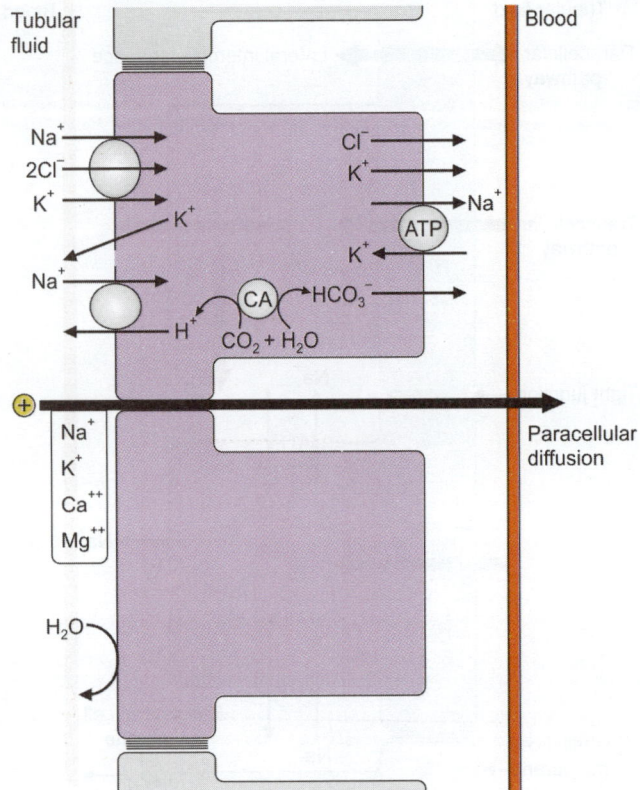

Fig. 8.13: Sodium (by symport and antiport mechanism) and chloride reabsorption and secretion of potassium and hydrogen ions in PCT

- From the interstitium, sodium enters the capillary accompanying the renal tubules by a passive process because of Starling's forces.

2. Glucose Reabsorption (Fig. 8.14)

- It occurs only in proximal convoluted tubule.
- It is brought about by symport mechanism.
- It occurs because of co-transport with sodium.
- It is by a secondary active transport as the energy spent for sodium reabsorption helps in binding of sodium to the carrier protein, which in turn facilitates the binding of glucose to the carrier.
- From the epithelial cell, glucose diffuses into the interstitium and from here it finally diffuses into the peritubular capillary blood.
- Normally glucose is not excreted in the urine and hence the glucose clearance value is 0 ml/min.
- The renal threshold for glucose is 180 mg% (Fig. 8.15) and the tubular maximum for glucose is 375 mg/min.

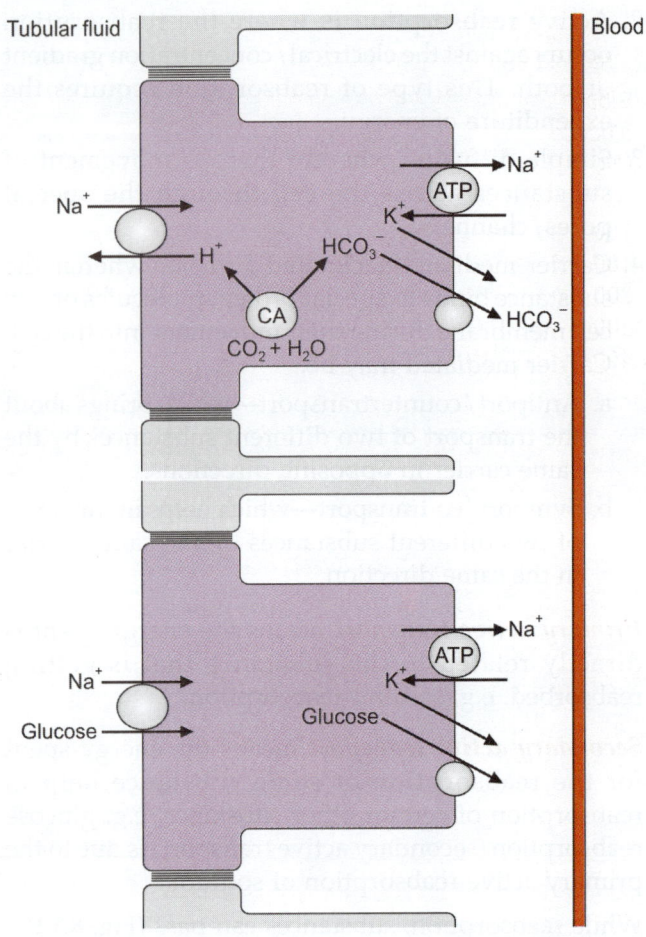

Fig. 8.14: The reabsorption of glucose by symport mechanism

Assuming that GFR is 125 ml/min, the following representative values (Table 8.4) can be taken to understand what would happen to the amount of glucose reabsorption in PCT and the amount of glucose excreted in urine for varying blood glucose levels.

Even though TmG for glucose is 375 mg/min and filtered load is less than TmG, still glucose starts appearing in the urine (renal splay) when the plasma glucose level exceeds 180 mg% is for the following reasons:

a. Though TmG is taken as 375 mg/min, all the two million nephrons will not have the same TmG.

b. The volume of filtrate formed in all the 2 million nephrons will not be the same.

Presence of glucose in the urine, the condition is known as glycosuria. Glucose starts getting excreted when blood glucose level exceeds the renal threshold of 180 mg%.

Table 8.4: Representative values used to drive home renal threshold and tubular maximum

Blood glucose (mg %)	Filtered load (mg/min)	Amount of glucose excreted (mg/min)	Amount of glucose re-absorbed (mg/min)
100	125	0	125
180	225	0	225
200	250	10	240
300	375	80	295
400	500	125	375

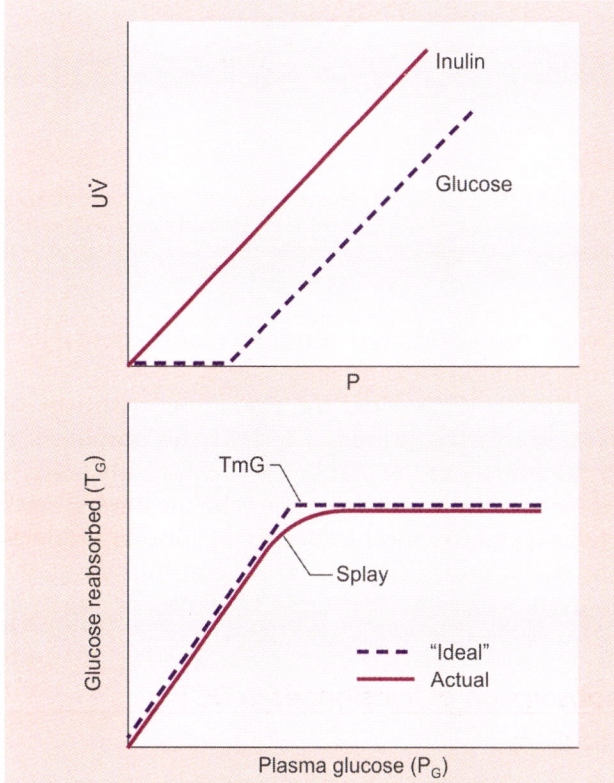

Fig. 8.15: Graph at the top showing the renal threshold for glucose when compared to inulin. Graph at the bottom showing the renal splay for glucose

One of the common conditions in which glycosuria occurs is diabetes mellitus. Other examples are alimentary and renal glycosuria.

3. Bicarbonate Reabsorption (Fig. 8.16)

- From the tubular lumen into the epithelial cell, bicarbonate enters as carbon dioxide and not as bicarbonate.

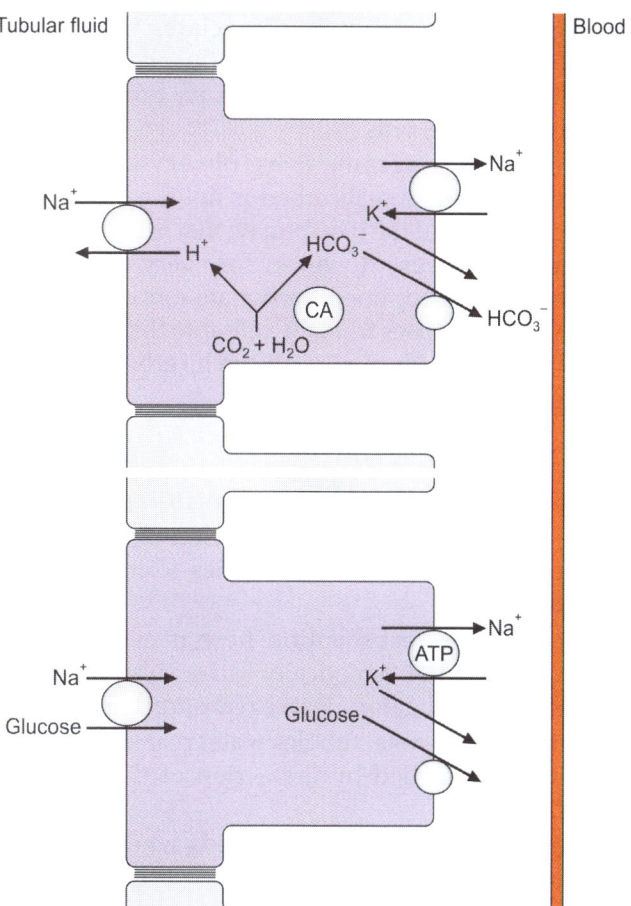

Fig. 8.16: The reactions involved in the process of bicarbonate reabsorption

- Inside the cell, carbon dioxide reacts with water in presence of carbonic anhydrase and brings about the formation of carbonic acid. This apart the carbon dioxide produced because of the metabolic activity of the cell also can react with water inside the cell to bring about the production of carbonic acid.
- This acid immediately dissociates into bicarbonate and hydrogen ion.
- Bicarbonate ion diffuses from cell into the interstitium and ultimately enters capillary accompanying the renal tubules.
- The hydrogen ion is secreted into the tubular lumen by antiport mechanism. During process of secretion of hydrogen ion, one sodium ion gets reabsorbed.
- The hydrogen ion that has entered the tubular lumen reacts with bicarbonate present in the tubular lumen and forms carbonic acid.

- This acid immediately dissociates into carbon dioxide and water under the influence of carbonic anhydrase present in the brush border of the tubular lining cells.

From the diagram, it is observed that the bicarbonate that is reabsorbed is not the bicarbonate that is filtered but the bicarbonate that is found within the epithelial cells. However, for every bicarbonate ion that is filtered, one bicarbonate ion is formed in the cells and diffuses from the cells into the peritubular capillary blood. Normally, all the bicarbonate that is filtered will be reabsorbed.

4. Water Reabsorption

- About 75% of filtered water is reabsorbed here.
- Will be secondary to reabsorption of osmotically active substance and hence tries to maintain the osmolality.
- Since water reabsorption here is secondary to reabsorption of osmotically active substances, it is known as obligatory water reabsorption.
- In this part of renal tubules water reabsorption will not be controlled by the action of the hormone ADH.

Obligatory water reabsorption is when reabsorption of water is:

- Secondary to reabsorption of some of osmotically active substances, like sodium, glucose.
- Primarily to maintain the osmolarity of plasma.
- Not influenced by the action of any of the hormones.
- Not affected by the body water content and ADH has no role to play in water reabsorption here.
- Obligatory water reabsorption occurs in proximal convoluted tubule only.

5. Urea

- Reabsorption occurs mostly in the proximal tubules.
- However, the amount of urea reabsorbed is limited when compared to other substances.
- Hence the urea clearance value is about 70 ml/min.
- Reabsorption occurs by a process of passive diffusion along concentration gradient.
- There is some amount of recycling of urea between the collecting duct, interstitium and the ascending limb of loop of Henle. This recycling helps in the concentration of urine. For concentration of urine

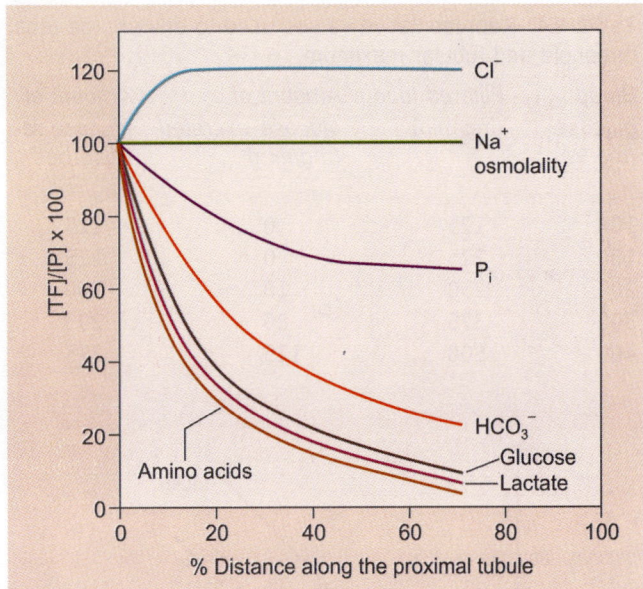

Fig. 8.17: In the graph, the concentration of various substances in the tubular fluid has been shown at the end of PCT when compared with the concentration at the beginning of PCT (which is nothing but plasma concentration)

to be brought about a hyperosmotic medullary interstitium has to be maintained.

Figure 8.17 indicating the concentration of substance in the tubular fluid when compared to plasma almost at the end of PCT. If the substance is reabsorbed, the line in the graph is below the 100 mark as the substance concentration in the tubular fluid has gone down and if the line in the graph is above the 100 mark, it means that there is relative increase in the concentration of the substance.

Reabsorption of Substances in DCT

1. Sodium

- It is influenced by the action of hormones aldosterone, atrial natriuretic peptide. Aldosterone hormone increases sodium reabsorption.
- It is by the antiport mechanism.
- Reabsorption will always be in exchange for either potassium or hydrogen ion that is secreted.
- It is also by an active process.

2. Calcium

- Reabsorption is always influenced by action of hormones PTH, calcitonin and 1, 25-DHCC.
- PTH and 1, 25-DHCC increase the reabsorption whereas calcitonin decreases the same.

3. Water

- Most of water reabsorption here is influenced by the action of hormone ADH.
- It is dependent on body water content. If the body water content is more, less water will be reabsorbed in DCT and collecting ducts.
- Reabsorption here will be independent of reabsorption of osmotically active substances.
- This type of reabsorption is known as facultative or facilitatory water reabsorption.

Facultative/Facilitatory Water Reabsorption

- It occurs in the distal convoluted tubules and collecting ducts.
- Here water reabsorption is independent of reabsorption of the other substances.
- The increase in the reabsorption will be due to the insertion of the water channels into the epithelial cells by the action of antidiuretic hormone.
- In the absence of ADH, there will be abnormal increase in the urine output, which can be as high as 22 L/day as against a normal value of 1–1.5 L/day.
- This type of diuresis is known as water diuresis.
- The extent of water reabsorbed is less when the body water content is more.

Diuresis

- Means an increased volume of urine output.
- Normally out of 125 ml of plasma filtered per minute, only 1 ml gets excreted as urine.
- In other words, per day urine output is about 1.5 L.
- When volume of urine excreted is more than normal this is termed as diuresis.

Osmotic Diuresis

- Here water excretion is secondary to the excretion of some of the osmotically active substances, like glucose (diabetes mellitus).
- Diuretics are drugs which will increase the quantity of urine formed and excreted.
- Commonly used diuretics are furosemide (lasix), ethacrynic acid and aldactone.

Water Diuresis

- Where the increased water excretion is due to faulty reabsorption of water especially in the distal parts of the renal tubules.

- One of the classical examples for this condition is deficiency of antidiuretic hormone (diabetes insipidus).
- A person can also have water diuresis when there is increased water intake.

Concentration of Urine

Concentration mechanism of urine: Depending on the body water content, the volume of water excreted from the body in the form of urine can be altered. Because of the operation of the countercurrent systems in the kidney, the concentration of the urine can be brought about.

In the kidney there are two countercurrent systems:

a. Countercurrent multiplier system contributed by the loop of Henle of the juxtamedullary nephrons

b. Countercurrent exchanger system contributed by the vasa recta.

There can be operation of these systems as countercurrent systems, due the fact that they possess the following criteria:

- Flow in the two limbs will be in opposite direction to each other.
- Flow in the two limbs will be parallel and close to each other.

Operation of the countercurrent system in these nephrons is because of the reason that there is a gradual increase in the osmolarity (Fig. 8.18) of the interstitium in the renal medulllary region reaching a peak of 1200 mOsm/L of water at the renal papilla due to the operation of the loop of Henle of juxtamedullary nephrons as countercurrent multiplier system. The loop of Henle of juxtamedullary nephrons is embedded in the hyperosmotic medullary interstitium and the length of these loops will be much when compared to the length of loop of Henle of cortical nephrons. The collecting ducts of all the nephrons pass through the medullary interstitium and contribute for concentration of urine by increasing water reabsorption. The water reabsorption at this part is due to action of antidiuretic hormone.

Countercurrent Multiplier

- During the process of concentration of urine, when the filtrate pass through the descending limb of loop of Henle of juxtamedullary nephrons, water keeps getting diffused from the tubule into the

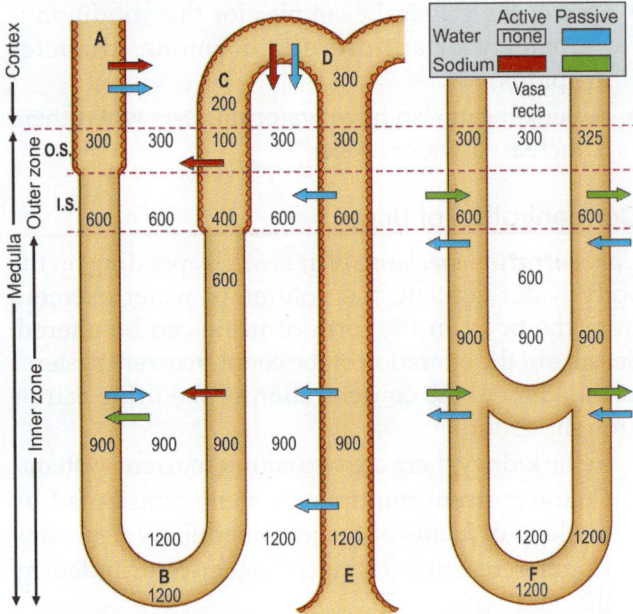

Fig. 8.18: The operation of countercurrent multiplier and exchanger mechanisms

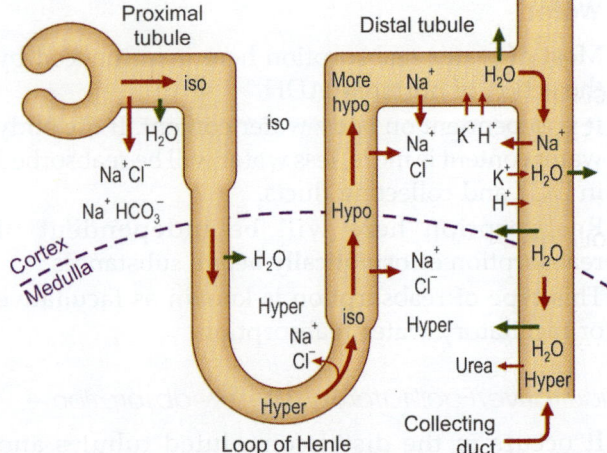

Fig. 8.19: Varying osmolarity of tubular fluid in the renal tubules of juxtaglomerular nephrons during the concentration mechanism of urine

interstitium (along the osmotic gradient) which is hyperosmotic.

- This ensures the gradual increase in the osmolality of the tubular fluid reaching equilibrium with the surrounding interstitium, due to a relative increase in the concentration of osmotically active substances in the tubular fluid. Because of this, a maximum of 1200 mOsm/L osmolality occurs in tubular fluid at the bend of the loop (Fig. 8.19).
- When the filtrate passes through the ascending part of the loop, the active co-transport of sodium, potassium and chloride into the interstitium gradually decreases the osmolality of the tubular fluid.
- The thick ascending limb of loop of Henle is impermeable to water.
- The osmolality of the filtrate reaching the beginning of distal convoluted tubules will be normally hypo-osmotic.
- Finally when this filtrate passes through the collecting duct, due to the action of antidiuretic hormone, water keeps getting reabsorbed and the urine will attain a higher osmolality.
- In addition to facilitating water reabsorption, anti-diuretic hormone will also help for urea to diffuse from the collecting duct into the interstitium. This later on diffuses into the ascending limb of loop of Henle along the concentration gradient.

- This recycling of urea contributes to the further increase in the concentration mechanism.

Countercurrent Exchanger

- Much like the loop of Henle of juxtamedullary nephrons, which is embedded in the hyperosmotic interstitium in renal medulla, the vasa recta, which accompany the renal tubules of these nephrons, are also exposed to this hyperosmotic situation (Fig. 8.20).
- Unlike the epithelial cells of renal tubules that are selectively permeable, the endothelial cell membrane lining the vasa recta is freely permeable.
- Because of this when plasma flows through the descending limb of vasa recta, there will be slight influx of ions like sodium, chloride and a simultaneous efflux of water into the interstitium.
- These processes ensure equilibration of osmolality of plasma with the interstitium.
- In the ascending limb, the reversal of the events bring about a decrease of the osmolality of plasma.
- Water gets diffused from the interstitium into the ascending limb and at the same time sodium, chloride diffuse out of the limb into the interstitium.
- This brings about a gradual decrease of the osmolality of the plasma in the ascending limb of vasa recta.
- Finally, the plasma leaving the vasa recta may have an osmolality of 325 mOsm/L as against an inflow plasma osmolality of 300 mOsm/L of water.

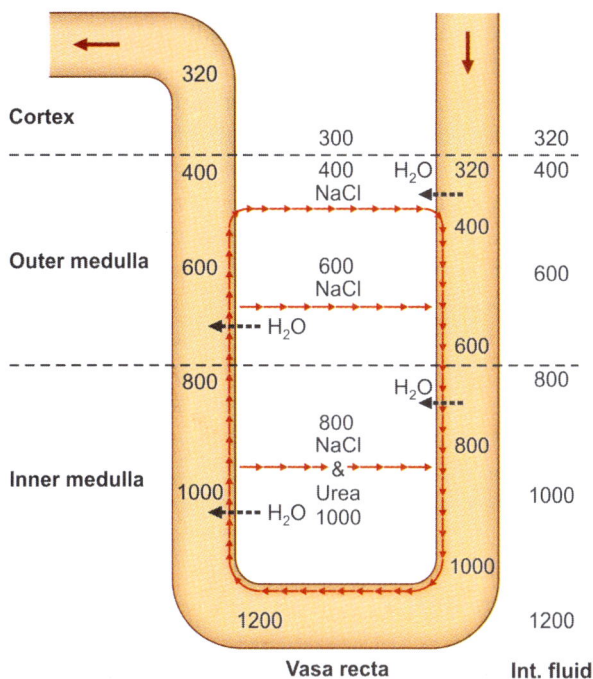

Fig. 8.20: Varying osmolarity of plasma in vasa recta during the concentration mechanism of urine

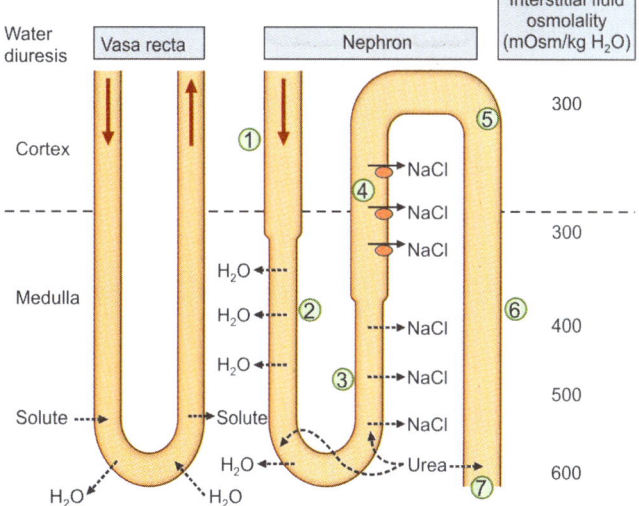

Fig. 8.21: Processes that are responsible to bring about water diuresis

In the above two diagrams, the movement of urea from the interstitium into the lumen of collecting duct or from lumen of collecting duct into the interstitium determines whether urine is diluted (Fig. 8.21) or concentrated (Fig. 8.22).

Secretion

Some of the substances are also secreted into the renal tubules at different parts. Hydrogen ion is secreted at almost all the parts of the tubules whereas potassium is secreted at distal convoluted tubules. Some amount of creatinine also gets secreted and hence the creatinine clearance value is more than glormerular filtration rate.

Diuretics are substances, which increase the urine output. Some of the commonly used diuretics are loop diuretics, spironolactone and acetazolamide. The loading of body with water can increase the urine output as well.

Regulation of pH by Kidney

• Though kidney comes into action slowly, it has got enormous power to regulate the pH more appropriately.

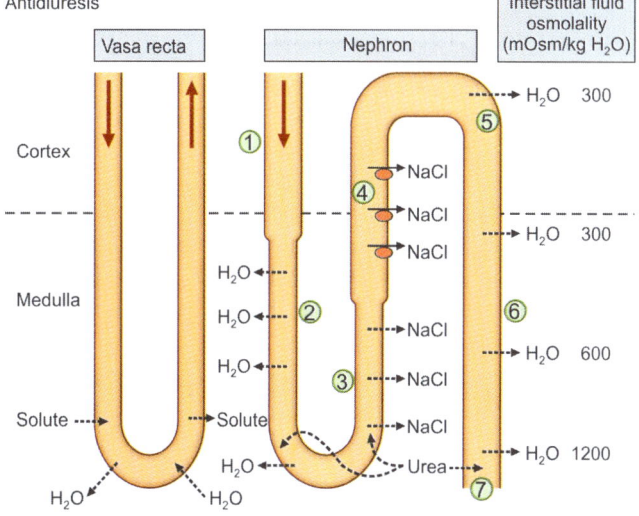

Fig. 8.22: Processes that are responsible to bring about antidiuresis

• It not only has the ability to excrete the non-volatile acids, but also has the ability to alter amount of bases excreted.
• Thereby, it helps in regulation of pH by taking care of both acids and bases of the buffer pair. The three buffer systems operating in the kidneys are (Fig. 8.23):
  a. Bicarbonate buffer system.
  b. Phosphate buffer system.
  c. Ammonia buffer system.

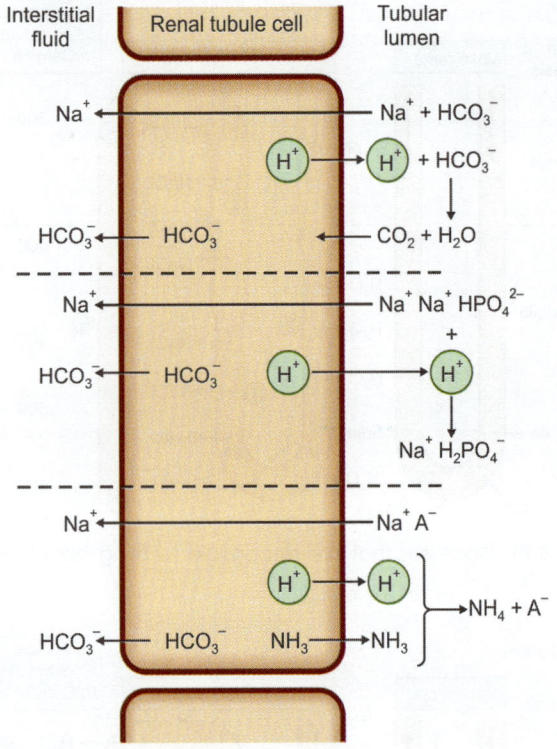

Fig. 8.23: Reactions involved during the buffering of hydrogen ions by renal tubules

Bicarbonate buffer system is most potent in the PCT and phosphate buffer system is more active in distal parts of nephrons. Ammonia buffer system operates equally in all the parts of renal tubules and among the three buffer systems; ammonia is the most efficient one. It is because the rate of ammonia secretion always parallels the rate of hydrogen ion to be excreted from the body. Most of the ammonia secreted is because of the metabolism of the amino acid glutamine. At any given time, the tubular fluid pH should never fall below 4.5, otherwise it impairs the functioning of the renal tubules and the secretion of the hydrogen ion by the renal epithelial cells cannot take place any more. Hence the ammonia buffer system operation prevents the pH from falling below 4.5.

Most of the times during 24 hours of the day, the urine pH is slightly acidic. It becomes transiently alkaline only after the heavy meal. This is termed as postprandial alkaline tide. After meal, the rate of secretion of HCl in stomach increases. Since bicarbonate enters blood from the parietal cells in exchange for chloride ions, the concentration of bicarbonate in blood increases. Hence, after meal,

kidneys excrete slightly more alkaline urine in order to restore the pH of blood.

As for bicarbonate is concerned, there is some amount of addition of new bicarbonate ion as well, because the carbon dioxide that is produced in the cells during the metabolic activity can be utilized for the synthesis of new bicarbonate ion. The new bicarbonate ion gets synthesized when hydrogen ion has to be secreted.

Hence, in acidosis, the kidneys secrete more and more of hydrogen ions and at the same time more amount of bicarbonate ions formed and added to the blood. So the ratio between bicarbonate and carbonic acid is brought back to normal 20:1. In acidosis, renal tubule cells also synthesize more amount of ammonia. This is made possible because of the activity of the enzyme glutaminase. Activity of this enzyme directly depends upon the rate of secretion of hydrogen ion.

Bicarbonate Buffer System Functioning

- In the tubular lumen, there are sodium and chloride ions.
- Inside the cell, carbon dioxide reacts with water in presence of carbonic anhydrase and brings about the formation of carbonic acid.
- This acid immediately dissociates into bicarbonate and hydrogen ion.
- The hydrogen ion is secreted into the tubular lumen by antiport mechanism. During process of secretion of hydrogen ion, one sodium ion gets reabsorbed.
- This hydrogen ion secreted should be prevented from reacting with chloride to form a strong acid namely hydrochloric acid.
- Hence the hydrogen ion that has entered the tubular lumen reacts with bicarbonate present in the tubular lumen and forms carbonic acid (H_2CO_3).
- This acid immediately dissociates into carbon dioxide and water and the enzyme for this reaction to take place is carbonic anhydrase and it comes from the brush border of the epithelial cells.
- This prevents drastic fall of pH of tubular fluid.
- Bicarbonate ion diffuses from cell into the interstitium and ultimately enters peritubular capillary blood.

Phosphate Buffer System

- Sodium dibasic phosphate will be filtered into the tubular fluid along with plasma.

- When hydrogen ion gets secreted, there will be reabsorption of one sodium ion coming from the sodium dibasic phosphate.
- This leads to soium dibasic phosphate getting converted into sodium monobasic phosphate with which the secreted hydrogen ion reacts to form NaH_2PO_4 and this will be excreted in the urine.
- As stated already, this system operates to a greater extent in the DCT and collecting ducts.

Ammonia Buffer System

- Ammonia is secreted in all the parts of renal tubules.
- Glutamine is converted to glutamic acid and ammonia.
- In the tubular lumen, the filtered sodium and chloride are present.
- When the tubular cells secrete hydrogen ion, in exchange for this there will be reabsorption of sodium ion leaving chloride in the tubular lumen.
- If the hydrogen ion reacts with chloride ion, it leads to the formation of a strong acid, namely hydrochloric acid.
- This has to be prevented. So when hydrogen ion is secreted, the same tubular cells also secrete ammonia into the tubular lumen.
- In the lumen, ammonia reacts with hydrogen ion to form ammonium.

- This ammonium later on reacts with chloride ion present in the tubular lumen to form ammonium chloride which is a neutral salt.
- So hydrogen ion will get excreted in the urine as ammonium chloride, which prevents the fall of pH below 4.5 in the renal tubules.

Acid-base Disorders (Fig. 8.24)

a. Metabolic acid-base disorder
b. Respiratory acid-base disorder
  - Metabolic acidosis—diarrhea, diabetes, failure of renal function
  - Metabolic alkalosis—vomiting, ingestion of antacids
  - Respiratory acidosis—impaired gas diffusion, respiratory depression, respiratory alkalosis—hyperventilation
  - Renal tubular acidosis
  - Paradoxical aciduria

Juxtaglomerular Apparatus (Fig. 8.25)

This is specialized structure in the kidney, which is composed of 3 different types of cells, namely:
- Specialized smooth muscle cells of the arteriolar walls—juxtaglomerular cells
- Specialized epithelial cells lining the distal convoluted tubules—macula densa

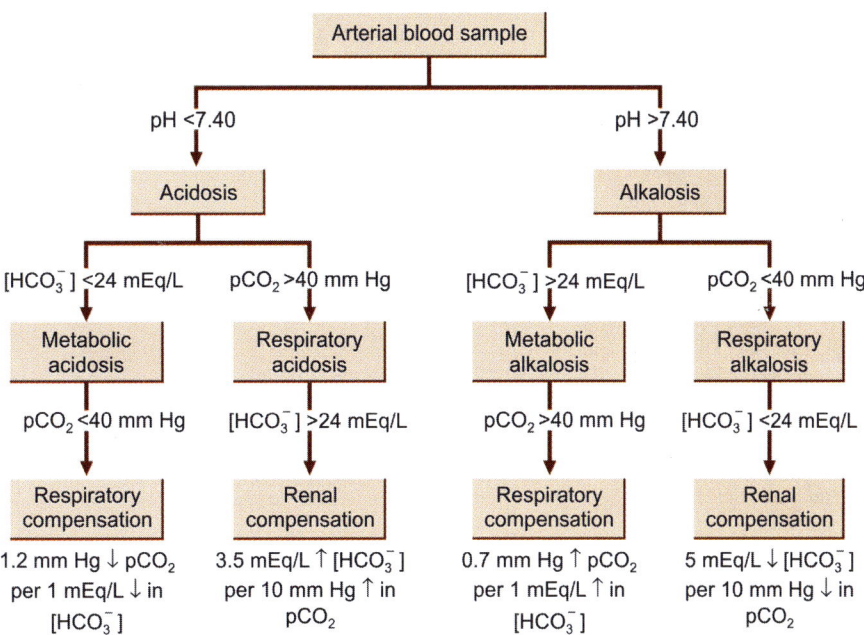

Fig. 8.24: Causes and compensatory changes in the body during acid-base imbalances

- Between the above two type of cells, there are certain other cells known as Lacis cells/mesangial cells.

The juxtaglomerular cells contain dense granules that contain renin. The macula densa acts as a sensor for sodium that is present in the lumen of distal convoluted tubule.

The juxtaglomerular apparatus (JGA) is concerned with the renin–angiotensin system. Renin secreted by the juxtaglomerular cells will act on angiotensinogen that is in circulation and converts it to angiotensin I. This further gets converted to angiotensin II by the action of the converting enzyme from the lungs. Some of the factors, which increase renin secretion are:

a. Na^+ depletion
b. Diuretics
c. Hemorrhage
d. Hypotension
e. Dehydration
f. Cardiac failure
g. Cirrhosis of liver

Factors affecting renin secretion

Stimulatory:
a. Increased sympathetic activity
b. Increased circulating catecholamines

Inhibitory:
a. Increased Na^+ and Cl^- reabsorption across macula densa
b. Increased afferent arteriolar pressure
c. Vasopressin

The actions of renin–angiotensin are:
- Stimulate the secretion of aldosterone hormone from the adrenal cortex
- It acts on the smooth muscle of blood vessels and brings about the vasoconstriction and thereby helps in the regulation of blood pressure.
- It also stimulates the thirst center and increases the release of ADH.
- Helps to bring about the autoregulation of the blood flow to the kidney.

Nerve Supply to Urinary Bladder and Urinary Tract (Figs 8.26 and 8.27)

- Comes from both the autonomic nervous system and somatic nervous system.
- All the nerves are mixed type (have both the afferent and efferent fibers).
- The fibers either take origin (efferent) from sacral segments (S2–S4) of spinal cord or carry impulses (afferent) to these segments.
- Pelvic nerve forms the parasympathetic component and hypogastric nerve is the sympathetic

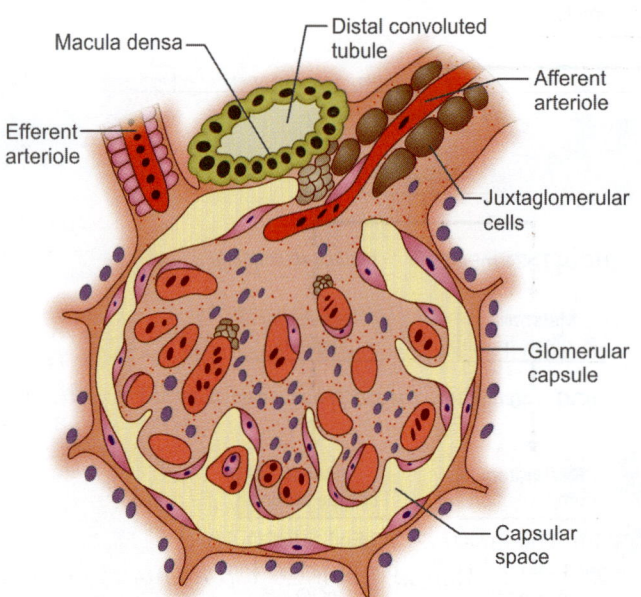

Fig. 8.25: Cells forming juxtaglomerular apparatus

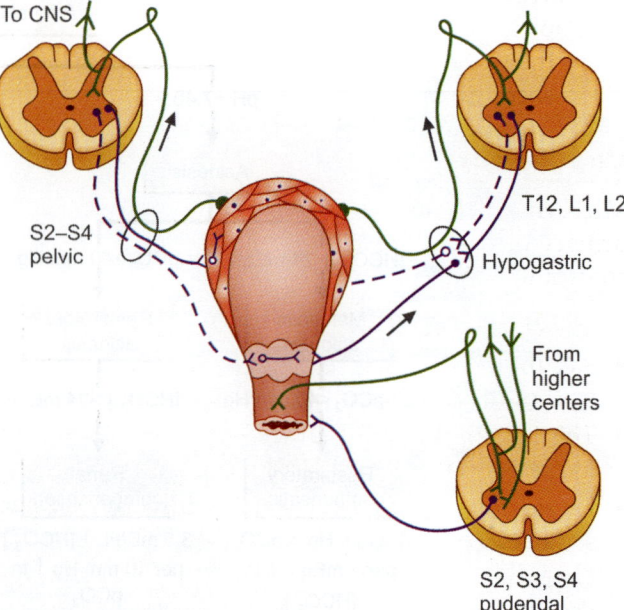

Fig. 8.26: Afferent and efferent innervation of the urinary tract

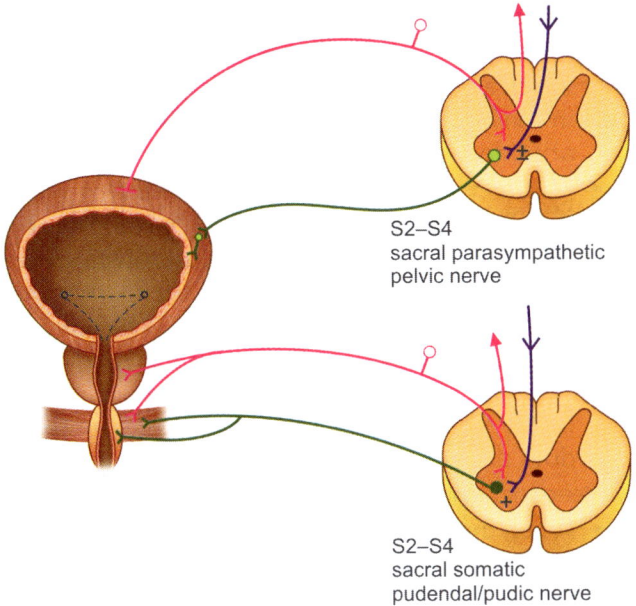

S2–S4
sacral parasympathetic
pelvic nerve

S2–S4
sacral somatic
pudendal/pudic nerve

Fig. 8.27: Motor innervation to urinary tract and the higher control over the spinal center

component supplying the urinary bladder. They are the two different limbs in the efferent components of the autonomic nervous system.

- The pelvic afferent carries the impulses from the stretch receptors present in the wall of the bladder and sympathetic afferent carries the pain impulses from the bladder.
- Urethra and external urethral sphincter are supplied by the pubic or pudendal nerves, which are the somatic nerves. They also take origin from the sacral segments (S2–S4) of spinal cord.

MICTURITION

Micturition is the periodic complete emptying of urinary bladder, which is normally under voluntary control in an adult.

At the time of voiding (micturition)

- Accumulation of urine in the bladder stretches the wall of the bladder.
- This in turn stimulates the stretch receptors present in the wall of the bladder.
- Pelvic afferent fibers carry the impulses to the sacral segments (S2–S4) of the spinal cord.
- Detrusor muscle, which is present in the wall of the bladder, gets the excitatory impulses through the pelvic efferent nerve (S2–S4).

- This brings about the contraction of the detrusor muscle. When the muscle is contracting the internal urethral sphincter relaxes and urine flows from the bladder into the urethra.
- Entry of urine into the urethra will stimulate the stretch receptors present in the urethra.
- The somatic afferent nerve fibers (pudic/pudendal) carry afferent impulses from here to the sacral segments of spinal cord.
- Somatic afferent impulses ultimately inhibit the efferent excitatory (pudic) nerves (S2–S4) supplying the external urethral sphincter (which is made up skeletal muscle).
- So the external urethral sphincter relaxes and the urine gets voided from the urinary bladder.
- Reinforcing impulses coming from the pontine centers to the spinal centers facilitate the spinal reflex and help to empty the bladder completely.

In the case of an adult, the higher centers can influence the activity of the spinal centers. The higher centers are present in cerebral cortex, hypothalamus, etc. In infants in whom the higher control is yet to establish on sacral segments of spinal cord. Because of this, the process of voiding is purely involuntary/reflex mechanism.

In the case of an adult, after complete transection of spinal cord micturition becomes a reflex act during the stage of recovery of reflex activity due to the loss of higher center control over spinal centers (as seen in paraplegics). This type of bladder is known as automatic bladder. Some of the other types of bladders are:

- Autonomous bladder in which the bladder will have got completely denervated.
- Atonic bladder is one in which there is loss of afferent innervation to the bladder (as seen in tabes dorsalis).

Incontinence is a condition in which the person is unable to bring about the complete voiding of urine as seen in normal individuals. There will be dribbling of urine but complete voiding will not occur as one event.

CYSTOMETROGRAM

Cystometrogram is graphical representation of the relationship between the volume of urine in bladder and the pressure in urinary bladder (Fig. 8.28).

This has been studied experimentally by introduction of double lumen catheter into the urinary bladder. Through one of the lumens, a known volume of isotonic saline will be introduced and the other lumen is connected to the manometer to record the pressure.

The configuration is due to plasticity property demonstrated by the smooth muscle present in the wall of the bladder and also because of the La Place law, which is obeyed by the bladder. According to the law, pressure developed in any spherical visceral structure is directly proportional to twice the tension (T) and inversely proportional to the radius (R).

$$P = \frac{2T}{R}$$

Explanation for the configuration of the graph:

1. Steep increase of pressure till about 150 ml:
   - When wall of the bladder get stretched, the stretching acts as a mechanical stimulus for smooth muscle.
   - This leads to contraction of the detrusor muscle.
   - This generates compressor force on the fluid present in the bladder.
   - The pressure rises. But when distension of the wall is maintained for sometime, the smooth muscle of the bladder instead of contracting, starts relaxing.
   - Hence it leads to a pressure drop for the same volume.

2. Pressure constancy between volume of 150 and 400 ml:
   - When about 150 ml of fluid has got accumulated in the bladder, the walls of the bladder will get unfolded in all the directions.
   - This increases the radii of the bladder.
   - Since pressure and radius have inverse relationship, the pressure is almost constant even though the volume of fluid in the bladder has got increased from 150 to 400 ml. As the bladder volume is increasing, T goes on increasing. But since the radius is also increasing the relationship of $2T/R$ remains the same and hence the P also does not get altered.

3. Steep increase of pressure beyond 400 ml (Fig. 8.29):
   - When the volume has reached about 400 ml, the walls of bladder have got distended almost optimally.
   - Beyond this volume when the walls are stretched, the over stretching of the walls of the bladder will steeply increase the tension developed.
   - Since pressure and tension have direct relationship, this will lead to a sharp increase of pressure development once again.

Composition of Urine

The normal constituents of urine will be Na^+, K^+, bicarbonate, urea, uric acid, creatinine, etc.

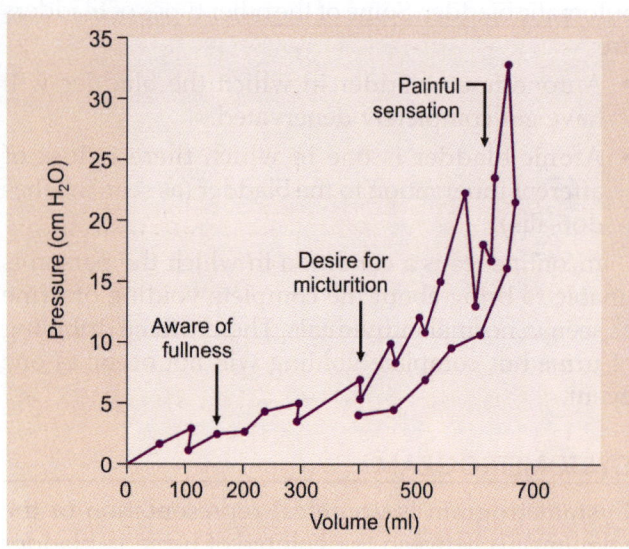

Fig. 8.28: Pressure–volume relationship of urinary bladder

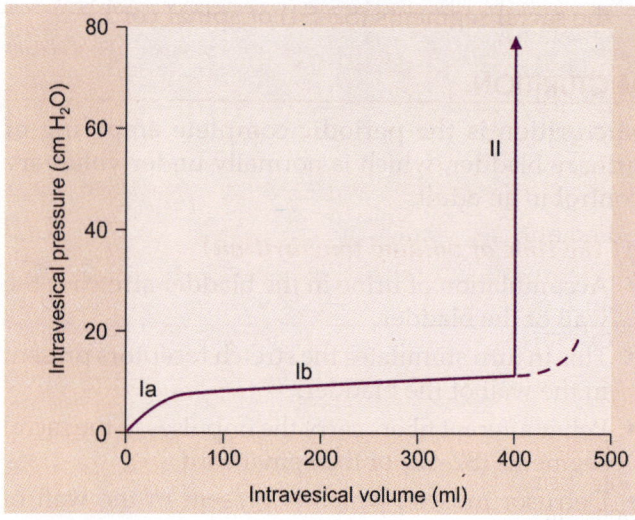

Fig. 8.29: Graph showing steep increase in pressure above 400 ml

- Abnormal constituents of urine are glucose, proteins, blood, bile salts, etc.
- In 24 hours sample of urine, specific gravity may range from 1005 to 1030 and urine of a normal person is slightly acidic most of the times.

Anuria means there is no urine formation/excretion whereas in oliguria the volume of urine formed decreases considerably.

Renal Failure (Table 8.5)

- Leads to the loss of function of kidney and hence the homeostasis of the body suffers.
- The person will not be able to survive, if remedial measures are not employed.
- The remedial measure may be temporary like the dialysis (hemodialysis or peritoneal) or permanent namely renal transplantation.

Renal Function Tests

Urine Analysis

1. *Physical examination* that is the volume assessment. In a normal adult, it is about 1500 ml per day. It is increased after meals and drinks and on exposure to cold. It is markedly decreased after excessive sweating. In pathological cases like diabetes mellitus, diabetes insipidus and in Conn's syndrome, it is markedly increased. In oliguric situations, like dehydration, hypovolemia, etc. urine volume is markedly decreased and in urinary tract obstruction there can be anuria also.
2. *Color and turbidity:* Urate precipitates in acidic urine on standing and makes the urine cloudy. Urate excretion increases in gout. Infection increases the pus cells and bacteria in urine and gives rise to cloudy appearance. Appears smoky in hematuria. Frothy in proteinuria. Milky in chyluria. Red-dark brown in porphyria. Red-dark brown black in hematuria.
3. *Specific gravity:* Normal range is about 1005 to 1025 and osmolality can be between 100 and 1200 mOsm/L. If the specific gravity is always around

1010 with osmolality on the lower side (300 mOsm/L), it is known as isosthenuria.

4. *pH:* It is normally slightly on the acidic side except for a short time after meals which is due to post-prandial alkaline tide. Consumption of alkali, impaired tubular acidification will give rise to alkaline urine.
5. *Chemical analysis:*
   a. Protein excretion in urine is almost nil (150 mg/day). Excretion of considerably more than the normal amount of protein excretion is called proteinuria. When glomerular permeability increases, large amount of proteins appear in urine (nephrotic syndrome, glomerulonephritis). Proteins also appear in urine, if tubular functions are impaired, e.g. Fanconi syndrome.
   b. Sugar: Glucose is absent in urine. Appearance of glucose in urine is known as glycosuria. The most common condition in which glucose appears in urine will be diabetes mellitus. It can also be due to some problem in kidney (renal glycosuria), etc. Lactose may appear in late pregnancy and lactation and pentose may after consumption of large quantities of plum, cherries and grapes.
   c. *Ketone* are normally absent in urine. Ketonuria occurs in diabetic ketoacidosis.
   d. Bile pigments: the normal excretory rate per day will be about 3 mg. Its excretion is increased in jaundice.
   e. Heme pigments are normally absent in urine. They appear in urine following intravascular hemolysis. They appear following crush injuries to muscles and in certain myopathies.
6. *Microscopic examination:*
   - Cellular casts are typically found in acute bacterial pyelonephritis.
   - Fatty acids are found in nephrotic syndrome.
   - Red cell casts are found in pathognomonic of glomerular bleeding.
   - Hyaline casts are structure less proteinous plugs seen in proteinuria.
   - Some of the common types of cells found in urine leukocytes, tubular epithelial cells and squamous cells.

Plasma composition: Neither plasma urea nor plasma creatinine rise until the GFR falls to a very low value. Once the GFR falls to as low as 30 ml/min, plasma

Table 8.5: Acute renal failure			
Variable	Prerenal	Renal	Postrenal
Urine osmolarity	>500	<350	<350
Urine Na	<10	>20	>40
Serum BUN/Cr	>20	<15	<15

creatinine value gets increased and is highly sensitive guide. Plasma urea level may be falsely high in dehydration, heart failure, nephrotic syndrome, high protein diet, gastrointestinal bleeding, etc.

GFR measurement: It is normally estimated by creatinine clearance value as creatinine is endogenously produced. Though its clearance value is slightly more than that of the inulin clearance value, in clinical practice, it forms one of easy tests to assess the GFR.

Diuretics (Fig. 8.30)

• Water	Inhibits ADH secretion
• Ethanol	Inhibits ADH secretion
• Antagonists of V2 receptors	Inhibits ADH action
• Osmotically active substances	Produce osmotic diuresis
• Xanthines	Decrease reabsorption of sodium and increase GFR

• Carbonic anhydrase inhibitors	Decrease H^+ secretion
• Loop diuretics	Inhibit Na^+–K^+–$2Cl$ in AL of LH
• Thiazides	Inhibit Na^+–Cl cotransport
• K^+ retaining diuretics	Inhibit Na^+–K^+ exchange

SKIN AND THERMOREGULATION

The normal temperature of body is around 37°C or 98.4°F. Since the human beings are homoeothermic animals, the temperature of the body should be maintained around the normal value for all the enzymatic activity to go on smoothly.

In our day-to-day life, there are so many ways the body will be producing heat, like (Fig. 8.31)
- Basal metabolism
- Specific dynamic action of food
- Muscular exercise
- Unconscious tensing of muscles
- Shivering.

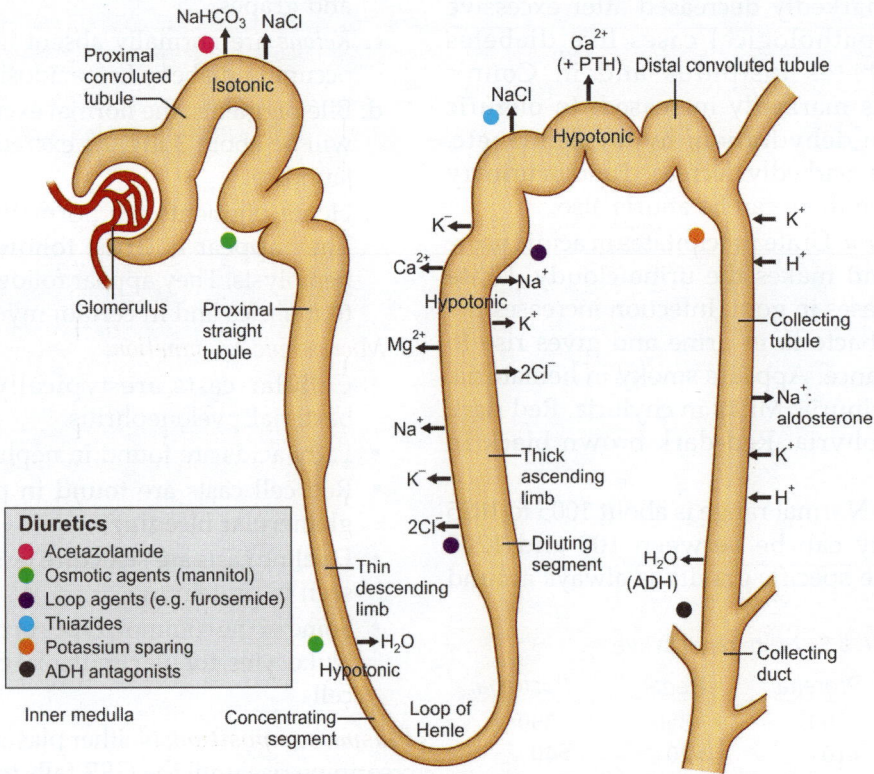

Fig. 8.30: The site of action of various diuretics

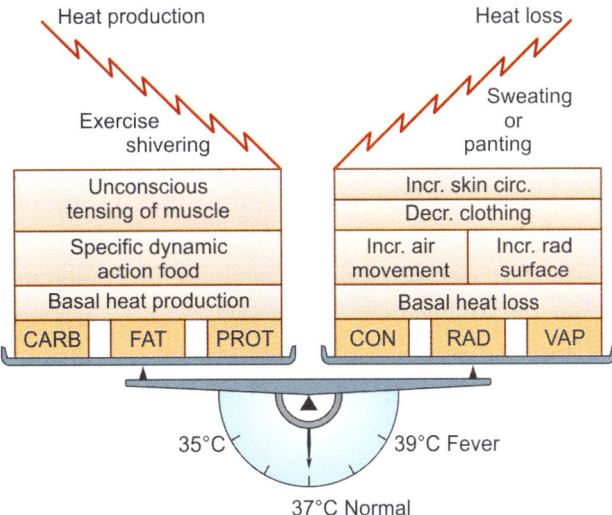

Fig. 8.31: Scale showing the various heat loss and heat gain mechanisms operating in the body while trying to maintain normal temperature

Likewise there are many ways by which heat can be lost from the body (Table 8.6):

a. Loss of heat from the body by physical mechanisms like:
   - Conduction
   - Convection
   - Radiation
   - Vaporization of water from the body (insensible perspiration).

Table 8.6: Partitioning of heat loss at various temperatures

Room temp	Radiation	Convection	Evaporation
Comfort 25°C	67%	10%	23%
Warm 30°C	41%	33%	26%
Hot 35°C	4%	6%	90%

b. Increase in cutaneous blood flow to facilitate the heat loss by above processes.

c. Exposure of body surface area to increase radiation heat loss.

d. Vaporization of sweat.

Thermoregulation

Mechanisms of heat gain/loss:
- Physical
- Physiological
- Behavioral

For regulation of body temperature, the centers are present in the hypothalamus and thermoreceptors are present in the skin (peripheral) and in the hypothalamus (central). The peripheral thermoreceptors sense the temperature of blood flowing through the skin as well as the ambient temperature, whereas the central thermoreceptors sense the temperature of the blood flowing through the hypothalamus. When body wants to lose heat the heat loss mechanisms become more active and heat gain mechanisms are inhibited and vice versa happen when the body wants to gain heat.

In the hypothalamus, there are heat gain and heat loss centers. The heat gain center is located in the posterior hypothalamus and heat loss center in the anterior hypothalamus. Apart from these two centers, there is also presence of biologic thermostat in the preoptic nucleus region of hypothalamus. A coordinated functioning of all these centers will help in the regulation of body temperature.

Efferent impulses from the hypothalamus through the sympathetic nerves reach the:
- Smooth muscle of blood vessels.
- Eccrine sweat glands present in the skin.
- Adrenal medulla to alter the secretion of the hormone catecholamine.

Apart from the role of nerves, there is alteration in the secretion of the hormones also during thermoregulation. The secretion of the hormones namely adrenaline, noradrenaline (catecholamine) and thyroxine gets altered. These hormones increase the metabolic rate of the body and hence known as calorigenic hormones.

The most common condition in which the body temperature increases (pyrexia) is in fever. Any infectious state usually results in onset of fever. When body temperature is more than 104°F, it is known as hyperpyrexia.

When body temperature is less than normal it is known as hypothermia. It can be accidental like accidents of ship on high seas, in temperate countries during the winter season when people do not have the proper shelter. In hospital set-up, hypothermia is induced during cardiac and neurosurgeries.

Skin

It is the outer most covering on the body. It performs many functions. Some of the important functions of the skin are:
- *Protection*—acts as a mechanical barrier between the subcutaneous tissues and the surrounding

environment and hence prevents the micro organisms invading the body.

- *Sense organ*—has many types of receptors, which help us to perceive the sensations like touch, pressure, pain, and temperature.
- *Thermoregulation*—is due to its ability to transfer heat from one body to another along the thermal gradient by various physical and also by physio-logical mechanisms. The sweat glands present in the skin have a vital role to play. Alteration in the skin blood flow and opening of arteriovenous anastomosis as the situation demands will also take place during thermoregulation.

- *Secretory*—apart from the sweat that is secreted by sweat glands, there is secretion of sebum by sebaceous glands, which is responsible for the maintenance of the smooth texture of the skin.
- *Absorption*—many of the lipid-based substances like creams, ointments, get absorbed through the skin.
- *Excretory*—some of the substances, like salts, urea and fatty substances, get excreted.
- *Endocrine* exposure of the skin to the UV light rays from the sun help for the endogenous production of vitamin D.

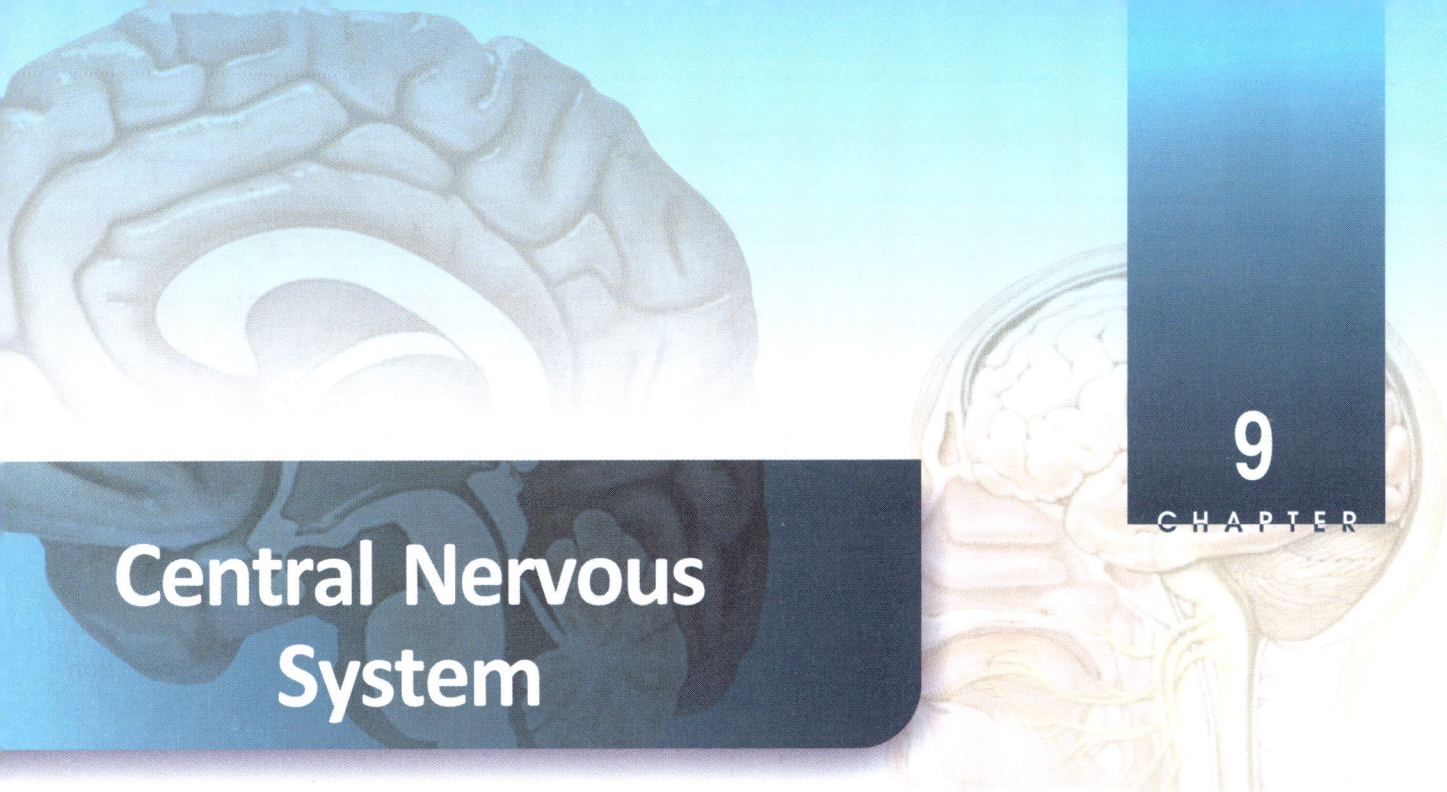

Central Nervous System

Activities taking place in our body have to be regulated. Regulation is brought about by 2 mechanisms:

1. Hormonal (slow regulation)
2. Neural (rapid regulation)

The nervous system is concerned with receiving impulse from various parts of body, interpret message received, analyze the event that is required to be brought about and send message accordingly to different parts of body for appropriate action.

The neurons present in brain and spinal cord are included under central nervous system, whereas neurons present outside central nervous system (that is neurons/nerve cells present in all different parts of body) are included under peripheral nervous system (PNS). Peripheral nervous system helps to establish communication between central nervous system and different parts of body. In PNS, both somatic and autonomic nervous systems are included (Fig. 9.1).

Various stimuli acting on different parts of body result in passing on information (afferent impulse) from different parts of body to CNS with the help of afferent nerve fibers of PNS. Likewise impulse generated by CNS will be conveyed to various parts of body with the help of efferent nerve fibers of PNS.

Stimulus: It is sudden change in internal or external environment. The strength of stimulus when is of certain magnitude, it brings about development of action potential in afferent nerve fiber. This impulse will convey information to CNS with the help of

afferent nerve fibers. The different types of energies (stimuli) constantly impinging on body will be:

- Mechanical stimulus (pressure, touch, vibration, etc.)
- Chemical stimulus
- Thermal stimulus
- Electromagnetic stimulus

Receptors

Certain specialized structures are present at the interface of stimulus and afferent nerve fibers. These specialized structures convert any type of energy into electrical energy or action potential in afferent fiber. This action is known as transduction. Hence receptors act as biologic transducers.

Some of these action potentials (electrical activities) in the afferent nerves on reaching brain come to our conscious perception. However, some electrical activities of the afferent nerves on reaching brain, like impulses from baroreceptors or movements in stomach, etc., do not come to our conscious perception.

Due to presence of receptors, CNS can exert its influence on:

1. Perception of stimulus
2. Regulation of many of the activity

When stimulus acts on receptor, there is some amount of electrical change occurring in receptor. This is known as receptor potential. When stimulus acts on a receptor, there is conformational change in the membrane of receptor, which increases permeability of membrane for Na^+. Hence there will be influx of

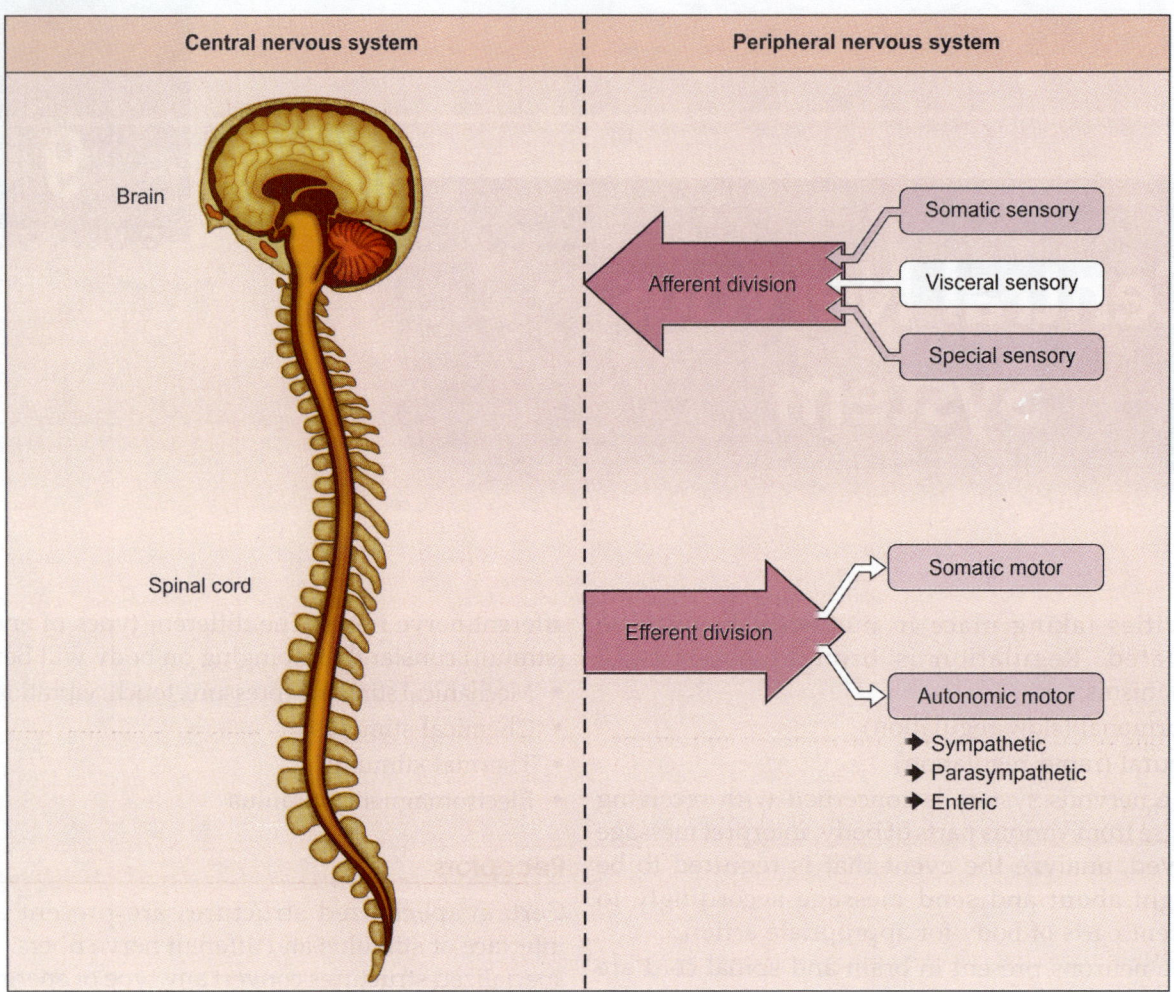

| Central nervous system | Peripheral nervous system |

Brain

Spinal cord

Afferent division
- Somatic sensory
- Visceral sensory
- Special sensory

Efferent division
- Somatic motor
- Autonomic motor
  - Sympathetic
  - Parasympathetic
  - Enteric

Fig. 9.1: Over view of CNS and PNS

Na$^+$ from ECF to ICF causes depolarization, and results in a graded potential called generator or receptor potential.

Receptor potential is a local potential. It is not an action potential. It cannot get conducted over long distance. Receptor potential is almost equal to end plate potential (EPP) of neuromuscular junction.

Receptor potential develops at specialized nerve endings or distinct bodies of afferent nervous system.

Genesis by conformational change in membrane of receptor which increases permeability of membrane for Na$^+$ ions from ECF to ICF. Therefore, there is generation of receptor potential.

Amplitude (Fig. 9.2): Directly related to strength of stimulus. Increase in strength of stimulus will increase amplitude of receptor potential unlike action potential which is all or none in nature.

Duration: Much more than the duration of action potential.

When the receptor potential moves towards 0 mV, electrical activity of receptor is said to be hypo-polarizing (depolarizing) type, and when potential moves away from 0 mV it is hyperpolarizing type. But as far as receptor potential is concerned, it is generally depolarizing type of potential. Apart from this, there are groups of receptors present in body which on getting stimulated get hyperpolarized and still bring about action potential. Photoreceptors of eye are classical example for this type of receptors.

Spread: Receptor potential cannot get conducted for long distance unlike action potential. Receptor

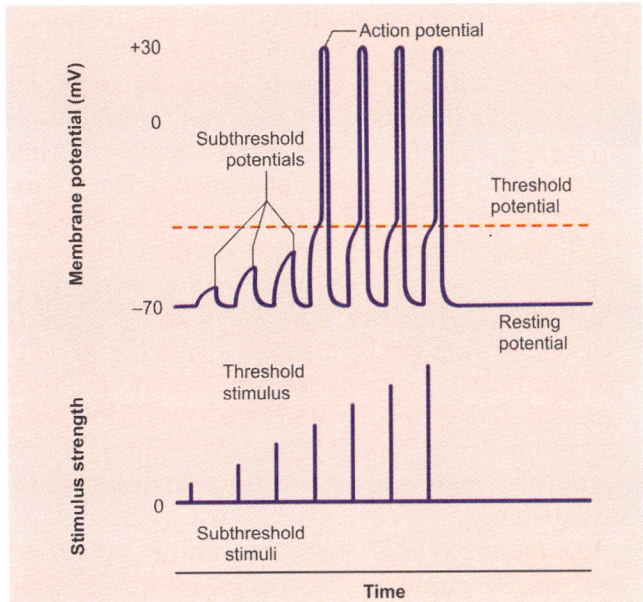

Fig. 9.2: Relationship between intensity of stimulus and receptor potential

potentials spread electrotonically to adjacent regions. As the potentials move away from site of stimulus and as time passes off, amplitude of receptor potential decrease exponentially in relation to space and time.

Classification of Receptors

Receptors can be classified based on different criteria.

Based on type of stimulus for which they respond, they can be classified into:

1. *Mechanoreceptors* (Fig. 9.3) respond for mechanical energy, like touch, pressure, vibration. These receptors are present in almost all parts of body. In skin, there are:
   - Merkel's disk
   - Meissner's corpuscle (touch receptors)
   - Pacinian corpuscle, etc.

   In visceral regions, are:
   - Barorceptors
   - Volume receptors
   - Auditory receptors, etc.

2. *Chemoreceptors* respond for chemical energy. Some of the examples for chemoreceptors are:
   - Taste receptors
   - Olfactory receptors
   - Carotid and aortic bodies
   - Osmoreceptors

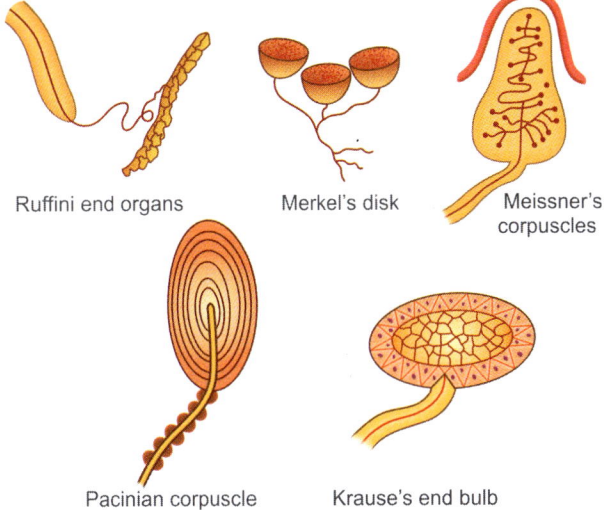

Fig. 9.3: Mechanoreceptors present in the skin

3. *Themoreceptors* get stimulated by warmth/cold energy. Thermoreceptors are present in skin (peripheral) and in hypothalamus (central).

4. *Nociceptors* respond for painful (noxious) stimulus. Naked nerve endings present in almost all parts of body act as nociceptors. Nociceptors are absent in central nervous system.

5. *Electromagnetic receptors* are present in eye. They respond for light rays (electromagnetic waves), e.g. rods and cones (photoreceptors).

Properties of Receptors

1. *Excitability* (Fig. 9.4): Since receptors are specialized nerve endings, they are in polarized state when not stimulated. On application of stimulus, change in

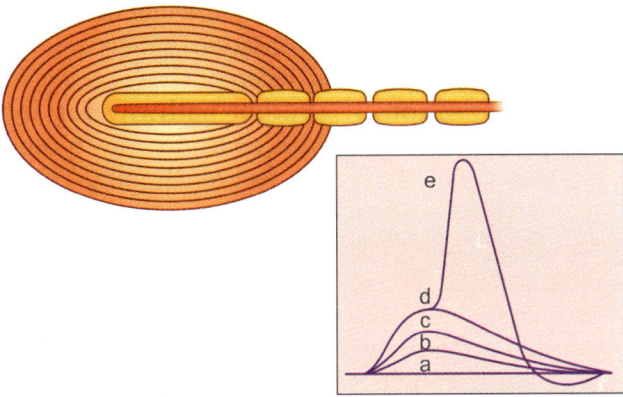

Fig. 9.4: Relatioship between intensity of stimulus and receptor potential in Pacinian corpuscle

polarized state occurs. This leads to development of receptor potential or generator potential. Receptor potential is one of the examples of local potential. When this potential reaches a critical value, there will be development of nerve action potential in the afferent fiber.

2. *Adequate stimulus* is just enough strength of stimulus to excite receptor for production of receptor potential which is sufficient enough to bring about development of an action potential in afferent fiber.

3. *Specificity:* Each group of receptor is specialized to respond for a particular type of stimulus very easily. However, the same receptors can get stimulated for some other type of stimulus provided; the strength of stimulus is very strong, e.g. photoreceptors are most sensitive to light but application of pressure on eyeball can also stimulate them.

Muller's law of specific nerve energy: Whenever receptor is stimulated with adequate strength of stimulus, there is development of action potential in afferent nerve fibers. This action potential reaches brain, and particular sensation is perceived.

However, configuration and amplitude of action potential whether coming from mechanoceptor or chemoreceptor, remains the same and reach the brain.

How is brain able to interpret when a person is feeling touch, or heat sensations, etc.?

There is some sort of conditioning taking place in CNS. For example, whenever touch receptor is stimulated, afferent impulse reaches cerebral cortex, sensation of touch is felt.

When impulse comes along a particular nerve fiber for months or years, the sensation brain is going to perceive is touch in case receptor stimulated is for touch sensation. If afferent pathway for this sensation is stimulated directly by any type of stimulus, still we always feel touch only. This is known as conditioning.

According to Muller's law, when afferent pathway is stimulated directly (by any type of stimulus that is mechanical or chemical or thermal in nature) sensation that is going to be felt is specific of the receptor from where it carries impulse. This is the basis to explain carpal tunnel syndrome, spondylitis, phantom limb, etc.

4. *Intensity discrimination:* Strength of stimulus applied can be assessed by magnitude of response from receptors which is in form of increased amplitude of receptor potential. An increased amplitude of receptor potential, increases the number of action potentials generated in afferent nerve fiber in unit time, as per Weber-Fechner law (as per this law, frequency of action potential produced in nerve fiber is directly proportional to log intensity of stimulus). Another way by which intensity discrimination can be made out is, as the strength of stimulus is increased, number of receptors stimulated will also increase (recruitment of receptors/recruitment of sensory units). This is because receptors also have different threshold for excitation.

5. *Adaptation:* When applied stimulus acts for a prolonged duration, some of receptors may stop responding in the course of time. So there will not be production of action potential in nerve fiber. There are some receptors that get adapted fast, e.g. olfactory receptors, and touch receptors in skin. Pain receptors will never ever get adapted.

The property of adaptation of receptor whether beneficial to body, depends on type of receptor that has got adapted. Baroreceptor adaptation is detrimental to body function as blood pressure cannot be restored to normal value during sustained hypertension.

Sensory unit is number of sensory receptors from which a particular afferent nerve fiber carries impulse. Recruitment of sensory units also helps for intensity discrimination.

SYNAPSE

Synapse can be defined as functional junction between parts of two different neurons. There is no anatomical continuity between two neurons involved in the formation of synapse.

At level of synapse, impulse gets conducted from one neuron to another due to release of neuro-transmitters, like ACh, noradrenaline, serotonin, etc.

The synapses, which require release of some chemical substance (neurotransmitter) during synaptic transmission, are termed as chemical synapses. In human body, almost all synapses are chemical type. Parts involved in a synapse are given in Fig. 9.5.

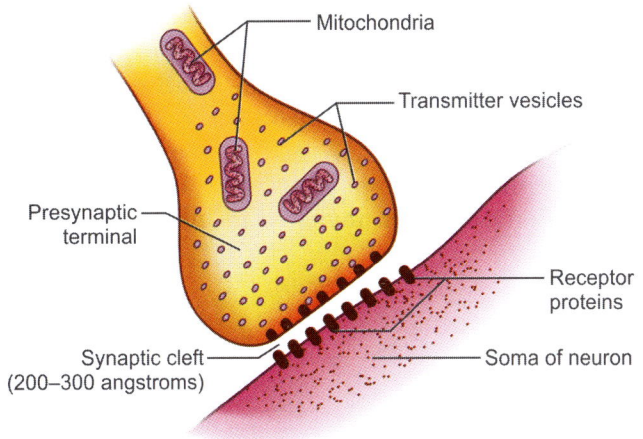

Fig. 9.5: Diagram of a typical chemical synapse

Labels: Mitochondria, Transmitter vesicles, Presynaptic terminal, Synaptic cleft (200–300 angstroms), Receptor proteins, Soma of neuron

Presynaptic region is mostly contributed by axon and postsynaptic region may be contributed by dendrite or soma (cell body) or axon of another neuron.

Accordingly, synapses can be of following types based on different parts of neuron involved information of synapse:

a. Axodendritic
b. Axosomatic
c. Axoaxonic
d. Dendritodendritic

Mechanism of Synaptic Transmission

a. Arrival of impulse
b. Depolarization of pre-synaptic region
c. Influx of calcium ions from ECF into presynaptic region
d. Release of neurotransmitter
e. Passage of neurotransmitter through synaptic cleft.
f. Binding of neurotransmitter to receptors on post-synaptic region.
g. Change in electrical activity of postsynaptic region. Depending on transmitter substance released, there can be generation of EPSP or IPSP (EPSP or excitatory postsynaptic potential or IPSP or inhibitory postsynaptic potential). If EPSP is produced, postsynaptic region becomes less negative and if IPSP is produced, postsynaptic region becomes more negative.
h. When EPSP reaches firing level, there will be generation of action potential in postsynaptic

region. EPSP is due to influx of sodium ion. If IPSP is produced, postsynaptic region becomes hyperpolarized and hence there will not be development of action potential in postsynaptic region. IPSP will be due to efflux of potassium ions or influx of chloride ions at postsynaptic regions.

Properties of Synapse

1. *One-way conduction (unidirectional conduction):* In chemical synapse, since neurotransmitter is present only in presynaptic region, impulse gets conducted from pre- to postsynaptic region only and not vice versa.
2. *Synaptic delay is for neurotransmitter to:*
   a. Get released from synaptic vesicles when action potential has reached presynaptic region
   b. Pass through synaptic cleft
   c. Act on postsynaptic region to bring about production of action potential in postsynaptic region.
   For all the above events to be brought about, some time is required. This is known as synaptic delay, which is normally about 0.5 msec at every synapse.
3. *Fatigability:* When synapses are continuously stimulated, after some time, due to exhaustion of neurotransmitter at presynaptic terminals, impulses fail to get conducted. This results in fatigue occurring at level of synapse. Fatigue is a temporary phenomenon. If some rest is given to neurons, resting facilitates resynthesis of neurotransmitter for further conduction of impulse across synapse.
4. *Convergence and divergence:* Impulses from one pre-synaptic nerve fiber may end on postsynaptic region of large number neurons and this is called as divergence. When nerve fibers of different pre-synaptic neurons end on a common postsynaptic neuron, this is known as convergence. In CNS, on an average about 10000 synapses are found on any one neuron.
5. *Summation:* When a stimulus of subthreshold strength is applied, there will not be development of action potential in postsynaptic region. But if many subthreshold stimuli are applied at pre-synaptic region, effects of these stimuli can get added up and lead to action potential development in postsynaptic region. This is known as summation.

There are two types of summation namely spatial and temporal. In temporal summation, presynaptic neuron stimulated will be same, but many stimuli are applied in rapid succession (timing of stimuli will be different, but place of stimulation will be same). In spatial summation, presynaptic neurons stimulated will be different but stimuli will be applied simultaneously (time of stimulation shall be same, but places of stimulation will be different) This is possible because of the property of convergence.

6. *Excitation or inhibition:* The impulse conduction across a synapse may either stimulate or inhibit activity of postsynaptic region. If there is stimulatory influence, then there will be production of action potential in postsynaptic neuron and if it has an inhibitory influence, then there is no action potential generation in postsynaptic region.

Synaptic Inhibitions

Examples of inhibition are:
- Postsynaptic inhibition (direct)
- Presynaptic inhibition
- Renshaw cell inhibition (feedback or recurrent)
- Reciprocal inhibition (feed forward)
- Lateral inhibition

Postsynaptic Inhibition

Events in postsynaptic inhibition:
- Arrival of impulse at presynaptic region
- Release of neurotransmitter
- Stimulation of internuncial neuron
- Action potential production in internuncial neuron
- Release of neurotransmitter from internuncial neuron
- Binding of neurotransmitter to receptors on postsynaptic region
- Influx of chloride ions into postsynaptic region
- Postsynaptic membrane becoming more negative (development of inhibitory postsynaptic potential or also known as IPSP)
- Hyperpolarization of postsynaptic region
- No action potential production in postsynaptic region.

Glycine substance is a classical example of inhibitory neurotransmitter at postsynaptic region. For example, when biceps muscle is contracting; there

will be associated relaxation of triceps muscle because of postsynaptic inhibition.

The mechanism of inhibition in all other types namely Renshaw cell (Fig. 9.6), lateral (Fig. 9.7) and reciprocal inhibitions (Fig. 9.8), will be like what has been explained for postsynaptic inhibition but orientation of neuron involved in inhibition will be different.

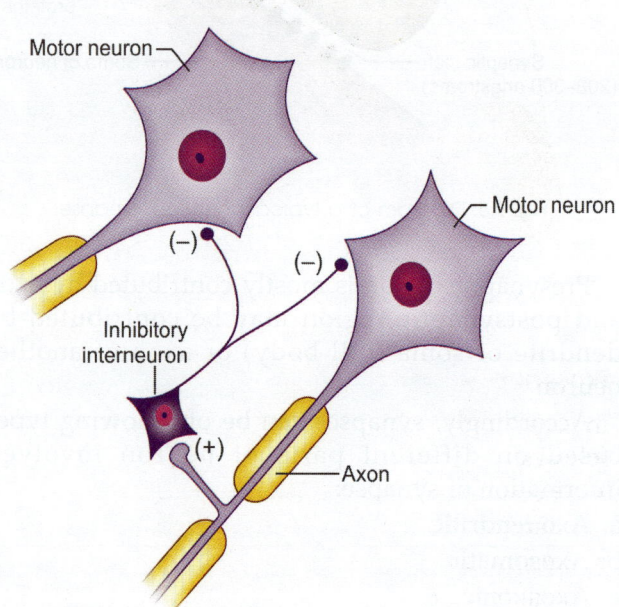

Fig. 9.6: Renshaw cell inhibition in central nervous system

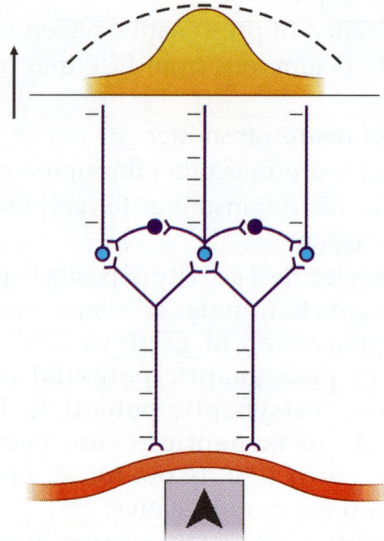

Fig. 9.7: Lateral inhibition in neuraxis

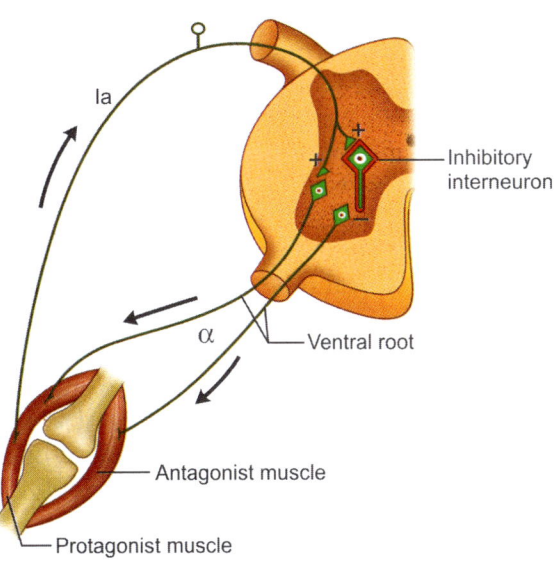

Fig. 9.8: Reciprocal inhibition and innervation

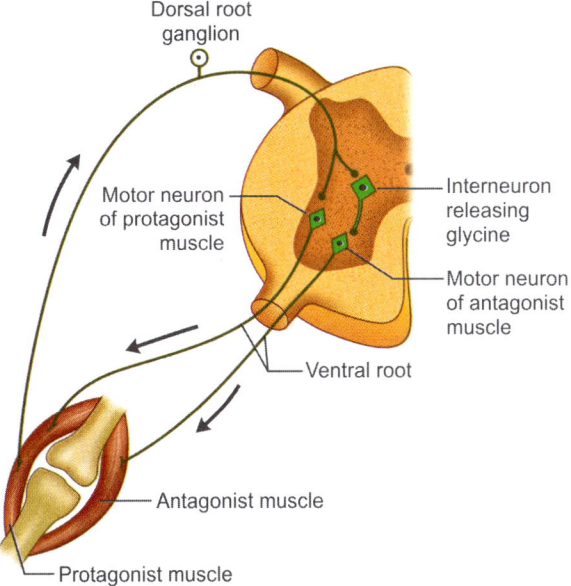

Fig. 9.10: Reciprocal inhibition

Presynaptic Inhibition (Fig. 9.9)

In presynaptic inhibition, the events occurring are as follows:

- The neuron ending on presynaptic terminal liberates neurotransmitter.
- Because of this, presynaptic terminal becomes less negative (because of influx of potassium ions)
- So the presynaptic terminal fails to remain in resting state.

Now when action potential reaches this presynaptic region, depolarization of presynaptic terminal will not be to the extent it normally occurs.

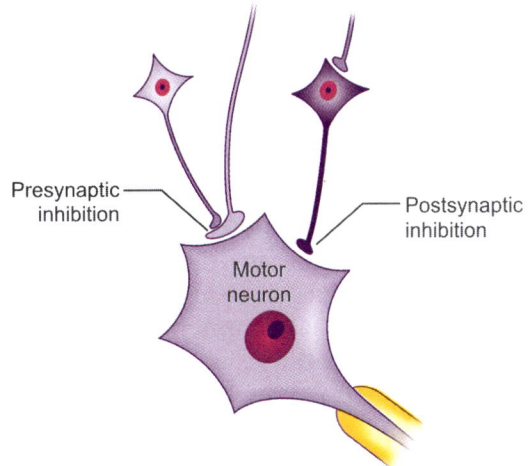

Fig. 9.9: Pre- and postsynaptic inhibitions

The amplitude of spike potential will be less than normal. When presynaptic neuron is kept in normal resting, during development of action potential, membrane potential will reach plus 35 mV from resting state of minus 70 mV. In which case, net change in potential will be about 105 mV. When action potential reaches a neuron which has been kept in a partially depolarized state (when membrane potential is made to be less negative), the net change in potential will be less than usual (will be less than 105 mV).

- This leads to release of less than normal amount of neurotransmitter from presynaptic terminals.
- Neurotransmitter on binding to receptors on postsynaptic region brings about development of EPSP.
- But the amplitude of EPSP will be less than normal and hence it will not be able to bring postsynaptic region to threshold state of stimulation.
- Because of this, there will not be production of action potential in postsynaptic region.

In reciprocal inhibition (Fig. 9.10), impulse from presynaptic terminal, will stimulate motor neuron supplying agonist muscle and through an internuncial neuron inhibits motor neuron supplying antagonist muscle.

Reflex

A reflex is defined as automatic/involuntary, stereotyped/repetitive, purpose serving or goal oriented response for afferent stimulation which can be internal or external.

For any reflex action to be brought about, basic reflex arc should be intact. The components of basic reflex arc are (Fig. 9.11):

a. Receptor
b. Afferent limb
c. Center
d. Efferent limb
e. Effector organ.

Center can be present either in brain or spinal cord. Damage to any part of basic reflex arc results in loss of reflex activity in that part of body.

Classification of reflexes may be done based on different criteria:

a. Unconditioned or conditioned reflex classification is based on whether the reflexes are present at birth. Unconditioned reflex is present by birth.
b. Monosynaptic or polysynaptic reflex is based on number of synapses involved in reflex arc. Stretch reflex is the only example for monosynaptic reflex in body.
c. Clinical classification is based on location of receptors which are involved in reflex action:
   1. Superficial reflexes—plantar, abdominal, corneal, etc.
   2. Deep reflexes—knee jerk, biceps jerk, ankle jerk, jaw jerk, etc.
   3. Visceral reflexes—Marey's reflex, micturition reflex, vomiting reflex, defecation reflex, etc.

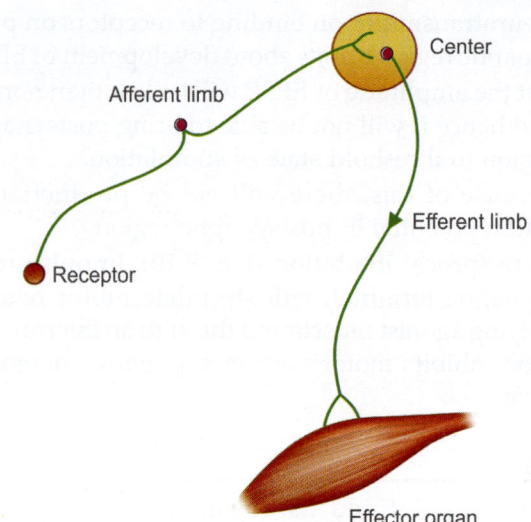

Fig. 9.11: Basic reflex arc

Properties of Reflexes

Many of the properties of synapses are also applicable for reflexes because in any reflex arc, there will be at least one synapse. Certain other specific properties, which are specific to reflexes, are after discharge is, even after stimulus is over, reflex response continues for prolonged duration. This is possible because of parallel and reverberating circuits in CNS. This is seen in flexion withdrawal reflex.

Habituation occurs when stimulus is benign (not harmful). For any benign stimulus, initially there will be response, but as stimulus is repeated, intensity of reflex response decreases and will be absent after sometime. Example for habituation is, ticking of a new clock; initially person may not get sleep due to this sound. But as person continues to stay in same environment, his sleep would not get affected in the course of time.

Sensitization is just opposite of habituation. When stimulus is dangerous or harmful, for subsequent exposure to same stimulus, intensity of reflex response will be much more. Some of the other properties of reflexes are:

• Irradiation
• Recruitment
• Rebound phenomenon
• Fractionation

Importance of knowledge of reflexes in clinical practice:

1. To differentiate between upper motor and lower motor lesions. In lower motor neuron lesions, all reflexes (superficial and deep) are lost, whereas in upper motor neuron lesions, all superficial reflexes are lost except plantar reflex which is Babinski +ve and deep reflexes are exaggerated. In cerebellar lesion, knee jerk (deep reflex) becomes pendular.
2. To assess level of lesion in CNS, e.g. if reflexes are normal in upper half of body but altered or absent in lower half of body, it can be concluded that lower half of spinal cord function is not normal.

Lower motor neuron is anterior horn cell (AHC) or corresponding cranial nerve motor nuclei with its axon. It forms the final common efferent pathway along which motor impulses reach any part of body.

There are two types of lower motor neurons, namely alpha and gamma motor neurons.

• The alpha motor neuron supplies extrafusal muscle fibers.

- Gamma motor neuron supplies contractile part (polar ends) of intrafusal muscle fibers.

Upper motor neuron (UMN) is any motor neuron which takes origin from cerebral cortex or subcortical regions and influence activity of the lower motor neuron. All descending tracts in general constitute extensions of upper motor neuron in spinal cord. They ultimately act on lower motor neuron.

Effect of Dorsal/Posterior/Afferent Nerve Sectioning

Dorsal nerve carries all sensory input from peripheral parts of body. It forms afferent part of basic reflex arc. Features are (in affected part of body):

a. Loss of all modalities of sensations in particular dermatome (if 3 consecutive nerve roots of spinal cord are involved) due to damage in afferent nerve fibers (Fig. 9.12).

b. Loss of all reflexes in the affected part of the body due to lesion in afferent part of basic reflex arc (Fig. 9.13).

c. Tone of muscle is lost or decreased due to damage to the alpha–gamma linkage pathway.

d. Voluntary movements are still present but not normal. This is because even though both lower and upper motor neurons are intact, there are no feedback signals from concerned part of body as afferent nerve has got damaged. These afferent signals are essential for coordination of movements.

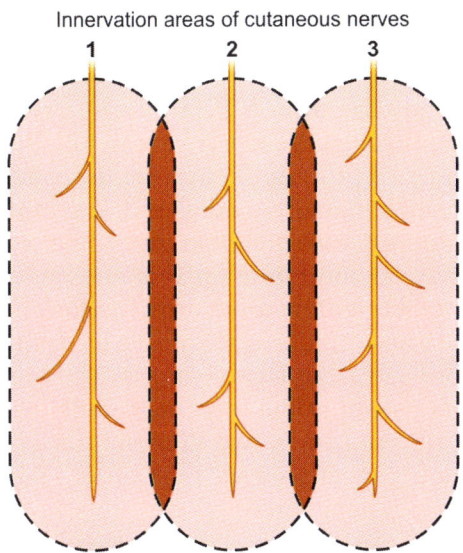

Innervation areas of cutaneous nerves

Fig. 9.12: Overlapping of the areas by the afferent nerves

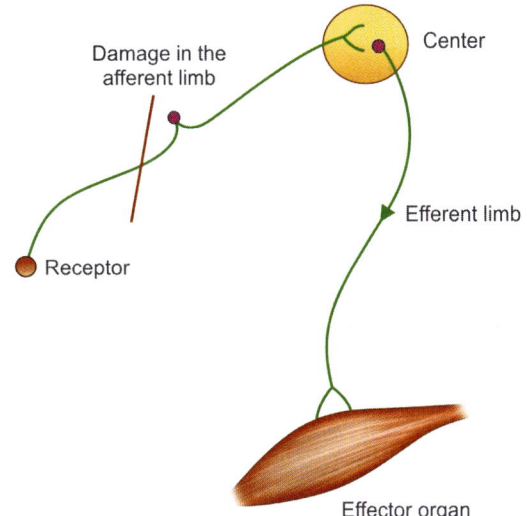

Fig. 9.13: Damage in the afferent limb of basic reflex arc

Due to loss of afferent feedback signals, there will ataxia (in-coordination of movements). This type of ataxia is termed as sensory ataxia.

e. Tissue damage and tropic ulcers due to loss of protective pain sensations.

Spinal Cord

The human spinal cord is made up 31 segments. From each of these segments, a pair of spinal nerves take origin. Hence there are 31 pairs of spinal nerves. Of 31 pairs:

- 8 belong to cervical segments
- 12 belong to thoracic segments
- 5 belong to lumbar segments
- 5 belong to sacral segments
- 1 belongs to coccygeal segment.

In a transverse section of spinal cord, in the central part will be H-shaped gray matter and this will be surrounded by white matter. The gray matter and white matter on either side have continuity through commissures (Fig. 9.14).

In the gray matter, nerve cell bodies are present whereas the white matter is composed of compactly packed nerve fibers in the form of tracts. The tracts which carry impulses from peripheral parts of body towards higher parts of CNS through spinal cord are called ascending tracts. Likewise, tracts which carry information from higher parts of CNS to motor neurons present in spinal cord are called descending tracts (Fig. 9.15).

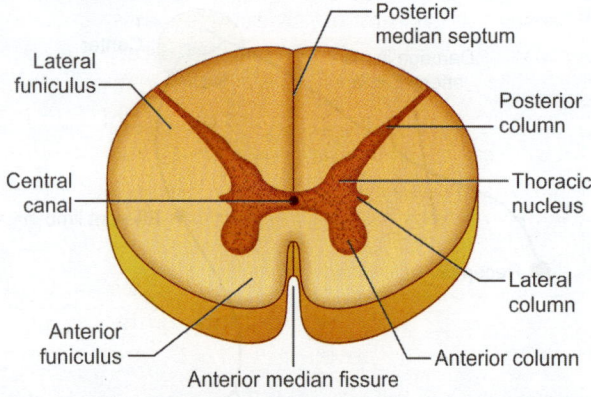

Fig. 9.14: Diagram of transverse section of spinal cord

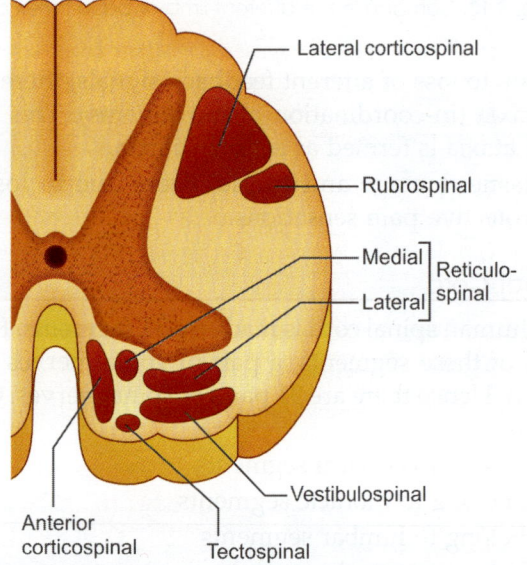

Fig. 9.15: Transverse section of spinal cord showing some of the important ascending and descending tracts

Structural and functional integrity of both gray matter and white matter areas is essential for normal functioning of nervous system. The cell bodies in gray matter area and tracts in white matter are both present in a bilaterally symmetrical way in spinal cord.

Ascending Tracts

- Carry information from spinal cord to higher parts of CNS.
- They are essential for sensory perception as impulses should reach brain from peripheral parts of body.

- Most of these tracts end in sensory areas of cerebral cortex.
- Some of the important ascending tracts are dorsal column tracts, lateral spinothalamic tract, anterior/ventral spin thalamic tract.

Dorsal Column Tract or Posterior Column Tract or Tract of Goll and Burdach or Fascicules Gracilis and Cuneatus

Sensations carried by these tracts are:
1. Fine touch
2. Tactile localization
3. Tactile discrimination (2 point discrimination)
4. Pressure sensation
5. Vibratory sensation
6. Proprioception or sense of position and joint movement and is also known as kinesthetic sensation.
7. Stereognosis

The above sensations from peripheral parts of body are carried by posterior column tracts to cerebral cortex. Nerve fibers carrying these sensations are A beta fibers. Receptors involved will be:
a. Merkel's disk
b. Meissner's corpuscle
c. Pacinian corpuscle
d. Ruffini's end organ
e. Receptors in and around joints

Touch sensation has dual pathways. Fine touch sensation is carried by posterior column tracts and crude touch sensation is carried by anterior or ventral spinothalamic tract.

From the receptors, A beta fibers carry impulse. When posterior nerve fibers reach spinal cord, the nerve trunk of posterior spinal nerve separates into two divisions, namely medial and lateral divisions between dorsal root ganglion and spinal cord. The fibers going to contribute for formation of posterior column tracts enter spinal cord through medial division. These fibers reach posterior funiculus of spinal cord and ascend up on same side of spinal cord. In the brainstem, at the level of medulla oblongata, these fibers synapse in two different nuclei, namely gracile and cuneate nuclei. First order neurons are posterior root ganglion cells.

The second order fibers take origin from the nuclei of gracile and cuneate and cross midline and to reach

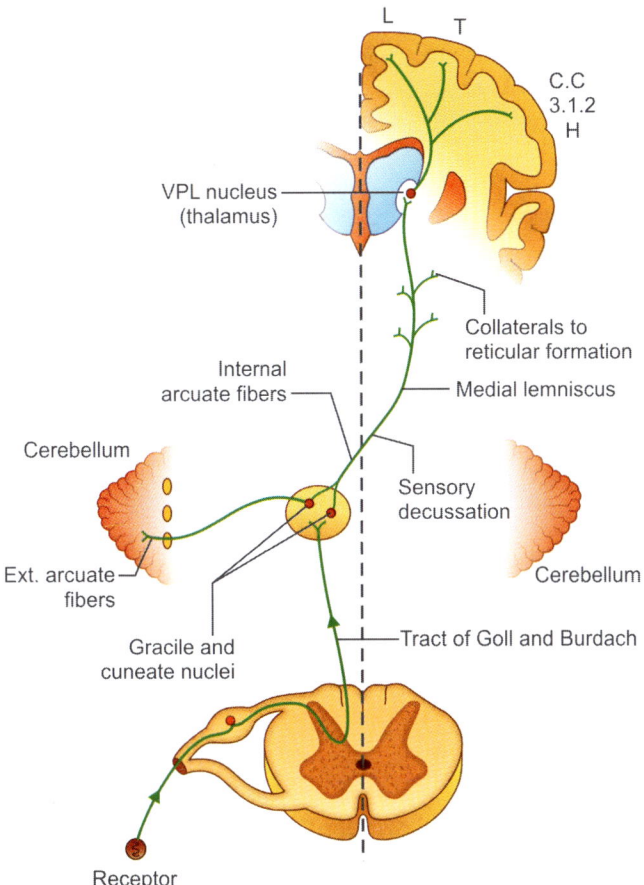

Fig. 9.16: Pathway carrying fine touch, tactile localization, etc. from peripheral parts of the body

impulses to cerbellum of same side by passing through inferior cerebellar peduncle. The internal arcuate fibers as they ascend up further to form medial lemniscus after crossing. Fibers of medial lemniscus synapse in ventroposterolateral nucleus present in thalamus. Neurons extending from gracile and cuneate nuclei to thalamus are called as second order neurons.

Fibers which take origin from ventroposterolateral nuclei pass through posterior limb of internal capsule to end in sensory area (3, 1, 2) of cerebral cortex (primary somesthetic area) present in postcentral gyrus. These fibers which end in cerebral cortex are known as thalamic/sensory radiation fibers and constitute third order neurons (Fig. 9.16).

Sensory Homunculus

In uncrossed tract, sacral segmental fibers will be medial most and cervical fibers will be lateral most. Knowledge of topographical arrangement afferent fibers in different ascending tracts is essential in certain spinal cord lesions especially when lesion is due to degeneration of tissue around spinal canal (syringomyelia).

Stereognosis: It is ability of person to identify some familiar/known objects even with closed eyes. The impulses for this sensation will be carried by posterior column tracts. The person is able to identify object based on:

- Shape
- Size
- Texture of object

Fine touch, tactile localization, and tactile discrimination, etc. from face.

opposite side. These fibers that cross are known as internal arcuate fibers (80%). Internal arcuate fibers will be contributing for sensory decussation. Approximately, 20% of fibers which takes origin from gracile and cuneate nuclei, do not cross midline and these are known as external arcuate fibers. They carry

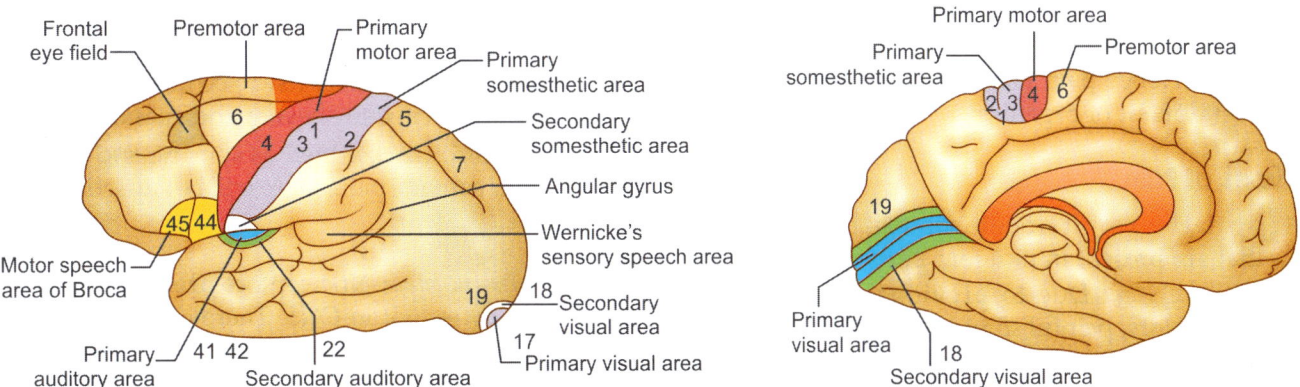

Fig. 9.17: Cerebral cortex showing some of the important areas

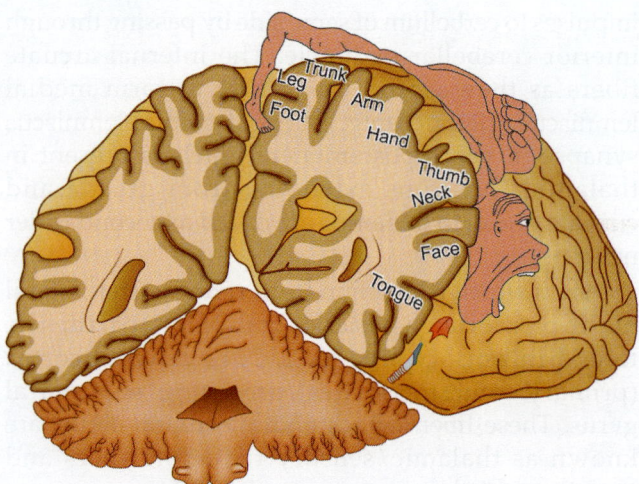

Fig. 9.18: Body representation in sensory cortex

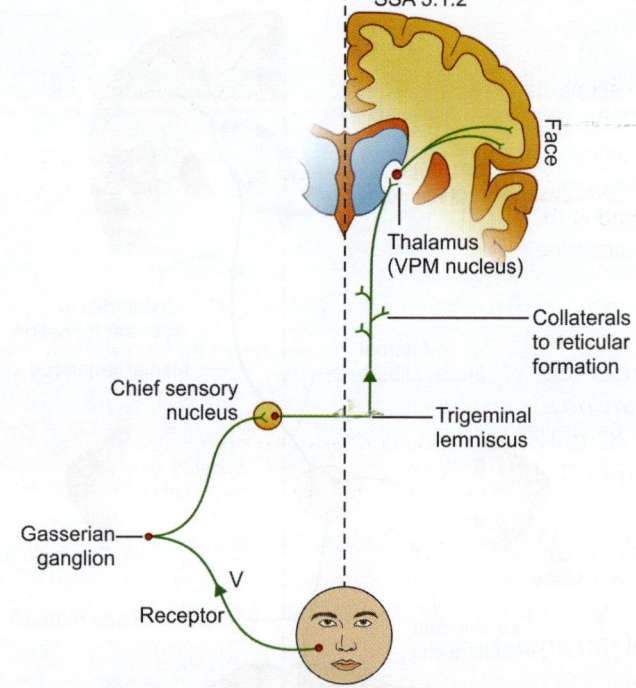

Fig. 9.19: Pathway for fine touch, tactile localization, etc. from face

Fibers carrying sensations from receptor belong to 5th cranial nerve (carry sensory fibers from face). These fibers reach Gasserian ganglion. From ganglion, fibers enter pons to synapse in chief sensory nucleus. From chief sensory nucleus, 2nd order fibers take origin and cross the midline to reach the opposite side. These fibers ascend upward as trigeminal lemniscus. They synapse in ventroposteromedial nucleus of thalamus.

From ventroposteromedial nucleus, 3rd order fibers originate. They end in lateral most part of cerebral cortex area number 3, 1, and 2 present in post-central gyrus where face is represented (Fig. 9.19).

Pain

Definition

Pain is a sensory experience, which normally evokes emotional responses and is associated with autonomic and somatic motor adjustments. Pain is experienced when there is damage or potential damage to any part of body. Hence pain is a "welcome" experience for the betterment of organism.

Types of Pain

1. *Nociceptive pain:* It is due to stimulation of nociceptors that are present in different parts of body.
2. *Hyperalgesia:* Due to previous sensitization of nociceptors, painful stimulus becomes all the more painful. If innocuous thermal or tactile stimulus evokes pain, it is known as allodynia and is due to hyperalgesia.
3. *Referred pain:* Pain from deep structures, like viscera, is not felt at site of viscera but is referred to some superficial part of the body that is away. This pain is poorly localized at site of origin.
4. *Neuropathic pain:* Pain occurs in absence of nociceptor stimulation. May be due to damage or irritation of peripheral nerves or in the pathway of pain in CNS. Accordingly, it may be referred to as peripheral or central pain.
   a. *Causalgia:* Area innervated by damaged peripheral nerve may develop severe pain and phantom limb is an example for this peripheral neuropathic pain.
   b. Thalamic lesion gives rise to central neuropathic pain, which is quite severe and spontaneous.

Pain can also be classified as somatic and visceral pain. Under somatic pain, there will be superficial and deep pain.

Receptors involved: Nociceptors are present in all parts of body except in CNS. There are two types of nociceptors, namely:

a. A δ mechanical nociceptors (fast pain)
b. C polymodal nociceptors (slow pain)

	Fast pain	Slow pain
	Table 9.1: Differences between fast and slow pain	
Receptors	A δ mechanical nociceptor	C polymodal nociceptor
Nerve fibers	A δ	C
Reticular formation	Get information along collaterals	Get information by multisynaptic pathway.
Thalamic nuclei	Ventroposteromedial	Intralaminar and midline involved
End in CC	Primary sensory area	Primary and other areas also
Localizing the site of pain	Very precise	Very poor

A δ nociceptors respond for mechanical stimuli, like pricking, crushing of skin, etc. and afferent fibers carrying impulses are A δ.

C polymodal nociceptors respond for all types of stimuli, like mechanical, chemical or thermal and afferent fibers which carry impulses belong to C group. Differences between fast and slow pain have been enumerated in Table 9.1.

Nociceptor stimulation is responsible for initiation of inflammation around area of pain and is known as neurogenic inflammation.

Causes for hyperalgesia: Any type of nociceptors may undergo peripheral sensitization after exposure to strong noxious stimulus. This would be the reason for hyperalgesia. Sensitization occurs due to release of certain substances like K^+, bradykinin, serotonin, histamine, etc.

Reason for hypersensitivity and other reactions at site of injury:

• Stimulation of nociceptors
• Impulses generated in the nerve fiber terminal
• Impulses travel along axon to CNS from concerned receptors that have got stimulated
• On reaching the branching area, impulses will also travel towards site of injury through other branches of nerve fiber
• These antidromically conducted impulses bring about release of substances like:
  a. Substance P
  b. CGRP (calcitonin gene-related peptide)
• The aforesaid agents along with substances liberated by damaged cells, platelets, mast cells, etc., lead to inflammation at site of injury.
• The inflammation leads to series of typical changes at site of injury, namely:
  a. Tumor/swelling/(neurogenic edema)
  b. Rubor/redness (due to increased blood flow)

c. Calor/warmth (due to heat production)
d. Dolor/pain (tenderness due to sensitization of pain receptors)

Pathway for Pain and Thermal Sensations from Peripheral Parts of Body

Receptors for pain and temperature are naked nerve endings which are present in almost all parts of body. The highest center for pain perception is thalamus. The impulses reaching sensory areas of cerebral cortex help for:

1. Precise localization of painful region.
2. Differentiate whether it is pricking pain, burning pain, etc.
3. Intensity discrimination of pain
4. Emotional reactions associated with pain.

Pain impulses are carried by two different groups of nerve fibers.

a. Fast pain is by A delta fibers
b. Slow pain is by C fibers

Nerve fibers of posterior root carrying pain impulses enter spinal cord through lateral division. Fast pain fibers synapse in neurons present in lamellae I and V in dorsal/posterior horn of spinal cord.

Slow pain fibers synapse in neurons present in lamellae I and II of dorsal horn. In general, fibers carrying pain and thermal sensations synapse in substantia gelatinosa Rolandi neurons present in posterior horn of gray matter. Hence, first order neurons extend from receptor to posterior horn of spinal cord.

From substantia gelatinosa Rolandi, second order fibers take origin and they cross midline in anterior gray and white commissure in front of spinal canal. After passing through commissure, fibers reach lateral funiculus of opposite side to form lateral spinothalamic tract. Fibers of lateral spinothalamic tract will then ascend up (Fig. 9.20).

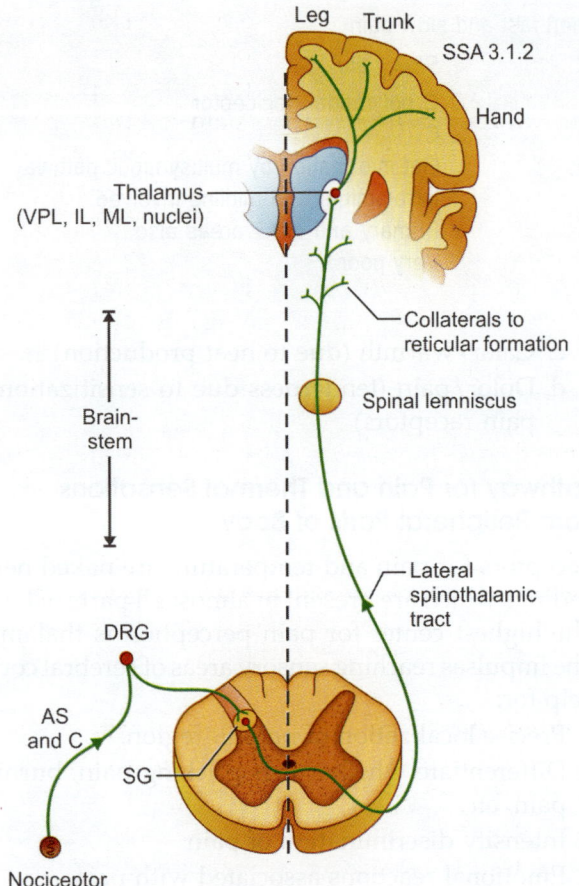

Leg Trunk

SSA 3.1.2

Hand

Thalamus
(VPL, IL, ML, nuclei)

Collaterals to
reticular formation

Brain-
stem

Spinal lemniscus

Lateral
spinothalamic
tract

DRG

AS
and C

SG

Nociceptor

Fig. 9.20: Pathway for pain and temparature sensation from peripheral parts of body

There are two types of fibers that form lateral spinothalamic tract; namely paleospinothalamic tract (spinoreticular tract) and neospinothalamic tract (spinothalamic tract). Spinothalamic/neospino-thalamic fibers synapse in ventroposterolateral nucleus of thalamus. The neospinothalamic tract fibers while passing through brainstem give collaterals to reticular formation present in this region.

The spinoreticular/paleospinothalamic tract fibers reach the reticular formation present in brainstem. In reticular formation of brainstem, these fibers have multisynaptic pathway. The fibers finally synapse in intralaminar and midline nuclei of thalamus.

From ventroposterolateral nucleus and from intralaminar and midline nuclei of thalamus, third order fibers take origin. All these fibers pass through posterior limb of internal capsule to reach cerebral cortex. Fibers coming from ventroposterolateral nucleus end in sensory cortex area no. 3, 1, and 2 only.

The fibers coming from midline and intralaminar nuclei end in sensory cortex area no. 3, 1, and 2 and also in almost all other parts of cerebral cortex.

Whenever fibers cross in spinal cord, sacral fibers come to occupy lateral most part and cervical fibers lie in medial most part. Arrangement of these fibers will be just opposite to fibers arrangement in posterior column tracts.

Pain and Temperature Sensation from Face

From receptor, A delta fibers and C group fibers take origin. Fibers belong to 5th cranial nerve that is trigeminal nerve. Fibers carrying pain and sensation from face enter brainstem at the level of pons. In pons, these fibers pass through chief sensory nucleus but they do not synapse, instead they descend downwards into upper part of cervical segments of spinal cord. Nucleus in which fibers end up is known as spinal nucleus of trigeminal nerve. Spinal nucleus of trigeminal nerve extends from lower part of pons to few upper segments cervical part of spinal cord. Second order neurons are constituted by fibers originating from spinal nucleus of trigeminal nerve. Fibers which have taken origin from this nucleus cross midline and ascend up though brainstem as trigeminal lemnisci.

The trigeminal lemniscus fibers synapse in ventro-posteromedial nucleus present in thalamus. From this nucleus, 3rd order fibers take origin and pass through posterior limb of internal capsule and end in cerebral cortex area no. 3,1, and 2 (sensory area of cortex) in lateral most part where face is represented (Fig. 9.21). Right half of face is represented in left cerebral hemisphere and vice versa.

Referred Pain

Pain in viscera is not felt at site of origin but felt in some superficial part of body which is remote or far away from site of origin of pain. Reason is, concerned visceral part of body takes origin from particular segment/dermatome in embryonic life from which superficial part of body also has taken origin. Examples for referred pain are plenty. Some of common ones are:

a. Ischemic heart pain is referred to inner part of left arm.
b. Pain in diaphragm is referred to tip of shoulder.
c. Pain in appendix is referred around umbilicus region.

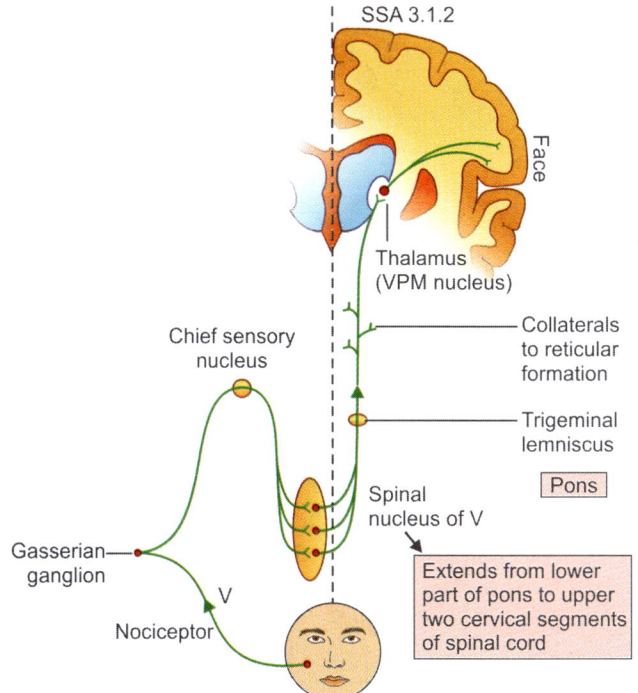

Fig. 9.21: Pathway for pain and temparature sensation from face region

Why should visceral pain get referred to superficial parts of body and not vice versa?

1. Pain always gets referred to superficial part of body of which has high density of receptors.
2. Superficial part of body gets represented quite distinctly in cerebral cortex when compared to visceral parts.
3. Till afferent fibers reach spinal cord, fibers from superficial and visceral parts are different. In neuronal axis of CNS, fibers from both superficial and visceral part synapse on common neuron and pathway continues up further like that.
4. Superficial parts of body are more prone to come across noxious stimulus when compared to visceral parts. Since in spinal cord and above, the pathway is common for both superficial and visceral pain, there will be some amount of "conditioning" that has taken place in cerebral cortex. Because of this, when pain is visceral in origin; it will be misinterpreted as if from superficial structures.

How can referred pain be explained?

Convergence theory: Skin is most prone to get damaged rather than visceral organs. When there is stimulation of pain receptors present in skin, impulse travels along cutaneous nerve to end on a second order neuron present in posterior horn of spinal cord. When there is stimulation of pain receptors present in viscera, impulse will go to spinal cord to end on same neuron on which somatic afferent nerve fiber has synapsed. In other words, because of convergence property of synapse, presynaptic fibers coming from different regions will be ending on common post-synaptic neuron. Impulses coming from either visceral or cutaneous region will be able to stimulate the second order neuron to threshold value. This results in production of action potential and the impulse is carried to cerebral cortex through lateral spino-thalamic tract. Sensory cortex interprets this impulse, as if coming from somatic area (skin).

Facilitation theory: Impulses coming along nerve fibers of visceral region may not be able to stimulate second order neuron to threshold value. So second order neuron gets stimulated only to sub-threshold value.

When there is mild stimulation of pain receptors (a mild pain) in cutaneous region, sensation of pain may not be normally perceived. It is because impulses coming along afferent fibers will not be able to stimulate second order neurons to threshold value. Hence person will not experience pain sensation.

Each of sub-threshold stimuli, if occur simul-taneously, effect of two sub-threshold stimuli on post-synaptic region gets added up (example for spatial summation). Because of these effects, facilitate firing of second order neuron to bring about development of an action potential.

Gate Control Theory of Pain

C group fiber entering spinal cord (slow pain) release substance P, which in turn stimulates substantia gelatinosa (SG) neurons (the gate) in spinal cord. Impulses from SG in turn stimulate 'P' cells. From 'P' cell, spinoreticular tract fibers take origin. Spino-reticular tract fibers carry slow pain sensation (Fig. 9.22).

When A δ fibers (fast pain) are stimulated, collateral from A stimulates 'I' cells in spinal cord. This neuron ('I' cell) later on inhibits SG and hence gate for slow pain gets closed. A δ fibers bring about stimulation of 'M' cells in spinal cord. From 'M' cells, fibers that are going to contribute for formation of neospinothalamic or spinothalamic tract take origin. This tract is concerned with conduction of fast pain impulses.

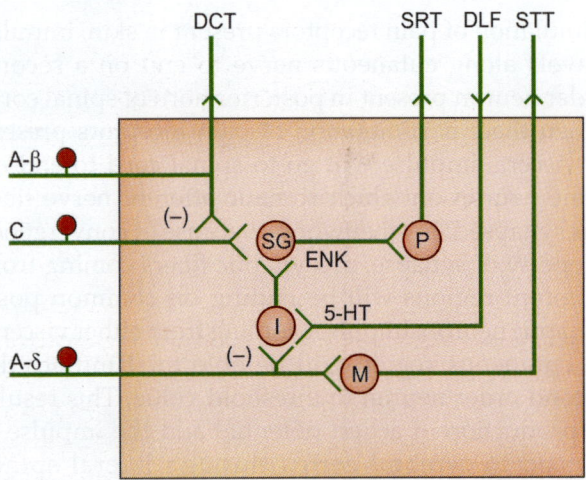

Fig. 9.22: Various cells involved in modulation of gate operation in the spinal cord (STT–spinothalamic tract, 5-HT–5 hydroxy-tryptamine, ENK–Enkephalin, DCT–Dorsal column tract, DLF–dorsolateral funiculus)

When there is massaging, and application of pain balms (leads to counter irritation), transcutaneous electrical nerve stimulation (TENS), acupuncture etc., A β fibers (which carry other sensations, like touch, pressure) get stimulated. They presynaptically inhibit (for details refer to presynaptic inhibition) fibers of C group ending on SG and does not allow opening of gate. Hence no impulse production in SG neurons. So person gets relief from pain.

Impulses coming along dorsolateral funiculus (DLF) release serotonin (5 HT). This neurotransmitter stimulates 'I' cells. 'I' cells now postsynaptically inhibit SG by releasing enkephalin (ENK). This leads to closing of gate and hence there will be no action potential production from SG cells.

Descending Analgesic System or Endogenous Analgesic System (EAS)

Neurons in periventricular gray (PVG) and periaqueductal gray (PAG) in midbrain (Fig. 9.23) have excitatory influence on nucleus raphe magnus (NRM) present in medulla oblongata.

The neurons of PVG and PAG are stimulated by impulses coming from cerebral cortex. This will be responsible for stress-induced analgesia in any life-threatening situation. PAG and PVG also get stimulated by ascending fibers (lateral spinothalamic fibers) which are carrying pain and thermal sensations.

Descending fibers pathway that take origin from NRM are termed as dorsolateral funiculus (DLF), and

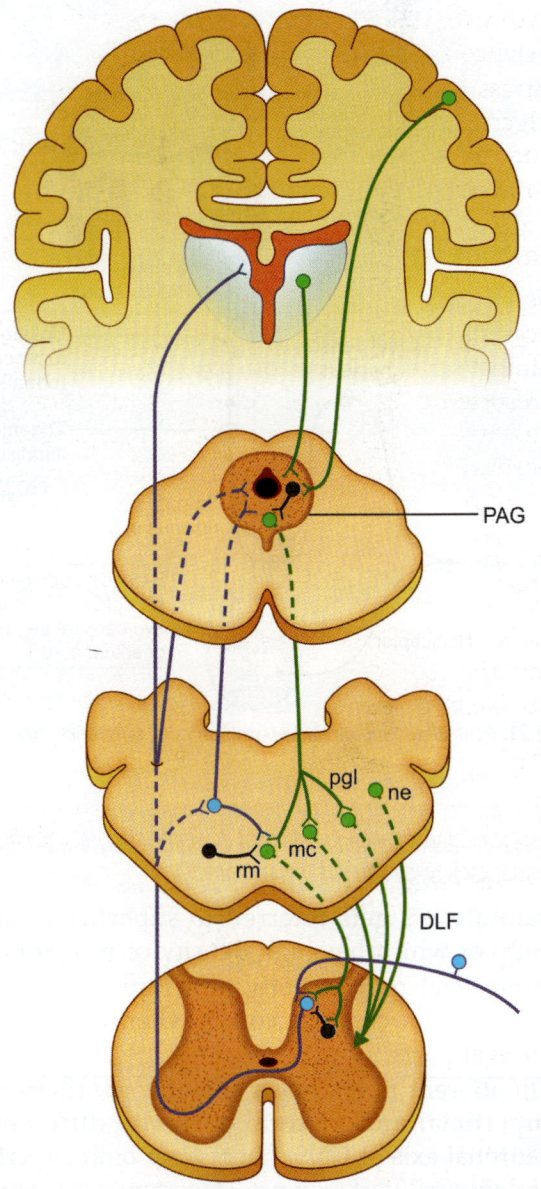

Fig. 9.23: Neurons in the brainstem involved in the descending analgesic system

they end on I cells present in dorsal horn of spinal cord. DLF fibers stimulate 'I' cells by releasing 5 HT and these 'I' cells subsequently inhibit SG (close the gate) by releasing enkephalin.

One of the groups of neurotransmitters liberated by EAS is termed as opioid peptides that include enkephalin, endorphin and dynorphin. Administering substances, like morphine, can augment activity of EAS. DLF fibers can also release neurotransmitters which are non-opioid in nature.

Administering naloxone can inhibit opioid substance mediated analgesic activity.

Stress can stimulate both opioid and non-opioid analgesic fibers as occurs during any emergency. This occurs in soldiers injured in battleground, athletes injured in sports events, etc.

Pain Relieving Surgical Procedures

When people suffer from intractable pain in certain cancerous conditions and when medical management is almost not helping, surgical methods may have to be resorted to. In such a situation, interruptions in pathway of pain may be of choice. In many of these procedures, either person does feel pain, or will not react to pain.

Interruption in pathway can be outside spinal cord, in spinal cord or even in higher parts of central nervous system. The pathway can be sectioned either outside spinal cord or in spinal cord more easily when compared to sectioning pathway in higher parts of CNS like in thalamus or cerebral cortex.

Some of the surgical procedures that can be employed when there necessity for interruptions in pathway is:

1. *Peripheral nerve sectioning:* Especially when somatic nerves sectioning is a must. One of the problems with this sectioning is, since there is complete sectioning of peripheral nerve, in affected part of body, there can be complete loss of sensations.

2. *Sympathetectomy:* From viscera, pain sensation from most of structures is carried by sympathetic afferent fibers. So relief from pain which is getting originated from viscera can be achieved by performing sympathectomy.

3. *Posterior rhizotomy* afferent nerves before they enter spinal cord, get separated into two bundles, namely lateral and medial divisions. Fibers of medial division will contribute for formation of posterior column tracts which carry fine touch, proprioception, etc. Fibers of lateral division contribute for formation of spinothalamic tracts. Hence by cutting lateral division alone, selective loss of pain, temperature and crude touch can be established in desired parts of body.

4. *Myelotomy:* In this procedure, fibers crossing midline in anterior gray and white commissure which are going to contribute for formation of lateral spinothalamic tract are cut off. This procedure is helpful especially when there is need to relieve pain on either side of body at particular regions.

5. *Anterolateral cordotomy:* In this procedure, there will be sectioning of lateral spinothalamic tract on any one side. Since lateral spinothalamic tract is present in lateral funiculus, selective lesion of this tract can be performed.

6. *Prefrontal lobotomy:* Here white matter connection of prefrontal lobe with other parts of cerebral cortex is cut off. Following this procedure, person can still feel pain, since thalamus is highest center for pain perception and impulses are reaching thalamus. But person's reaction to pain will be absent.

Pathway for Crude Touch from Peripheral Parts of Body

Crude touch sensation from peripheral parts of body is carried by anterior spinothalamic tract. Receptors involved are free nerve endings and nerve fibers which carry these impulses are A beta.

From receptor A beta fibers which carry impulses enter spinal cord through lateral division of dorsal nerve root. These fibers synapse in nucleus proprious. From nucleus proprious, 2nd order fibers take origin, cross the midline in anterior gray and white commissure in front of central canal. These fibers after crossing reach white matter in anterior funiculus and ascend up as anterior/ventral spinothalamic tract. While passing through brainstem, anterior spino-thalamic fibers give collaterals to reticular formation. Fibers finally reach ventroposterolateral nucleus of thalamus and synapse. From this nucleus the 3rd order fibers take origin, pass through posterior limb of internal capsule to end in cerebral cortex area no. 3, 1, and 2 in postcentral gyrus.

Motor System Overview

The movements of various parts of body should not only be executed, but also must be very much coordinated. It is not just voluntary movement that needs to be controlled; there should be proper regulation even in the case of reflex activities as well. For efficient execution and control over movements, it is essential that different parts of brain are able to exert their influence over motor neurons present in various parts of body. Different parts of brain that have major role to play in initiation and smooth control over movements of body are:

1. Cerebral cortex—motor areas especially for voluntary and skilled movements.
2. Reticular formation present in brainstem
3. Cerebellum
4. Basal ganglia
5. Red nucleus
6. Vestibular nucleus, etc.

The impulses that originate in these parts of brain (upper motor neurons) will be reaching lower motor neurons present in brainstem and spinal cord (Fig. 9.24). Since lower motor neurons of brainstem are very much in the vicinity of many of controlling parts, there are no separate well-defined bundles of nerve fibers which have to traverse long distance. On the other hand, bundles of nerve fibers from brain which have to control activity of lower motor neurons of spinal cord are quite distinct and have to traverse long distance to reach lower motor neurons. Bundle of nerve fibers which are descending through brainstem reach spinal cord to exert their influence on lower motor neurons are termed as descending tracts. For any part of body to execute smooth movements, it is very essential that structurally and functionally both upper and lower motor neurons should be intact. Some of the important descending tracts are (Fig. 9.25):

1. Lateral corticospinal tract
2. Anterior or ventral corticospinal tract

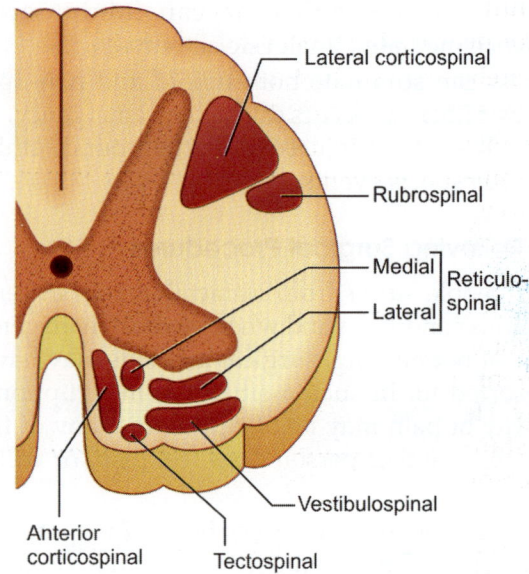

Fig. 9.25: Some of the important ascending and descending tracts in spinal cord

3. Rubrospinal tract
4. Reticulospinal tract
5. Vestibulospinal tract, etc.

The above mentioned tracts can be broadly classified into pyramidal and extrapyramidal tracts. Tracts involved in pyramidal group are lateral and anterior pyramidal tracts. But for these two, all other descending tracts are included under extrapyramidal tracts. Descending tracts are present either in lateral or anterior funiculus in spinal cord.

Lateral and anterior corticospinal tract: A large number of fibers take origin from motor areas present in motor cortex in the frontal lobe. Nerve fibers which take origin from motor cortex but influence lower motor neurons present in brainstem regions are termed as corticonuclear or corticobulbar fibers. These fibers regulate activity of nuclei from where motor cranial nerves take origin.

Rubrospinal tract: It takes origin from red nucleus present in midbrain and influences activity of lower motor neurons present in spinal cord.

Reticulospinal tract: This tract takes origin from reticular formation present in brainstem and exerts control over lower motor neurons of spinal cord.

Vestibulospinal tract: This tract takes origin from motor component of vestibular nucleus present in

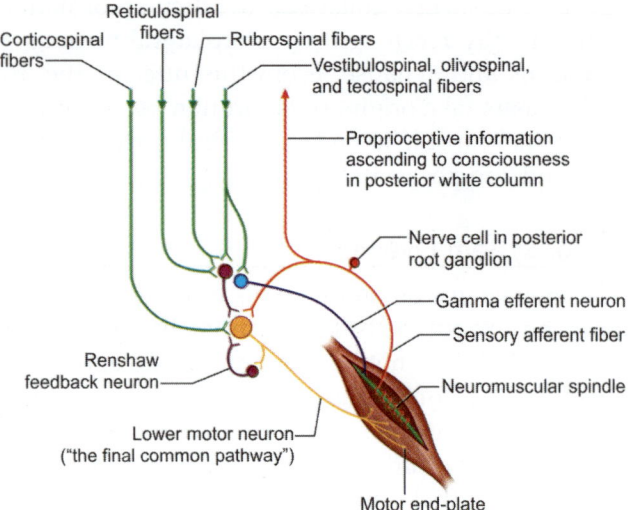

Fig. 9.24: Influence of various fibers on the anterior horn cell (motor neuron) that controls the activity of the muscle

medulla oblongata and exerts control over lower motor neurons of spinal cord (Fig. 9.26).

Cerebellum has no direct control over lower motor neurons of either brainstem or spinal cord. However, cerebellar role in smooth movement is very much warranted. Cerebellar influence over lower motor neurons is indirect. Cerebellum control over lower motor neuron is mediated through either motor cortex or red nucleus or reticular nucleus or vestibular nucleus (Fig. 9.27).

Motor function cannot be smooth in the absence of afferent impulses coming from peripheral parts of body. Hence during any movements, there would be constant bombarding of afferent impulses from different parts of the body (Fig. 9.28) to areas of brain, like cerebellum, vestibular nucleus, sensory areas of cerebral cortex, etc. This type of feedback influence facilitate smooth movements.

Another way to classify descending motor pathways will be lateral motor system versus medial motor system.

The lateral pathways end directly on motor neurons or interneuronal groups in lateral parts of spinal cord gray matter, whereas medial pathways excite motor

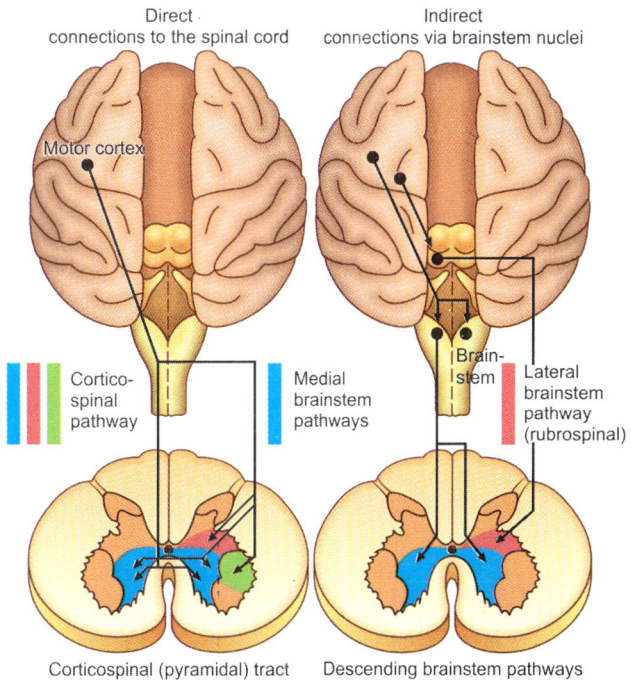

Fig. 9.26: Control over the spinal motor neurons by cerebral cortex and subcortical regions

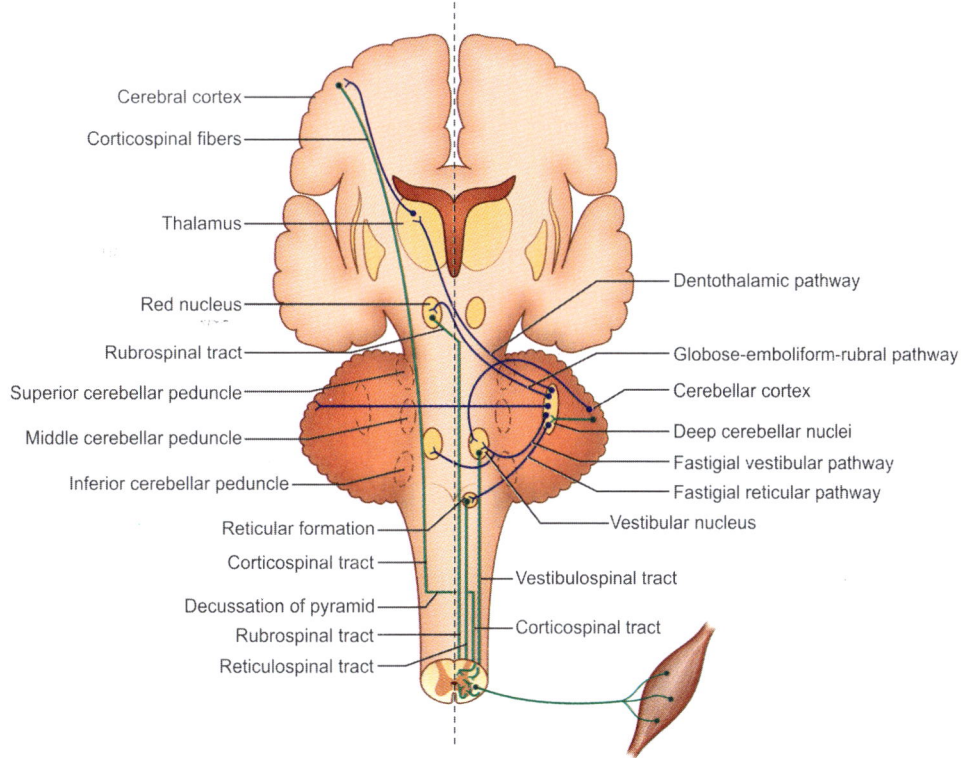

Fig. 9.27: Influence of cerebellum and other higher parts of CNS over the anterior horn cell action in spinal cord

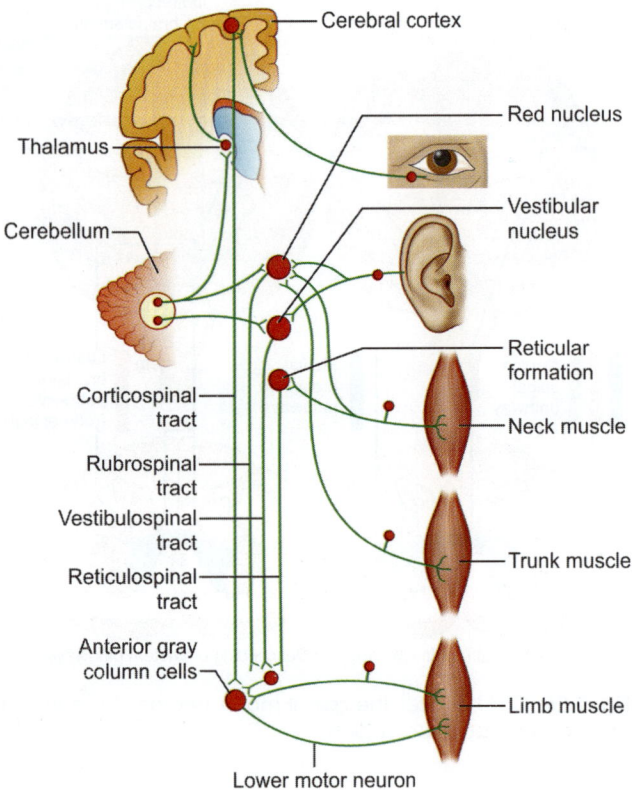

Fig. 9.28: Afferent impulses from peripheral parts of body reaching CNS that are necessary for smooth activity to be brought about

- In motor cortex, body representation is upside down (Fig. 9.29).
- The motor cortex exerts contralateral control that is, right half of body activity is controlled by left cerebral cortex and vice versa.
- Representation is not for individual muscles but for movements. Movements are brought about by involvement of group of muscles.

In precentral gyrus, there are special cells present, namely Betz cells or pyramidal cells. These cells contribute for origin of pyramidal tract in addition to neurons present in premotor cortex and sensory cortex.

Axons of these fibers converge towards internal capsule to form corona radiata. Corona radiata fibers as they approach internal capsule get compactly packed. In internal capsule, fibers pass through anterior two-thirds of posterior limb and genu.

In brainstem, cranial nerve motor nuclei are present. When pyramidal tract fibers pass through brainstem, some of these fibers synapse on motor nuclei of cranial nerve. Pyramidal tract fibers influencing cranial nerve nuclei 3, 4, 6 are called as corticonuclear fibers and those fibers influencing cranial nerve nuclei 5, 7, 9, 10, 11, and 12 are called as corticobulbar fibers.

In lower part of medulla oblongata, majority of pyramidal tract fibers (80–85%) cross midline to reach opposite side. Crossing of fibers is known as motor deccussation. Fibers after crossing descend down as lateral corticospinal tract (LCST), and remaining fibers which have not crossed the midline descend down in

neurons directly. They also influence reflex arcs that control fine movements in distal limbs apart from supporting musculature in proximal limbs.

The medial pathways end on motor neurons in the medial ventral horn or interneuronal groups present in this part of gray horn. These interneurons connect bilaterally with motor neurons that control axial musculature and thereby contribute for balance and posture. They also contribute to control of proximal limb muscles.

Pyramidal Tract

- This tract is also known as corticospinal or cerebrospinal tract.
- The tracts included in pyramidal tract are lateral and ventral or anterior corticospinal tract.
- The tracts take origin from cerebral cortex present in precentral gyrus area no. 4. In addition to this, fibers also take origin from premotor cortex area no. 6 and 8 and some of the fibers also take origin from sensory cortex area no. 3, 1, and 2.

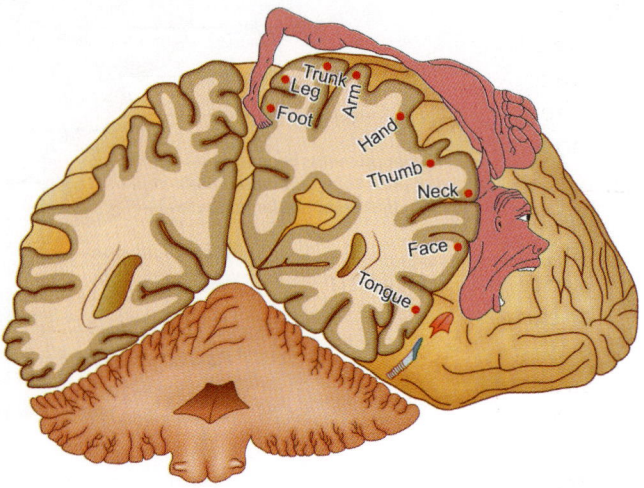

Fig. 9.29: Body representation in the motor cortex

spinal cord as anterior/ventral corticospinal tract (ACST/VCST).

In the anterior horn of spinal cord, lower motor neurons (LMN) are present. Lateral corticospinal tract fibers which are located in lateral funiculus of spinal cord along their course, end on LMN at every segmental level. Many fibers end directly on LMN and some of them may end through an internuncial neuron.

Anterior corticospinal tract fibers descend down in anterior funiculus of spinal cord. Just like lateral corticospinal tract fibers, fibers of anterior corticospinal tract also synapse on LMN present in anterior gray matter. Just before ending on LMN, many of anterior corticospinal tract fibers cross midline to end on LMN present in opposite half of spinal cord. However, some fibers end on LMN present in anterior gray matter on same side. About 95% (about 85% will have crossed in medulla oblongata and another 10% will cross at every segmental level) of pyramidal tract fibers control activity of LMN present in opposite half of spinal cord. It is because of this, 95% of pyramidal tract fibers will control activity of LMN of opposite side.

Functions of Pyramidal Tract

1. *Voluntary motor activity* in any part of body is because of pyramidal tract. Whenever there is damage to pyramidal tract, most of voluntary movements in distal parts of body will be lost. Loss of voluntary control over muscles activity is known as paralysis.

2. *It is also concerned with regulation of skilled movements* like playing a piano, hand writing, modulation of voice, etc. Hence, it plays an important part whenever refine or precision is required for movement.

3. *Regulates muscle tone:* Pyramidal fibers have excitatory influence on LMN (inhibitory influence on LMN will be because of extrapyramidal fibers). Hence, if there is pure pyramidal tract lesion, loss of excitatory influence leads to decreased muscle tone and hypotonia results. But in clinical situations, pure pyramidal tract lesions are quite rare. Apart from damage to pyramidal tract, there will be damage to extrapyramidal fibers also. Because of this, rather than hypotonia, hypertonia is seen in most of UMN lesions.

Effects of Lesion to Pyramidal Tract at Different Levels

1. *Unilateral lesion in internal capsule:*
   a. Loss of voluntary movement in opposite half of body that is contralateral hemiplegia. But some muscles escape paralysis. Muscles which do not get affected are muscles of upper half of face on opposite side, muscles of trunk and back (axial group of muscles). Muscles which have escaped effect have bilateral representation in motor cortex. All features (refer differences between UMN and LMN lesions) of upper motor neurons are observed in affected part of body.
   b. In addition to motor fibers since sensory fibers are also passing through internal capsule, sensations in opposite half of body will be lost. So there will be contralateral hemianesthesia, homonymous hemianopia (field of vision (in one eye temporal field and in the other eye nasal field are affected), but hearing would not get affected much since hearing has bilateral pathways.

2. *Crossed hemiplegia:* It is seen in a patient when there is lesion in one half of pons. Since pyramidal tracts are yet to cross, there will be contralateral hemiplegia (UMN lesion) in the other parts of body. In addition to this, cranial nerve motor nucleus of 7th nerve is damaged. Because of this, muscles of face are paralyzed on same side (LMN lesion).

3. *A complete transection of spinal cord above level of C3 segment* will lead to paralysis in whole body except in face. Person cannot survive due to respiratory paralysis because of involvement of both diaphragm and intercostal muscles (since phrenic fibers take origin from cervical segments 3, 4 and 5).

4. *Complete transection at C6 or C7:* There will be quadriplegia (paralysis of all 4 limbs). Muscles of face and diaphragm will not be paralyzed. Since diaphragm is not paralyzed, person is able to breath on his own (diaphragmatic breathing).

5. *If there is unilateral sectioning in spinal cord around C6 segment,* it leads to hemiplegia on same side. It is because majority of fibers have already crossed midline at medulla oblongata.

6. *Section at T12 segment:* If there is transaction of spinal cord at this level, lower limb muscles supplied by lumbosacral segments on both sides are paralyzed. Hence results in paraplegia. If lesion is only on one side above origin of lumbosacral

plexus, there is paralysis of only one of lower limbs on affected side. Hence results in monoplegia.

Characteristic Features in UMN and LMN Lesions

Lower motor neuron refers to anterior horn cell or corresponding cranial nerve motor nuclei and its axon. There are two types of LMN, namely gamma (γ) and alpha (α) motor neurons. Special feature of LMN is it forms final common efferent pathway from CNS to any part of body.

Upper motor neuron takes origin from cerebral cortex or subcortical regions and exerts influence over LMN.

Differences between upper and lower motor neuron lesions have been enumerated in Table 9.2.

Features of Reaction of Degeneration

1. *Alteration in chronaxie:* For galvanic current (long duration current), there will slow sluggish movement (worm-like movement). For faradic current, there will not be any response.
2. *Fibrillation:* Involuntary contraction of individual muscle fibers occurs. This can be made out by EMG.

3. *Fasciculation:* Involuntary contraction of a group of muscle fibers will also be present.

Muscle Tone Maintenance and Regulation

How are structures in muscles organized to bring a proper control over movement of muscles?

It is basically due to stretch reflex. This reflex is an example for deep reflex. The functional integrity of muscle is maintained as long as stretch reflex is normal. The details of stretch reflex are as follows:

- Receptors in muscles are muscle spindle (intrafusal fiber), which is arranged parallel to extrafusal fiber (Fig. 9.30). The extrafusal fiber contains contractile unit of muscle namely sarcomere. In addition to muscle spindle, another receptor present in muscle is tendon end organ (Fig. 9.31).
- The intrafusal fibers are of two types, namely nuclear bag fiber (attached to extrafusal fiber) and nuclear chain fiber which is attached to nuclear bag fiber (Fig. 9.32).
- In nuclear bag fiber, dilated central region is known as equatorial zone. This part acts as receptor area and part has many nuclei.

Table 9.2: Features of UMN and LMN lesions

Feature	UMN lesion	LMN lesion
Extent of paralysis	Widespread (large number of muscles are involved)	Restricted to a few muscles supplied by particular LMN.
Tone	Increased muscle tone and hence hypertonia (it is because usually UMNs have inhibitory influence on LMN activity)	Complete loss of muscle tone or atonia (complete loss of influence on muscles to contract)
Type of paralysis	Spastic paralysis	Flaccid paralysis
Resistance to passive movements	Present. Because of this it leads to clasp knife rigidity. Resistance will be experienced up to certain limit and beyond this point resistance is lost completely.	No resistance throughout passive movement. Hence flaccid paralysis.
Reflexes	Deep reflexes are exaggerated due to loss of inhibitory influence on lower motor neurons. All superficial reflexes are lost except plantar reflex which will be Babinski +ve	Both superficial and deep reflexes will be lost due to damage in efferent pathway of basic reflex arc.
Wasting of muscles	Not seen unless there is disuse atrophy	Will be seen and this leads to atrophy of muscles. Muscle mass decreases.
Regeneration	Not possible because neurons of CNS cannot regenerate due to absence of neurilemma	Possible if nerve fiber has got damaged. If anterior horn cells have got affected, then there will not be any regeneration.
Reaction of generation	Not present	Present
Fasciculation and fibrillation	Not present	Present

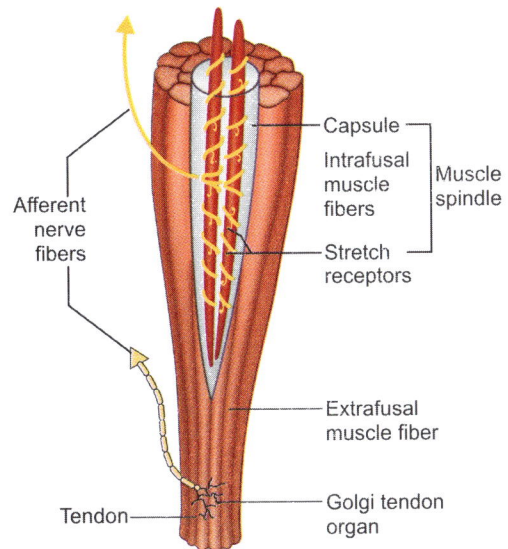

Fig. 9.30: Arrangement of intrafusal and extrafusal fibers

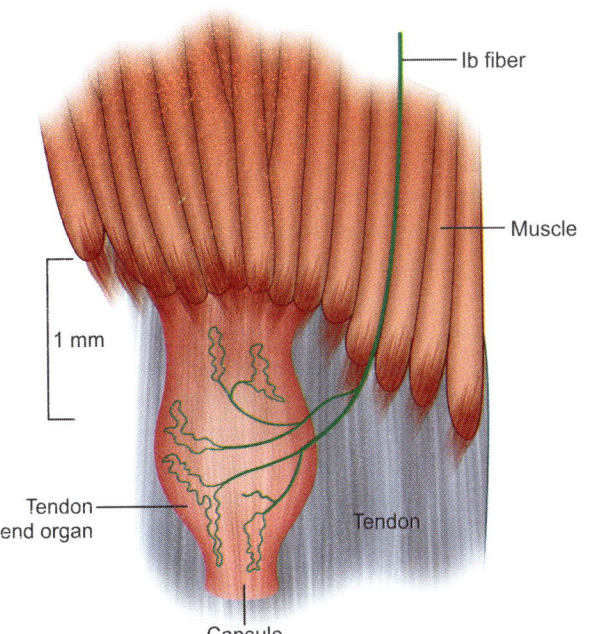

Fig. 9.31: Serial arrangement of tendon end organ with the extrafusal fiber

- In nuclear chain fiber, nuclei are arranged serially.
- Ia primary afferent fibers carry information from central portion of both nuclear bag and nuclear chain fibers.
- Nuclear chain fiber has another afferent nerve supply coming from II (secondary) afferent fibers.

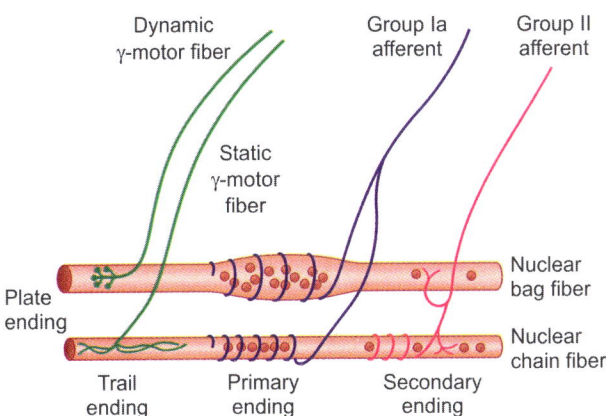

Fig. 9.32: Nuclear bag and nuclear chain fibers with the innervations

- The polar region (peripheral regions) of intrafusal fibers has contractile elements which are supplied with static γ efferent.
- Also there are dynamic γ efferent fibers supplying predominantly to nuclear bag fiber.

Role of muscle spindle with respect to functioning of extrafusal fiber (EFF): Extrafusal fiber (EFF) refers to muscle fiber contraction that brings about various actions in body.

EFF gets motor nerve supply from spinal cord through alpha motor neuron, whereas motor neuron supplies polar region of intrafusal fiber (IFF).

Afferent innervation to intrafusal fibers: Ia primary afferent fibers carry impulses from nuclear chain and nuclear bag fibers.

IIa secondary afferent fibers carry impulses from nuclear chain fibers (Fig. 9.32).

Whenever EFF is stretched, primary afferent fibers are stimulated due to stretching of equatorial zone of intrafusal fibers. Primary afferent fibers carry afferent information from IFF about both, the amount of stretch of IFF, and velocity or rate at which stretch is taking place.

II afferent fibers are able to detect amount of stretch only.

Tone of muscle is partial state of contraction of muscle even at rest or resistance exerted for passive movement.

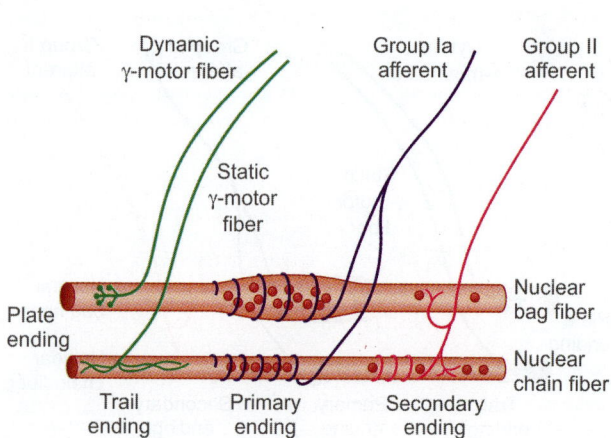

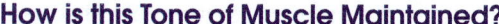

Fig. 9.33: Afferent and efferent innervations of muscle spindle

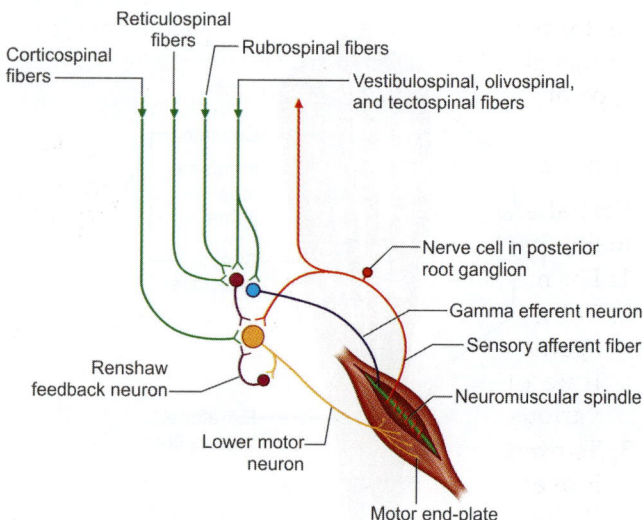

Fig. 9.34: α-γ linkage in the regulation of muscle tone

How is this Tone of Muscle Maintained?

Anterior horn of spinal cord has both α and γ motor neurons. Supraspinal influences from cerebral cortex and subcortical regions act on γ motor neuron present in anterior horn of spinal cord. The γ efferent fibers when carry impulses (Fig. 9.33) to IFF bring about contraction of polar ends of IFF (as they have contractile elements). This leads to stretch/distortion of equatorial zone of IFF. When this happens, receptors present at equatorial zone of IFF get stimulated. This leads to production of action potentials which is carried to spinal cord through Ia primary afferent fibers. These afferent impulses in turn stimulate alpha motor neuron in anterior horn of spinal cord. When alpha motor neuron is stimulated, it brings efferent impulses to sarcomere of EFF, giving rise to contraction of EFF. As IFF is attached parallel to EFF, when the muscle contracts, stretching of IFF will decreases. Since stretching of equatorial zone is decreased, receptors in muscle spindle will not be stimulated any more. This brings about no action potential development in afferent fiber. Because of this, impulses going to spinal cord along Ia fibers is decreased. When there are no impulses along Ia fibers, stimulation of alpha motor neuron also stops (Fig. 9.34). Now muscle starts relaxing. This type of alternating contraction and relaxation goes on continuously and is responsible for maintenance of muscle tone.

This whole mechanism is known as α-γ linkage. Some of impulses from higher parts of CNS may predominantly stimulate alpha motor neuron and some may stimulate γ neuron only.

Increase in the tone of muscle is seen whenever there is mid collicular section. Increase in muscle tone in this situation is due to increased γ discharge. This is known as *Sherrington's animal* or condition is also known as decerebrate rigidity. If posterior nerve root is also sectioned (deafferentation) in decerebrate rigidity, tone of muscles is decreased. Decrease in muscle tone now is due to interruptions in α-γ linkage (that is Ia primary afferents are unable to carry impulses to spinal cord through posterior nerve to stimulate alpha motor neurons).

Pollock-Davis animal is due to increased stimulation of alpha motor neurons and results in rigidity. When there is ischemia of cerebellum it results ischemic decerebration. This type of rigidity will not be lost by deafferentation (that is sectioning of posterior nerve roots). It is because in this condition increased muscle tone is due to hyperactivity of alpha motor neurons itself and not due to gamma motor neuron hyperactivity.

Stretch Reflex

This reflex is an example for monosynaptic reflex. Passive stretch does not involve γ motor neuron. Tapping on tendon of the muscle, brings about stimulation of stretch (muscle spindle) receptors as intrafusal fibers (IFF) are arranged parallel to extrafusal fibers. Impulses from stretch receptors of IFF reach spinal cord along Ia fibers. They stimulate alpha motor neurons present in spinal cord and this in turn brings about contraction of EFF. While eliciting this type of reflex passive stretch of IFF occurs.

Functional Significance of α-γ Linkage

Partial state of contraction that is tone has to be maintained even at rest. This tone is important:

1. For maintenance of postural balance even at rest
2. To maintain/facilitate load effect acting on body against gravity that is while threading a needle, tone of muscle should be maintained during various skilled activities.
3. To exert damping effect—after intended movement is over, contractions of muscle should not continue. It should be stopped immediately. If contractions do not stop instantaneously, it will bring about oscillations in that part of body. It is because of this reason, in UMN lesions, knee jerk gets exaggerated. In cerebellar lesions, knee jerk becomes pendular.

If dorsal nerve root is sectioned, afferent impulses are not able to reach CNS. Therefore, α-γ linkage is broken. This will also lead to oscillation movements or physiological tremors. The α-γ linkage provides a feedback mechanism for smooth movement in any part of body.

Inverse Stretch Reflex

- This reflex is an example for polysynaptic reflex.
- The receptors involved are Golgi tendon organs (tendon end organ)
- Golgi tendon end organ is arranged serially with extrafusal fibers.
- In an inverse stretch reflex, concerned muscle relaxes.
- Reflex operates when muscle is in isometric contractile state, that is length of muscle remains same but tension (due to contraction) in muscle is increased.
- When muscle contracts isometrically, there is no change in length of muscle but tendon of muscle gets pulled at either ends like what is seen in arm wrestling or tug of war, etc.
- If this pulling is beyond certain limit, tendon might snap and get detached from bone/muscle.
- In order to avoid snapping of tendon or rupture of muscle fibers, muscle is released by a reflex mechanism.

Reflex pathway involved: Due to sudden excessive stretching, Golgi tendon end organ gets stimulated, afferent impulses are carried to spinal cord Ib fibers. When impulses reach spinal cord, they stimulate activity of internuncial neuron present between afferent fiber and alpha motor neuron. Stimulation of internuncial neuron in turn brings about inhibition of alpha motor neuron. Hence there will be no more excitatory impulses to EFF of muscle. This leads to relaxation of muscle. The tension in the muscle decreases. This prevents muscle from getting damaged.

Hence this reflex is a protective reflex. The inverse stretch reflex is an example for autogenic inhibition.

Withdrawal Reflex

- When a noxious stimulus is applied to any part of body, there will be a reflex withdrawal of that part of body away from stimulus.
- This is a protective reflex as it prevents further damage by removing that affected part of body from source of stimulus.
- When noxious stimulus is applied, nociceptors are stimulated.
- This brings about production of action potentials in afferent nerve fibers.
- Fast pain is carried by A δ fibers.
- The afferent impulses on reaching spinal cord stimulates motor neuron supplying flexor group of muscles and inhibit motor neurons supplying extensor group of muscles.
- This brings about withdrawal of part of body away from source of noxious stimulus.
- This reflex is also an example for polysynaptic reflex.

Crossed Extensor Reflex

- In the case of humans, it is more pronounced in lower limbs since human beings are biped unlike most of animals which are quadrupeds.
- In the case of human beings whenever noxious stimulus is applied to one of the lower limbs, crossed extensor reflex can be elicited.
- Due to noxious stimulus, limb which is getting injured flexes reflexly thereby bringing about withdrawal flexion reflex and at same time contralateral limb becomes extended.

- The purpose of flexion of affected limb is to prevent further damage and opposite limb has to be extended in order to maintain posture and equilibrium of body.
- Receptors involved are nociceptors (pain receptors).
- Afferent impulses reach spinal cord through small diameter (A delta) fibers.
- These afferent impulses on reaching spinal cord stimulate motor neurons supplying flexor muscles on same side. In addition to this, they also inhibit through an internuncial neuron the motor neurons supplying extensor group of muscles on same side. This brings about flexion of affected limb.
- These afferent impulses also affect motor neurons supplying muscles of opposite limb. Afferent impulses stimulate activity of motor neurons supplying extensor muscles and through internuncial neuron.
- This leads to extension of opposite limb. This is how posture and equilibrium can be maintained even on one limb.
- Stimulation of agonist muscle and inhibition of antagonist muscle is an example for reciprocal inhibition.

Plantar Reflex

- This is one of the examples for superficial reflex.
- In UMN lesions, all superficial reflexes are absent except plantar reflex which will show Babinski +ve sign.

- In LMN or afferent nerve lesions, plantar reflex will be absent since there is damage to basic reflex arc.
- When sole of foot is firmly stroked from lateral side and continued up to area below toes, normally there will be plantar flexion of all five toes. This forms a normal plantar response (Fig. 9.35).
- When plantar response is Babinski +ve type, there will be dorsiflexion of great toe and fanning out of other toes (Fig. 9.35). This type of response is normally seen in UMN lesion particularly in pyramidal tract lesion in which all superficial reflexes are absent except plantar reflex. Babinski +ve sign can be seen in normal infants also till the age of one to one and half years. In infancy, it occurs due to incomplete myelination of pyramidal tract. Babinski +ve sign is also seen in normal adults especially when they are dreaming (during REM sleep), and in person who is in state of coma.

Effects of Hemisection of Spinal Cord (when only one-half of spinal cord is sectioned) (Fig. 9.36)

Features of effects of hemisection of spinal cord have been tabulated in Table 9.3.

Dissociated anesthesia: It is a condition in which in a particular part of body, certain sensations are retained, and certain sensations are lost. Dissociated anesthesia is seen in:

a. Hemisection of spinal cord below the level of lesion

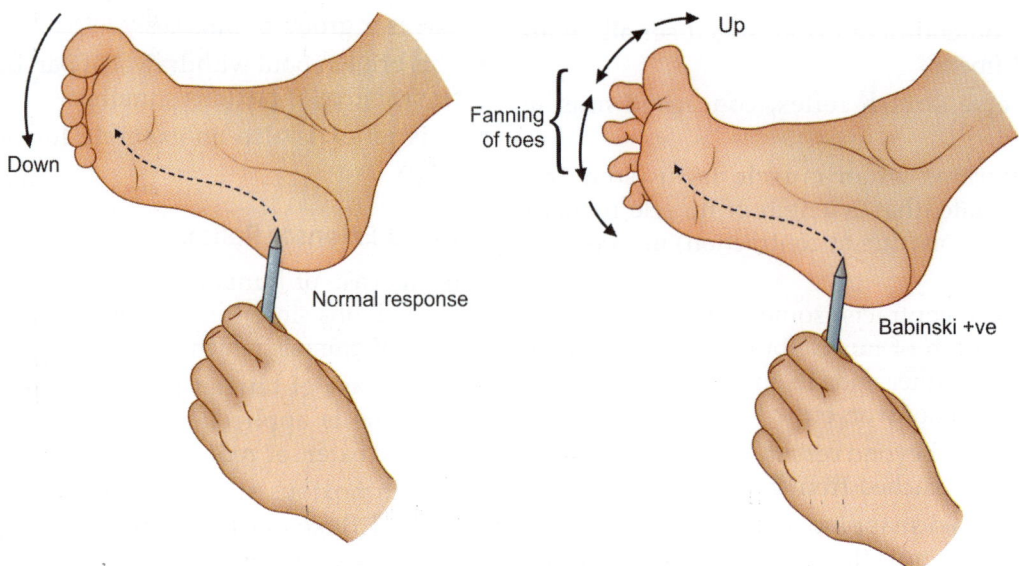

Fig. 9.35: Normal plantar response and Babinski +ve

Table 9.3: Effects of hemisection of spinal cord	
Same side	*Opposite side*
Changes seen below the level of lesion	
Pain and temperature sensations remain intact as lateral spinothalamic tract carrying impulses cross and ascend up on contralateral half of spinal cord	Pain and temperature sensation is lost as lateral spinothalamic tract carrying from opposite half of body is damaged
Postural and other sensations are lost as posterior column tract fibers have not crossed but will cross only at level of medulla oblongata	Postural and other sensations are normal as posterior column tract which carry these impulses up ipsilaterally and has not got damaged
UMN type of paralysis because descending tracts are damaged	Normal because descending tracts are not damaged
At the level of lesion	
All sensations are lost in a dermatome, if 3 consecutive spinal nerves are damaged	Sensations will be normal
LMN lesion due to damage to anterior horn cells	Motor functions will be normal
Above the level of lesion	
Hyperesthesia due to irritation of sensory nerve fibers	No hyperesthesia

b. Syringomyelia—pain and temperature is lost bilaterally but other sensations are retained in the affected parts of the body.

c. Tabes dorsalis—postural sensations are lost but pain and temperature is retained in the affected parts of the body.

Effect of Complete Transection of Spinal Cord

It may occur due to accidental injury (motor vehicle, sports accidents), gunshots wound, stab injury to spinal cord. In these types of injuries, spinal cord will be cut into two different parts. Signs and symptoms are seen below level of lesion in both halves of body.

Effect on Skeletal Muscles

- When spinal cord is transected completely (for example at the level of T6 that is mid-thoracic level) part of body supplied below spinal segment T6 is affected. There will be complete paralysis of skeletal muscles in lower parts of body. So no voluntary movements are possible in both lower limbs. Person suffers from paraplegia. Paraplegia results when there is transaction of spinal cord occurs anywhere above lumbosacral plexus origin but below the level of brachial plexus.

- If lesion is at level of C6 or C7, upper and lower limbs get paralyzed and hence result in quadriplegia (paralysis of all four limbs).

Effect on Blood Pressure (BP)

- If lesion is at T6 or anywhere between T6 and sacral segments, fall of blood pressure limited. Fall of blood pressure is not much since sympathetic nerves function above the level of section will be normal.

- If lesion is above T1, there will be severe fall of blood pressure since all lateral horn cells are separated from vasomotor center which bring facilitatory impulses to lateral horn cells (sympathetic fibers take origin from LHC of thoracolumbar segments). There will be complete loss of vasomotor tone.

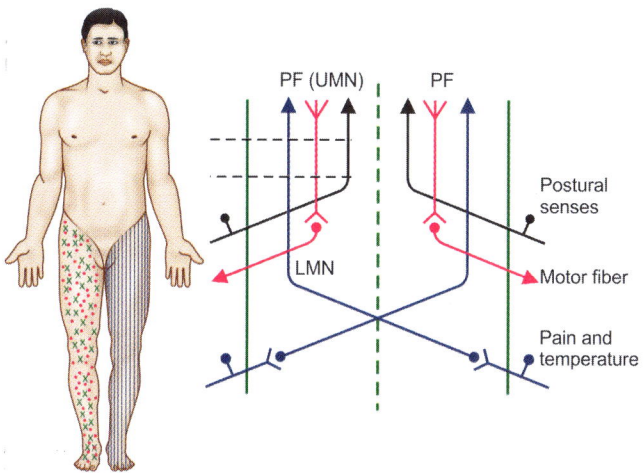

Fig. 9.36: Effect of hemisection of spinal cord

Effect on Respiration

- If lesion is above C3, it leads to instantaneous death due to paralysis of all muscles of respiration.
- If lesion is below C5, diaphragmatic respiration continues, only intercostal muscles get paralyzed. (Intercostal muscles are supplied by nerve coming from T1 to T10 segments of spinal cord.)

Consequences of Complete Transaction of Spinal Cord

1. Stage of spinal shock
2. Stage of recovery of reflex activity
3. Stage of reflex failure.

Spinal Shock

- Lasts for about 1–6 weeks in human beings.
- Duration of spinal shock is directly related to hierarchy/evolution of the animal. In frogs, spinal shock lasts for few minutes only (1–2 min).

Features observed during stage of spinal shock: Signs and symptoms are seen below level of lesion in either side of body.

1. Loss of all sensations in affected parts of body as all ascending tracts are damaged.
2. Motor neurons which are required for motor activities in muscles are affected. Therefore, there will be loss of all voluntary movements in affected parts of body giving rise to flaccid type of paralysis.
3. Reticulospinal tract is damaged, so no excitatory influence to LHC in thoracolumbar segments. This brings about loss of vasoconstrictor influence on smooth muscles of blood vessels. Arterioles get dilated and blood pressure falls (especially diastolic blood pressure). As mentioned earlier, extent of fall of blood pressure depends on level of transection. In addition to vasodilatation, venous return will also get decreased due to dilation of veins (loss of venomotor tone). Pooling of blood in venous system occurs. Decreased venous return affects cardiac output and contributes to fall in systolic blood pressure.
4. There will be complete loss of muscle tone due to no impulses from motor neurons to the muscles.
5. There will be loss of all types of reflexes (superficial, deep and visceral) even though reflex arc is intact. It is because motor neurons of spinal cord are under constant excitatory influence from higher parts of CNS. When supraspinal facilitatory influences are suddenly withdrawn, motor neurons of spinal cord undergo functional depression. Reflexes will be lost completely resulting in a state of areflexia. Functional depression of motor neuron is known as diaschiasis.
6. Position of lower limbs will be determined by gravity and the part of body suffers from stagnant hypoxia and cyanosis occurs.
7. When lesion is above T6 segment, all visceral sensations are also lost. Reflexes, like micturition, defecation, etc., will be lost during this stage of spinal shock. But some amount of urine may dribble out at times. This occurs because of over flow incontinence.
8. Bedsores and ulcers: Fall of blood pressure and pressure contact of part of body with area of support, brings about compression of blood vessels. This leads to decreased blood flow to tissue. Tissues suffer from stagnant hypoxia and this result in atrophy of tissues resulting in bedsores, loss of secretions, etc.

When a patient is in a state of spinal shock, if proper care is not taken, he may not go to 2nd stage that is stage of recovery of reflex activity. Hence management of patient during stage of spinal shock is crucial.

Managing of patient during stage of spinal shock period:

1. When there is accumulation of urine in urinary bladder it may lead to infection. Therefore, bladder has to be catheterized to drain urine continuously. This prevents over distension of bladder and minimizes infection.
2. Administration of rectal enema to remove feces.
3. Bedsore development should be minimized not only to prevent tissue damage and bleeding, but also to prevent any infection. Infections of urinary tract and lungs are prevented by suitable antibiotics.
4. Certain drugs, like amphetamines, which have ability to stimulate motor neurons of spinal cord may be given.

Stage of Recovery of Reflex Activity

- During this stage, voluntary motor activity will not be regained because in CNS regeneration of nerve fibers is not possible. Therefore, descending tracts nerve fibers cannot get regenerated.

- There is no recovery of sensations as ascending tract nerve fibers also cannot regenerate.
- Lateral horn cells function is recovered to a certain extent. Regain of sympathetic activity leads to increase of vasomotor tone and rise of blood pressure.
- There will be functional recovery of lower motor neurons. Because of this, reflex activity is possible, but not normal. Only spinal reflexes recover.
- Visceral reflex also get recovered. Micturition reflex becomes completely automatic even in adults but complete evacuation of bladder would not take place. This will be due to loss of reinforcing influences from pons over sacral segments of spinal cord. So there will be retention of some urine in bladder.
- Defecation reflex also recovers but it too becomes completely an automatic reflex even in adults.

Somatic reflexes observed will be:

a. *Flexor withdrawal reflex:* Motor neurons supplying flexor group of muscles recover earlier. So muscle tone is regained in flexor compartment first. Because of this, withdrawal reflex can be elicited. Most of the times limbs are held in flexion. Hence this is known as paraplegia in flexion.

b. Later on, extensor group of muscles start recovering (these muscles have a delayed recovery as compared to flexor muscles). So reflexes can also be elicited in extensor compartment. Now limbs will be in extended position. This is known as paraplegia in extension.

c. *Coitus reflex:* After complete transaction, impulses from higher centers, like cerebral cortex, are unable to reach nerves supplying reproductive organs. Hence any erogenic thought will not bring about erecting of penis. But such people can still have erection of penis and coitus reflex responses when there is physical stimulation of glans penis. During coitus reflex, there will be curling up of skin around scrotal sac, stiffening of penis, erection, engorgement of penis with blood due to dilation of vessels, and at times ejaculation of seminal fluid.

Mass reflex (pathological reflex): Whenever skin on medial upper part of thigh is scratched, there will be flexion of limb, contraction of abdominal muscles, rise in arterial blood pressure, sweating, reflex micturition and defecation. Mass reflex will be due to irradiation of afferent impulses into many segments of spinal cord and heightened excitability of spinal motor neurons.

Stage of Reflex Failure

Sometimes, even when a person has gone into stage of reflex recovery of reflex activity, it can still suddenly get into a stage of reflex failure. Some volume of residual urine will always be present in urinary bladder, which can lead to infection of bladder either due to constant presence of urine or bedsores, etc. These infections may be more generalized, and later may affect blood pressure. Fall in blood pressure affects normal functioning of kidney and leads to renal failure. Thus internal environment (homeostasis is impaired). All these may lead to failure of heart and nervous system function and can lead to death.

Cerebellum

Cerebellum is also termed as little brain. Present in the posterior part of cranial fossa below occipital lobe.

Connected to other parts of brainstem by three pairs of peduncles, namely:

1. Superior peduncle
2. Middle peduncle
3. Inferior peduncle

In cerebellum, there is a lot of white matter just like in cerebral cortex. Deep below the white matter many nuclei of cerebellum are present. They are:

1. Dentate
2. Emboliform
3. Globose (the nucleus emboliform and globose together sometimes refer to as nucleus interpositus)
4. Fastigial

Special Features

a. Though cerebellum receives a lot of afferent inputs fibers of proprioceptors from various parts of body, conscious perception of sensation will not be possible.

b. It cannot exert its control directly over LMN. However, influence from cerebellum on LMN is essential for proper co-ordination of any movement.

c. Unlike cerebral cortex that controls activity of contralateral half of body, cerebellum controls motor activity of ipsilateral half of body.

d. Apart from nuclei, we find Purkinje, granular, basket, and Golgi cells are also present. There is lot of connection between these various cells.

Divisions of Cerebellum (Fig. 9.37)

Formed by important parts (anatomically):
1. Anterior lobe
2. Flacculonodular lobe
3. Posterior lobe
4. Vermis

Phylogenetically (i.e. depending on order of development during evolution), cerebellum is subdivided into:
1. Archicerebellum (primitive)
2. Paleocerebellum (old)
3. Neocerebellum (newest)

Functionally cerebellum is subdivided into (Fig. 9.38):
1. Flocculonodular lobe (corresponds to archicerebellum) also known as vestibulocerebellum
2. Vermis and part of cerebellum immediately lateral to vermis on either side in anterior and posterior lobes is known as spinocerebellum.

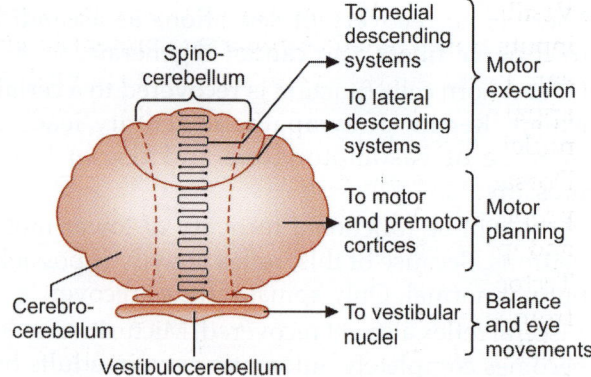
Fig. 9.38: Functional divisions of cerebellum

3. Most lateral part of cerebellar hemisphere is known as cerebrocerebellum / corticocerebellum. This part is very highly developed in human beings.

Connections of Cerebellum (Fig. 9.39)

Afferent Connections

Cerebellum has a lot of afferent inputs coming from proprioceptors (receptors involved in sense of position and movement). However, when impulse reaches cerebellum, it will not come to conscious perception.
a. The proprioceptive inputs from head and neck region reach cerebellum through cuneocerebellar tract.

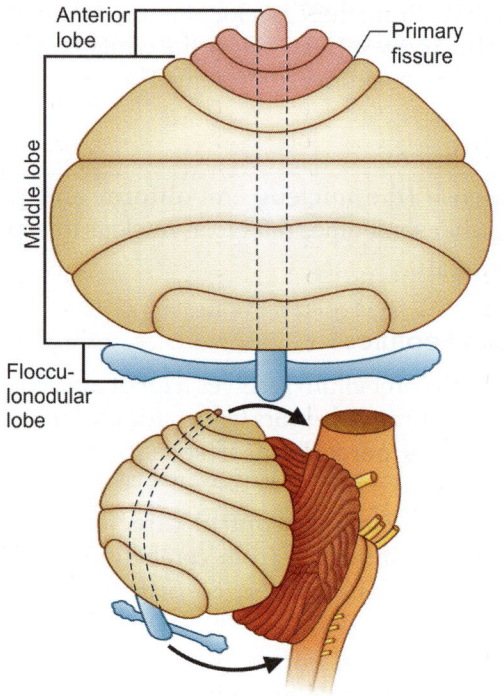
Fig. 9.37: Different lobes of cerebellum

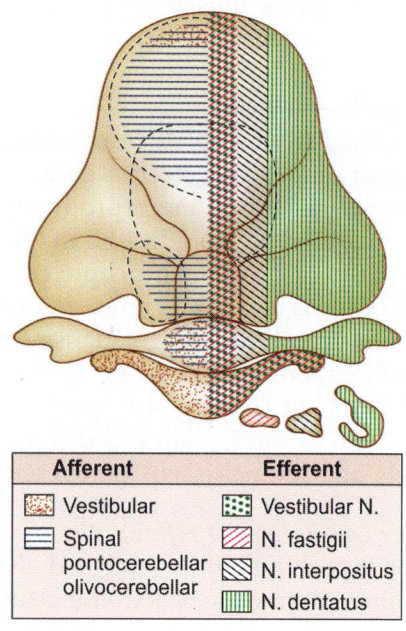

Afferent	Efferent
Vestibular	Vestibular N.
Spinal pontocerebellar olivocerebellar	N. fastigii
	N. interpositus
	N. dentatus

Fig. 9.39: Afferent inputs and efferent outputs of cerebellum

b. Vestibulocerebellar pathway carries proprioceptive inputs from vestibular apparatus present in inner ear. Proprioceptive impulses from vestibular apparatus reach cerebellum through vestibular nuclei present in brainstem.

c. Dorsal and ventral spinocerebellum tracts carry proprioceptive impulses from both contralateral and ipsilateral sides of various parts of body.

d. Tectocerebellar pathway carries afferent impulses from superior and inferior colliculi of tectum of midbrain. This colliculus receives afferent inputs from visual and auditory areas.

e. Olivocerebellar tract takes origin from inferior olivary nucleus. Inferior olivary nucleus receives afferent proprioceptive inputs from almost all parts of body.

f. Also there are corticopontocerebellar fibers which come from motor and premotor (area number 4 and 6) areas of cerebral cortex.

Efferent Connections

The cerebellum can exert its influence either on nuclei in brainstem or neurons present in motor and pre-motor areas of cerebral cortex through the following efferent connections namely:

1. Cerebellovestibular
2. Dentatorubrothalamocortical
3. Cerebelloreticular, etc.

Cerebellum has no direct influence on LMN present in spinal cord. But, influence on LMN of spinal cord is through various descending tracts that take origin from brainstem regions (Fig. 9.40).

Functions of Cerebellum

1. *Regulation of posture and equilibrium:* Flocculonodular lobe is involved in this function. It receives afferent inputs from vestibulocerebellar tract and proprioceptors from all over the body.

Afferent inputs coming to flocculonodular lobe are processed, and efferent impulses from cerebellum are sent to vestibular and reticular nuclei present in brainstem. From these nuclei, impulses are sent to lower motor neurons through vestibulospinal and reticulospinal tracts. Impulses coming from flocculonodular lobe control activities of axial (midline trunk) muscles and proximal limb muscles (muscles which attach limb to trunk part of the body).

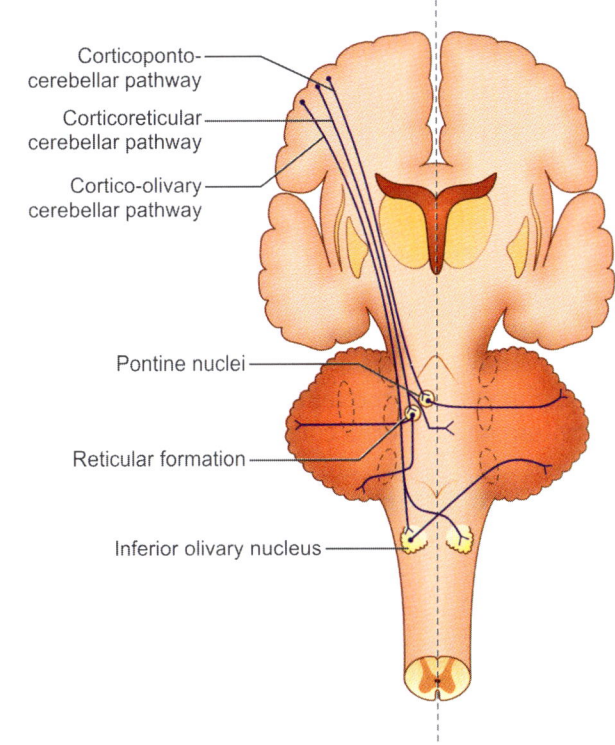

Corticoponto-cerebellar pathway

Corticoreticular-cerebellar pathway

Cortico-olivary cerebellar pathway

Pontine nuclei

Reticular formation

Inferior olivary nucleus

Fig. 9.40: Cerebellar influence on the neurons in brainstem region

Hence cerebellum has an important role to play in maintenance of posture and equilibrium.

2. Also controls activities of extraocular muscles which control eye movements through medial longitudinal bundle. This bundle controls activity of 3, 4, and 6 cranial nerve motor nuclei. Thus flocculonodular lobe of cerebellum helps in fixing gaze/vision. Even though position of head is fixed, we can move eyeballs to focus on any particular object/subject that we want to see.

3. Cerebellum also brings about coordination of movements. For smooth movements to be brought about, there will be involvement of three groups of muscles. They are:

a. Agonists/protogonists—directly involved in performing a movement.

b. Antagonists—muscle group involved in opposing movements are made to relax.

c. Synergistic—not directly involved but needed for coordination of smooth movement.

In cerebral cortex, only movements are represented and not individual muscles.

During coordination of movement, the following characteristic features have to be taken care off:

a. Force generated during movement
b. Rate of movement
c. Range of movement
d. Direction of movement

If there is an error in any one or all of characteristics, there is said to be in-coordinated movement (ataxia). Ataxia is characteristic feature in cerebellar lesion and this is called as motor ataxia. Ataxia can also occur due to some sensory deficits in which case it is called as sensory ataxia (posterior or afferent nerve root lesion, thalamic syndrome).

Coordination of movement is possible because cerebellum acts as servo comparator.

Whenever impulses are sent from motor and pre-motor areas of cerebral cortex to LMN, a copy of the command is sent to cerebellum through the cortico-pontocerebellar pathway (Fig. 9.41).

Cerebellum behaves as a servo comparator. Movements are initiated in the body due to impulses coming to part of body through corticospinal tracts. A copy of the command sent to LMN by cerebral cortex is also sent to cerebellum through cortioponto-cerebellar pathway. During every step of movements, proprioceptive impulses arising from muscles and joints are sent back to cerebellum from the part of body that is involved in movement. These inputs keep informing cerebellum about various aspects of movement that is taking place (like degree of movement, direction, force, etc.).

If movement is not according to motor command, cerebellum compares command for intended movement with the movement that is going on (afferent inputs will be informing about this) and any rectification of error is faithfully relayed back to motor cortex through dentato-rubro-thalamo-cortical pathway. This leads to modification/rectification of movements so that target is reached accurately.

4. Cerebellum also helps in maintenance of muscle tone: Vestibulocerebellum influences activity of vestibular nucleus and pontine reticular formation. Spinocerebellum influences activities of nuclei present in brainstem. Rubrospinal, vestibulospinal and pontine reticular formation extend their influence over LMNs present in spinal cord. The efferent impulses coming from cerebellum through these nuclei are generally excitatory to LMNs. Because of this, if there is cerebellar lesion it leads to hypotonia (decreased muscle tone).

5. Cerebellum also has a role to play in learning and memory especially some of movements which are to be excelled for a short time by repeated trials.

Features of Cerebellar Lesion

1. Imbalance in posture and equilibrium
2. Incoordination of movements
3. Hypotonia
4. Knee jerk gets affected (pendular knee jerk)
5. Dysarthria
6. Nystagmus

Applied Aspects

Vestibulocerebllar damage: Unsteady gait/posture. The person will have drunken gait (feet far apart from each other).

Control of subconscious associated movements will be absent, for example, swinging of arms while walking will be absent.

Ataxia or incoordination of movement is also seen: Incoordination leads to features, like

a. *Dysmetria:* Rate of movement (it may over shot or under shoot the target). Unable to gauge length of movement efficiently.

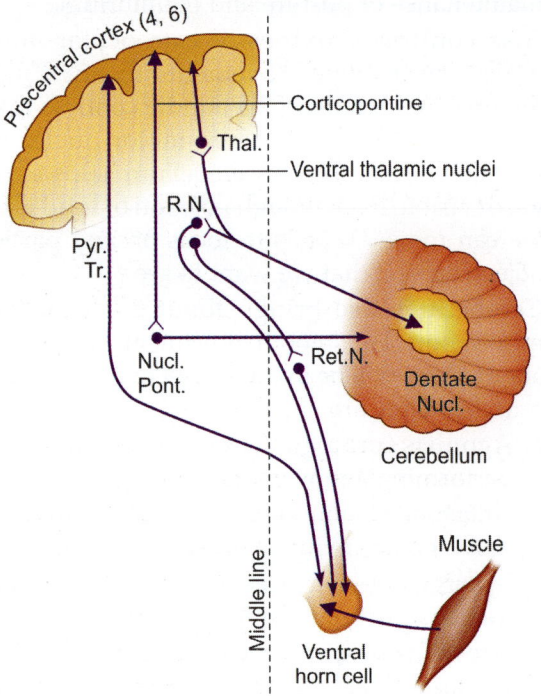

Fig. 9.41: Closed circuit connection between motor cortex and cerebellum

b. *Adiadochokinesia:* Inability to perform rapid alternating movements (alternatively supinating and pronating the palm, or flexion and extension fingers, etc.) cannot be brought about.

c. *Decomposition of movement:* When one has to perform any complex movement involving many joints, normally the movement can be quite brisk and smooth. But when there is in-coordination or ataxia, complex movement will occur, but in steps and slowly, that is movement at each joint will be performed as a separate entity one after the other.

d. *Dysarthria:* Speech is also affected. Speech is usually a complex movement involving articulation of lips, laryngeal muscles, tongue, etc. In cerebellar lesion, slow staccato speech is observed that is a single word is broken into many syllables.

Tremors: As long as the person is at rest, tremors will be absent. Tremors are seen when any voluntary movement starts and the intensity of tremors increase during the course of movements. So these are known as intention/kinetic tremors.

Knee jerk is an example of deep reflex. When knee jerk is elicited in a person suffering from cerebellar lesion, the knee jerk becomes pendular. Muscle tone will be less than normal that is hypotonia in the case of human beings.

Tests for Cerebellar Lesion

- Test for muscle tone and tremors
- Stand with eyes closed
- Walking along a straight line
- Finger nose test
- Heel knee test
- Knee jerk test—look for pendular jerk.

Basal Ganglia

- It is composed of nuclear groups present in sub-cortical region.
- Like cerebellum, this ganglia is involved in muscular activity.
- Differences between cerebellum and basal ganglia are:
  a. Cerebellum receives proprioceptive impulses from peripheral part of body but basal ganglia have no proprioceptive inputs.
  b. Cerebellar impulses coming to cerebral cortex come mainly to motor and premotor areas but

influences from basal ganglia go to almost all areas of cerebral cortex.

c. Many nuclei in brainstem are influenced by cerebellum whereas influence of basal ganglia on brainstem is limited.

Basal ganglia is composed of the following nuclei:

1. Caudate nucleus
2. Putamen
3. Globus pallidus
4. Red nucleus
5. Substantia nigra
6. Subthalamic nucleus (body of Luys)

Caudate nucleus and putamen together is called striatum.

Putamen and globus pallidus together is known as lentiform nuclei.

Gobus pallidus is composed of two different parts namely globus pallidus externa and globus pallidus interna.

Substantia nigra is also made up two parts—pars reticulata and pars compacta.

Connections of Basal Ganglia

There is a closed circuit connection: There is a lot of mutual influence between various nuclei of basal ganglia.

Striatum receives afferent inputs from motor and premotor areas of cerebral cortex. From striatum impulses, efferent impulses reach pars reticulata of substantia nigra. Efferent impulses from striatum also reach globus pallidus.

- Striatum to substantia nigra—striatonigral pathway
- Striatum to globus pallidus—striatopallidal pathway.

From pars compacta region, efferent connection going to striatum is known as nigrostriatal pathway. The neurotransmitter released by this pathway is dopamine. From globus pallidus, impulses go to subthalamic nucleus. Impulses will also come back to globus pallidus (efferent) from subthalamic nucleus. Also, efferent impulses from subthalamic nucleus will reach pars reticulata of substantia nigra.

From globus pallidus, impulses (efferent) come to centromedian, ventroanterior and ventrolateral nuclei of thalamus. From centromedian nucleus, efferent impulses reach striatum. From ventrolateral,

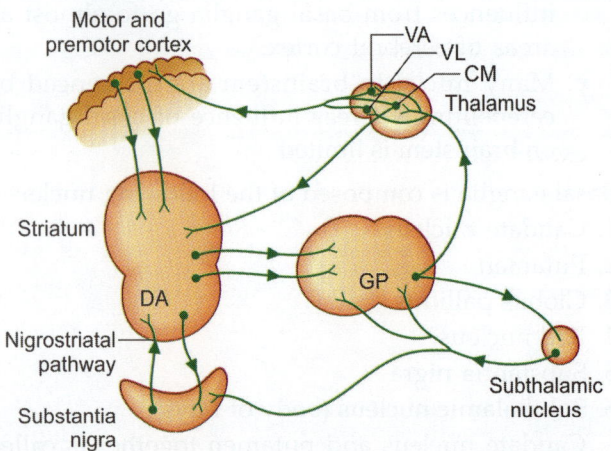

Fig. 9.42: Closed circuit diagram of basal ganglia connections with motor and premotor cortex

ventroanterior and centromedian nuclei impulses are relayed back to motor and pre-motor areas of cerebral cortex. So whole of basal ganglia connection is like a closed loop (Fig. 9.42).

The neurotransmitters involved in basal ganglia activity are (Fig. 9. 43):

1. Dopamine
2. GABA
3. Glutamate
4. Substance P
5. ACh

One of the most important neurotransmitters is dopamine.

Functions of Basal Ganglia

Planning and programming of movements: Cortico-striato-pallido-thalamo-cortical tract (which is a closed loop circuit) brings impulses from motor and pre-motor cortex to nuclei of basal ganglia and after processing are relayed back to motor and premotor cortex. Because of this connection, there is proper coordination of muscle activity at every step of movement. But unlike cerebellum, basal ganglia cannot function as servo comparator; because there are no afferent inputs to nuclei of ganglia from different parts of body.

Controls subconscious-associated movements, like swinging of arm while walking; nodding of head during conversations; various facial expressions; gestures; and modulation of voice, etc. Caudate nucleus is especially important for this function; it facilitates subconscious-associated movement.

Provides postural background for any movements that is during movements it is not only particular joint that has to take part directly in intended movement, but also other joints must be held in proper position to facilitate smooth movement. Globus pallidus has important role to play for this activity.

Regulation of muscle tone: Basal ganglia influences can reach certain area in brainstem and alter activity of neurons present in red nucleus, reticular formation, etc. From these areas, impulses are sent to lower motor neurons through rubrospinal and reticulospinal tracts to regulate the muscle tone.

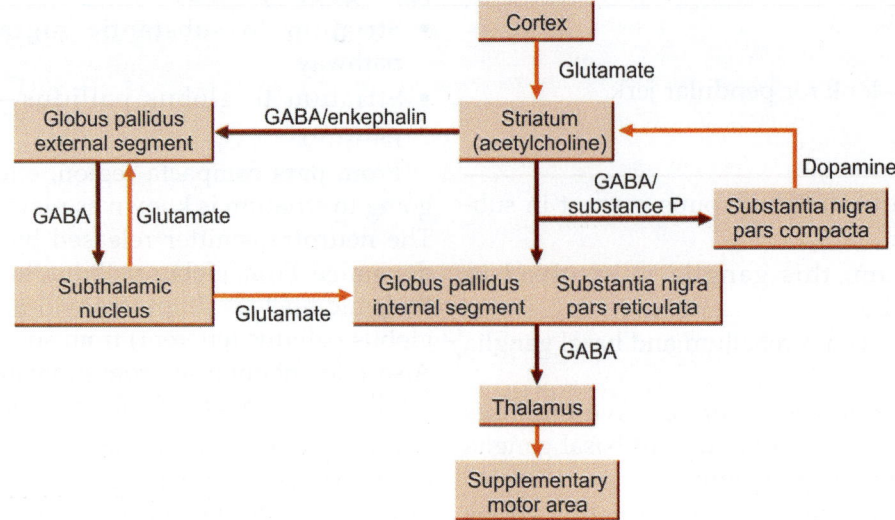

Fig. 9.43: Neurotransmitters' profile at different regions of basal gangalia

In lower animals in which motor cortex is not developed, basal ganglia performs role of motor cortex. And hence it has important role to play in all voluntary movements.

Conditions associated with problems in different nuclei or connections of basal ganglia dysfunction:

- Parkinsonism
- Ballism
- Hemiballism
- Huntington's chorea
- Athetosis

Parkinsonism

Nigrostriatal pathway is important in this aspect. The neurotransmitter released by this pathway is dopamine. If this tract is not functioning properly, it leads to Parkinsonism or paralysis agitans or Parkinson's disease

Features of Parkinsonism

1. *Hypertonia:* Increase in muscle tone in both flexor and extensor group of muscles. There will be an abnormal increase of muscle tone, which gives rises to rigidity.
2. *Rigidity:* Rigidity can be of two types, namely cogwheel rigidity and lead-pipe rigidity. In lead-pipe rigidity, during the course of passive movements rigidity is experienced throughout the course of movements without any release phenomenon, for e.g. flexion of elbow is not possible. The whole arm will move as one piece. In cog-wheel rigidity, the resistance and release phenomenon alternate in installments and hence passive movements would be possible in steps. The abnormal increase of muscle tone both in flexor and extensor group of muscle makes it difficult to elicit deep reflexes.
3. *Tremors* are also seen, unlike in cerebellar region, there will be static/resting tremors. As long as person is at rest, fine tremors are more prominent in distal parts of body. But as soon as person starts some voluntary movement, tremors disappear. One of the ways tremors get manifested will be in the form of pill rolling movements (rubbing thumb against index finger).
4. *Akinesia (bradykinesia)* (Kinesia means movement): These patients can hardly initiate any voluntary movement. Because of this, they continue to be in a particular posture for long hours. Upper and lower limb joints are usually kept in flexion—universal flexion.
5. *Loss of automatic associated movements:* They will also lose automatic associated movements, like facial expressions, modulation of voice, bodily expressions, etc. (in the form of gestures, facial expressions). Hence, they shall have mask like face (expression less face). These patients try to walk in short steps as if they are trying to catch their center of gravity after every step.

Treatment

Giving L-dopa, which is precursor of dopamine. Unlike dopamine, which cannot cross blood–brain barrier, L-dopa can cross blood–brain barrier and gets converted to dopamine in basal ganglia to exert its influence.

Nowadays, transplantation of a part of fetal adrenal medullary tissue is also being tried since from adrenal medulla there is secretion of dopamine. This would make treatment easier for prolonged durations. Future research will no doubt focus on this potential for human embryonic stem cells to play such a therapeutic role.

Reticular Formation

Reticular formation is phylogenetically oldest part of brain developed very well in the case of higher animals. It is not an anatomical structure but more of a physiological entity.

The reticular formation extends throughout the brainstem. It gets extended on cephalic side to thalamus and hypothalamus and on caudal side it can extend up to cervical segments of spinal cord as well.

In the brainstem reticular formation, nerve cell bodies are scattered within the meshwork of nerve fibers/reticulum. Many of these cell bodies are grouped together as nuclei, and have definite functions. The reticular formation extending in neuraxis/brainstem is divided into medial division and lateral divisions. These divisions have bilateral symmetrical arrangement.

Connections (Figs 9.44 and 9.45)

Afferent Connections

- All sensory pathway (special or general senses), along their way to cerebral cortex, give out a number of branches that is collaterals to reticular formation. So afferent collaterals from many ascending tracts including that from special sensations go to reticular formation and keep feeding afferent information to this area.

- Motor and premotor cortices also have afferent connections to reticular formation.
- Afferent impulse also comes from certain nuclei of basal ganglia.
- Afferent impulses come from nuclei of cerebellum
- Afferent impulses also come from vestibular nucleus in brainstem.

Efferent Connections

- Reticulospinal tracts that take origin from medullary and pontine reticular formation carry

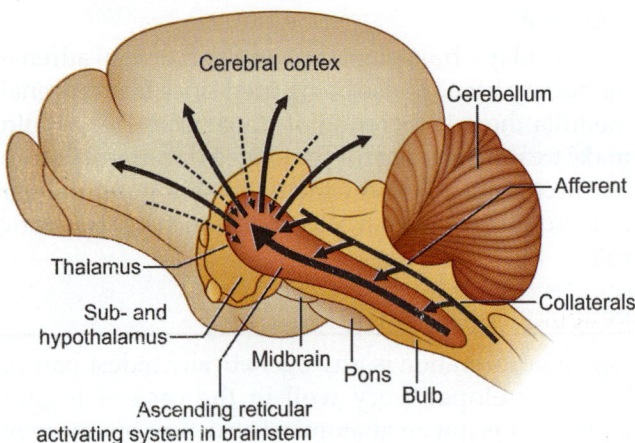

Fig. 9.44: Some of the important afferent and efferent connections of brainstem reticular formation

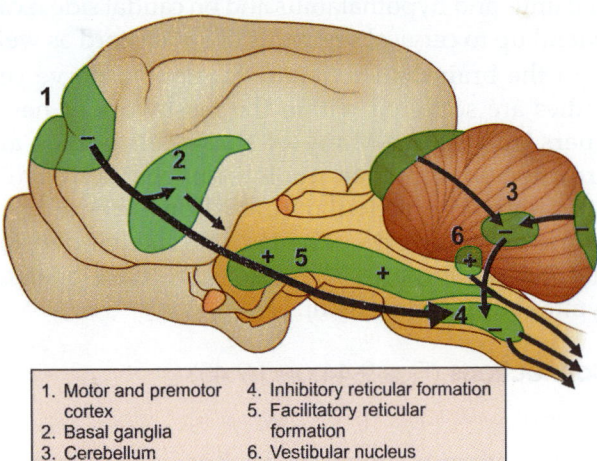

1. Motor and premotor cortex
2. Basal ganglia
3. Cerebellum
4. Inhibitory reticular formation
5. Facilitatory reticular formation
6. Vestibular nucleus

Fig. 9.45: Some of the important afferent and efferent connections of brainstem reticular formation

impulses to anterior horn cells present in spinal cord.

- Another reticulospinal tract connects brainstem reticular formation with lateral horn cells of spinal cord present in thoracolumbar region. These lateral horn cells give rise to sympathetic nerves responsible for vasomotor tone, venomotor tone, etc.
- Ascending reticular activating system: Reticular formation sends efferent impulses to almost all areas of cerebral cortex through ARAS.

In the diagram (Fig. 9.45) descending tracts numbered in black color are reticulospinal tracts which would descend down into spinal cord. And numerals indicate:

1. Cerebral cortex (motor and premotor cortex)
2. Basal ganglia
3. Cerebellum
4. Inhibitory area of reticular formation
5. Facilitatory area of reticular formation
6. Vestibular nucleus

Functions

1. *Visceromotor function:* There are many centers present in brainstem, like vasomotor center; deglutition center, respiratory center, etc. which have influence over functioning of autonomic nerves in body. Thereby they have role to play in regulation of heart rate, blood pressure, GI tract motility and secretion, etc. The impulses from these centers reach autonomic nerves present in spinal cord through reticulospinal tract.

2. *Somatomotor function:* Reticular formation present in brainstem is very important for this function. The pontine reticular formation sends excitatory impulses to gamma motor neurons controlling muscle tone whereas influence from reticular formation of medulla oblongata on same motor neurons will be inhibitory. The impulses from regions of pons and medulla reach anterior horn cells present in spinal cord through reticulospinal tracts. Under normal conditions, activity of medullary regions is dominant because inhibitory area of medulla is constantly stimulated by impulses coming from cerebral cortex, basal ganglia, cerebellum, etc. Hence, inhibitory influence has dominant role to play. If there is a mid-collicular section (transection between superior and inferior colliculi), it will cut off majority of the inhibitory

inputs exerted (from cerebral cortex and basal ganglia) over the reticular formation in medulla oblongata. In addition to this, now pontine facilitatory reticular formation influence becomes unopposed. Because of this, it results in a condition know as decerebrate rigidity. In this condition, there will be severe increase in muscle tone throughout the body, especially so in muscles present in extensor compartment.

3. *Somatosensory:* Modulation of all sensations. All sensory pathways from general sensations or special sense organs reach reticular formation either through collaterals or through multisynaptic pathways. The reticular formation in turn is connected to most of the parts of cerebral cortex. These sensory inputs when processed and sent to cerebral cortex would result in alteration of behavior of individual. It is because of this, for same type of stimulus, reaction of individual varies depending on factors, like:
   a. Place of stimulation
   b. Time of stimulation
   c. Mental state of individual at the given time, etc.
   Because of above reasons, the way the person reacts to situations varies.

4. *Ascending reticular activating system (ARAS) has role to play in arousal, alertness, and sleep state (AR–arouse,*

A–alert, S–sleep). Impulses discharged from reticular formation reach thalamus; hypothalamus before reaching cerebral cortical region. The pathway involved is ARAS. The frequency of impulse discharge in this pathway determines state of activity of brain. ARAS activity would bring about alterations in the pattern of EEG recordings. The activity of ARAS can be influenced by substances, like anesthetics, tranquilizers, sedatives, etc.

5. *Modulation of pain:* From nucleus raphe magnus present in reticular formation of brainstem, dorsolateral funiculus takes origin. This tract has ability to alter activity of the gate that is involved in modulation of pain sensation. The neurotransmitter liberated by this tract is 5-hydroxytryptamine (refer to gate control theory of pain and descending analgesic system).

Vestibular Apparatus (Fig. 9.46)

- Vestibular apparatus is present in inner ear
- The three important parts of vestibular apparatus are utricle, saccule and semicircular canals.
- There are three semicircular canals on the both sides and function as pairs.
- The three semicircular canals are termed as:
  a. Anterior canal (superior)

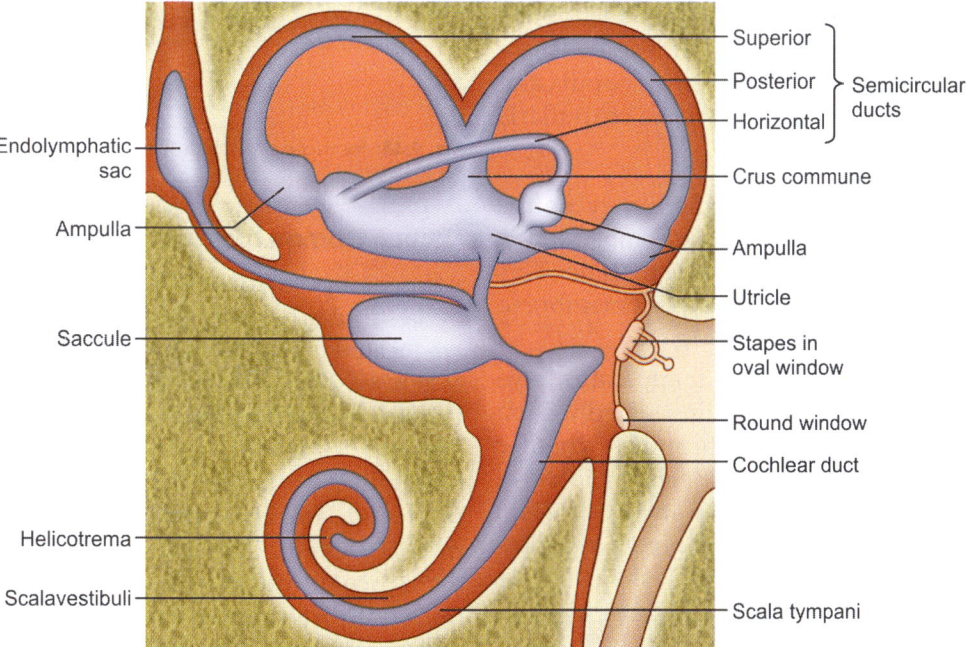

Endolymphatic sac
Ampulla
Saccule
Helicotrema
Scalavestibuli

Superior
Posterior } Semicircular ducts
Horizontal
Crus commune
Ampulla
Utricle
Stapes in oval window
Round window
Cochlear duct
Scala tympani

Fig. 9.46: Parts of vestibular apparatus

b. Posterior canal

c. Horizontal canal (lateral)

- The anterior semicircular canal of one side and posterior canal of the opposite side are placed in the same plane and similarly other two pairs also.
- Whether in utricle or saccule or in three semicircular canals, receptors are present. These receptors are mechanoceptors in nature.
- These receptors are termed as proprioceptors.
- Receptors are present in dilated portions of semi-circular canals termed as ampulla.
- Vestibular division of VIII cranial nerve carries impulses from vestibular apparatus to brain (afferents).

Receptors: Receptors get stimulated when there is:

a. Linear acceleration or deceleration

b. Angular acceleration or deceleration

c. Rotation of head

When there is dorsiflexion or ventriflexion of the head, receptors present in utricle gets stimulated. When there is movement of head sideways, receptors present in saccule get stimulated. Rotation of head along long axis of body brings about stimulation of receptors present in semicircular canals.

Crista ampullaris: They are present in semicircular canals. The receptors are known as hair cells. They are present over a ridge. Hairs of these cells are embedded in gelatinous substances called cupula and together with hair cells is called cristae ampullaris (Fig. 9.47).

Otolith organ: In utricle and saccule, the receptors are present on a ridge. The hair cells are embedded in a gelatinous matrix namely otolith membrane. This membrane is rich in calcium salts. Otolith membrane with hair cells is known as otolith organ.

The hair cells present in vestibular apparatus have many hairs. There will be one kinocilium and direction of bending of this kinocilium determines whether receptor is stimulated or not. In case stereocilia move away from kinocilium, receptor is inhibited (Fig. 9.48). So there is differential stimulation of receptor depending on movement of cilia.

From receptors, afferent inputs are carried to central nervous system by vestibular division of vestibulocochlear nerve.

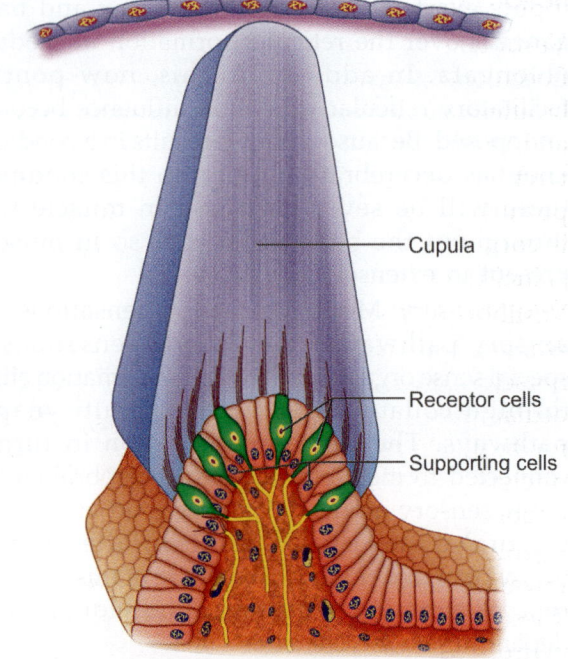

Fig. 9.47: Details of crista ampullaris

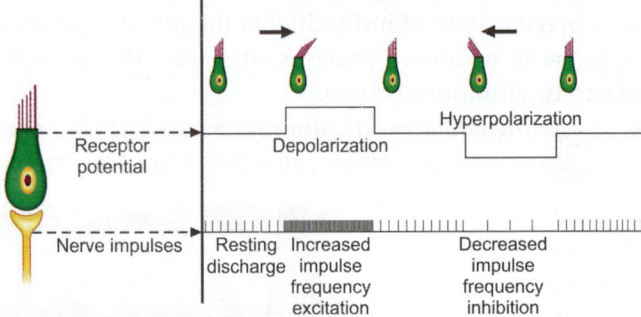

Fig. 9.48: Increased or decreased impulse discharge from the receptor based on the directional movement of the stereocilia

Neural Communication

Afferent inputs from vestibular apparatus are carried by vestibular nerve fibers. Cell bodies of these fibers are located in Scarpa's ganglion. From here, impulses reach vestibular nucleus present in brainstem. Impulses are carried to cerebellum (to flocculonodular lobe or vestibulocerebellum) through vestibulo-cerebellar pathway. From vestibular nuclei of brainstem, impulses are also sent to cranial nerve motor nuclei of 3rd, 4th and 6th nerves supplying extra-ocular muscles. In addition to this, vestibular nucleus in brainstem is also connected to lower motor neurons present in spinal cord through vestibulospinal tract which carry motor impulses.

Functions of Vestibular Apparatus

1. Vestibular nucleus in brainstem is connected to flocculonodular lobe of cerebellum through both by afferent and efferent fibers as vestibulocerebellar and cerebellovestibular tracts, respectively. This tract has functional importance in maintenance of posture and equilibrium. Any postural imbalance is corrected in cerebellovestibular and vestibulo-spinal tracts.

2. Vestibular nucleus of brainstem is connected to 3rd, 4th, and 6th cranial nerves supplying extraocular muscles. Because of this, coordination of extra-ocular muscles is brought about while it is required for fixing gaze on a particular object. So if this nucleus is damaged, it can lead to nystagmus (inability to fix gaze).

3. Vestibular nucleus of brainstem is connected to lower motor neurons through vestibulospinal tract. These nuclei send motor impulses to lower motor neuron of spinal cord. And through this connection, it plays role in maintenance of muscle tone.

Derangement of functioning of vestibular apparatus is seen in Meniere's syndrome. Not only is vestibular apparatus affected, but cochlea function is also affected.

Features of Meniere's syndrome are:
1. Vertigo is illusion of movement
2. Nystagmus
3. Ataxia

During motion sickness, there will be excessive stimulation of vestibular apparatus, e.g. when traveling across rough sea, in a plane, when taking a hair pin bend, during a train journey the person complains of vertigo, vomiting, nystagmus, etc.

Cerebrospinal Fluid (CSF)

- Apart from neuronal tissue, blood and CSF will be present in cranial vault.
- CSF forms interstitial fluid in CNS or tissue fluid of CNS.
- CSF presents inside ventricles of brain, in central canal of spinal cord and in subarachnoid spaces (space present between arachnoid and pia mater).
- Three layers namely dura mater, arachnoid mater and pia mater cover brain (Fig. 9.49).
- On an average about 150 ml of (100–200 ml) CSF is present in human beings.

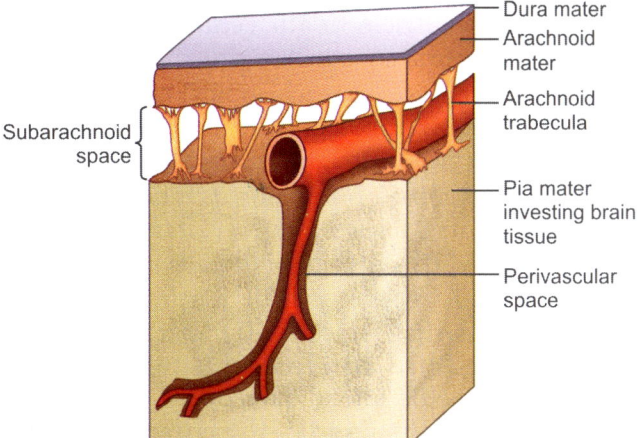

Fig. 9.49: Coverings of brain and subarachnoid space

- It gets turned over about 4 times a day (600 ml of CSF is formed in per day).
- There should be constant formation and absorption, in order to maintain volume at 150 ml and this maintains CSF pressure (intracranial tension).

Composition of CSF and Other Properties

1. Clear, colorless, transparent fluid
2. Alkaline in nature
3. Around 0.3 ml of CSF is produced/min
4. Specific gravity 1.005
5. Water—99.13%
6. Solids—0.87 %
7. K^+ = 3.00 mEq, whereas plasma has 5.0 mEq
8. Cl^- = 114.0 mEq whereas plasma has 100 mEq
9. *Glucose:* 60 mg% whereas plasma has 60–90 mg%
10. *Proteins:* 20 mg% whereas plasma has 6–8 gm%

In brain, there are four ventricles. They are two lateral ventricles (one each in cerebral hemispheres) and third and fourth ventricles. Choroid plexuses present more abundantly in lateral ventricles than in 3rd or 4th ventricles. These choroid plexuses (capillary network) are main source of formation of CSF. CSF is formed by two different processes, namely active secretion and ultrafiltration.

a. Active secretion is brought about by choroid plexus.
b. Ultrafiltration or dialysis is brought about by blood vessels that are present in ventricular regions

Circulation of CSF

- From lateral ventricles, CSF reaches 3rd ventricle through foramina of Monroe.

- From 3rd ventricle to 4th ventricle, it reaches through cerebral aqueduct or aqueduct of Sylvius.
- From 4th ventricle, it reachesspinal canal through foramen of Magendie and into subarachnoid spaces throughout CNS through foramina of Luschka.

CSF formed gets absorbed after its function is over. Most of CSF gets absorbed into arachnoid villi and granulations which dip into subdural venous sinuses.

Subarachnoid spaces can be reached either by lumbar or cisternal puncture. Lumbar puncture is preferred because cisternal puncture requires insertion of needle into subarachnoid spaces near brainstem region. In the process, there are chances of brainstem neurons getting damaged. It is much easier to perform lumbar puncture to get a sample of CSF for diagnostic purposes.

Lumbar Puncture

A special needle is introduced from posterior aspect into subarachnoid spaces of spinal cord between L3 and L4 vertebrae. Between L1 and L2 vertebrae, spinal cord ends and, therefore, when needle is introduced between L3 and L4 vertebrae injury to spinal nerves is prevented (Fig. 9.50).

Significance

- To obtain a sample of CSF for chemical, physical and histological examination.

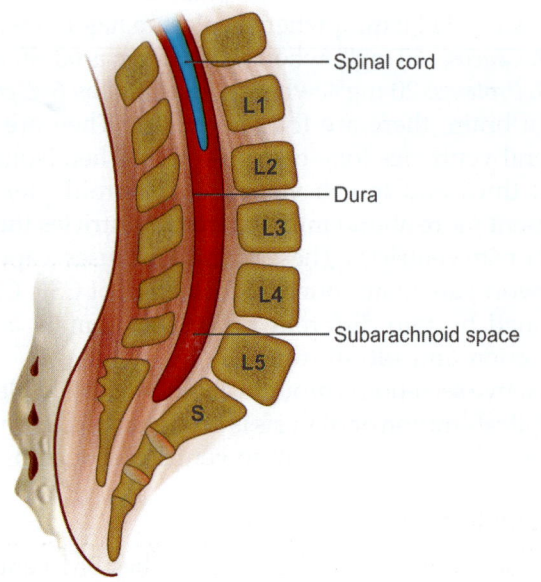

Fig. 9.50: The extension of spinal cord and subarachnoid space

- Measure intracranial tension and if intracranial tension has increased, some amount of CSF can be removed to decrease tension. However, while relieving raised intracranial tension by lumbar puncture; there are chances of herniation of brain. This should be borne in mind before lumbar puncture is desired to relieve raised intracranial tension.
- To inject antibiotics that cannot pass through blood brain barrier.
- To induce spinal anesthesia.

Functions of CSF

1. CSF provides buoyancy effect to brain. Normal weight of brain is about 1500 gm. Because of buoyancy effect provided by CSF, the effective weight of brain is reduced to about 50 gm. This facilitates maneuverability of head over neck region. Weight of brain acts on lumbar region because CSF extends into spinal cord along the course of vertebral column. From vertebral column, it gets radiated to ground along support legs provide to body. So the person would feel 50 gm out of total weight of 1500 gm. Total weight does not decrease only effective weight borne by head is reduced by almost 30 times.
2. Acts as an effective interstitial fluid so that exchange of substances can take place between blood and brain tissues.
3. Interstitium of brain (microenvironment in brain) is maintained so that excitability of neuronal tissue is achieved and properly maintained.
4. Acts as shock absorber: Prevent damage to neuron in CNS because any damage to neurons in CNS is almost irreparable. When there is any impact on cranium, since brain is suspended in fluid environment of CSF, CSF acts as water cushion. The impact on head is dissipated to wider area and thereby direct impact on underlying brain tissue is minimized.
5. Tries to maintain contents of intracranial cavity as constant (relative volume of blood, neuronal tissue and CSF). Cranial vault is made of bony structures and hence cranial cavity volume is fixed. In this fixed volume, neuronal tissue, blood and CSF are present. If there is an increase or decrease in volume of either neuronal tissue or blood, corresponding changes in volume occupied by CSF is brought about.

Blood–Brain Barrier

When trephan blue (an acidic dye) is injected into blood all tissues of body get stained except for certain regions in brain tissue. There is a barrier preventing diffusion of dye from blood into brain tissues and this barrier is known as blood–brain barrier.

- Present in CNS.
- Provides protection to maintain constant internal environment in CNS.
- Tight junctions at adjacent endothelial cells of brain capillaries contribute for formation of blood–brain barrier.
- In addition to this, foot process of astrocytes reinforces this barrier.
- Some of regions of CNS which are devoid of this barrier are (hypothalamus region):
  i. Posterior pituitary
  ii. Area postrema
  iii. Organum vasculosum of lamina terminals
  iv. Subfornical organ

Area postrema, organum vasculosum of lamina terminalis and subfornical organ are together called as circumventricular organs.

In newborn infants, blood–brain barrier is not completely developed. It is developed completely only after birth. In about 1 ½ to 2 years of life, it is developed completely.

Hence during postpartum jaundice (neonatal), bilirubin can get deposited on neurons in basal ganglia resulting in kernicterus.

Knowledge of blood–brain barrier is important for doctors because while administering certain drugs they should know whether the drug has ability to cross the barrier to reach neurons in CNS in order to bring about actions.

Hydrocephalus is a condition in which there will be abnormal accumulation of CSF in skull leading to enlargement of head.

Internal/non-communicating hydrocephalus is where one of foramina for passage of CSF into ventricles is blocked. This leads to dilation of ventricle.

When subarachnoid villi are blocked, it is known as communicating or external hydrocephalus. This can lead to atrophy of brain, mental weakness and convulsions.

Thalamus

- It forms major part of diencephalon.
- It is strategically placed between tracts and cerebral cortex. Thalamus forms medial boundary for internal capsule.
- In thalamus, there are many nuclei.
- Also included in thalamus are medial and lateral geniculate bodies.
- It is either in anterior, medial and lateral group, there are some specific nuclei. In Y-shaped structure, the non-specific nuclei.

Nuclei in Thalamus

a. Specific projection nuclei
b. Non-specific projection nuclei

From specific projection nuclei, impulses are sent to discrete areas of cerebral cortex and from non-specific projection nuclei, impulses are sent to almost all areas of cerebral cortex. Some of the important specific projection nuclei are:

a. Ventroposterolateral nuclei (VPL)
b. Ventroposteromedial nuclei VPM)
c. Ventrolateral nuclei (VL)
d. Ventroanterior nuclei (VA)
e. Centromedian nuclei (CM)
f. Medial geniculate body (MGB)
g. Lateral geniculate body (LGB), etc.

Intralaminar nucleus (ILN), pulvinar nucleus and midline nucleus (MLN) are grouped under non-specific projection nuclei.

Some of the important afferent and efferent connections along with the nueleus involved have been shown in Table 9.4.

Functional Aspects of Thalamus

1. It acts as a relay station for almost all sensory input except for olfactory impulses (pathway or tract does not relay here). But these days it is also mentioned that even olfactory sensations is relayed in thalamus.

2. It acts as a relay station between cerebral cortex and cerebellum and also for impulses from basal ganglia. It helps in normal co-ordination of movements and also helps to maintain normal muscle tone.

3. Ascending reticular activity system (ARAS) is important for emotional reactions. ARAS fibers during the course to reach cerebral cortex do get relayed inthalamic nuclei.

Table 9.4: Connections of thalamus (afferent and efferent)

Afferent	Nuclei	Efferent
Posterior column tract/medial lemniscus	VPL	Cerebral cortex area 3,1,2
Lateral spinothalamic tract	VPL	Cerebral area no. 3,1,2
Spinoreticular tract	ILN and MLN	Primary and secondary sensory area
Anterior spinothalamic tract	VPL	Area no. 3,1,2 on cerebral cortex
Taste pathway	VPM	Cerebral cortex area no. 3,1,2
Optic tract	LGB	Cerebral cortex area no. 17,18,19
Auditor pathway	MGB	Cerebral cortex area no. 41, 42 and 21, 22
All the above tracts are associated with sensory pathway, but there are connections from motor components as well		
Dentato thalamo	VA, VL	Cerebral cortex area no. 4,6
Globus pallidus and substantia nigra of basal ganglia	VA, VL and CM	Almost all parts of cerebral cortex
Brainstem reticular formation	ILN, MLN	Almost all parts of cerebral cortex
Mammillothalamic tract	Anterior nucleus	Limbic lobe, entorhinal cortex

4. Anterior thalamic nuclei is responsible for recent memory.

5. Seat for subcortical pain sensations. Even if sensory cortex is removed we are able to feel pain sensations. Localization and differentiation of different modalities of pain and intensity discrimination is not possible, if impulses do not reach cerebral cortex area no. 3, 1, 2. So for better localization, intensity assessment, discriminate between different types of pain and also to bring about balanced emotional reactions during painful situation, impulses must reach cerebral cortical areas.

Thalamic Syndrome

When thalamogeniculate branch of posterior cerebral artery is infarcted (blocked), there will be degeneration of posterior and ventral group of nuclei due to non-supply of oxygen and nutrition. Characteristic features of this syndrome are:

1. Loss of all sensations mediated by tract of Goll and Burdach as these tracts synapses in VPL nucleus of thalamus.

2. Pain is still felt as pain impulse also reaches ILN and MLN through spinoreticular tract. This pain is poorly localized and threshold for pain is increased. However, when once threshold is crossed, there will be excruciating pain.

3. Light touch, exposure to cold may sometimes bring about perception of pain.

4. Over reaction for pain sensation: In a normal person, extent of emotional reaction is always proportionate to intensity of pain. In these individuals, there will be exaggerated emotional reactions for pain.

5. Motor disturbances: Impulses coming from cerebellum and basal ganglion get relayed in ventral group of nuclei. Since these nuclei are damaged, it leads to in-coordination of movements and results in ataxia.

6. Tone of muscle decreases and there can be muscular weakness.

7. Epicratic sensations: Epicratic sensations are more refined or synthetic sensations, like tactile localization, tactile discrimination, stereognosis, fine touch, etc. All these sensations are lost in thalamic syndrome.

8. Protopathic sensations: These are more primitive, not refined sensation, e.g. pain temperature, and crude touch. They will be intact in thalamic syndrome.

Hypothalamus

- *Hypothalamus:* Forms a part of diencephalon.
- Oldest structure in CNS
- Forms a part of limbic system
- Weighs about 10 gm
- Made up of number of nuclei
- Said to control/regulate almost every function in body. It is responsible for maintenance of homeostasis.

Some of important nuclei in hypothalamus (Fig. 9.51):

1. Preoptic nuclei
2. Anterior hypothalamic nuclei
3. Posterior hypothalamic nuclei
4. Ventromedial nuclei of hypothalamus
5. Lateral hypothalamic nuclei
6. Supraoptic nuclei
7. Paraventricular nuclei
8. Mammillary body
9. Suprachiasmatic nuclei, etc.

Connections of Hypothalamus

Some important afferent and efferent connections of hypothalamus are given in Fig. 9.52 and Table 9.5.

Afferent Connections

These various nuclei of hypothalamus bring a lot of afferent input/connections which are:
- Visceral and somatic inputs through ascending tracts
- Olfactory pathway or olfactory tract (medial fore brain bundle)
- Corticohypothalamic (from neocortex, i.e. frontal lobe) tract
- Hippocampus (via fornix)
- Amygdalo-hypothalamic (via stria terminalis)
- Thalamohypothalamic (from midline nucleus of thalamus)
- From tegmentum of midbrain

Efferent Connections

- Hypothalamohypophyseal tract
- Mammillothalamic tract (connects mammillary body to anterior thalamic nuclei)
- Mammillotegmental tract (connects mammillary body to tegmentum present in midbrain)
- Connected to vital centers in brainstem motor neurons in spinal cord.

The above mentioned are neural tracts—but hypothalamus is connected to anterior pituitary gland through hypothalamohypophyseal portal system (vascular connection).

Functional Aspects of Hypothalamus

1. Regulation of Body Temperature

Preoptic nucleus of hypothalamus acts as biologic thermostat. This thermostat is normally set to maintain a temperature of 37°C. In addition to this, anterior hypothalamus acts as heat loss center and posterior hypothalamus as heat gain center. Concerted activity of all these centers will help in regulation of body temperature.

Information about state of temperature in different parts of body reaches the nuclear areas through lateral spinothalamic tract which carry pain and temperature information from peripheral thermoreceptors. In addition to this, in hypothalamus itself there are thermoreceptors which are termed as central

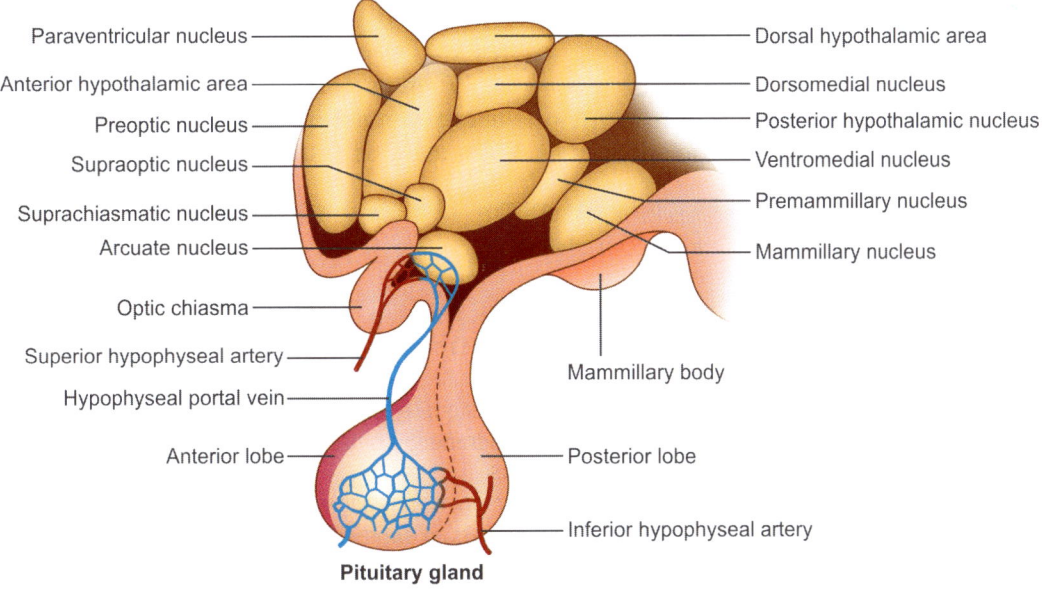

Fig. 9.51: Some important nuclei of hypothalamus

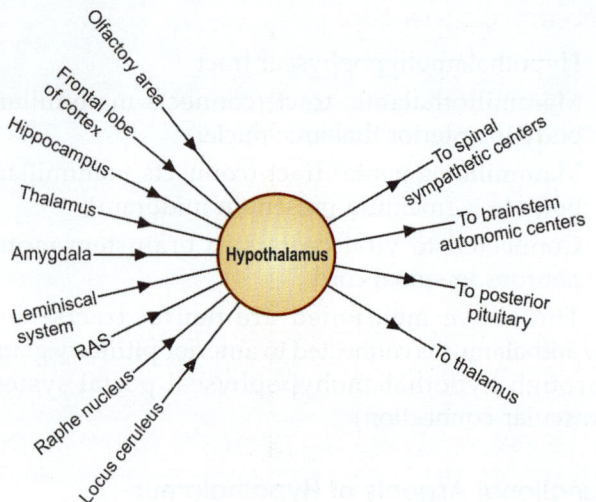

Fig. 9.52: Some important afferent and efferent connections of hypothalamus

thermoreceptors. These receptors sense temperature of blood flowing through hypothalamus.

Depending on temperature of body (fever) or if body is exposed to altered temperature, hypothalamus tries to influence restoration of body temperature by bringing about alterations in autonomic, endocrine, sweat gland activity and behavioral changes. These will ultimately ensure maintenance of body temperature.

Resetting of biological thermostat to a high temperature is very detrimental to body. Hence when person is having severe temperature (as during high fever) applying cold packs on the forehead is done in order to prevent resetting of thermostat.

2. Regulation of Food Intake

Ventromedial and lateral hypothalamic nuclei regulate food intake. Ventromedial nucleus acts as satiety center and lateral hypothalamic nucleus as hunger center. These two nuclear regions have role to play in glucose homeostasis in body. In whole of brain for cells to utilize glucose insulin is not necessary. But for cells of ventromedial nucleus for their glucose utilization, insulin is necessary. Hence in diabetes mellitus when insulin is unable to exert action, there is impairment of glucose homeostasis.

The lateral hypothalamic nucleus area which acts as hunger center is a tonically active center. Normally this center activity is inhibited by impulses coming from ventromedial nucleus. In diabetes mellitus, when ventromedial nucleus activity is decreased or lost, inhibition on hunger center is lost (disinhibition). This leads to polyphagia.

If hunger center is destroyed, person suffers from aphagia: don't eat at all.

If hunger center is over stimulated, person suffers from hyperphagia/polyphagia, person keeps eating more and more.

If satiety center is destroyed, it results in hyperpolyphagia and leads to hypothalamic obesity (Fig. 9.53).

3. Regulation of Body Water Content

The lateral hypothalamic nuclear area also acts as thirst center. In addition to this, in hypothalamus there is presence of osmoreceptors which sense osmolality of plasma flowing through hypothalamus. When body water content is decreased, thirst center gets stimulated and person drinks water and thereby there would be replenishment of body water.

When osmolality of plasma is increased, it brings about stimulation of osmoreceptors due to the process of exosmosis. Osmoreceptors stimulation in turn leads

Tract	Afferent/ efferent	Description
Medial forebrain bundle	A, E	Connects limbic lobe and midbrain via lateral hypothalamus
Fornix	A, E	Connects hippocampus to hypothalamus, mostly mammillary bodies
Stria terminalis	A	Connects amygdala to hypothalamus, mostly mammillary bodies
Mammillary peduncle	A	Connects brainstem to lateral mammillary nuclei
Dorsal noradrenergic bundle	A	Axons of noradrenergic neurons projecting from locus ceruleus to dorsal hypothalamus
Serotonergic neurons	A	Axons of serotonin secreting neurons raphe nuclei to hypothalamus
Retinohypothalamic fibers	A	Optic nerve fibers to suprachiasmatic nuclei from optic chiasm
Mammillothalamic tract of Vicq d'Azyr	E	Connects hypothalamus to reticular portions of midbrain
Hypothalamohypophyseal tract	E	Axons of neurons in supraoptic and paraventricular nuclei

Table 9.5: Principal pathways to and from the hypothalamus

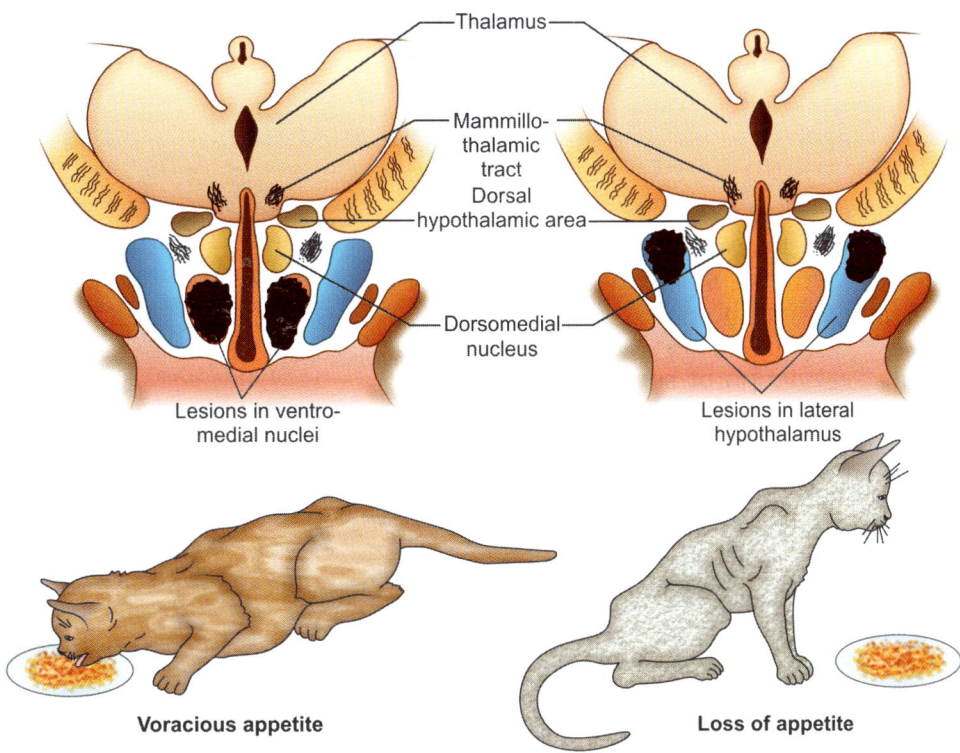

Fig. 9.53: Effect of destruction of ventromedial and lateral hypothalamic nuclei on the appetite in cat

to stimulation of supraoptic nuclear regions of hypothalamus and bring about an increase in amount of secretion of ADH. ADH in turn brings about conservation of body water by enhancing water reabsorption from distal convoluted tubule and collecting ducts in kidney. This leads to decreased volume of urinary output, increased retention of water and correction of crystalloid osmotic pressure/osmolality.

4. Highest Center for Autonomic Nervous System

Hypothalamus is known to act as head ganglia of autonomic nervous system. Both sympathetic and parasympathetic activity would be regulated by hypothalamus. Stimulation of various parts of hypothalamus is known to alter heart rate, blood pressure, respiration, etc. Stimulation of posterior hypothalamus increases heart rate and blood pressure and stimulation of anterior hypothalamus does the converse. Also influences GI secretion and motility and contraction of urinary bladder.

5. Endocrine Control

Almost all hormonal secretions in body are regulated by hypothalamus. Anterior pituitary gland which secretes many of the tropic hormones is constantly under influence of releasing factors or release-inhibiting factors secreted by hypothalamus. These factors are secreted from median eminence region of hypothalamus. These factors reach anterior pituitary gland through hypothalamohypophyseal portal system to exert their actions on anterior pituitary.

In addition to above, posterior pituitary hormones are synthesized in supraoptic and paraventricular nuclear regions of hypothalamus. The hormones reach posterior pituitary gland through hypothalamo-hypophyseal tract and get released from here to circulation.

Since hypothalamus controls most of hormonal secretions in body, it has role to play in growth, metabolism of various substances and hence controls homeostasis.

6. Role in Reproduction

Hypothalamus also controls secretion of gonadotropic hormone secretions from anterior pituitary gland which in turn control growth and function of gonads. Gonads are responsible for secretion of sex hormones and gametogenesis. Because of these reasons, hypothalamus is essential for normal reproductive/sexual activity.

7. Influence on Sleep, Arousal and Alert State

The impulses from ascending reticular activating system during their course to reach cerebral cortex do relay in various nuclei of hypothalamus. From hypothalamus, the onward transmission of impulses is regulated by a center which regulates sleep, arousal state of individual. Destruction of some of these neurons in hypothalamus induces permanent sleep suggesting existence of a sleep center in hypothalamus.

8. Acts as a Biologic Clock

The suprachiasmatic nucleus region of hypothalamus is believed to act as biologic clock. This nucleus keeps track of time inside the body. Tracking time is essential as many of activities in body do get altered based on time with respect to:

a. 24 hours in a day which is known as circadian rhythm/diurnal variation.
b. Number of days of a month and this is known as circalunar rhythm.
c. Number of years in life of an individual and this rhythm is known as circannual rhythm.

9. Role in Emotional State and Learning

Many of changes that occur in the body during various emotional states, like anger, fear, sorrow, anxiety, etc., are being controlled by neurons present in hypothalamus. In addition to this, hypothalamic neurons also form part of limbic system and thereby have role in learning, motivation, etc.

In nutshell, functions of hypothalamus can be remembered with following pneumonic—SEAT[2]

S: Sleep, sexual activity

E: Emotion, endocirne

A: Autonomic nervous system, appetite

T: Thermoregulation, thirst

Limbic System

It is part of brain which includes cingulate gyrus, septal nuclei, hippocampus and amygdala (Fig. 9.54).

Functionally hypothalamus is intimately associated with limbic lobe. Functions of limbic system are:

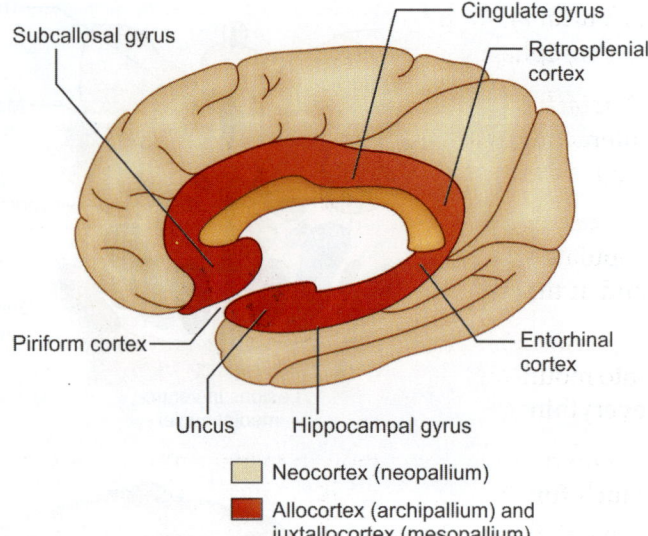

Fig. 9.54: Parts of limbic system

1. *Role in emotion:* Different emotions produce different sets of behaviors. Emotional expressions during rage, sex drive, affection and pleasure are all different. Amygdala stimulation is known to induce fear and anxiety behavior in human beings.

2. *Sexual behavior:* Sexual activity has different components namely sex drive (urge to copulate), sex behavior and act of copulation. Sex behavior is due to both neural and endocrine components.

3. *Reward and punishment:* Lateral hypothalamus, septum, median forebrain bundle, etc., are reward areas. If an electrode placed in any one of these regions in an animal and if animal is placed in a specially designed box namely Skinner's box, the animal repetitively presses the pedal to have sensation of pleasure. This is because stimulation of reward area brings about a sensation of pleasure. On the other hand, if electrode is placed in punishment area, stimulation of this area leads to punishment.

4. *Motivation:* It appears that conditions which result in stimulation of reward areas produce motivation to do a job.

Klüver-Bucy Syndrome

Bilateral temporal lobotomy leads to:

a. Placidity
b. Hypersexuality
c. Hyperorality

d. Viusal agnosia

e. Omniphagia

Placidity: The animal loses sense of fear and start interacting with any creature without usual fear or aggressive reaction.

Hypersexuality: Sexual drive is increased and tries to copulate with an animal of same sex or opposite sex and at times even with inanimate objects.

Hyperorality: Tries to put anything and everything into mouth and thereby tries to examine anything and everything.

Visual agnosia: Even though visual pathway is very much functional, animal may dash against an object since analysis of visual impulses has been totally lost.

Omniphagia: Eats anything and everything.

Electroencephalogram (EEG)

1. Electroencephalogram is recording of summated electrical activity of neurons of brain with help of surface electrodes placed on scalp.
2. During surgery, electrodes may be placed directly on cortex of brain and recording thus obtained is known as electrocorticogram.
3. Pair of electrodes is used, placed over different parts of scalp like frontal, parietal, temporal and occipital areas.
4. Recording can be bipolar or unipolar.
5. Recording obtained are summated electrical potentials of very large number of cortical neurons.
6. Amplitude of EEG recordings depends on whether discharge from neurons is synchronous in which case amplitude will be large, if asynchronous, amplitude will be small.

Rhythms

1. *α rhythm:* Recorded when person is awake, eyes closed, not concentrating or thinking.

Klüver-Bucy syndrome

1. Visual—agnosia
2. Oral tendency
3. Hypermetamorphosis
4. Placidity
5. Omnisexuality
6. Omniphagia

a. This rhythm is also known as Burger rhythm.

b. Best recorded from occipital and parietal lobe areas.

c. Frequency will be about 8–13 cps

d. Amplitude will be about 50 microvolts

2. *β rhythm:* Recorded when person opens eyes or starts thinking or working out some mathematical problems.

a. Best recorded from frontal or parietal lobe areas

b. Frequency 13–30 cps

c. Voltage will be about 20 microvolts

d. It is also known as alpha block or desynchronization

3. *Theta waves*

a. Recorded in a child.

b. Occurs when a person is in light sleep

c. Frequency 4–7 cps

d. Amplitude 10 microvolts

4. *Delta waves*

a. Occurs when a person is in deep sleep.

b. Frequency 0.5–4 cps

c. Amplitude will be about 100 microvolts

d. Suggests highly synchronized activity of cortical neurons.

Amplitude of EEG recordings depend on a number of factors, like:

a. Synchronized or desynchronized activity of neurons in brain

b. Fall in blood glucose level

c. Decrease of body temperature

d. Decreased cortisol level in circulation

e. Increased tension of carbon dioxide in circulation

Source of EEG

It is due to current flow in fluctuating dipoles formed on dendrites of cortical cells and cell bodies (Fig. 9.55).

Mechanism of desynchronization: Stimulation of reticular formation of midbrain tegmentum, and of non-specific projection nuclei of thalamus brings about desynchronization of EEG.

Activity of ARAS can be increased by:

1. Afferent impulses coming from various ascending tracts.
2. Afferent impulses coming from organs of special senses.

3. Afferent impulses coming from superior transverse temporal gyrus and orbitofrontal cortex (cortico-fugal fibers). Through these fibers, intercortical events can bring about arousal (emotional aspect can bring about arousal).

Clinical Significance of EEG

1. Diagnosis of epilepsy, like grand mal or petit mal.
2. Brain death
3. Subdural hematoma
4. Space occupying lesions
5. Changes are also seen when blood glucose level falls/fall in steroid levels in circulation.

Autonomic Nervous System

It is the part of nervous system, which regulates functioning of visceral organs. Two different limbs of autonomic nervous system are sympathetic and parasympathetic nervous system components.

Sympathetic takes origin from lateral horn cells of thoracolumbar segments of spinal cord whereas parasympathetic takes origin from cranial (in brain) and sacral (in spinal cord) regions. In parasympathetic component, nerves included are cranial nerves 3, 7, 9 and 10 and also pelvic nerve from sacral segments of spinal cord (Fig. 9. 56).

- Centers for autonomic nervous system are present in hypothalamus.
- The anterior hypothalamus controls activity of parasympathetic and posterior hypothalamus that of sympathetic nerves.

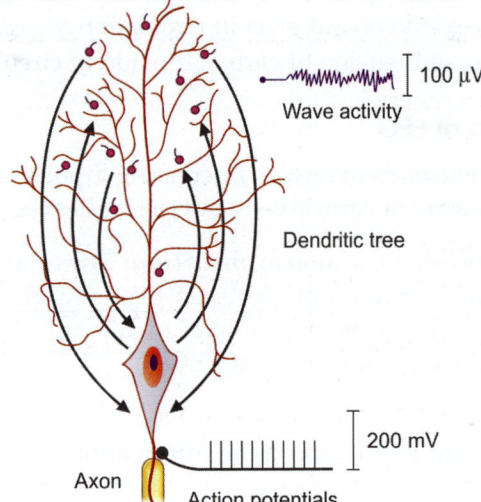

Fig. 9.55: Flow of current in dendritic tree

- In any autonomic nervous system pathway, there are two neurons along efferent pathway. The preganglionic and postganglionic. The neurotransmitter at pre- and post-ganglionic regions in parasympathetic part is acetylcholine. In sympathetic, at preganglionic region, it is acetylcholine whereas in post-ganglionic region in most of parts of body it is noradrenaline. In some parts, at the post-ganglionic region of sympathetic nervous system, the neurotransmitter liberated is ACh.
- Acetylcholine can act through nicotinic or muscarinic receptors present in pre- and post-ganglionic regions respectively.
- Noradrenaline can act through alpha or beta receptors.
- Alpha receptors are of two types namely alpha 1 and alpha 2 and likewise even beta receptors are of two types namely beta 1 and beta 2.

Blockers for Various Receptors

Nicotinic receptors can be blocked by:
- Hexamethonium
- Pentolinium

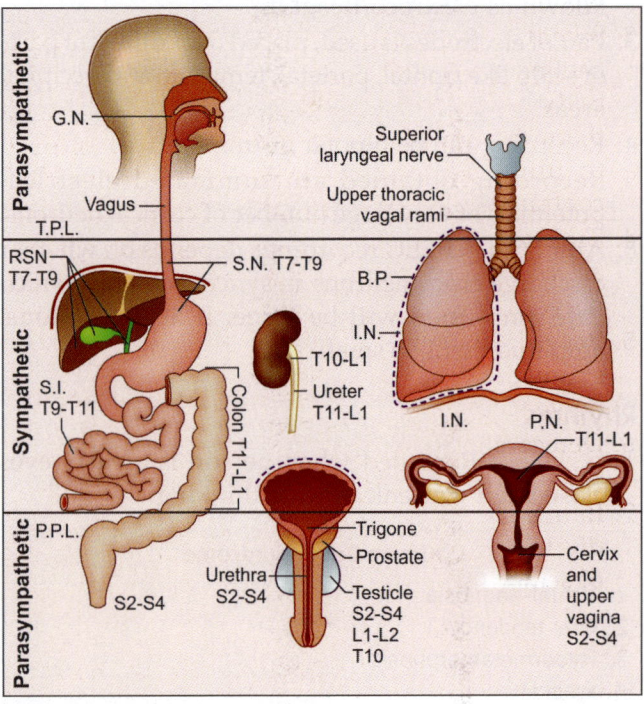

Fig. 9.56: Parts of the body that are influenced by sympathetic and parasympathetic activity

Muscarinic receptors can be blocked by:
- Atropine
- Scopolamine

Alpha receptors blockers are:
- Phenoxybenzamine
- Phentolamine

Beta receptors can be blocked by:
- Propranolol
- Atenelol

All involuntary organs/structures in the body have dual innervations. But some exceptions are:
1. Adrenal medulla
2. Eccrine sweat glands
3. Vascular smooth muscles
4. Juxtaglomerular apparatus.

Functions of Autonomic Nervous System

1. Regulation of functions of visceral organs, like heart, gastrointestinal tract, etc., and thereby help to regulate heart rate, blood pressure and gastro-intestinal secretion and motility.
2. In lungs, bring about bronchodilation when acts through sympathetic nerve and vice versa effect, when parasympathetic nerve is acting.
3. Sweat glands are supplied by sympathetic cholinergic fibers and are involved in regulation of body temperature. In addition to this, during thermoregulation, goose pimples are formed due to piloerrection which is brought about by contraction of erector pilorum muscle.
4. Secretions from adrenal medulla are regulated by activity of sympathetic nerves (pelvic splanchnic nerve).
5. In eyes, pupillary dilation is by sympathetic nerve stimulation and constriction by parasympathetic nerve stimulation.
6. Defecation and micturition are possible due to activity of parasympathetic nerves stimulation.
7. In male reproductive system, errection of penis is due to parasympathetic stimulation and ejaculation of semen is because of sympathetic nerve activity.

Sleep and Wakefulness

Sleep is an altered state of consciousness during which some of body functions are depressed and some others activated.

Sleep and coma: A person who is in sleep can be aroused by tapping and a person who is in a state of coma cannot be aroused even by a painful stimulus.

Sleep can be a slow wave sleep (NREM) or a rapid eye movement (REM) sleep. Usually these two types of sleep are seen one following the other. And such 5 to 7 cycles alternate during entire sleeping hours.

Based on EEG recordings during sleep, slow wave sleep is divided into four stages, namely stage 1 to stage 4. Stages 1 and 2 will be light sleep; stages 3 and 4 will be deep sleep stages (Fig. 9.57). This sequence is followed when a person continues to sleep, but EEG recording suddenly changes to high frequency, low amplitude waves showing brain is alert during REM sleep even though person is in a state of deep sleep—therefore, this is known as paradoxical sleep. This is usually associated with rapid eye movements and dreams. Hence it is often called REM sleep.

Age and sleep patterns: Duration of sleep declines with age. A newborn spends most time in sleep; at least 50% of this duration is of REM type of sleep.

In puberty, duration of sleep is reduced. Approximately 25% of this duration is of REM type. After the age of 60, total duration of sleep is markedly reduced. The duration of REM sleep is almost negligible. At this age, most of time is spent in stages 1 and 2 (light sleep). Barbiturates which are commonly used as sleeping pills suppress stages 3 and 4 of sleep. It also suppresses REM sleep.

Progressive changes in EEG: Slow wave sleep—stage 1, low voltage high frequency wave resembling that of alert state.

Stage 3—appearance of sleep spindles and low frequency, high voltage waves.

Stage 4—very high voltage waves with a marked decrease in frequency refer to as delta waves (Fig. 9.58 and Table 9.6).

Importance of REM sleep: Suppressed emotions will be vent out during this sleep and hence normalize the balanced activity of neurons. If this cannot occur, person becomes highly irritable and complains of insomnia and this may lead to pure psychosis.

A newborn needs no teaching as to how to suckle. It has learnt the same during its REM sleep in uterus.

Theories of Sleep

Passive theory: Experimental evidences show that when all sensory inputs to ARAS are cut off, ARAS

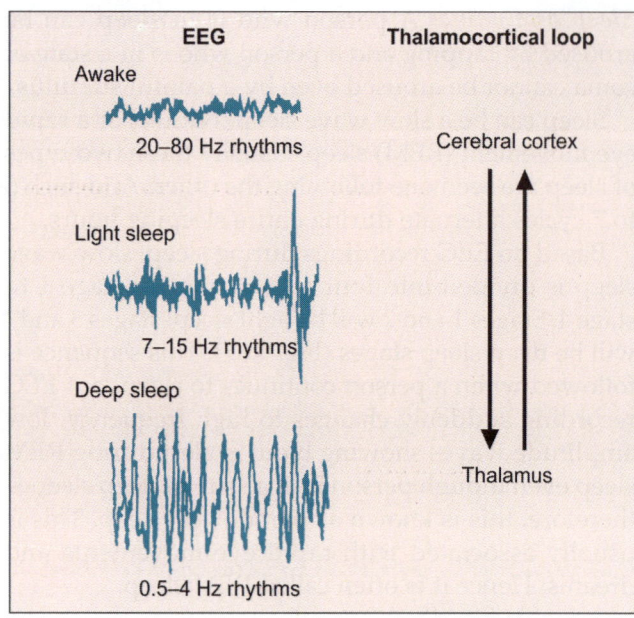

Fig. 9.57: EEG patterns in light and deep sleep

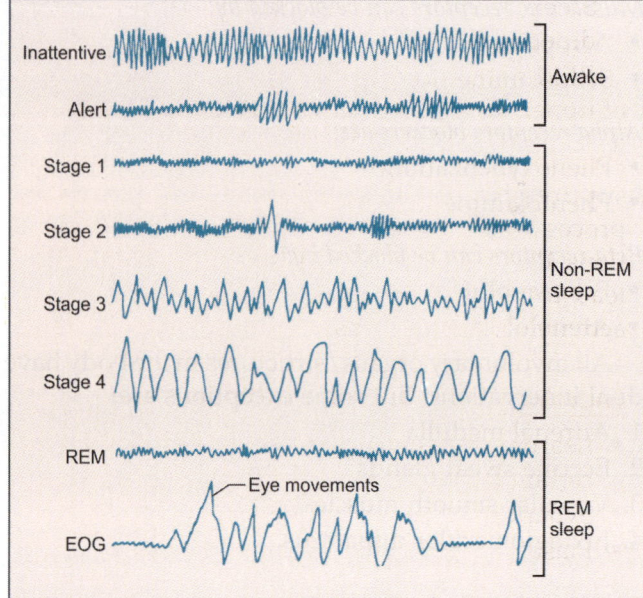

Fig. 9.58: Changes in EEG during different stages of sleep and REM sleep

activity markedly decreases resulting in decreased activity of cortical neurons and hence resulting in sleep.

Present view: Process which results in sleep is an active one. Stimulation of:

a. Raphe nucleus
b. Nucleus of tractus solitarius
c. Preoptic and suprachiasmatic nuclei in hypothalamus result in sleep.

Impulses from raphe nucleus go up to thalamus, reticular formation and all parts of cerebral cortex, hypothalamus and limbic system.

Transmitter substance involved is 5 HT (drugs that block synthesis of 5 HT, the animal cannot sleep). But there are some reservations about involvement of 5 HT, because when a sample of CSF is obtained during sleep, there was no increase of 5 HT in CSF. Further

research has shown that muramyl dipeptide may be a candidate, interleukin associated with bacterial infections may also be substance.

When there is lesion in raphe nucleus, suprachiasmatic nucleus, and anterior hypothalamus, inhibition on ARAS are removed and animal will be in arousal state throughout. Sleep inducing areas of brain include:

a. Raphe nucleus
b. Nucleus of tractus solitarius
c. Suprachiasmatic nucleus and preoptic nucleus

And also stimulation of cutaneous nerve fibers (inducing sleep in babies)

Neurotransmitters involved:

1. Raphe nucleus—5 HT, slow wave sleep
2. Preoptic nucleus—5 HT, REM sleep

Table 9.6: Differences between slow wave sleep and REM sleep

Slow wave sleep	REM sleep
Increased parasympathetic activity	----------------
Decreased heart rate, BP, respiration	Irregular EEG
Increased GI motility, papillary constriction	Showing alert state
Decreased muscle tone, change in body posture	Brain metabolism increased by 20%
Not associated with dreams	GI movements completely stopped, muscle tone is highly decreased; penile errection may be present, eyeballs show rapid movements

3. Sleep producing substances are—muramyl dipeptide (MDP), interleukin I

REM sleep is due to release of ACh from neurons of upper ARAS. This activates many parts of brain.

Physiological importance of sleep: Prolonged suppression of sleep will result in disruption of process of thinking, followed by behavioral alterations. Person becomes more irritable and at time may lead to psychosis. Sleep restores natural balanced activity of CNS neurons.

Learning and Memory

- Learning is alteration in behavior consequent to certain experiences
- Synaptic function is very essential
- Plasticity of synapse is involved.

Types of Learning

1. ***Imitation learning:***
   - Imitating people, sounds or situations around you.
   - Occurs early in life without much of thinking.
2. ***Associative learning*** *is of two types, namely:*
   a. *Classical conditioning* in which to start with an unconditioned stimulus is coupled with a neutral stimulus to elicit a reflex action. After repeated training with schedule (that is unconditioned stimulus and neutral stimulus when paired in an orderly manner), when neutral stimulus alone is presented, there would be reflex response for neutral stimulus. This can be explained based on Pavlovian study on dogs:
   i. On day 1, he rang the bell (neutral stimulus), and after sometime he presented food (unconditioned stimulus) to dog. The reflex response was salivary secretion (unconditioned reflex).
   ii. This schedule that is ringing bell, and after few minutes of pause, presentation of food, is continued for few days at specific time.
   iii. After few days, bell is rung but food is not presented, but still come across reflex salivary secretion in dog. This response is now known as conditioned reflex (conditioned response).
   iv. During the course of training, when neutral stimulus was coupled with unconditioned stimulus, dog starts associating sound of bell to getting food following sound. Hence it starts responding to sound by secreting saliva even before food is presented.
   v. When neutral stimulus (sound) is coupled with unconditioned stimulus (food), in the course of time one is able to generate response (secretion of saliva) for neutral stimulus alone. The neutral stimulus is termed as conditioned stimulus and response thus obtained for conditioned stimulus is known as conditioned reflex (response).
   b. *Instrumental conditioning:*
   - Instrumental conditioning was first demonstrated by Skinner and he used a specially designed box for this study known as Skinner's box.
   - In this experiment, animal is trained to keep pressing pedal inbox either to avoid certain punishment or to get some reward like food pellets or water, etc.
   - Initially animal is trained to perform task and after few sessions of training, animal starts performing task moment it is transferred to box.

Either avoiding punishment or getting reward when a particular task is done can be seen in human beings also. When you perform certain tasks, you either get some punishment like scolding and you try to avoid the same. At times, you get some reward when you perform certain tasks (parent presenting a vehicle to their child for excellent grades in academics).

MEMORY

- Memory is the ability to recall/retrieve stored information at a later date.
- There are many parts of brain that are involved in memory.
- Some of the important parts involved are hypothalamus, amygadala, thalamus, etc.
- Recent memory—anterior thalamic nucleus is involved.
- When there is sensory registration, memory comes into play.
- When stimulus acts on body or brain for more than 1 second, registration of sensory information occurs.
- This sensory registration gradually gets converted to primary memory (Fig. 9.59).

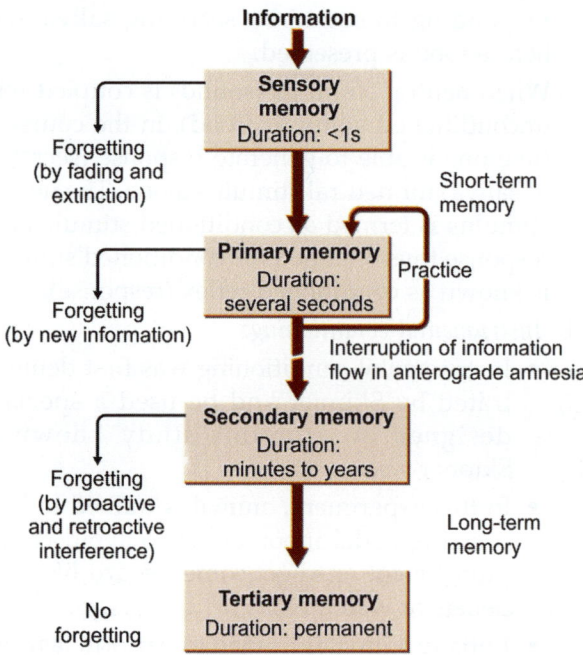

Fig. 9.59: The process of consolidation of memory

- Depending on whether information is essential, it is stored for varying periods of time (long or short).
- When constant rehearsal goes on, the primary memory gets converted to secondary memory. In secondary memory stage, information can be stored for few months to few years. There would be constant erasing of stored information, if it is not retrieved.
- After a few years, old information is erased and new information is stored. Some of old information stored may get erased and is replaced by some new information.
- Under constant rehearsal, secondary memory is converted to tertiary memory which lasts for life and there is no erasing of this information even when it is not recalled often, e.g. your place of birth, school you attended to as a child, etc.

Amnesia

- Loss of memory
- There are two different types, namely:
  a. Retrograde
  b. Anterograde
- In retrograde amnesia after some shock or accidents, information stored prior to accident or incident will be lost.

- In anterograde amnesia, after particular incident (shock or accident) new memory consolidation cannot be brought about but old information is retained.

Cerebral Cortex

1. Frontal Lobe

It has area 4, 6—motor and premotor area, 4S suppressor area, 8-frontal eye field. In prefrontal lobe, areas 9–12 are present. Areas 44, 45 are called Broca's area of speech and this area is present in dominant/categorical hemisphere only (Fig. 9.60).

Functions

- It gives origin to pyramidal tract which is necessary for all voluntary movement and also for skilled movements. Area no. 8 function is essential for accommodation for near vision.
- About 40% of communication between individuals is verbal. Areas 44 and 45 have role to play for verbal communication. When these areas are damaged person cannot talk but can understand spoken language.

2. Parietal Lobe

It has areas 3, 1, 2 termed primary sensory areas and areas 5, 7 called association areas (Fig. 9.61). In primary sensory areas, body representation is contralateral, upside down and extent of representation of body is not dependent on anatomical size of body but on functional importance.

Functions (Fig. 9.62)

- Function of primary sensory area is to help perception of all general sensations. In addition to this, areas also help in perception of taste sensation.
- Association areas help in analysis of all generation sensations and taste sensation.
- Areas 3, 1 and 2 also contribute for formation of pyramidal tract that is involved in voluntary movements.

3. Occipital Lobe

It has areas 17, 18 and 19. Area no. 17 is termed primary visual area and 18 and 19 are called as visual association areas. Fovea centralis part of retina has wider area of representation and relay in occipital lobe

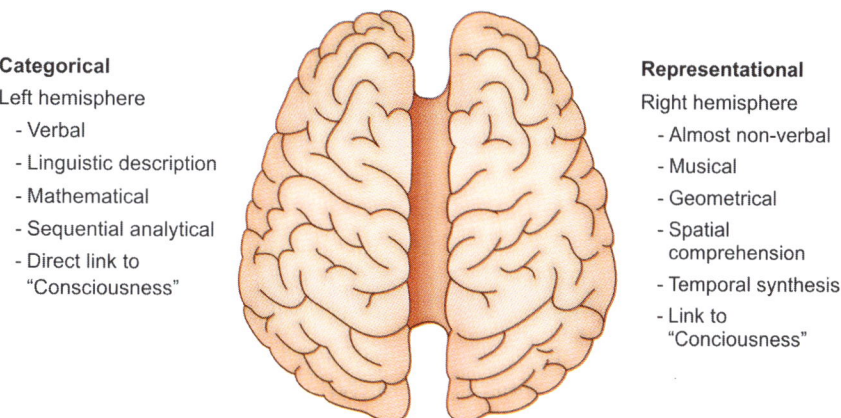

Categorical

Left hemisphere
- Verbal
- Linguistic description
- Mathematical
- Sequential analytical
- Direct link to "Consciousness"

Representational

Right hemisphere
- Almost non-verbal
- Musical
- Geometrical
- Spatial comprehension
- Temporal synthesis
- Link to "Conciousness"

Fig. 9.60: The functional diffentiation in the two different hemispheres

of opposite side also. Hence fovea centralis has bilateral representation

Functions

Area no. 17 helps in perception of visual sensation. Areas 18 and 19 help for analysis of vision that is perceived. If there is lesion in occipital lobe of one side, it leads to homonymous hemianopia that is loss of nasal field of vision in one eye and temporal field of vision in opposite eye. In certain homonymous hemianopia, macular sparing may occur due to bilateral representation of macula lutea (fovea centralis).

4. Temporal Lobe

The lobe has areas 41, 42 which are termed as primary auditory areas and also areas 21 and 22 called auditory

association areas. In posterior part of superior temporal gyrus, one more area is present and this is called Wernicke's area. Wernicke's area is the general association area and is present in dominant (categorical) hemisphere only.

Functions

- Areas 41 and 42 help for perception of sounds heard and areas 21 and 22 for analyzing details of sound and give meaning for the sound.
- Impulses from sensory (general) area, visual (general) area, and auditory (general) area reach Wernicke's area (Fig. 9.63). When there is damage to this part, person in unable to understand spoken and written language and leads to sensory aphasia. Person can talk but cannot comprehend language (spoken or written)

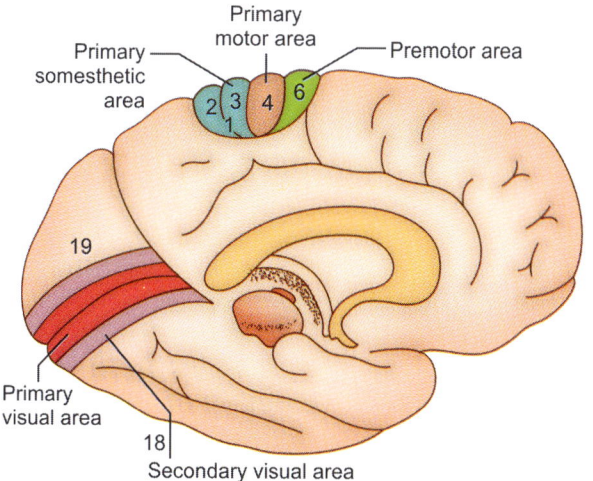

Fig. 9.61: The imortant sensory and motor areas of cerebral cortex

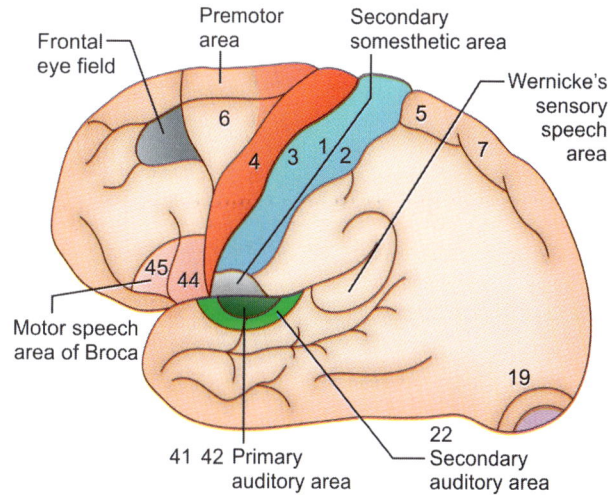

Fig. 9.62: Important areas in cerebral cortex that are involved in various functions

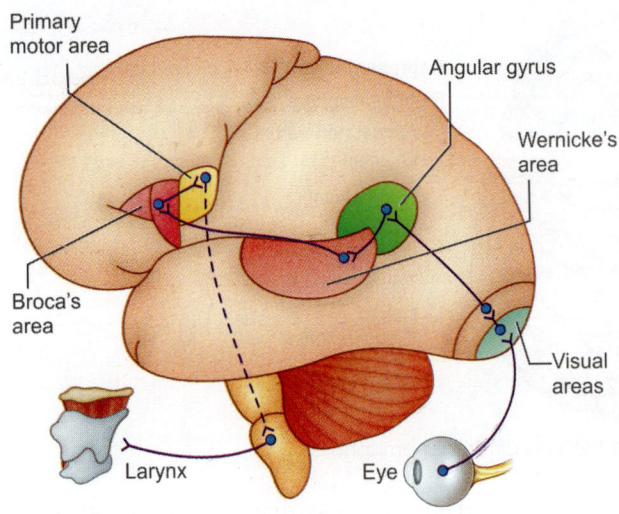

Fig. 9.63: Various influences on Wernike's area

Functions of Prefrontal Lobe

1. It has role in learning and memory
2. It is important to maintain moral sense and appropriate social behavior.
3. It has important role to play for balanced emotional reactions.
   Functions were studied only after damaging that is after prefrontal lobotomy.

Features of Prefrontal Lobotomy

1. *Flights of ideas*
   - No correlation between statements and action
   - Random thoughts
2. *Euphoria*
   - False sense of well-being prevails
   - Feeling of conquering world
3. *Memory impairment*
4. *Alterations in social behavior*
   - For examples, act friendly to snakes
   - Act unfriendly with humans
5. *Lack of initiative*
   - No urge or attempt to bring about activities
   - No interest to perform certain tasks
   - Laid back attitude, i.e. lethargy
6. *Emotion*
   - No restraint on emotions
   - May demonstrate temper tantrums
   - Balanced emotional reactions are lost
7. *Loss of orientation of space and time*
   - Unable to comprehend where they are or what time it is.
8. *Impairment of moral sense*
9. *Perseveration*
   - Keep doing same task with no rhyme or rhythm
   - Keep doing same task over and over again (repeated performance of same task).

(Pneumonic to remember prefrontal lobe altered functions after prefrontal lobotomy: FEMALE LIP)

Special Senses

10

C H A P T E R

VISION

Eye subserves the most important function that is vision. The receptors involved are the rods and cones. The rods have a low threshold; respond to light intensity as low as one photon unit. They are for scotopic vision (dim light vision). With this vision, neither the details of an object nor the color of the object can be made out.

The other type of receptors are the cones. They are responsible for photopic vision (bright light vision). The borders, and shape of the objects are clearly made out including the color of the objects is made out properly.

The Layers of the Eye (Fig. 10.1)

Eye has three layers. The outer sclera is a fibrous protective layer. Anteriorly, it continues as the transparent cornea. Cornea forms an important refractive media of the eye. It contributes about 40D powers for refraction. It is a highly sensitive structure; free nerve endings are receptors present in the cornea. Stimulation of these receptors will give rise to corneal reflex, the response being closure of the eyes.

The middle layer is the choroid layer. This is a highly vascular and pigmented layer. The blood vessels that supply this layer also supply the receptor layer of the retina. The pigment that is present here plays an important role in vision. The light rays after stimulating the receptors get absorbed by the pigment that is present in the choroids. This prevents scattering

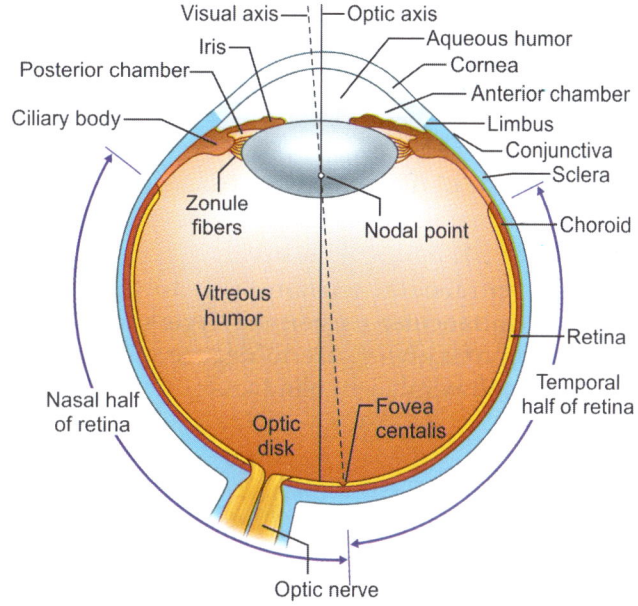

Fig. 10.1: Different layers, namely sclera, choroid and retina of eye

of the light rays and, therefore, improves vision. Anteriorly, this continues as the ciliary body and iris. The ciliary body has ciliary processes and ciliaris muscles. The ciliary processes play important role in secreting aqueous humor (Fig. 10.2).

Aqueous humor presents in the anterior and posterior chambers of the eye (Fig. 10.3). The fluid secretion is an active process. It serves many useful functions.

1. Supplies nutrition to the avascular structures of the eyes, namely the lens and the cornea.

289

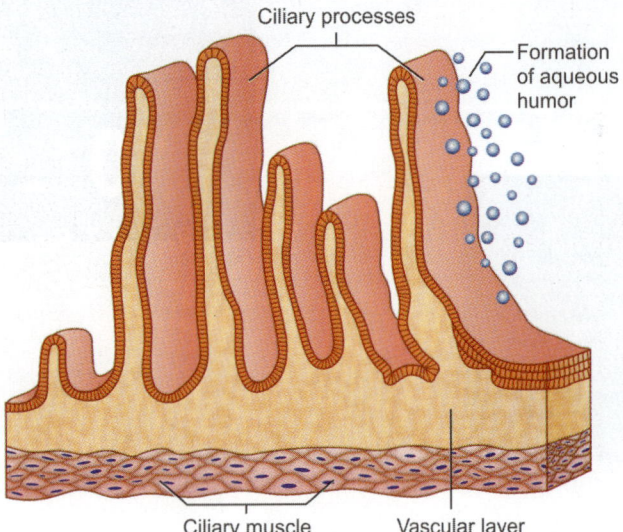

Fig. 10.2: Ciliary processes and aqueous humor

2. It maintains the intraocular pressure normally about 12 to 20 mm Hg.
3. Helps to drain the metabolic waste, produced by the lens.
4. It forms one of the refractive media of the eye.
5. Helps to maintain the shape of the eyeball and, therefore, the optics of the eye.

Raised intraocular tension leads to glaucoma. Increased intraocular tension may press up on the visual receptors giving rise to degeneration of the receptors, and permanent blindness.

Ciliary muscle is involved in the process of accommodation. A person who is looking at a distant object, suddenly starts looking at a nearby object, in order to focus the nearby object exactly on the retina, the diopteric power of the lens must be increased. The ciliary muscles contract, the suspensory ligaments relax and the tension in the ligaments is reduced. Therefore, the anterior curvature of the lens becomes more convex. This increases the lens power by about 14 diopters in a young person. In addition to this, two other changes are also taking place when a person accommodates for near vision. They are: the pupil constricts and the eyeball is rotated medially which facilitates the eyes converge towards the point of regard.

Iris (Fig. 10.4) is the pigmented portion of the eye that can be seen from the front. The color of the eye depends on this. It surrounds an aperture of the pupil. The pupillary size may vary from 1 mm to about 8 mm when it is fully dilated. The iris has two different types of muscle fibers. One, the circular muscle fibers known as the constrictor pupillae fibers that are innervated by the parasympathetic nerve fibers which take origin from the Edinger-Westphal nucleus, course along the oculomotor nerve, relayed in the ciliary ganglion cells. The postganglionic fibers supply the constrictor muscle fibers. Stimulation of these fibers will give rise to pupillary constriction.

The other type of muscle fibers is radially running the dilator muscle fibers. They receive motor nerve

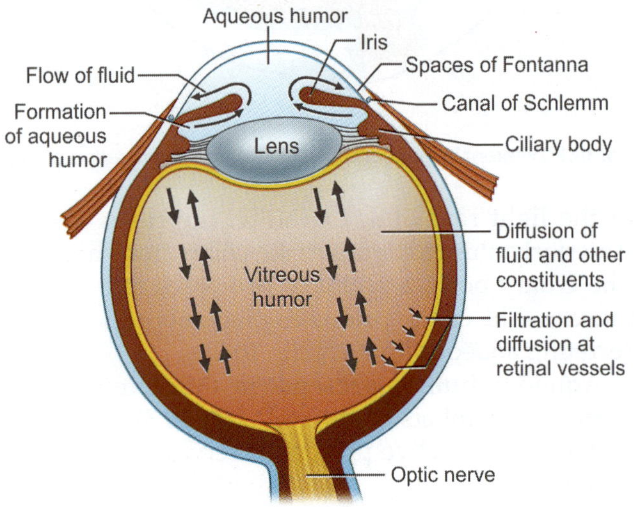

Fig. 10.3: The circulation of aqueous humor through posterior and anterior chambers

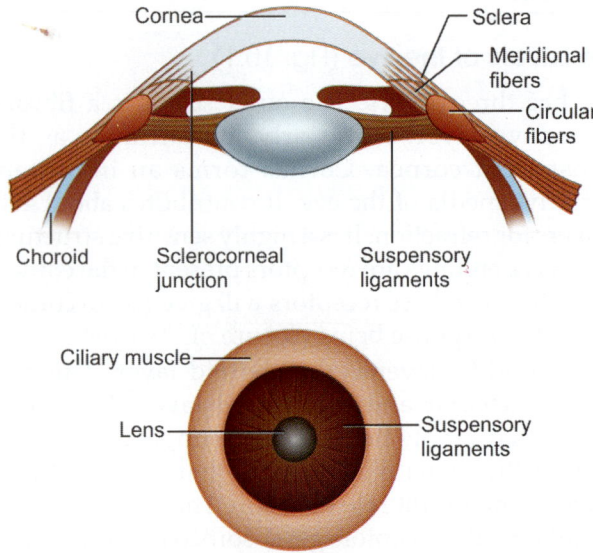

Fig. 10.4: The lens, suspensory ligament and ciliaris muscle

supply from the sympathetic fiber. These fibers take their origin from the lateral horn cells of T1 segment of the spinal cord, synapse at the superior cervical ganglion cells. The postganglionic fibers travel along the blood vessels and supply the dilator muscle fibers. Stimulation of these fibers will give rise to pupillary dilatation. When a bright light is thrown on to the eye or when a person is looking at a near object the pupil constricts. Pupillary constriction will serve three important functions.

1. It minimizes the amount of light entering into the eye.
2. It increases the depth of focus.
3. It minimizes the chromatic and spherical aberrations, which two types of physiological refractory errors.

Retina

The inner most layer of the eye is the retina. It is the neural layer of the eye. The visual receptors are present in this layer. It extends anteriorly to the ora serrata. On the posterior aspect slightly medial to the posterior pole of the eyeball is the area at which the

optic nerve leaves the eyeball. This area has no visual receptors; because of which even if the light rays fall on this part images cannot be formed and, therefore, known as the blind spot. Here the retinal artery enters the retina and the vein leaves the retina.

The blind spot can be seen through an ophthalmoscope. The central portion of the blind spot is depressed known as physiological cupping. Whenever the intracranial tension is increased, the cup becomes less shallow. A greater depression may be seen in optic atrophy, a degenerative condition of the ganglion cell layer of the retina.

Slightly lateral to the posterior pole of the eyeball is the most sensitive part of the retina, known as the fovea centralis. The acuity of vision is the highest here. Any specific object which is looked at, the image of the specific object is formed here.

The outer most layer of the retina is the pigment layer (Figs 10.5 and 10.6). When the light rays enter the eye, they stimulate the rods and cones and then they are absorbed by the pigment layer of the retina. This prevents scattering of the light rays. Preventing the scattering of light rays improves the clarity of the

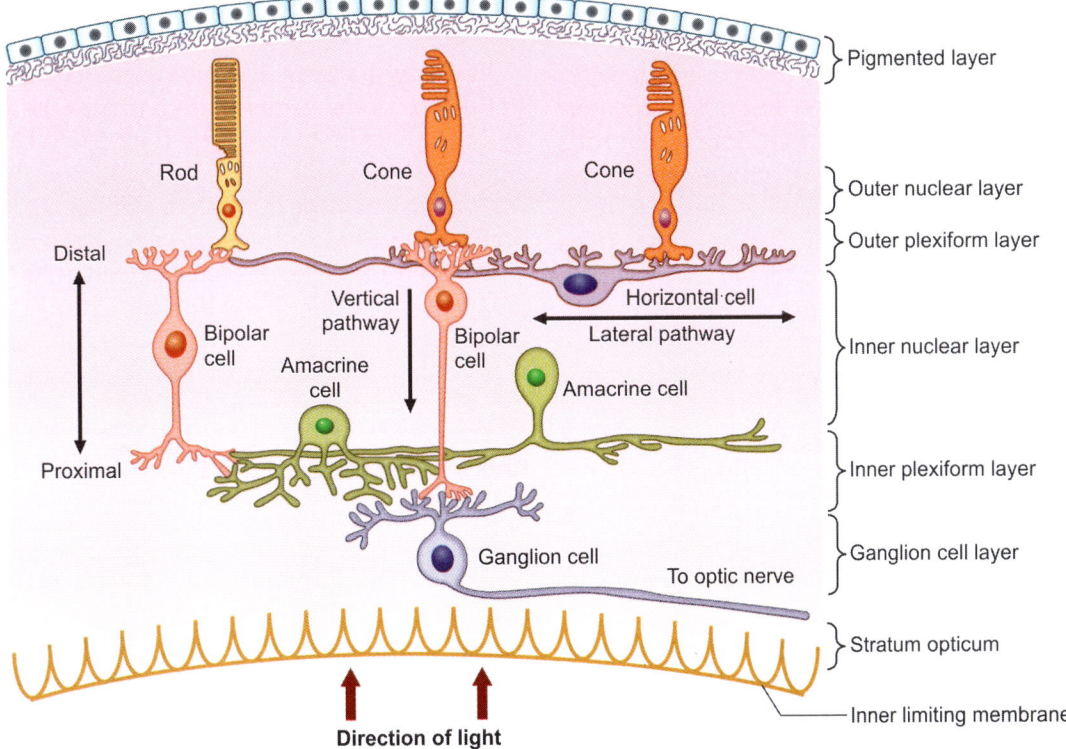

Fig. 10.5: Different layers of retina and the direction of penetration of light rays

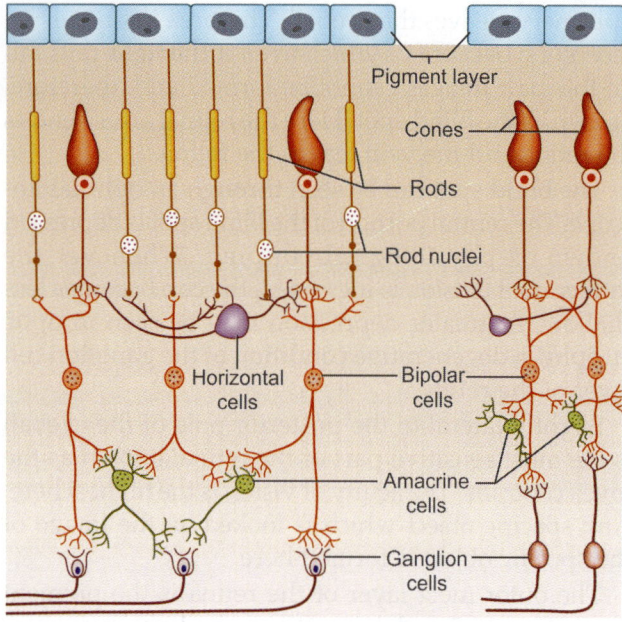

Fig. 10.6: Different layers of retina with the various cell types

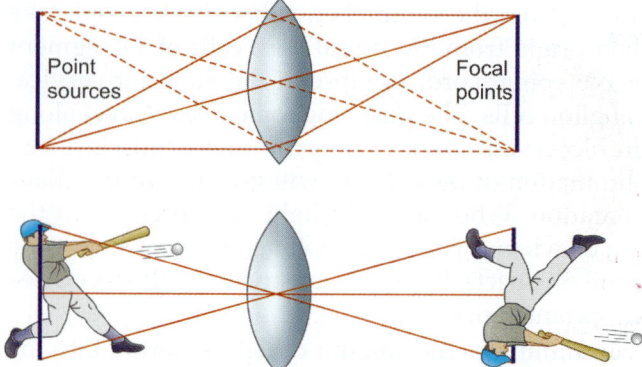

Fig. 10.7: Source of light and image formation on the retina

visual image. Pigment layer is also responsible for phagocytosis of the old disks in the outer segments of the rods. It may also store vitamin A, which plays important role in the resynthesis of rhodopsin, the visual pigment.

The next layer in the retina is the receptor layer. There are about 120 million rods and 6 million cones in the retina. They differ in shape and structure; their distribution in the retina also varies (diagram of rods and cones; Fig. 10.6). In the fovea centralis, only cones are present. These cones are special cones. The cone density is highest here. The ratio between the cones and the ganglion cell is 1:1. Fovea is the thinnest part of the retina. Most of the layers of the retina are pushed to the side and, therefore, when light rays fall, the rays directly fall on the receptor layer. This part of the retina has the widest area of representation in the occipital cortex. Because of these reasons, the acuity of vision is highest in fovea centralis.

Rods are not present in the fovea. The maximum number of rods seen at about 20 degrees outside the fovea. From there onwards, the rod concentration falls towards the periphery of the retina.

The outer segments of the rods contain the photosensitive pigment rhodopsin. This is synthesized by the inner segment of the rods and stored in the outer segments in the disks. When light falls on the receptors, the pigment gets bleached. This initiates the

neural mechanism that is responsible for vision. The disks containing the photosensitive material getting pushed towards the periphery, and they are replaced by the newer disks. Accumulation of the older disks, if not removed, will give rise to retinitis pigmentosa, resulting in visual deterioration.

The human eye can be compared to a camera. The camera has a lens system through which the light rays can pass; the objects can be focused on to the photo film. The distance between the film and the lens can be adjusted so as to focus the objects exactly on the photo film. The size of the aperture in the camera can be varied.

In the human eye, the biological lens corresponds to the lens of the camera, the retina to the photo film and the aperture to the pupil (Fig. 10.7). The distance between the lens and the retina cannot be altered. Instead to focus a near object or a distant object exactly on the retina the diopteric power of the lens is altered. When a far off object is being looked at, the biconvex lens becomes thinner, the diopteric power of the lens is reduced. On the other hand, when a nearby object is looked at, the biconvex lens becomes more convex, its' diopteric power is increased.

Refractory Media of the Eye

The cornea, the vitreous humor, the lens and the aqueous humor form the refractory media of the eye (Fig. 10.8). The human eye has a total refractory power of 60 diopters. Most of the refraction occurs in human beings at the air–cornea interface. If the refractory index of air is taken as 1, the refractory index of the cornea is about 1.38. The refractory power of the cornea is about 40 diopters. Lens has a refractory power of 20 diopters. During accommodation for a

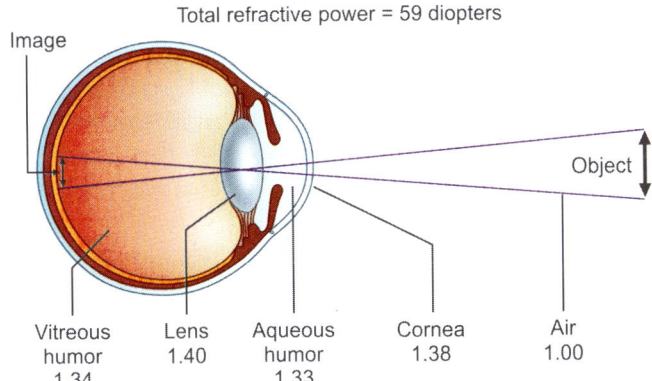

Total refractive power = 59 diopters

Fig. 10.8: Refractive indices at different parts in eye. Maximal bending of light rays occurs at air–corneal interphase

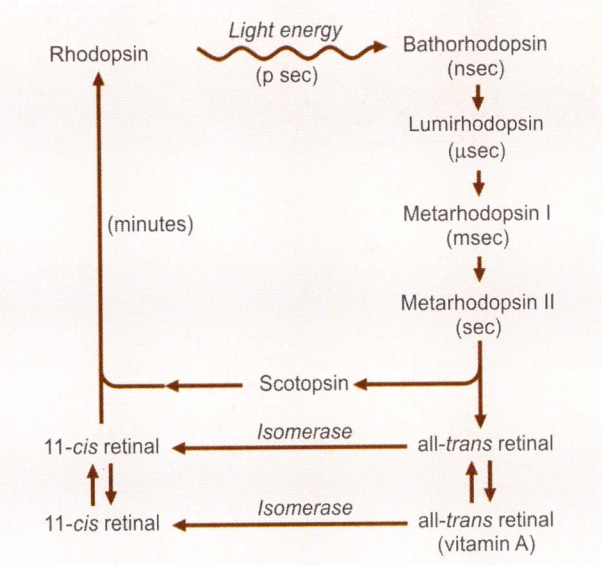

Fig. 10.9: The rhodopsin cycle

near object, the refractory power of the lens can be increased further by about 14 diopters. This depends on the age of the individuals. As age advances, refractory power decreases. At the age of 60, it may be reduced to only 2 diopters.

Far vision is the farthest distance an individual can see, and it is at infinity. Sun, moon and stars can be seen, if a person's vision is not obstructed.

Near vision is the nearest distance at which objects can be clearly seen. It is about 25 centimeters from the eyes at the age of 20 years. As age advances, the near vision recedes and at the age of 60 years it will be about 80 cm. This condition is known as presbyopia (Table 10.1).

Resynthesis of Rhodopsin (Fig. 10.9)

The all-*trans* retinal that is formed is converted to 11-*cis* form by an enzyme known as retinal isomerase. This can combine with scotopsin and resynthesize rhodopsin. In the presence of vitamin A, the resynthesis of rhodopsin can occur. If a person is suffering from vitamin A deficiency, it will result in

Table 10.1: Distance from eyes at which near point will be at different age of the person

Age (yrs)	Near point (cm)	Amplitude of accommodation (D)
10	9	11–14
20	10	10
30	12.5	8
40	18	5.5
50	50	2
70	100	1

night blindness. This vitamin deficiency will damage the receptors permanently may give rise to blindness.

There are three different types of cones containing three different types of cone pigments. Not only they are the receptors for bright light vision, they are also the receptors for color vision. The three primary colors associated with three cones are blue, red and green. Stimulation of these receptors equally will produce the white color. If they are stimulated in different proportions, different shades of colors are produced.

Visual Pathway and Effect of Lesions at Different Levels

Visual Pathway or Optic Pathway (Fig. 10.10)

This pathway is essential for the impulses that have got originated in the retina to reach cerebral cortex for conscious perception of the image.

The schematic events that occur during the perception of vision will be:

1. Light rays falling on the retina
2. Stimulate the photoreceptors on retina
3. Afferent impulses are generated in the optic nerve fibers
4. The nasal half of the retinal fibers cross the midline at optic chiasma and beyond optic chiasma, there is formation of optic tract. This tract contains fibers coming from the temporal half of same side retina and nasal half of the contralateral retina.

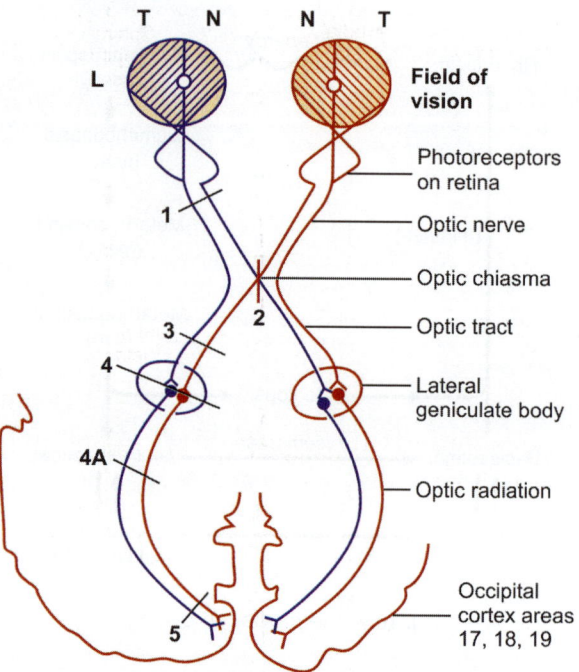

Fig. 10.10: The visual pathway and probable common sites of lesions (1-5)

5. Impulses reach lateral geniculate body and relayed here.
6. From the lateral geniculate body or the lateral geniculate nucleus, the geniculocalcarine tract or optic radiation fibers take origin.
7. These fibers pass through the posterior limb of internal capsule. While traversing as optic radiation, the fibers form a loop forward in the temporal lobe as Meyer's loop.
8. Optic radiation fibers relay in the occipital cortex area no. 17, which is known as primary area for vision. Impulses will also go to areas 18 and 19. These areas are known as visual association areas. The analytical part of the vision is brought about by the visual association areas.

Effect of Lesion at
Different Levels in Visual Pathway

1. Optic nerve damage (Fig. 10.10, no.1) (unilateral) leads to complete blindness of the affected eye, because the afferent fibers are unable to carry impulses along the visual pathway.
2. Optic chiasma damage (Fig. 10.10, no.2) (medial side) brings about bitemporal hemianopia. In this condition, there will be loss of temporal field of

vision in both the eyes. This condition is also an example for heteronymous hemianopia, that is, in this condition the left half of visual field of left eye and right half of visual field of right eye will be lost. One of the conditions in which this occurs is when there is enlargement of pituitary gland (acromegaly).
3. Unilateral optic tract lesion (Fig. 10.10, no.3) leads to homonymous hemianopia. In this condition, there will be loss of temporal field of vision in one eye and nasal field of vision in the opposite eye. In other words, there will be loss of either the left or right visual fields in both the eyes. For a right side homonymous hemianopia to occur there should be lesion in the left optic tract and vice versa for left side homonymous hemianopia.
4. Lesion any where beyond the optic tract untill occipital cortex and if it is unilateral and extensive (Fig. 10.10, no.4 and 4A), may lead to homonymous hemianopia. If the lesion is more restricted, it may lead to quandrantanopia.
5. If there is an extensive lesion in occipital cortex of one side (Fig. 10.10, no.5), then it may lead to homonymous hemianopia with macula sparing. That is, if the image gets focused on the macula, the person is still able to see. Macula sparing occurs because of the following reasons:
   a. Macula region has extensive area of representation and hence damage to occipital cortex may not affect the whole of macula area representation.
   b. Geniculocalcarine tract fibers, just before termination in the occipital cortex, a few of the fibers will cross over to the opposite side as well to end in occipital cortex of opposite side. It is because of this, there is bilateral representation for macula fibers.
   c. It is believed that some of the macula fibers do not accompany the classical optic pathway, but go to occipital cortex separately along the midline to relay in occipital cortex.

Visual field: It is the extent of external world that can be seen when vision is fixed on particular object. Normally it is tested separately for each of the eye. For monocular vision, the field of vision will be:
a. Nasal about 40°
b. Temporal about 140°
c. Upper about 40°
d. Lower about 40–60°

The extent of field of vision is influenced by bony prominences.

Methods to determine field of vision
1. Perimetry that is using a perimeter.
2. Confrontation method.

Accommodation and Light Reflexes

Accommodation is the process by which an eye is able to focus the images of a distant object or a nearby object exactly on the retina. Such an eye is known as an emmetropic eye.

When eyes are getting accommodated to near vision, this is termed as accommodation to near vision and reflex is known as near reflex or conventionally speaking is known as accommodation reflex. There will be three important changes taking place in visual system when eyes are getting accommodated to near vision. They are:

1. The sphincter pupillae muscle contracts, thereby pupillary aperture size is decreased.
2. The lens becomes more convex, this increases the diopteric power of the lens. The diopteric power of the lens is increased by about 14 diopters in young persons.
3. The medial rectus muscles on both the sides contract, the eyeballs converge, the visual axis meet at the corresponding points, this prevents diplopia or double vision.

Constriction of pupil brings about:
a. Decreased amount of light entering the eye.
b. Prevents spherical and chromatic aberrations by allowing the light rays to pass through nodal point.
c. Increases the depth of focus (Table 10.2).

Curvature of lens increase results in increasing the diopteric power of lens, so that the diverging rays are made to converge.

Convergence of eyeballs will allow the light to get focused on corresponding points in the two eyes. This prevents diplopia or double vision.

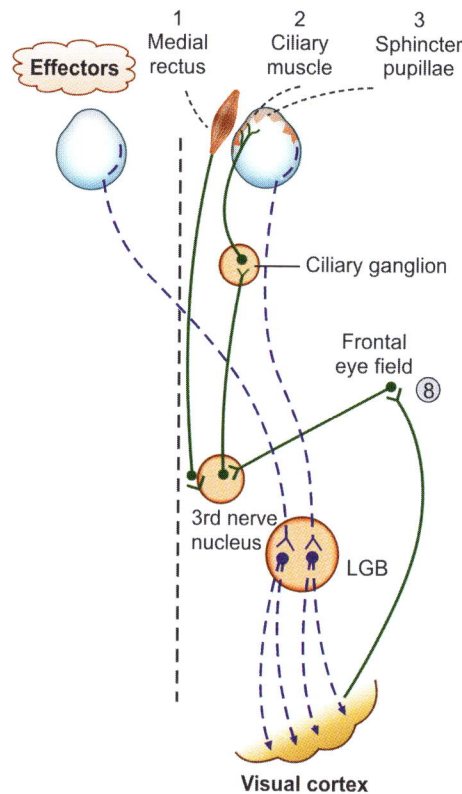

Fig. 10.11: Pathway for accommodation reflex

Pathway involved (Fig. 10.11): Impulses arising from the retina made to reach the visual cortex through the optic pathway. From visual cortex, impulses are relayed to the prefrontal eye field area number 8. Nerve fibers arising from area no. 8 are relayed to the autonomic and somatic nuclei of the third cranial nerve. The parasympathetic fibers carry these impulses to the ciliary muscles as well as the constrictor muscle fibers. Impulses are carried to the medial recti through the somatic part of the third cranial nerve.

Emmetropia is one which is capable of focusing the parallel rays of light originating from a far object on the retina without the help of any accommodation (that is without changing the diopteric power of lens).

Range of Accommodation

In a normal eye, far point is infinity. Near point is about 15 cm at the age of 20 years. The near point recedes as age advances. The difference between the far point and near point is called as range of accommodation.

Table 10.2: Depth of focus		
Pupil diameter	Depth at infinity	Depth at 1 metre
1 mm	from infinity to 1.25 m	5.0 m to 56 cm
2 mm	from infinity to 2.33 m	1.8 m to 70 cm
3 mm	from infinity to 2.94 m	1.5 m to 75 cm
4 mm	from infinity to to 3.57 m	1.4 m to 78 cm

Amplitude of accommodation: The change in the diopteric power of lens when a person looking at a distant object suddenly looks at a near object.

For far object, it is about 18D.

For near object, it is about 36D.

Therefore, the amplitude of accommodation will be about 36–18 = 18D.

Light reflex: When a beam of light is suddenly thrown on the eye, there will be reflex constriction of pupil. This is known as light reflex. Light reflexes are of two types namely direct light reflex and an indirect light reflex. The indirect light reflex is also known as consensual light reflex. Throw a beam of light on one eye, the pupil on that side constricts. This is the direct light reflex. Through a beam of light on one eye, the pupil on the opposite eye also constricts. This is the indirect light reflex. The center for the light reflex is the pretectal nucleus in the midbrain. The impulses for pupillary constrictor muscle fibers come along the oculomotor nerve fibers (Fig. 10.12).

Argyll Robertson pupil: This is a clinical condition wherein the light reflex is absent but the accommodation reflex is retained. In this condition, there will be atrophy of the muscles of the iris, the pupillary margin becomes irregular and mydriatic, the pupil reacts very slowly. One of the clinical conditions wherein it occurs is neurosyphilis. In this condition, the pretectal nucleus in the midbrain is damaged. Pretectal nucleus is the center for light reflex (Fig. 10.13). Damage to the center will lead to loss of light reflex.

Visual acuity is the ability of the eyes to distinguish two points as two separate points. It is the shortest distance at which two lines can be separated and still be perceived as two lines. It is highest at the region of fovea centralis that has large concentration of cone pigments only. Visual acuity is more for photopic vision than for scotopic vision.

Visual acuity can be tested for both far and near visions. For distant vision testing, Snellen's chart is used whereas for testing near vision the chart used will be Jaeger's. The result for the distant vision testing is expressed as a fraction, wherein the numerator of the fraction is fixed (i.e. 20 feet away where the patient is made to remain), and the denominator is greatest distance from the chart at which a normal individual can read the smallest line. When the fraction is more

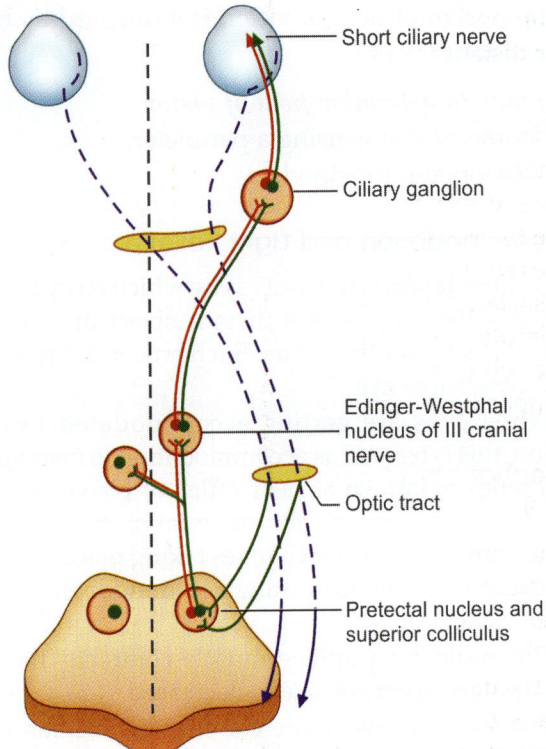

Fig. 10.12: Pathway for light reflex

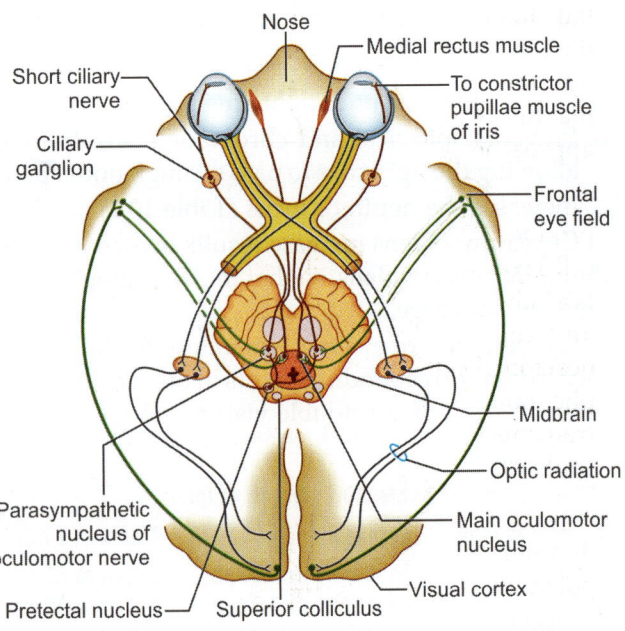

Fig. 10.13: Composite diagram showing pathways for both light reflex and accommodation reflexes

than one, it means that the person's acuity is better for distant vision.

Neurophysiological Basis of Vision

There are three different types of cones containing three different types of cone pigments. Not only they are the receptors for bright light vision, they are also the receptors for color vision. The three primary colors associated with three cones are blue, red and green. Stimulation of these receptors equally will produce the white color. If they are stimulated in different proportions, different shades of colors are produced.

Mechanism of Hyperpolarization of the Receptors

The inner segment of the rods continually pumps sodium ions from inside of the rod to the outside. This creates negativity inside the rods. The outer segment of the rod, where disks are located is leaky to sodium in the dark. Therefore, the positively charged sodium leaks back to the inside of the rods and there by neutralize much of the negativity on the inside of the rods (Fig. 10.14). Normally the rods have a resting membrane potential of about minus 40 mV.

When the rods are exposed to light, the permeability of the outer segment to sodium is completely blocked; the sodium that is pumped out fails to enter in. This creates a greater negativity on the inner side of the rods. The greater the amount of light entering greater is the negativity created. At maximum light intensity, the membrane potential approaches –70 to –80 mV.

Neural functions of the retina: The hyperpolarization produced is conducted electrotonically to the bipolar cell layer of the retina. The horizontal cells connect laterally between the synaptic bodies of the rods, cones and the bipolar cell bodies. The output of the horizontal cells is always inhibitory. This leads to the phenomenon of lateral inhibition. This helps in the transmission of visual patterns with proper visual contrasts.

Bipolar cells: Some of these cells undergo depolarization; some other cells undergo hyper-polarization when the signals reach these cells.

Amacrine cells response are different. One type of cells respond at the onset of the visual signals and the response dies quickly. The other type responds at the

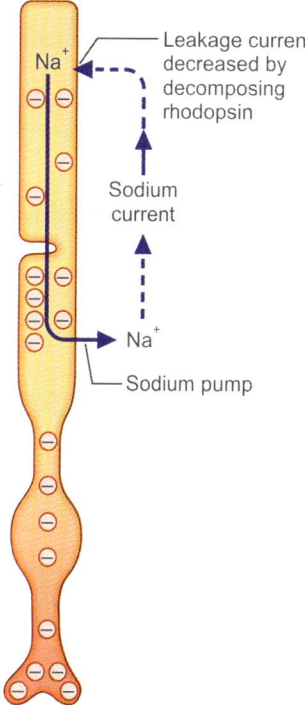

Fig. 10.14: Continual movement of sodium from and into the receptor

offset of the signals, again these responses die quickly, a third type of amacrine cells respond both at the onset and at the offset of the stimulus. Some of the amacrine cells are stimulated to the movement of a spot across the retina in a specific direction.

Responses from the ganglion cell layer of the retina: The number of ganglion cells is about 1.6 million in the retina. Thus an average of 60 rods and 2 cones converge on each ganglion cell. Ganglion cell responds by producing action potentials.

Three different types of ganglion cells are known. They are W, X and Y cells.

W cells: They are about 40% of the ganglion cells. They are small cells, they transmit signals at a very slow velocity of 8 meters/sec. They receive their signals mostly from the rods. They have broad fields of vision. They are especially sensitive to detect directional movements in the visual field.

The X cells are highest in number and are about 55% of the total. They are of the medium size; transmit signals at about 14 meters/sec. They receive impulses from a small field. They receive signals from cones and are responsible for the transmission of color vision.

The Y cells are the largest of all the cells. They transmit signals at a fast rate of about 50 meters/sec. They pick up signals from larger areas of the retina. They respond to rapid movements or rapid changes in light intensity.

Responses from the ganglion cells: The axons of the ganglion cells form the optic nerve fibers. The ganglion cells respond to the incoming signals by producing action potentials. These cells produce impulses at a steady rate of 5 to 40/sec whether they are stimulated or not. The signals coming from the receptors modify this background firing. Some of the cells respond by firing more number of impulses when light signal is on. When the light is turned off they stop producing impulses. These cells are known as on-off cells; their response is known as on-off responses. There are other ganglion cells. They are inhibited when the light is turned on and their signal discharge is increased when the light is turned off; they are known as off-on cells and their response is known as off-on responses.

Different colors excite different ganglion cells. On the other hand, if the three cones which are responsible for the three primary colors stimulate the same cone, a white color is appreciated. Color differentiation may begin at the retina itself. It is further analyzed at the level of the brain.

From the ganglion cells, the impulses reach the lateral geniculate body. It serves two important functions namely:

1. It acts as a relay station from the optic tract to the visual cortex. This neural body is made up of six layers. Layers 2, 3 and 5 receive signals from the temporal half of the ipsilateral retina whereas layers 1, 4 and 6 receive impulses from the nasal half of the contralateral retina.

2. The second major function of the lateral geniculate body is to gate the impulses to the visual cortex. Not all the impulses that reach the retina are allowed to reach the visual cortex. Most of the unimportant signals are prevented from reaching the cortex.

From the lateral geniculate body, the visual impulses reach the occipital cortex. Area number 17, the primary visual area, and from here they go to the secondary areas (areas 18 and 19; Figs 10.15 and 10.16). In area 17, the entire retina has a topographical representation. The macula has the largest area of

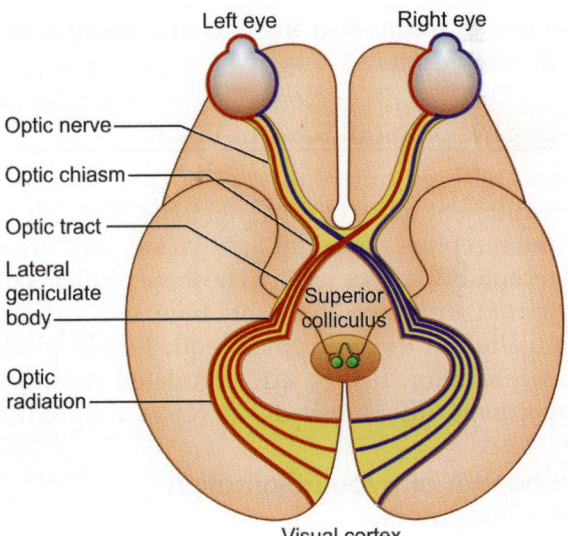

Fig. 10.15: Optic pathway fibers ending in visual cortex

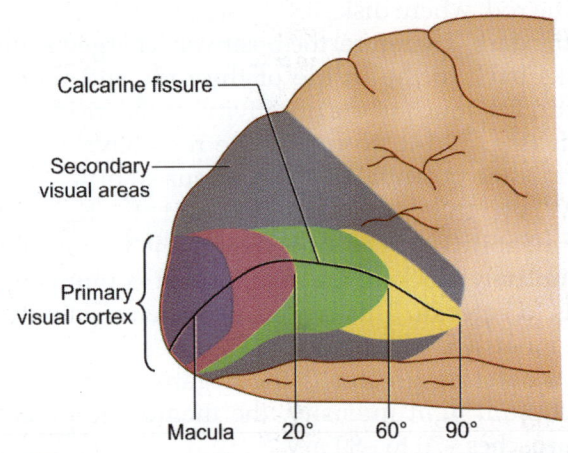

Fig. 10.16: Visual cortex with primary and secondary visual areas

representation. This area is also represented bilaterally. The upper part of the retina is represented on the upper lip of the calcarine sulcus and the lower half of the retina is represented at the lower lip of the calcarine sulcus.

The primary visual area has six layers in the cortex. The geniculocalcarine fibers mainly terminate in layer 4 of the cortex. The action potentials arising from the X and Y ganglion cells reach this part of the cortex and they are relayed both vertically upwards and downwards to the deeper and superficial layers of the cortex.

The neurons in the visual cortex are arranged in vertical columns. Each column is made up of 1000 or

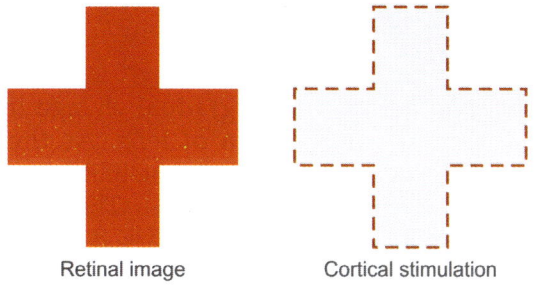

Retinal image   Cortical stimulation

Fig. 10.17: The margin of cortical neurons that are stimulated maximally

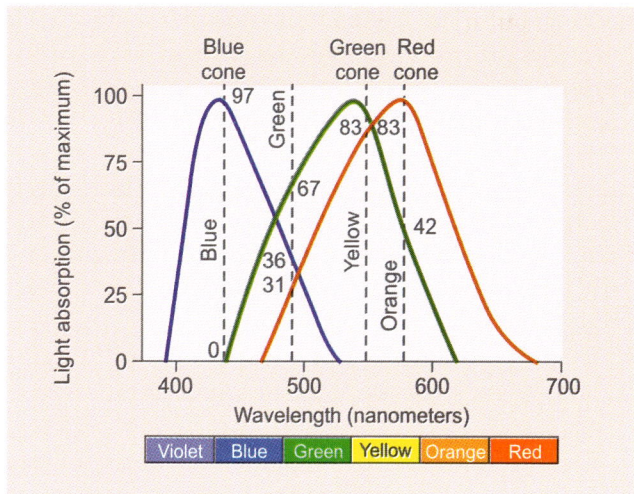

Fig. 10.18: The wavelength of different colors

more neurons and each one forms a functional unit. Impulses coming from the retina are further analyzed here.

Interspread with the primary visual columns are special columns of cells Color blobs. They are particularly activated by color signals. And they analyze the color signals.

When a person is looking at an object, the neurons that lie at the contrasting borders are maximally stimulated (Fig. 10.17). Some of the columns respond to vertical lines and some others to horizontal lines. Removal of the primary visual cortex will produce loss of conscious vision that is blindness.

Photochemistry of Color Vision

Three cones are responsible for three primary colors, namely the blue, the green and the red colors. They contain three separate pigments. These three cones respond maximally at three different wavelengths of light (Fig. 10.18), the blue at 445 nm, the green at 535 nm, and the red at 570 nm. When all the three cones are stimulated to equal proportion, it will produce white color but when they are stimulated to different extent by a given wavelength, it produces different shades of colors. This theory of color vision is known as the trichromatic theory.

Out of the three cones, one may be missing. This leads to color blindness. Commonly, it is the red cone that is missing. The term used for this type of color blindness is protonopia. On the other hand, if the missing cone is the green, the term used is duetranopia. Very rarely the blue cone may be absent. When cones for a particular color is absent, the person will try to make out the color of a given object with the help of the remaining two cones. This will lead to defective color identification.

Color defect is seen in families. The men are the sufferers and the females are the carriers. The gene responsible for the color vision (dominant gene) is present on the X chromosome and since a female has two X chromosomes (one having normal dominant gene and the other having recessive gene), they are rarely color blind. In the population about 8% of men are color blind and usually for red. In some of these cases, the red cone may be present but it may be weak. The terms used are protonopia and protonomaly. When only one cone is present the person is unable to differentiate colors, he can make out only black and white. They are known as monochromates.

Color blindness is tested by using Ishihara's chart (Fig. 10.19), and Edridge green color perception lantern.

Dark Adaptation and Light Adaptation

A person who is standing in a brightly lit area suddenly moves into a dark room, the person sees

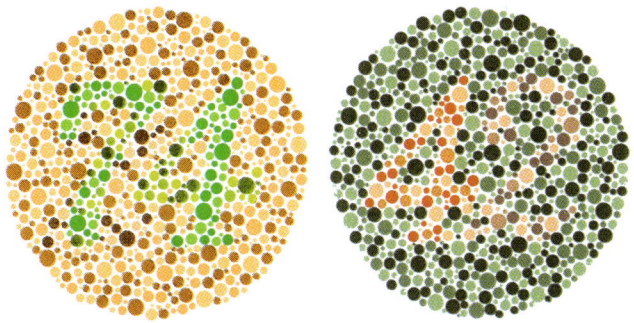

Fig. 10.19: One of the plates in the Ishihara's chart

nothing, but if he spends some time in the dark area, his vision improves. The mechanism involved is known as dark adaptation. For complete dark adaptation, it takes about 40 minutes (Fig. 10.20). During this time, the sensitivity of the retina is increased by few thousand folds. The enzymatic reactions occur in the cones are much faster and therefore the cone adaptation occurs to start with, and will be followed by rod adaptation. The factors influencing dark adaptation are:

1. The duration the person has spent in bright light.
2. The intensity of the light to which the person is exposed.

The duration for dark adaptation can be minimized by using red goggles when the person is working in the bright light. The red goggles prevent the bleaching of the cone pigment, therefore, as soon as the person gets into the dark room he will be able to see. Deficiency of vitamin A will increase the time required for dark adaptation.

When a person comes out from a dark room to a brightly lit area since the light is too bright to start with there will be too much of a glare and he will not be able to see. But within about 5 minutes, his vision becomes clear. This is known as light adaptation.

Refractive Errors

Physiological errors are:
• Spherical aberration

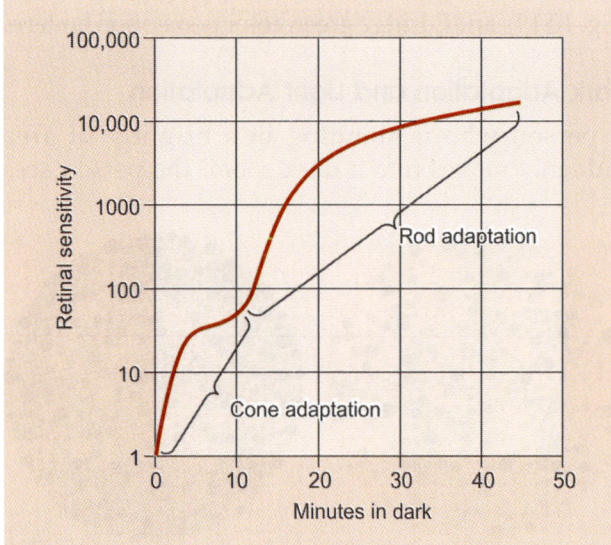

Fig. 10.20: Time required for dark adaptation of cones and rods

• Chromatic aberration
• Presbyopia.

Presbyopia: defect due to gradual change in the structure and composition of lens. As the age advances, the person complains of inability to see the near objects, like reading a newspaper. The near point gradually recedes. This is due to marked decrease in the amplitude of accommodation.

At the age of 60 years, amplitude of accommodation is reduced to about 1D from about 18 D. The physiological changes in the lens that is responsible for this disorder will be due to:

a. Decrease in water content of lens.
b. Sclerosis of cortical portion of lens.

The above change usually starts around the age of 45 years. Convex or bifocal (one part for near vision and the other part for far vision) lens is used to correct this defect.

Pathological Errors of Refraction

Myopia

• Short sightedness.
• Person can see near objects but not far objects.
• May be due to abnormal increase in the length of eyeball.
• Parallel rays from distant object are focused in front of retina, whereas the light rays from near objects are focused on the retina.
• Hence the person will have blurred vision of far objects.
• The amplitude of accommodation is markedly decreased. Hence the far point can be infinity but is up to a particular range only.
• Correction is done by using concave lens (Fig. 10.21). The lens brings about divergence the light rays coming from the far object before the rays fall on the eye. So the rays are able to get focused on retina now.

Hypermetropia

• Long sightedness.
• Person can see far objects but not near objects.
• It is due to decrease in the length of the eyeball.
• The parallel light rays coming from far object come to focus behind retina. So the vision gets blurred. By using the accommodative power, the light rays are made to focus on retina. Constant contraction

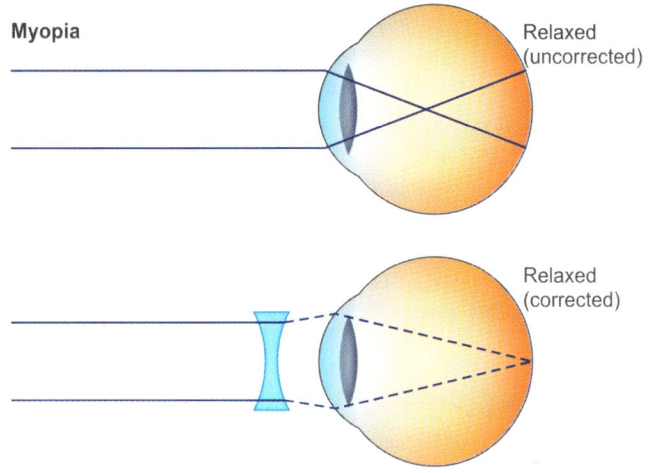

Myopia
Relaxed (uncorrected)
Relaxed (corrected)

Fig. 10.21: Myopic condition corrected by biconcave lens

of ciliaris muscle leads to hypertrophy of the muscle. The constant contraction of the ciliaris muscle leads to headache. Convergence of the eyeballs may give rise to certain amount of squint.
- Correction is done by using convex lens (Fig. 10.22). The lens will bring about the convergence of light rays from far object before the rays fall on the eye.

Astigmatism

- It is a condition in which light rays are not brought to sharp focus on the retina.

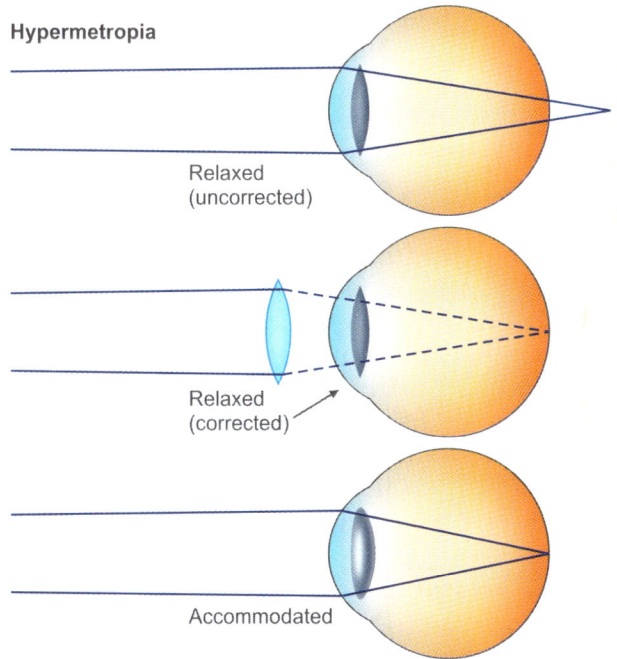

Hypermetropia
Relaxed (uncorrected)
Relaxed (corrected)
Accommodated

Fig. 10.22: Hypermetropia corrected by using biconvex lens

- The curvature in the different meridians (horizontal or vertical) of the visual appratus will not be same.
- It will be due to difference in the meridians either with cornea or lens. Most often the problem is with cornea.
- Even in any normal person, there is some amount of error in the meridians but does not produce obvious defect or error.
- Astigmatism is corrected by using cylindrical lens.

Horner's Syndrome

It is a clinical condition. The lesion responsible for this syndrome is at the superior cervical ganglion affecting the sympathetic fibers. The signs and symptoms are:
a. Dropping of the upper eye lid (ptosis)
b. Pupillary constriction (meiosis)
c. Absence of sweating in the affected region (anhydrosis)
d. Flushing on the affected half of the face and
e. Absence of ciliospinal reflex.

There can be enophthalmos as well. The eyeball appears to be pushed into the orbital socket. There will be absence of ciliospinal reflex that is no dilatation of pupil on pinching of skin over the neck region.

HEARING OR AUDITION

Ear has two important functional components:
1. Cochlea the hearing part containing receptor for hearing is located here
2. The vestibular part having semicircular canals, the utricle, and the saccule are present here.

The receptor in these is responsible for the maintenance of equilibrium and posture.

Function of ear in general for hearing and also act as a direction detector.
a. Important protective role
b. It modulates once own voice.

Ear has three parts the outer, the middle and the inner ear. The outer ear has the pinna, in lower animals this can move which helps in detecting the direction of sound waves. Sound waves which are captured by the pinna pass through the external auditory canal and vibrate the tympanic membrane. The auditory tube is directed medially, downwards and forwards. The skin around the tube has lots of ceruminous glands which on exposure forms the ear wax. The direction of the external auditory tube as well as the

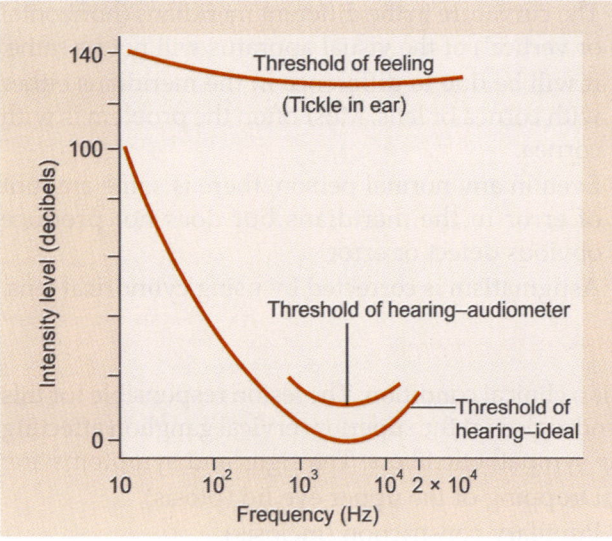

Fig. 10.23: Audibility curve graph

ear wax protects the tympanic membrane from injuries.

The tympanic membrane is a fibrous structure. Its main function is to act as a resonator. Sound waves make the membrane vibrate. Tympanic membrane has a surface area of 68 sq mm. When the frequency of the sound wave is less than 2000 cps the entire membrane vibrates. If the frequency is more than 2000 cps, the membrane vibrates in segments; approximately 75% of the membrane vibrates.

Figure 10.23 (graphical representation) showing the relationship between the frequency of sound waves and the intensity of the sound. It shows that the sound frequencies between 2000 and 4000 cps are heard with the lowest intensities.

Middle Ear

Contents of the Middle Ear

The middle ear contains three bony ossicles namely the malleus, the incus and the stapes. These ossicles articulate with one another. The long process of the malleus articulates with the short process of the incus and forms a lever system. The handle of malleus is attached to the tympanic membrane and the foot plate of the stapes is attached to the oval window. Through this mechanism, the vibrations of the tympanic membrane are conducted to the inner ear. The middle ear is also connected to the pharynx through the pharyngotympanic tube (Eustachian tube/auditory tube).

There are two small muscles in the middle ear. They are the tensor tympani and the stapedius. The tensor tympani when contracts make the tympanic membrane tense. The contraction of the stapedius pulls the foot plate of the stapes outwards. Both of these actions decrease the conduction of sound waves into the inner ear. Functions of the middle ear:

1. Impedance matching
2. Static pressure equilibration
3. Protective function—acoustic reflex (attenuation reflex)
4. Acts as a physiological filter.
5. Because of the impedance matching, it forms the preferential route of conduction.

1. *Impedance matching:* As the sound waves are passing through the air medium, through the ear ossicles into the fluid medium of the internal ear, because it has to vibrate the fluid, a certain amount of sound energy is lost. This will give rise to a decrease in the sound intensity and the significance of the sound may be lost. The mechanism involved in minimizing the loss of sound energy is known as impedance matching.

The mechanisms involved are:

a. When the frequency of the sound wave is more than 2000 cps, only 75% of the tympanic membrane is thrown into vibration which is about 58 mm². The foot plate of the stapes is about 3.2 mm². The pressure applied over a larger surface area of the tympanic membrane is getting converged on to a much smaller area in the oval window. This magnifies the pressure acting on the oval window by about 14 to 17 times.

b. The handle of the malleus is longer than the short process of the incus and they articulate with each other forming a lever system. Because of this lever mechanism, there is an additional magnification by about 1.3 times. Therefore, the total magnification increased is by about 17 to 21 folds. Thus the loss of sound energy is minimized. If this mechanism fails, the person will have a hearing deficit of approximately 10 to 20 dB.

2. *Static pressure equilibration:* For the proper functioning of the tympanic membrane as a vibrator, the pressure on either side of the membrane must be kept equal. Atmospheric

pressure is the one which acts on the tympanic membrane from outside. Since the middle ear is connected to the pharynx, the pressure in the middle ear is also made equal to the atmospheric pressure. Normally, the pharyngotympanic tube is kept closed. Whenever the pressure in the middle ear falls, the tube opens up connecting the middle ear to the pharynx and the pressure is equalized. If the fall in the pressure in the middle ear is too much as it can happen when an unconscious person is brought to the sea level, there is a possibility that the tympanic membrane may rupture. This results in a loud noise being followed by signs and symptoms of shock.

3. *Protective function:* Explosive noises may damage the very fine structures of the inner ear. Within a matter of 15 to 17 milliseconds (the latent period), the two small muscles in the middle ear contract. The tympanic membrane is pulled inwards and the foot plate of the stapes is drawn outwards. This results in decreased amount of sound waves reaching the inner ear. This protects the finer structures present in the cochlea. This reflex is known as the tympanic reflex. This reflex can be initiated even by the ticking sounds of a time piece. In paralysis of the facial nerve, the stapedius muscle is paralyzed. Hence, the protective mechanism is lost and these patients complain of painful hearing—hyperacusis.

4. *It acts as a physiological filter:* It allows the transmission of speech frequency and prevents the transmission of noise frequency. The axis of rotation of the foot plate of the stapes gets changed and it prevents the transmission of noises.

5. *Preferential route of conduction:* There are two routes through which the sound waves can be conducted to the inner ear. One of the routes will be through the bone conduction and the other being the ossicular conduction (air conduction). Since, impedance matching is available only for ossicular conduction, this route of conduction forms the preferential route of conduction.

The Inner Ear

This part lodges two important structures, namely the cochlea and the vestibular apparatus. The cochlea is the hearing part of the inner ear (Fig. 10.24).

The cochlea is a coiled structure about two and a half circle. The cochlea is divided into three compart-

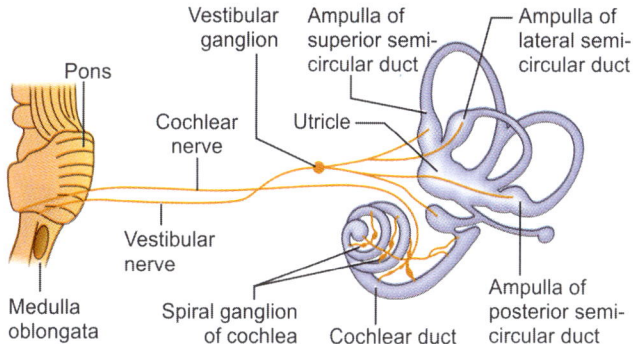

Fig. 10.24: Inner ear showing cochlea

ments by two membranes namely the basilar membrane and the Reissner's membrane. The upper compartment is scala vestibuli, the middle is scala media and the lower scala tympani. The scala vestibuli and scala tympani contain perilymph, the composition of this fluid resembles that of ECF and the scala media contains endolymph, the composition of which resembles that of ICF.

The receptors for hearing are the organ of Corti (hair cells) present on the basilar membrane. There are two types of hair cells namely, the outer row of hair cells, arranged in three rows and a single row of inner hair cells. The outer row of hair cells is test tube-like, whereas the inner row of cells is flask-like (Fig. 10. 25). Signals produced by these receptors are carried by the cochlear division of the eighth cranial nerve. These receptors also receive efferent nerve supply. These fibers take origin from the olivary nucleus (olivocochlear bundle of nerve fibers). Overlying the hair cells is the tectorial membrane. The hairs on the hair cells are actually embedded in the substance of the tectorial membrane.

Cochlea

The cochlea is the hearing part of the inner ear. The cochlea is a coiled structure about two and a half circle. The cochlea is divided into three compartments by two membranes, namely the basilar membrane and the Reissner's membrane. The upper compartment is scala vestibuli, the middle scala media and the lower scala tympani (Fig. 10.26). The scala vestibuli and scala tympani contain perilymph, the composition of this fluid resembles that of extracellular fluid and the scala media contains endolymph, the composition of which resembles that of intracellular fluid.

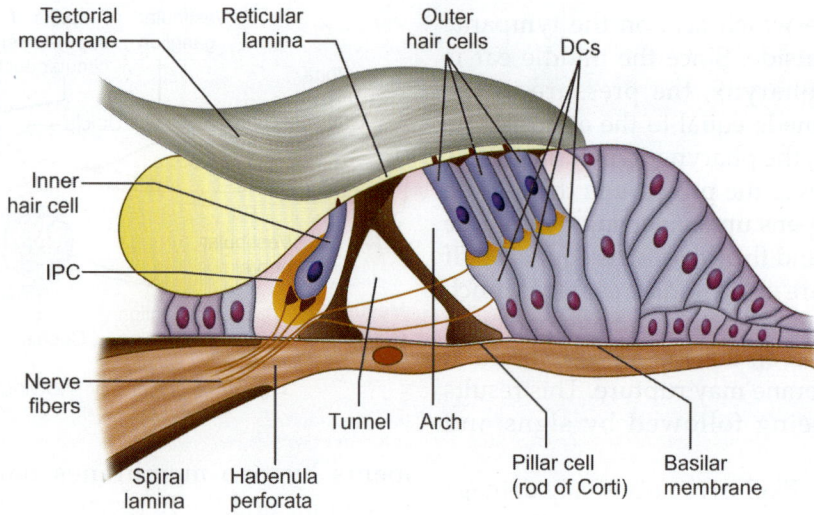

Fig. 10.25: Details of organ of Corti

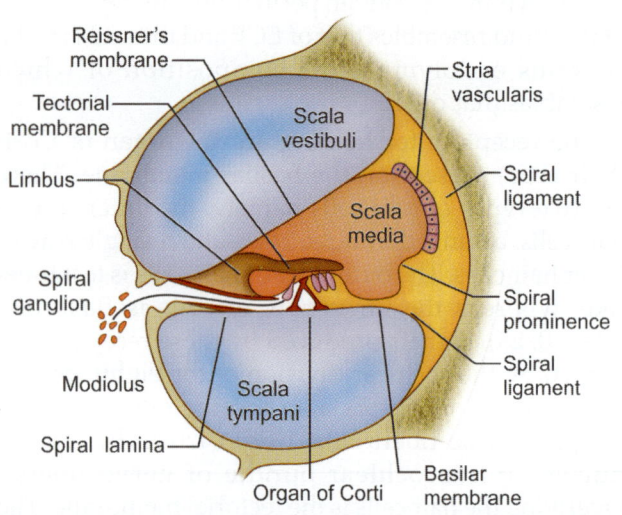

Fig. 10.26: The scala and the three important membranes

Resistance offered by Reissner's membrane is extremely small as it is a thin delicate membrane. Reissner's membrane stretches from the upper surface of the spiral lamina to the bony wall of the canal a little above the attachment of the basilar membrane.

Basilar Membrane

Basilar membrane is attached to the spinal lamina to the outer wall of the canal. There is no tension in the fibers maintaining the basilar membrane.

1. If a cut is made in the basilar membrane, no gaping is seen in the membrane showing the fibres are not taut or kept under tension.

2. Basal part of basilar membrane is narrow and width is gradually increased upwards to the apex. Basilar membrane is about 32 mm long.

3. Rods of Corti form the supporting pillars. The height of these rods are increased from base to apex, and the rods of Corti are present on the basement membrane.

There are certain differences between the base and apical part of cochlea (Fig. 10.27). They are with respect to:

a. Breadth
b. Thickness of membrane
c. Response to frequencies

The receptors for hearing are the organ of Corti (hair cells) present on the basilar membrane. There are two types of hair cells namely, the outer row of hair cells, arranged in three rows and a single row of inner hair cells. The outer row of hair cells is test tube-like, whereas the inner row of cells is flask-like. Signals produced by these receptors are carried by the cochlear division of the 8th cranial nerve (Fig. 10.28). These receptors also receive efferent nerve supply. These fibers take origin from the olivary nucleus (olivocochlear bundle of nerve fibers). Overlying the hair cells is the tectorial membrane. The hairs on the hair cells are embedded in the substance of the tectorial membrane. The hairs of the hair cells are bathed in endolymph present in scala media.

When the sound vibrations are transmitted through the foot plate of the stapes to the inner ear, the fluid medium is set into motion (Fig. 10.29). This in turn

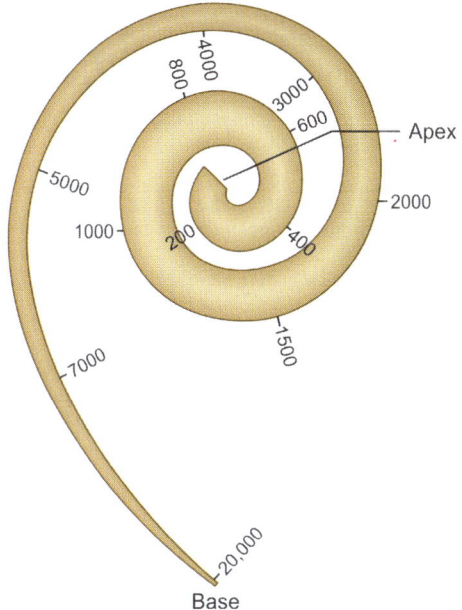

Fig. 10.27: Different parts of cochlea that are tuned to respond maximally for a particular frequency and the variation in the width

moves the basilar membrane, which later on moves the tectorial membrane. The shearing motion of the tectorial membrane bends the hairs of the receptor cells.

Mechanism of Stimulation of Receptors in Cochlea

1. Movement of oval window.

2. Disturbance of fluid in scala vestibuli.
3. Movement of Reissner's membrane.
4. Disturbance of fluid in scala media.
5. Movement of tectorial membrane.
6. Shear motion on the hair of hair cells due to movement of tectorial membrane
7. Stimulation of receptor cells (Fig. 10.29).

This brings about the production of receptor potentials known as cochlear microphonic potentials. The amplitude of the microphonic potentials depends on the intensity of the impinging sound waves. Greater the intensity, greater is the amplitude of the microphonic potentials. The cochlear microphonic potentials are nothing but the local potentials and hence have almost all the properties of local potential. These cochlear microphonic potentials in turn bring about the development of action potentials in the auditory nerve fibers. Further:

1. The disturbance of fluid in the scala media also brings about movement of basilar membrane.
2. Leads to disturbance of fluid present in scala tympani
3. Movement of round window

There should be movement of the round window in an appropriate direction when the oval window moves. This is essential because, in the cochlea the fluid is present and this fluid is incompressible. If fluid is unable to get disturbed, there will not be scope for the stimulation of receptors since the receptors for hearing are nothing but mechanoceptors.

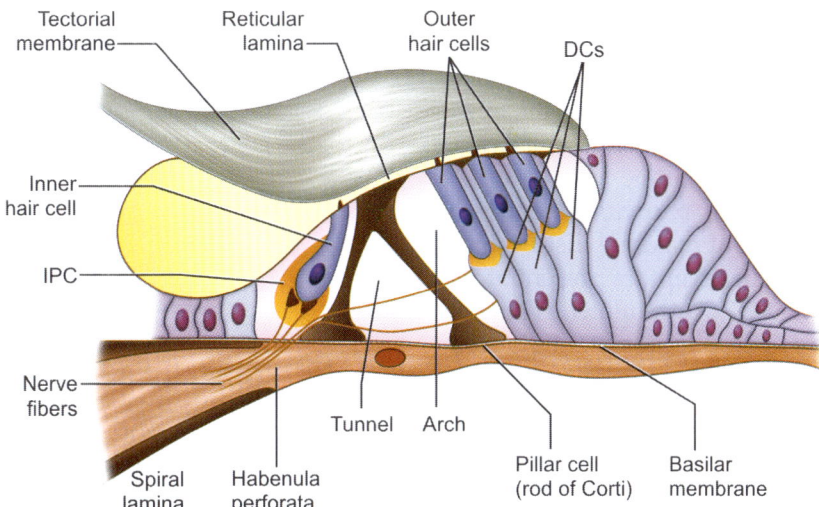

Fig. 10.28: Afferent cochlear nerve fibers from the hair cells

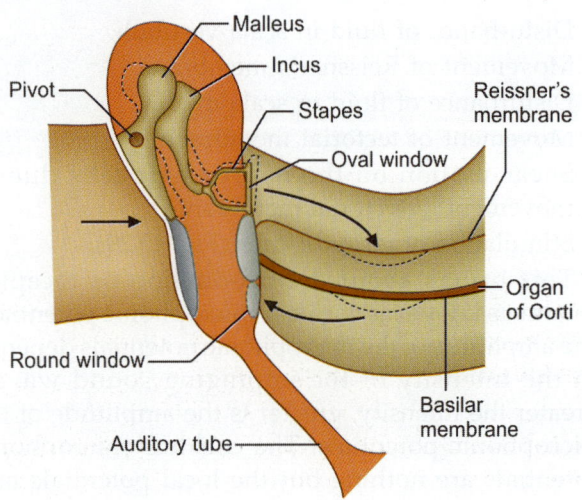

Fig. 10.29: The conduction of sound waves from outer ear into inner ear mediated through the ear ossicles of the middle ear.

Theories of Hearing

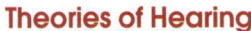

1. Resonance theory.
2. Traveling wave theory.
3. Place theory.

The basilar membrane is about 31 mm long and its width increases gradually from the base to the apex. Depending on the frequency of the sound waves, different parts of the membrane is displaced to varying extent. For low frequency, the apical portion of the membrane gets displaced to a greater extent stimulating those receptors. For higher frequency sounds, the basal part of the membrane gets displaced stimulating those receptors. Whenever there is disturbance in the fluid medium of cochlea, a wave of disturbance originates from the base of cochlea irrespective of the pitch of the sound. This wave as it traverses from the base towards the apex, the amplitude of wave goes on increasing till it comes across a point on the basilar membrane which is tuned to respond maximally for that particular frequency (Fig. 10.30). Beyond the area of maximal disturbance, the wave dies out. Hence the receptors present at the site of maximal disturbance get stimulated. This fact is proved by recording microphonic potentials from different parts of the basilar membrane and also directly observing the movement of the membrane. Frequency analysis of the sound waves is, therefore, partly made at this level itself. Further analysis is made by the auditory cortex when these impulses reach the cortex.

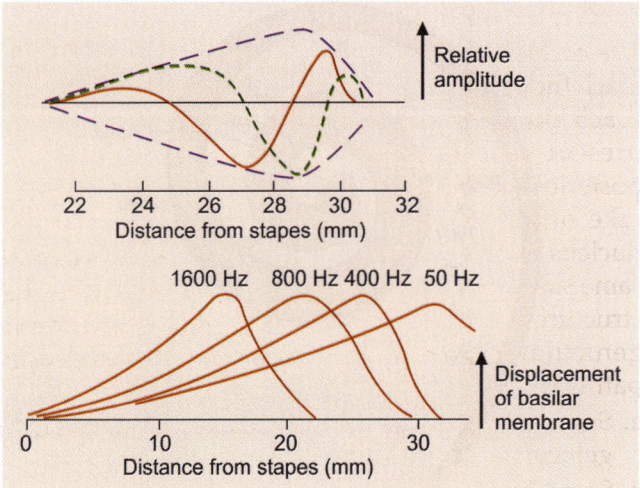

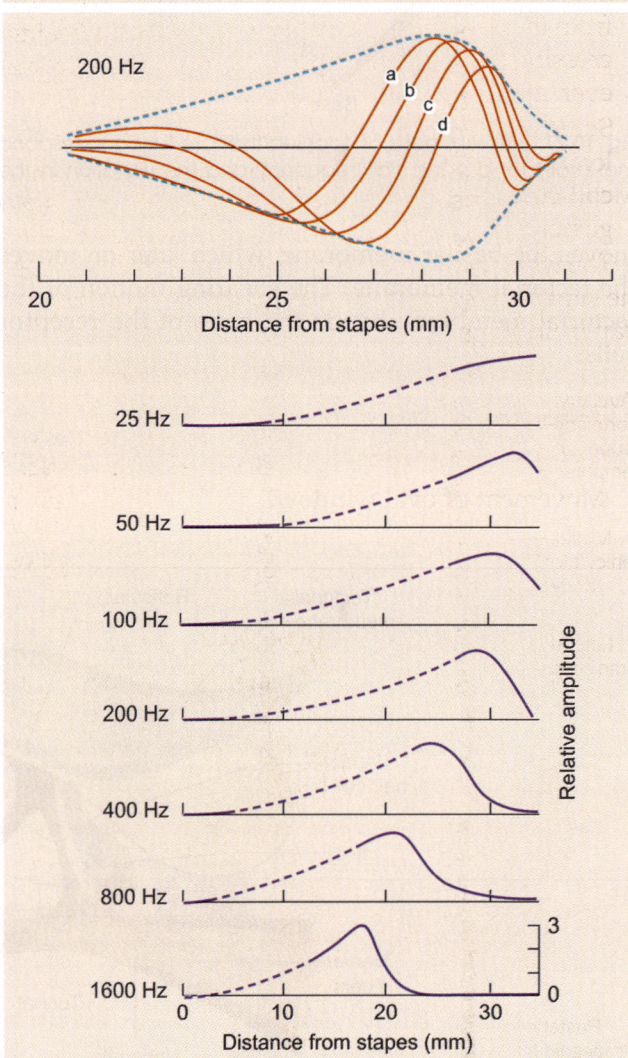

Fig. 10.30: The maximal displacement of basilar membrane for a particular frequency of sound

Auditory Pathway (Fig. 10.31)

The cochlear afferent nerve fibers from the receptors reach the spiral ganglion. From the ganglia, the fibers reach the anterior and posterior cochlear nuclei present in the brainstem and synapse. From the posterior and anterior cochlear nuclei, nerve fibers take origin and synapse in the superior olivary nucleus and posterior nucleus of trapezoid body of same side as well as on the opposite side. From these structures, nerve fibers taking origin reach the medial geniculate body through any of the following pathways:

a. Some of the fibers directly reach the medial geniculate body and synapse.
b. Some fibers synapse in the inferior colliculus and from there reaches the medial geniculate body. The crossing of the fibers to the opposite side can occur even at inferior colliculus.
c. Some other fibers synapse in the nucleus of lateral leminscus. From here, the fibers reach the inferior colliculus and synapse and finally reach medial geniculate body.

The whole bundle of nerve fibers taking origin from the superior olivary nucleus and posterior nucleus of trapezoid body is known as lateral lemniscus. The lateral lemniscus gives out collaterals that feed information to the reticular formation present in the brainstem.

From the medial geniculate body, fibers taking origin are called as auditory radiation fibers. Auditory radiation fibers pass through the posterior limb of internal capsule to reach the auditory cortex present in the superior temporal gyrus.

Auditory Cortex

In the auditory cortex (superior transverse temporal gyrus), there are two important areas:
   i. Primary auditory area (area no. 41, 42)
   ii. Association auditory area (area no. 21, 22)

The primary auditory area is connected to medial geniculate body. The association area is connected to the primary auditory area. Fibers from primary auditory area convey information to the association area. The association area also receives fibers directly from the thalamus. The individual tone and frequency is represented in the auditory cortex that has tonotopic representation.

Intensity of sound discrimination: It is similar to intensity discrimination in general sensory physiology. Intensity of sound discrimination can be explained by:
1. Recruitment of receptors
2. Weber-Fechner law

Direction Analysis

The laterality of the sound can be discriminated by:
1. Time lag in the stimulation of receptors present in two different ears. In the ear which is directed towards the source of sound, there will be stimulation of receptors few milliseconds earlier than the stimulation of receptors present in the opposite ear.
2. Decrease in the amplitude of the sound in the opposite ear as the sound waves while reaching the opposite ear will strike against the hard bones of the cranium and would lose some amount of sound energy because of this.

Types of Deafness

1. Conductive type
2. Perceptive type
3. Central type

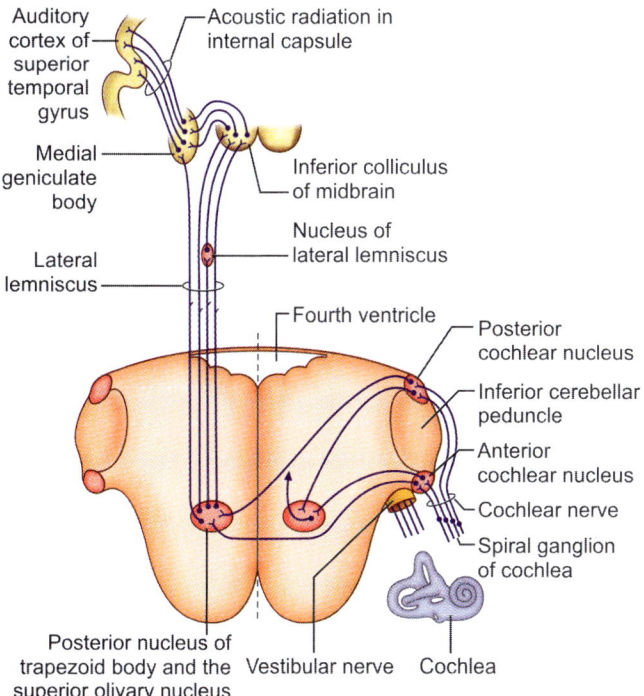

Auditory cortex of superior temporal gyrus
Acoustic radiation in internal capsule
Medial geniculate body
Inferior colliculus of midbrain
Lateral lemniscus
Nucleus of lateral lemniscus
Fourth ventricle
Posterior cochlear nucleus
Inferior cerebellar peduncle
Anterior cochlear nucleus
Cochlear nerve
Spiral ganglion of cochlea
Posterior nucleus of trapezoid body and the superior olivary nucleus
Vestibular nerve
Cochlea

Fig. 10.31: The details of the auditory pathway

1. Conductive type—due to:
   a. Accumulation of wax in the auditory meatus.
   b. Damage to tympanic membrane.
   c. Damage to ear ossicles.
2. Perceptive type—due to:
   a. Site of lesion mainly the receptors, e.g. prolonged listening of rock music.
   b. May be due to tumor arising from the auditory nerve fibers compressing the other fibers.
   c. Toxicity of certain drugs (anti-malarial drugs), quinine and streptomycin (anti-TB drugs).
3. Central type—very rare.

Tests Employed to Detect Hearing Impairment

Audiometry: The recording is called audiogram.

Ear phones are placed over the subject's ear and one ear is tested at a time. Subject is connected to instrument. Gradually, there will be increased frequency of sound. The intensity of the sound applied corresponds to the standard intensity this is reported as normal or represented as 0 db.

If the findings of the study are graphically represented and is around zero line, the subject is supposed to be normal.

Conductive and perceptive types of deafness can be differentiated by the audiometry.

Gross difference between bone conduction and ossicular conduction: If ossicular conduction is affected to a greater extent, it means that it is a conductive type of deafness and in such person bone conduction is better than ossicular conduction. In perceptive deafness, both bone and ossicular conduction are affected to the same extent. Audiometry enables to ascertain the:
1. Type of deafness—conductive or perceptive
2. Extent of the loss

Tests Conducted to Ascertain the Type of Deafness

1. *Rinne's test:* Place the vibrating tuning fork on the mastoid process and ask the subject if he can hear. For accurate result, do not allow the subject to move. Subject is asked to tell when he is unable to hear. When he is unable to hear, transfer the tuning fork from mastoid process to the front of the ear and if subject is able to hear it means that ossicular conduction is better than bone conduction.

2. *Weber's test:* Strike a tuning fork and place the vibrating tuning fork on the forehead of the patient. Subject must be able to hear equally in both the ears. If he hears better in the right ear, it may be due to:
   a. Conductive type of deafness in right ear
   b. Perceptive type of deafness in left ear

In conductive type of deafness, when Weber's test performed, the subject is able to hear better on the affected side. In perceptive type of deafness, subject is able to hear better on the normal side.

Presbyacusis is the hearing loss that is due to old age. In aged people, the ability to hear higher frequencies decline.

Chemical Senses

Taste Receptors and Olfactory Receptors

Activity in these receptors concerned with visceral function, i.e. concerned with food intake thus they are classified under visceral receptors. They can be also termed as chemoreceptors as they respond to chemical changes.

Differences between Taste and Smell Sensations

1. The pathway involved in olfaction does not pass through the thalamus. All the other sensory pathways pass through the thalamus.
2. The olfaction sensation has no neocortical projection—it is a very primitive type of sensation.

These two sensations play a vital role in food intake.

In lower animals, the olfactory receptors also play other important roles in:
   i. Sexual instinct
   ii. Detection of enemies—protective role

TASTE/GUSTATION

Receptors are present in taste buds (Fig. 10.32), situated in the tongue, soft plate, epiglottis and certain regions of the pharynx.

Microvilli project from one end of the pole. Central portion of dorsum of tongue is devoid of papillae (Fig. 10.33).

Afferent Nerve Supply

- Anterior two-thirds of tongue—chorda tympani branch of facial nerve
- Posterior one-third of tongue—glossopharyngeal
- Epiglottis, pharynx, etc.—vagus

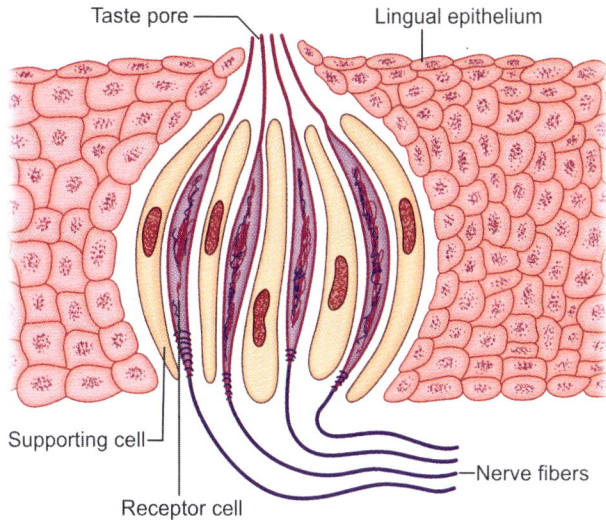

Fig. 10.32: Cell types in a taste bud

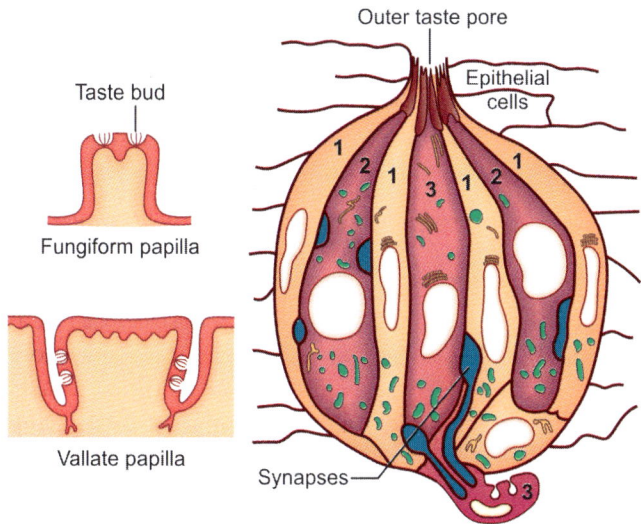

Fig. 10.33: Fungiform papilla and vallate papilla

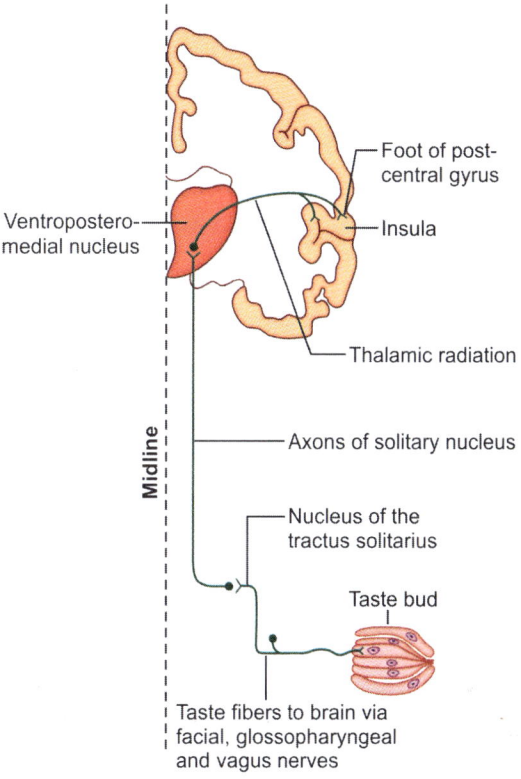

Fig. 10.34: Pathway for taste sensation

Pathway for Taste (Fig. 10.34)

Afferent fibers (7th, 9th, and 10th) join to form the tractus solitarius. The nerve fiber end over nucleus of tractus solitarius. Nerve fibers arising from nucleus of tractus solitarius cross to opposite side and ascend up along with the medial lemniscus to terminate in the posteroventromedial nucleus of thalamus. Nowadays, it is said that the pathway does not cross, but reaches the thalamus of the ipsilateral side.

From thalamus, the 3rd order neuron fibers that have taken origin end in cerebral cortex (area 3, 1, 2) in the general sensory region. The fibers terminate in the lower region of the sensory area of cortex which is the area of representation for the face.

The 4 primary/basic modalities of taste sensations are:
1. Bitter
2. Sour
3. Sweet
4. Salt

A taste bud may respond to any one or more than one as well. Taste buds at the:
a. Side of tongue respond best for sour.
b. Tip of tongue respond best for sweet.
c. Middle and tip tongue respond best for salt.
d. Back of tongue respond best for bitter.

One theory says that taste buds are covered by polyelectrolyte field. Therefore, this particular field has electrical charges arranged in a specific fashion. When food is taken, there is alteration in the changes of the membrane. These receptors covered by a protein membrane covering certain amount of receptor site. This region brings about alteration in the changes in the membrane and lead to production of action potentials.

Simultaneous Contrast and Successive Contrast

Simultaneous contrast: Over the ½ of tongue apply salt solution. Over the other ½ apply a sweet solution. The sweet solution becomes much sweeter.

Successive contrast: Apply sweet and salt solutions one after another. The sweet solution appears much sweeter.

Taste Blindness

Taste blindness occurs in about 30% of the cases but not for all substances. When low concentration of phenylthiocarbamide (PTC) is applied in normal individual, it gives sour taste. In 30%, it does not give rise to any taste. These individuals are said to be taste blind. This is due to Mendelian recessive gene.

Ageusia means loss of taste sensations and dysgeusia refers to difficulty to perceive the taste sensation.

SENSE OF SMELL (OLFACTION)

Like taste sensation, smell is also a chemical sensation. For taste, the substance must be in soluble form, and for smell it must be in gaseous form.

Olfactory Sensation

1. Impulses do not pass through thalamus.
2. Impulses do not pass to neocortex (no neocortical representation).
3. Receptors are first order neurons in this case and in other sensations the first order neurons are in the posterior root ganglion.

The olfactory receptors are bipolar in nature. The dendrites have an expanded end called olfactory rods. Over this surface area, a number of cilia projecting upwards. They act as antenna. About 10–20 million receptors are present in the nose. The supporting cells secrete some sort of mucus. The cilia are found within the mucous layer.

Olfactory area is confined to a small area (500 mm^2) in nose in human beings. Human beings are considered as microsomatic. Lower animals have a wide area of representation in the cortex. In macrosomatic animals, olfactory sensation plays protective role and sexual instinct.

In the olfactory bulb, two different types of neurons are seen:

1. Majority—mitral cell
2. Minority—tufted cell

Axon from tufted cells crosses to the opposite side by passing through anterior commissure. They end in the olfactory bulb of the opposite side through the olfactory tract of opposite side. Some of the fibers pass through the intermediate olfactory striae and end in the anterior perforated substance and region of diagonal band. From here they are relayed to the limbic system and hypothalamus.

Axons from most of the mitral cells pass through the lateral olfactory striae and go to prepyriform cortex (Fig. 10.35).

Amygdaloid nuclear complex and periamygdaloid region form the higher centre for smell.

Mechanism of Stimulation of Receptors

The substances have a particular odor (odoriferous substance) gets dissolved in the mucus.

Normally, as you breathe in, the substance entering the nostrils will not reach the olfactory region. When some eddy currents are produced and then only

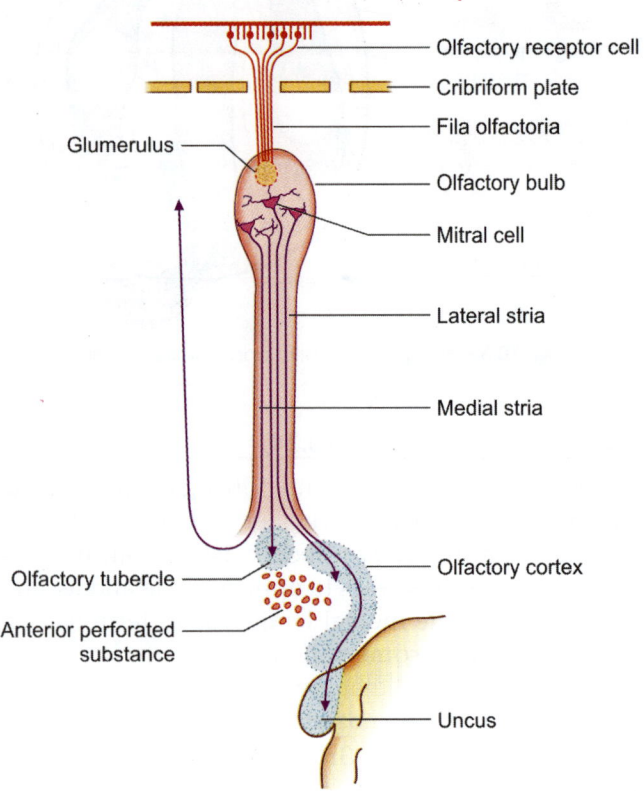

Fig. 10.35: The olfactory pathway

substances are able to reach the olfactory region and stimulate the receptor. Sniffing brings about production of eddy currents. Odoriferous substances should get dissolved in the water and lipid lining of the membrane and if it does so, it can stimulate the receptors more effectively.

Adaptation of these receptors is extremely fast. Receptors show adaptation only for a particular odor.

Abnormalities of Olfactory Sensation

1. *Anosmia:* Loss of sense of smell, e.g. common cold.
   Reasons for anosmia:

   a. During the inflammatory condition, the mucus lining is inflamed. The edematous cells compress the nerve fibers. Hence, from the receptor, thus impulses cannot be transmitted.

   b. Fracture of ethmoidal bone.

   c. Tumor pressing upon olfactory nerve fibers.

2. *Parosmia:* Altered/perverted sense of smell sensation, e.g. hysteria.

3. *Hyperosmia:* Smell and taste sensation greatly increased in adrenal cortical insufficiency. It also occurs in raised intracranial pressure, etc.

Index

1-25 DHCC 186
17 alpha hydroxylase deficiency 167
21 beta hydroxylase deficiency 167
2-3 DPG 106

A band 45
Abdominal pump 63
ABO system 24
Absolute refractory period 42
Accessory organs of sex 190
Acclimatization 115
Accommodation reflex 295
Acetylcholine 43
Achalasia cardia 126
Achlorhydria 133
Achondroplasia 156
Achrodextrin 123
Acidosis 4
Acinus 119
Acromegaly 156
ACTH 151
Actin 45
Action potential 33
Adaptation 238
Addison's disease 166
Adenohypophysis 153
ADH 157
Adiadochokinesis 267
Adrenal cortex 161
Adrenergic receptors 168
Adrenogenital syndrome 166
Aerophagia 127
After-load effect 78
Ageusia 310
Agglutination 23
Agglutinin 23
Agglutinogen 23
Agonist muscle 265
Agranulocyte 13
Air conduction 303
Akinesia 269
Albumin 2
Albumin-globulin ratio 2
Aldehyde oxidase 169
Aldosterone 161
Alimentary glycosuria 181
Alkalosis 4
All or none law 42

Alpha 1 receptors 168
Alpha 2 receptors 168
Alpha block 281
Alpha cells 177
Alpha motor neuron 258
Alpha-gamma linkage 258
Alveolar epithelial cells 100
Alveolar ventilation 96
Alveoli 94
Amenorrhea 190
Aminoglutethimide 165
Aminopyridine 57
Ammonia buffer system 226
Amnesia 286
Amphetamine 262
Amplitude of accommodation 296
Amygdala 280
Anaphylactic shock 89
Androgen 162
Androgen binding protein 194
Androstenedione 162
Anemia 5
Anemic hypoxia 114
Aneuploidies 209
Angiotensin I 93
Angiotensin II 93
Angiotensinogen 93
Anosmia 310
ANP 29
Antagonist muscle 265
Anterior chochlear nucleus 307
Anterior corticospinal tract 255
Anterograde amnesia 286
Anterograde catheterization 79
Anterograde transport 35
Anterolateral cordotomy 251
Antiallergic action 164
Anticholinesterases 44
Anticoagulants 21
Antigen 16
Antihemophilic factor 20
Anti-inflammatory action 163
Antiport 219
Anuria 231
Aortic body 73
Aortic nerve 73
Aphagian 278
Apnea 116

Apneustic breathing 111
Apneustic center 110
APUD cells 132
Aquaporins 158
Aqueduct of Sylvisus 274
Aqueous humor 289
ARAS 271
Archicerebellum 264
Archnoid mater 273
Area postrema 275
Argyll Robertson pupil 296
Arrhythmia 55
Artificial respiration 117
Asphyxia 112, 116
Astigmatism 301
Astrocytes 34
Ataxia 243
Atelectesis 99
Atonic bladder 229
Atrial diastole 68
Atropine 133
Audiometry 308
Auditory pathway 307
Auerbach plexus 118
Augmented histamine test 134
Auriculotemporal nerve 120
Auscultatory method 80
Autocatalytic reaction 138
Autocrine 149
Autoimmune 153
Autonomic nervous system 282
Autonomic nervous system blockers 283
Autonomous bladder 229
Autoregulation of blood flow 92
Autorhythmicity 51
Axon 34
Axon telodendrion 43
Axonotemesis 40

Babinski +ve 260
Bainbridge reflex 74
Baroreceptors 73
Basal body temperature 201
Basal ganglia 267
Basilar membrane 304
Basophil 13
Basophilia 15
Basophilic 8

Bathmotropic effect 73
Belching 127
Beneficial effect 48
Beta 1 receptors 168
Beta 2 receptors 168
Beta cells 177
Betz cells 254
Bicarbonate buffer system 30
Bicarbonate reabsorption 221
Bickel's pouch 130
Bile pigment 141
Bile salt 141
Bilinogen 11
Bilirubin 11
Bilirubin glucuronide 11
Biliverdin 11
Bioamplifier system 20
Biologic clock 280
Biosynthesis of adrenal cortical
    hormones 161
Biot's breathing 116
Biphasic action potential 39
Bipolar cell 33
Bitemporal hemianopia 294
Bleeding time 18
Blind spot 291
Blood buffers 30
Blood coagulation 19
Blood gas barrier 102
Blood glucose level 177
Blood group 23
Blood indices 10
Blood pressure 79
Blood–brain barrier 275
BMR 172
Bohr's effect 106
Botulinum toxin 44
Bowman's capsule 211, 214
Bradycardia 72
Bronchi 94
Bronchial asthma 101
Bronchioles 94
Buccal stage 124

Cachetic state 18
Caisson's disease 116
Calcitonin 188
Calcium reabsorption 222
Calorigenic agent 170
Capillary dynamics 3
Capillary fluid shift mechanism 28
Carbamino compound 107
Carbon dioxide dissociation curve 108
Carbonic anhydrase 107
Cardiac catheterization 79
Cardiac cycle 67

Cardiac index 75
Cardiac muscle 51
Cardiac output 75
Cardiac sphincter 126
Cardinal symptoms of diabetes mellitus 180
Cardioinhibitory center 73
Cardiogenic shock 89
Cardiomegaly 157
Cardiovascular shock 89
Carotid body 73
Carotid sinus 73
Carpopedal spasm 187
Carrier-mediated transport 219
Cascade reaction 20
Castration
    after puberty 197
    before puberty 197
Catecholamine 168
Caudate nucleus 267
Causalgian 246
CCK-PZ 136
Cell membrane bound receptor 151
Cellular immunity 16
Central chemoreceptors 112
Central nervous system 235
Central thermoreceptors 233, 278
Cerebelloreticular tract 265
Cerebellovestibular tract 265
Cerebellum 263
Cerebral aqueduct 274
Cerebral circulation 86
Cerebral cortex 286
Cerebrospinal fluid 273
Cervical mucus 201
Chemoreceptors 73
Cheyne-Stokes breathing 116
Chief/peptic cell 128
Chime 137
Chloride shift 108
Cholecystography 143
Choleglobin 11
Cholegogue 142
Choleretic 142
Cholesterol esterase 136
Cholinesterase 43
Chondrogenesis 155
Chorda tympani 120
Chorda tympani syndrome 124
Chorionic villi 202
Choroid plexus 273
Christmas disease 23
Christmas factor 20
Chromophils 153
Chromophobes 153
Chronaxie 36
Chronological age 155

Chvostek's sign 187
Chyluria 231
Chymotrypsin 138
Chymotrypsinogen 136
Ciliaris muscle 290
Ciliary body 289
Cimetidine 133
Circadian rhythm 164
Classical conditioning 285
Clearance concept 214
Clearance value 213
Clinical significance of EEG 282
Clot retraction 19
Clotting time 22
CNS ischemic response 83
Coagulation factors 19, 20
Cochlea 301
Cochlear microphonics 305
Cog-wheel rigidity 269
Coitus reflex 263
Colectomy 147
Colloid 171
Colloidal osmotic pressure 3
Color blindness 299
Color vision 297
Colorimetry 10
Competitive inhibitors 44
Compound action potential 40
COMT 169
Conditioned reflex 122
Conducting system of human heart 54
Conduction blocks 67
Conduction deafness 308
Conductivity 36
Cones 289
Congenital adrenal hyperplasia 167
Congenital hypothyroidism 174
Conn's syndrome 166
Connections of hypothalamus 277
Constipation 147
Constrictor pupipllae 290
Contraception 205
Contraceptive methods 205
Convergence 239
Convergence theory 249
Coordination of movement 265
Copper T 205
Cornea 289
Cornification 201
Coronary blood flow 87
Corpus albicans 200
Corpus luteum 200
Cortical nephrons 212
Corticobulbar fibers 254
Corticonuclear fibers 254
Corticopontocerebellar tract 265

Corticospinal tract 252
Corticosterone 161
Corticotropes 153
Cortisol 161
Counter-current
    exchanger 223
    multiplier 223
Creatinine 215
Cretinism 174
CRH 153
Cricopharygeal sphincter 126
Crista ampullaris 272
Critical closing or opening pressure 59
Cronotropic effect 73
Crossmatching 25
Crossed extensor reflex 259
Crossed hemiplegia 255
Cryptorchidism 197
Cuneate nuclei 244
Cushing's syndrome 166
Cyanide poisoning 115
Cyanosis 114
Cystic duct 140
Cystometrogram 230
Cytosolic receptor 151
Cytotoxic T cell 16

Dark adaptation 300
Dead space volume 96
Deafferentation 258
Decompression sickness 116
Defecation
    reflex 147
Deglutition
    center 124
Dehydroepiandrosterone 161
Delta cells 177
Dendrite 33
Dentate nucleus 263
Dentatorubrothalamocortical tract 265
Deoxycorticosterone 161
Deoxyribonuclease 136
Depolarization 39
Depolarizing blockers 44
Detrusor muscle 229
Deuterium 28
Dextran 215
Diabetes
    inspidus 160
    mellitus 180
Diaphragm 96
Diaphragmatic breathing 255
Diarrhea 148
Diaschiasis 262
Diastasis 70
Diastolic pressure 79

Dicoumarol 21
Diffusing capacity 103
Diffusion coefficient 103
Digitalis 51
Dihydrotestosterone 191
Dihydroxyphenylalanine 168
Diiodotyrosine 171
Dilator pupillae 292
Diltiazim 57
Diopteric power 290
Distensibility 51, 52
Diuresis 223
Diuretics 232
Diurnal variation 152
Divergence 239
Dopamine 168
Dorsal column tract 244
Dorsolateral funiculus 250
Down regulation 151
Down's syndrome 209
Dromotropic effect 73
Duct of Santorini 136
Duct of Wirsung 136
Ducts of Rivinus 120
Duetranopia 299
Duodenocolic reflex 146
Dura mater 273
Dwarfism 156
Dynorphin 250
Dysarthria 267
Dysbarism 116
Dysmetria 266
Dysphagia 127
Dyspnea 115

Early normoblast 8
Eccrine sweat glands 233
Ectopic beat 55
Edema 4
Edinger-Westphal nucleus 290
EDTA 21
Effect of complete transaction of spinal cord 261
Effect of dorsal nerve root sectioning 243
Effect of hemisection of spinal cord 260
Effect of lesion in pyramidal tract 255
Effective filtration pressure 215
Effective renal plasma flow 213
Effector organ 242
Einthoven's law 65
Einthoven's triangle 65
Electrical axis of heart 67
Electrocardiogram 64
Electroencephalogram 281
Electromagnetic receptors 237
Electrophoresis 3

Emboliform nucleus 263
Emmetropia 295
End diastolic volume 76
End plate 43
End plate potential 43
End systolic volume 76
Endocrine 149
Endogenous analgesic system 250
Endolymph 304
Endometrium 200
Endorphin 250
Endosmosis 6, 279
Enkephelin 250
Enterogastric reflex 136
Enterogastrone 132
Enterohepatic circulation 141
Enterokinase/enteropeptidase 138
Enzyme substrate reaction 20
Eosinopenia 15
Eosinophil 13
Eosinophilic 8
Eosinophilia 15
Ependymal cell 34
Epinephrine/adrenaline 168
Epiphyseal plate 155
Equatorial zone 256
Equilibrium potential 37
Erlanger and Gasser classification 35
Erythroblastosis fetalis 26
Erythrocyte 8
Erythrodextrin 123
Erythropoiesis 6
Erythropoietin 9
Esophageal stage 124
ESR 5
Essential endocrine gland 50
Estrogen 200
Evan's blue 27, 75
Eve's rocking method 117
Exchange transfusion 27
Excitability 33
Excitation–contraction coupling 46
Exophthalmos 175
Exosmosis 279
Expiratory center 110
Expiratory reserve volume 100
External arcuate fibers 245
External intercostals muscle 96
External respiration 94
External urethral sphincter 229
Extrafusal fibers 257
Extraction ratio 213
Extrinsic system 19

F cells 177
Facilitation theory 249

Factors affecting regeneration 42
Facultative water reabsorption 223
Famotidine 134
Far vision 293
Fasciculation 256
Fasciculus gracils and cuneatus 244
Fastigial nucleus 263
Features of prefrontal lobotomy 288
Feedback circuit for regulation of BP 84
Fertilization 190
Fibrillation 256
Fibrinogen 2
Fibrinolysis 21
Fick's law 102
Fick's principle 75
Filtered load 217
Filtration fraction 216
Filtration membrane 214
Finger ergography 48
Flacculonodular lobe 264
Flexor withdrawal reflex 263
Follicular phase 199
Foramen Luschka 274
Foramen Monro 274
Formen Magendie 274
Fovea centralis 291
Fractional test meal 134
Fractionation 242
Frolish dwarf 156
Frontal lobe 286
FSH 151
Functional residual capacity 100
Functions of autonomic nervous system 283
Functions of basal ganglia 268
Functions of CSF 274
Functions of hypothalamus 277
Functions of placenta 202
Functions of thalamus 275
Furosemide 232

G cell 128
Galactorrhea 157
Gamete 190
Gamma motor neuron 258
Ganglion 33
Gasping 111
Gasserian ganglion 246
Gastric emptying time 135
Gastric fistula 131
Gastric lipase 128
Gastric pits 127
Gastrin 127
Gastrocolic reflex 146
Gastroileal reflex 145
Gastropancreatic reflex 139
Gastroscopy 131

Gate control theory of pain 249, 250
Gelatinase 129
Gestation/taste 309
Gigantism 157
Gilbert's syndrome 12
GIP 136
Globose nucleus 263
Globulin 2
Globus pallidus 267
Glomerular filtration rate 214
Glomerulonephritis 217
Glucagon 177
Glucocorticoid 162
Gluconeogenesis 178
Glucose reabsorption 220
Glucuronyl transferase 11
Glycine 240
Glycogenesis 178
Glycogenolysis 178
Glycosuria 180
GnRH 153
Goiter 176
Goldman equation 38
Gonad 190
Gonadal dysgenesis 208
Gonadotropes 153
Gracile nuclei 244
Graded potential 37
Granulocyte 13
Graves' disease 175
GRH 153
Growth hormone 153
Gynacomastia 157

H band 45
Habituation 242
Hageman's factor 20
Haldane's effect 108
Half-life of hormone 152
Hamburger's phenomenon 108
Hashimoto thyroiditis 175
hCG 203
HCl 127
HCS 206
Heart blocks 55
Heart rate 71
Heidenhain's pouch 130
Helicobacter pylori 134
Helper T cell 16
Hematocrit/(PCV) 1
Heme 10
Heme-heme interactions 106
Hemianopia 157
Hemodialysis 231
Hemoglobin 10
Hemolysis 6
Hemophilia 23

Hemostasis 18
Heparin 16
Hepatic stage 6
Hering-Brueur reflex 111
Hermophroditism 208
Heteronymous hemianopia 294
Hippocampus 280
Hirschsprung's disease 147
Hirsutism 157
Histamine 16
Histotoxic hypoxia 115
Hollander's test 134
Homeostasis 211
Homonymous hemianopia 294
Hormone 149
Horner's syndrome 301
Humoral immunity 16
Hunger center 278
Hunger pangs 136
Hyaline membrane disease 100
Hydrocephalus 275
Hyperacusis 303
Hyperalgesia 246
Hyperbilirubinemia 12
Hypercapnia 116
Hyperchlorhydria 133
Hyperglycemia 177, 179
Hyperkalemia 67
Hypermetropia 300
Hyperorality 281
Hyperosmia 311
Hyperparathyroidism 187
Hyperphagia 278
Hyperpigmentation 167
Hyperplasia 155
Hyperpyrexia 233
Hyperreflexia 187
Hyperthyroidism 176
Hypertonia 269
Hypertrophy 155
Hyperventilation 116
Hypochlorhydria 133
Hypoglycemic action 177
Hypokalemia 67
Hypoparathyroidism 187
Hypothalamohypophyseal portal system 153
Hypothalamohypophyseal tract 157
Hypothalamus 276
Hypothermia 233
Hypothyroidism 176
Hypovolemic shock 8
Hypoxia 114
Hypoxic hypoxia 114

I band 45
I cell 249

Iatrogenic 153
Idioventricular rhythm 55
IgA 16
IgD 16
IgE 16
IgG 16
IgM 16
Immunity 16
Immunization 17
Immunoglobulins/gamma globulin 1
Impedance matching 302
Incontinence 229
Incus 302
Inhibin 194
Inotropic agents 78
Inspiratory center 110
Inspiratory reserve volume 100
Instrumental conditioning 285
Insulin 177
Insulin-dependent diabetes mellitus 180
Insulin-like growth factor 154
Integer of velocity of flow 59
Intensity discrimination 238
Intercostals nerves 110
Intermediate normoblast 8
Internal arcuate fibers 245
Internal intercostals muscle 96
Internal respiration 94
Internal urethral sphincter 229
Internuncial neuron 240
Intra-alveolar pressure 98
Intrafusal fibers 256
Intraocular tension 290
Intrapleural pressure 98
Intraocular pressure 290
Intrinsic factor 9
Intrinsic system 19
Inulin 215
Inverse stretch reflex 259
Iodide trapping 171
Iodinase 171
Ionotopic effect 73
IPSP 240
Iris 289
Iron 9
Irradiation 242
Irreversible shock 90
Ishihara's chart 299
Islets of Langerhans 177
Isohydric principle 31
Isomaltase 123
Isometric contraction 46
Isopotential line 39
Isoproterenol 57
Isotonic contraction 46
Isovolumetric ventricular contraction 69

Isovolumetric ventricular relaxation 70
IUCD 205

Jaundice 11
Jugular venous pulse 71
Juvenile diabetes 179
Juxtaglomerular apparatus 228
Juxtamedullary nephrons 212
Juxtaglomerular cells 85, 228

Kallmann's syndrome 210
Karl Landsteiner's law 24
Kasper Hauser syndrome 156
Ketoconazole 165
Ketone bodies 177
Kidney 211
Kinocilium 272
Klinefelter syndrome 208
Kluver-Bucy syndrome 281
Korotkoff's sounds 80
Kyphosis 157

L channels 57
L tubule 45
La Place law 230
Lacis cells 228
Lactation 157, 206
Lactotropes 153
Lamina propria 119
Laminar flow 81
Laplace's law 135
Laron dwarf 156
Laryngeal muscle spasm 185
Lashing movement 145
Late normoblast 8
Latent tetany 187
Lateral corticospinal tract 255
Lateral inhibition 240
Lateral lemniscus 307
Lateral spinothalamic tract 247
L-dopa 269
Lead pipe rigidity 269
Lead system in ECG 64
Learning and memory 285
Lesser superficial petrosal nerve 120
Leukocytes 13
Leukopenia 15
Leukocytosis 15
Leydig cells 192
LH 151
Ligand gated channels 43
Light reflex 296
Limbic system 280
Lipase 136
Lipogenesis 179
Lipogenetic agent 179
Lipolysis 179

Lippe's loop 205
Liver function tests 12
Local potential 38
Loop diuretics 232
Lower motor neuron 242
Lumbar puncture 274
Lung compliance 99
Luteal phase 199
Lymph 29
Lymphocyte 13
Lymphocytopenia 15
Lymphocytosis 15

M cell 249
M line 45
Macrocytic 10
Macrophage 15
Macula densa 228
Macula sparing 294
Malleus 302
MAO 169
Marey's law 73
Mass peristalsis 146
Mass reflex 263
Mastication 124
Maturation factors 9
Maximum ejection 69
Mean arterial pressure 79
Mean corpuscular hemoglobin (MCH) 9
Mean corpuscular hemoglobin concentration (MCHC) 9
Mean corpuscular volume (MCV) 9
Mechanics of respiration 96
Mechanoceptors 237
Medial lemniscus 245
Megacolon 147
Megaloblastic pattern 8
Meisserner's plexus 119
Meissner's corpuscle 237
Memory T cell 16
Menarche 190
Meniere's syndrome 273
Menopause 190
Menstrual cycle 198
Merkel's disc 237
Mesoblastic stage 6
Metabolic acid-base disorders 227
Metabolic acidosis 32
Metabolic alkalosis 32
Metahypophyseal diabetes 155
Metanephrine 168
Microcryoscopy 218
Microcytic anemia 9, 10
Microglia 34
Microphage 15
Micropipette technique 218

Micturition 229
Mid-collicular section 258
Milk ejection reflex 160
Mineralocorticoid 162
Mixed nerve 40
Mixing movements 135
Monocyte 13
Monocytosis 15
Monoiodotyrosine 171
Monophasic action potential 38
Monoplegia 256
Monosynaptic reflex 242
Monro-Kellie doctrine 87
morning sickness 204
Morphine 250
Motor decussation 254
Motor neuron 34
Motor unit 44
Mountain sickness 115
Mucopolysaccharides 173
Muller's law 238
Mullerian duct 191
Mullerian inhibiting substance 191
Multiunit smooth muscle 49
Multipolar cell 33
Muscle fatigue 48
Muscle spindle 256
Myasthenia gravis 44
Myelin sheath 34
Myelinated nerve fibers 34
Myelinogenesis 35
Myeloid stage 6
Myelotomy 251
Myenteric plexus 118
Myoepithelial cell 160
Myogenic theory 93
Myometrium 160
Myopia 300
Myosin 45
Myxedema 174

Naloxone 251
Nasogastric tube 131
Near vision 293
Neck cells 127
Negative feedback 152
Neocerebellum 264
Neoplastic 152
Neospinothalamic tract 248
Neostigmine 44
Nephritic syndrome 217
Nephrolithiasis 217
Nephron 211
Nerst equation 37
Nerve injuries 40
Nerve trunk 33

Neuro-endocrine reflex 160
Neurogenic shock 89
Neuroglia 34
Neurohypophysis 157
Neuroma 42
Neuromuscular blockers 43
Neuromuscular junction 43
Neuromuscular transmission 43
Neuron 33
Neurontemesis 40
Neuropathic pain 246
Neuropraxia 40
Neutropenia 15
Neutrophil 13
Neutrophilia 15
Nigrostriatal pathway 267
Nociceptive pain 246
Nociceptors 237, 246
Nodal delay 55
Nodal rhythm 55
Nodes of Ranvier 35
Non-insulin dependent diabetes mellitus 180
Non-myelinated/unmyelinated 34
Non-respiratory function 95
Norepinephrine/noradrenaline 168
Normetanephrine 168
Normoblastic pattern 8
Normocytic 10
NREM sleep 283
Nuclear bag fiber 256
Nuclear chain fiber 256
Nuclear receptor 151
Nucleus interpositus 263
Nucleus raphe magnus 250
Nystagmus 273

Obligatory water reabsorption 222
Obstructive lung disease 101
Occipital lobe 287
Oculocardiac refle 74
Olfactory sensation 310
Oligocythemia 5
Oligodendroglia 34
Omniphagia 281
One way conduction 239
Oogenesis 199
Opioid peptides 250
Optic chiasma 293
Optic radiation 294
Optic tract 294
Organ of Corti 303
Organification 171
Organum vasculosum 275
Osmolality 159
Osmoreceptors 159, 279
Osmotic diuresis 223

Osteoclasts 186
Osteocytes 186
Osteomalacia 188
Oval window 302
Ovarian cycle 199
Overt tetany 187
Ovulation 200
Oxygen dissociation curve 106
Oxygenated blood 104
Oxyphil cells 185
Oxytocin 157

P cell 249
P wave 66
P50 107
Pacemaker region 53
Pacinian corpuscle 237
PAH 213
Paleocerebellum 264
Paleospinothalamic tract 248
Palpatory method 80
Pancreatectomy 140
Pancreatic polypeptide 177
Paracellular 219
Paracrine 149
Paradoxical aciduria 227
Paralytic salivary secretion 122
Parosmia 311
Paraplegia 256
Parathormone 185
Parathyroid gland 185
Paraventricular nucleus 157
Parietal lobe 286
Parietal/oxyntic cell 128
Parkinsonism 269
Parotid gland 119
Partial pressure of carbon dioxide 107
Partial pressure of oxygen 104
Parturition reflex 161
Pavlov's pouch 130
Pelvic nerve 229
Pendular movement 145
Pentagastrin 134
Pepsin 127
Pepsinogen 128
Peptic ulcer 134
Percentage saturation of hemoglobin 10, 105
Perceptive deafness 308
Periaqueductal grey 250
Perilymph 304
Periodic breathing 116
Peripheral chemoreceptors 111
Peripheral nervous system 235
Peripheral resistance 59
Peripheral thermoreceptors 233
Peripheral utilization of glucose 178

Peristalsis 126
Peristaltic rush 145
Peritoneal dialysis 231
Periventricular grey 250
Permissive action 162
Pernicious anemia 9
pH regulation 30
Phagocytosis 15
Pharyngeal stage 124
Phenylalanine 168
Pheochromocytoma 170
Phonocardiogram 71
Phosphate buffer system 31
Phospholipase 136
Photopic vision 289
Phrenic nerve 96, 110
Physiologic jaundice 12
Physostigmine 44
Pia mater 273
Pill rolling movements 269
Placenta 202
Placidity 281
Plantar reflex 260
Plasma cells 16
Plasma thromboplastin antecident 20
Plasminogen 22
Plasticity property 230
Plasticizer action 46
Platelet plug 18
Platelets or thrombocytes 17
Pleura 96
Pneumocytes 100
Pneumotaxic center 110
Poiseuille-Hagen formula 61
Polar ends 257
Pollock-Davis animal 258
Polychromatophilic 8
Polycythemia 2
Polypeptide chain 10
Polyphagia 177
Polysynaptic reflex 242
Polyuria 177
Positive feedback 152
Posterior cochlear nucleus 307
Posterior rhizotomy 251
Post-partum jaundice 275
Postsynaptic inhibition 240
Potassium glycocholate 141
Potassium taurocholate 141
Potentials 37
Potentiating action 172
PQ segment 66
P-R interval 66
Precentral gyrus 254
Precocious pseudopuberty 210
Precocious puberty 210

Prefrontal lobotomy 251
pregnancy diagnosis tests 203
Preload effect 78
Premature contraction 52
Preoptic nucleus 279
Presbyacusis 308
Presbyopia 300
Presynpatic inhibition 240
Primary active transport 219
Primary amenorrhea 192
Primary memory 286
Primary oocyte 199
Primary organ of sex 190
Primary purpura 18
Primary response 17
Proaccelerin 20
Procarboxypeptidase 136
Proconvertin 20
Proelastase 136
Proerythroblast 8
Progeria 156
Progesterone 200
Prognatism 157
Prolactin 152
Proliferative phase 200
Properties of cardiac muscle 51
Proprioceptors 244
Prostate gland 197
Protein buffer 31
Protein C 22
Protein S 22
Proteinuria 231
Prothrombin 2
Prothrombin time 23
Protodiastole 70
Protonopia 299
Ptyalin 120
Puberty 190, 191
Pudic nerve 229
Pulmonary circulation 50
Pulmonary ventilation 96
Pulse pressure 80
Pupil 290
Purkinje fibers 55
Purpura 18
Putamen 267
Pyogenic infection 15
Pyramidal tract 254
Pyrexia 233

QRS complex 66
Q-T interval 66
Quadriplegia 261
Quantal summation 44

Radioimmunoassay 152
Range of accommodation 295

Ranitidine 134
Reabsorption 218
Reaction of degeneration 256
Receptive relaxation 135
Receptors 235
Reciprocal inhibition 240
Red nucleus 267
Reduced ejection 70
Referred pain 246
Reflex 241
Reflex arc 242
Refractory period 52
Refractory index 293
Refractory media 292
Regeneration 41
Regulation of BP 81
Regulation of pH by kidney 225
Reisserner's membrane 304
Relative refractory period 42
REM sleep 283
Renal blood flow 212
Renal fraction 212
Renal glycosuria 181
Renal splay 220
Renal threshold 219
Renal tubular acidosis 227
Renal tubules 211
Renin 85
Renin–angiotensin mechanism 85
Renin–angiotensin theory 93
Rennin 128
Renshaw cell inhibition 240
Repolarization 39
Residual volume 100
Resonance theory 306
Respiratory acid-base disorders 227
Respiratory acidosis 31
Respiratory alkalosis 31
Respiratory distress syndrome 100
Respiratory function 95
Respiratory membrane 102
Respiratory rate 96
Resting membrane potential 37
Restrictive lung disease 101
Reticular formation 269
Reticulocyte 8
Reticulospinal tract 252
Retina 291
Retrograde amnesia 286
Retrograde catheterization 79
Retrograde transport 35
Reversible shock 90
Reynold's number 59
Rh system 24
Rheobase 36
Rhodopsin 292

Rhythmic segmentation 144
Ribonuclease 136
Rickets 188
Rigidity 269
Rinne's test 308
Rods 289
Rouleaux formation 5
Rubrospinal tract 252
Ryle's tube 131

SA node 53
Saccule 271
Sacoplasmic triad 45
Safe period 206
Salivary amylase 121
Saltatory or leaping conduction 35
Sarcomere 45
Sarcoplasmic reticulum 45
Satiety center 278
Scala media 304
Scala tympani 304
Scala vestibuli 304
Schwann cell 34
Scotopic vision 289
Second messenger 151
Secondary active transport 219
Secondary memory 286
Secondary oocyte 199
Secondary response 17
Secondary sexual characteristics 190
Secretin 133
Secretion 218
Secretogogue 133
Secretomotor fibers 121
Secretors 24
Secretory phase 200
Semen 196
Semicircular canal 271
Seminal vesicle 197
Seminiferous tubules 197
Sensory decussation 245
Sensory homunculus 245
Sensory neuron 34
Septicemic shock 89
Serotonin 18
Serous coat 118
Sertoli cells 194
Serum 21
Servo comparator 266
Sex differentiation 190
Sham feeding 130
Shear rate 58
Shear stress 58
Sheehan's syndrome 157
Sherrington's animal 258
Sialorrhea 123

Sick sinus rhythm 55
Significance of ECG 67
Simultaneous contrast 310
Sinus arrhythmia 72
Sinus nerve 73
Sinus rhythm 55
Skeletal muscle pump 63
Skinner box 280
Sleep and wakefulness 283
Sliding filament theory 46
Smooth muscle 49
Sodium glycocholate 141
Sodium reabsorption 219
Sodium taurocholate 141
Somatomedin C 154
Somatomotor function 270
Somatosensory function 271
Somatostatin 177
Somatotropes 153
Spatial summation 249
Specific gravity 2
Specificity 238
Spectrophotometer 152
Spermatogenesis 193
Spermatogonium 193
spermicides 205
Sphygmomanometer 80
Spinal nucleus of trigeminal nerve 248
Spinal shock 262
Spinocerebellar tract 265
Spirogram 100
Spleen 30
Squirting movement 135
SS 153
ST segment 66
Stagnant hypoxia 114
Standard bipolar limb lead system 64
Stapes 302
Starling's hypothesis 29
Starling's law 48
Stem cell/haemocytoblast 8
Stenson's duct 120
Stercobilinogen 11
Stereognosis 245
Sterocilia 272
Stimulus 33
Stop flow technique 218
Strength duration curve 36
Stretch reflex 258
Stroke volume 76
Stuart-Prower factor 20
Subarachnoid spaces 273
Subdural venous sinuses 274
Subfornical organ 275
Sublingual gland 119
Submandibular gland 119

Substance P 249
Substantia gelatinosa rolandi 247
Substantia nigra 267
Subthalamic nucleus 267
Subthreshold 38
Successive contrast 310
Succinylcholine 44
Summation 239
Super female 209
Superficial reflex 242
Supraoptic nucleus 157
Suprachiasmatic nucleus 280
Surfactant 100
Suspensory ligaments 290
Sylvester's method 117
Sympathectomy and blood flow 62
Sympathetectomy 251
Sympathetic nerve supply to ventricle 72
Symport 219
Symptomatic purpura 18
Synapse 33, 238
Synaptic delay 239
Synaptic transmission 239
Synaptic vesicles 43
Synergistic muscle 265
Syringomyelia 245
Systemic circulation 50
Systole and diastole in cardiac muscle 67
Systolic pressure 79

T tubule 45
T wave 66
Tabes dorsalis 261
Tachycardia 72
Taste blindness 310
Taste pathway 309
Tectocerebellar pathway 265
Tectorial membrane 304
Temporal lobe 287
Tendon end organ 256
Tertiary memory 286
Testis 192
Testosterone 191
Tetanus 48
Thalamic syndrome 276
Thalamus 275
Theca interna 200
Theories of sleep 284
Thermodilution method 76
Thermogenic action 202
Thermoregulation 233
Thermostat 278
Thiazides 232
Thoracic pump 63
Threshold stimulus 33
Thrombin 20

Thrombocytopenia 17
Thrombocytosis 17
Thrombomodulin 22
Thyrocalcitonin 170
Thyroid binding albumin 172
Thyroid binding globulin 172
Thyroid binding prealbumin 172
Thyroid function tests 174
Thyroid storm 177
Thyrotropes 153
Thyroxine 170
Tidal volume 96
Timed vital capacity 101
Tissue fluid pressure theory 93
Tissue metabolite theory 93
Tissue plasminogen activator 22
Tissue thromboplastin 20
Tone of muscle 257
Total lung capacity 101
Total renal plasma flow 213
Trachea 94
Tract 33
Tract of Goll and Burdach 244
Tractus solitarius 309
Transcellular 219
Transmembrane potential 37
Traveling wave theory 306
Tremors 267
TRH 153
Trigeminal lemniscus 246
Triiodothyronine 170
Trisomy 13 209
Trisomy 18 209
Trisomy X 209
Trophoblast cells 202
Tropic hormone 15
Tropomyosin 46
Troponin 46
Trousseaus's sign 187
Trypsin 138
Trypsinogen 136
TSH 151
Tubectomy 206
Tubocurarine 44

Tubular maximum 219
Tunica adventitia 57
Tunica intima 57
Tunica media 57
Turbulent flow 81
Turner's syndrome 208
Tympanic membrane 302
Tympanic plexus 120
Tympanic reflex 303
Tyrosine 168

Ultrafiltration 214
Unconditioned reflex 122
Unipolar lead system 64
Unipoloar cell 33
Universal donor 25
Universal recipient 25
Up regulation 151
Upper esophageal sphincter 126
Upper motor neuron 243
Urea reabsorption 222
Ureter 211
Urethra 211
Urinary bladder 211
Urobilinogen 11
Urokinase 22
Utricle 271

V_1 receptors 159
V_2 receptors 158
Vagal tone 73
Vagovagal reflex 136
Vagus nerve supply to ventricle 72
Valsalva maneuver 147
Vasa recta 213
Vasectomy 206
Vasoconstrictors 60
Vasodilators 60
Vasomotor center 59, 81
Vasopressin 157
Vasovagal syncope 55
Venomotor tone 63
Venous return 62
Ventilation perfusion ratio 101
Ventricular diastole 68

Ventricular muscle 50
Ventricular muscle fiber action potential 56
Ventricular systole 68
Verapamil 57
Vermis 264
Vertigo 273
Vestibular apparatus 271
Vestibulocerebellar pathway 265
Vestibulospinal tract 252
VIP 122
Virilism 166
Vis a fronte 63
Vis a tergo 63
Visceral reflex 242
Visceral smooth muscle 49
Visceromotor function 270
Viscosity 4
Visual acuity 296
Visual agnosia 281
Visual field 294
Visual pathway 293
Vital capacity 101
Vitamin B_{12} 9
VMA 168
Voltage-gated channels 43
Volume receptors 159
Vomiting 148

Wallerian degeneration 40
Water diuresis 223
Water reabsorption 222
Weber's test 308
Wharton's duct 120
Withdrawal method 206
Withdrawal reflex 259
Wolffian duct 191

Xanthenes 232
Xerostomia 123
XYY male 209

Z line 45
Zona fasciculata 161
Zona glomerulosa 161
Zona reticularis 161